Clinical Linguistics

In memory of a dear friend
Jacqueline Elizabeth Henry (née McCormick)
23.3.1971 ~ 24.1.2001

Clinical Linguistics

Louise Cummings

EDINBURGH UNIVERSITY PRESS

© Louise Cummings, 2008

Edinburgh University Press Ltd
22 George Square, Edinburgh

Typeset in 11/13 Ehrhardt MT and Gill Sans
by Servis Filmsetting Ltd, Manchester, and
printed and bound in Great Britain by
Antony Rowe Ltd, Chippenham, Wilts

A CIP record for this book is available from the British Library

ISBN 978 0 7486 2076 0 (hardback)
ISBN 978 0 7486 2077 7 (paperback)

The right of Louise Cummings
to be identified as author of this work
has been asserted in accordance with
the Copyright, Designs and Patents Act 1988.

Contents

List of Figures and Tables

Figures

Tables

Acknowledgements

I wish to acknowledge with gratitude the assistance of the following people and organisations: Kathy Sulik, Karlind T. Moller, InHealth Technologies, Mayer-Johnson LLC and the Cleft Palate Foundation, for their permission to use a number of the illustrations that appear in this book; the Tennessee Craniofacial Center, for its donation of *The Craniofacial Surgery Book*; Roger Bromley, Liz Morrish and John Tomlinson, for their provision of a sabbatical and rearrangement of teaching duties; John Wells, for advice on phonetic fonts and Sarah Edwards of Edinburgh University Press, for accommodating my numerous requests as the book developed. The assistance of each of these individuals and organisations has been invaluable.

Much of the research for this book was undertaken while I was a Visiting Fellow in the Centre for Research in the Arts, Social Sciences and Humanities (CRASSH) at the University of Cambridge. I am grateful to the Director of CRASSH, Mary Jacobus, for her support and encouragement. During my time at Cambridge, Wolfson College provided me with an environment that was particularly conducive to conducting research. I extend my gratitude to its President and Fellows.

The task of writing a book is made more manageable when one receives the assistance of others. I particularly wish to thank Judith Heaney for her careful preparation of the manuscript. I am also grateful to her husband Stewart for his work on the numerous diagrams in the following pages. Jo Mills of the Clifton Audio-Visual Unit at Nottingham Trent University reproduced the embryology images in chapter 2 and I extend my gratitude to her. Roberta Davari-Zanjani has assisted me at various stages with the scanning of diagrams and I thank her for not growing tired of my endless requests. The assistance of

Sian Griffiths and other staff in the Clifton Library of the university is also gratefully acknowledged.

Finally, I have been supported in this endeavour by family members and friends who are too numerous to mention individually. I am grateful to them for their kind words of encouragement during my many months of writing.

Preface

In recent years, some remarkable developments have taken place in our knowledge and management of communication and swallowing disorders in children and adults. Some of these developments have come about through work in medical disciplines: for example, the study of the genetics of specific language impairment. Other developments are the result of technological progress in fields such as computer science and medical diagnostics. One need only consider the phenomenal growth that has recently occurred in augmentative and alternative communication to appreciate the significance of such progress for the management of clients with severe communication disorder. Similarly, the dysphagia clinician and voice therapist rely heavily on these technological achievements in their assessment and treatment of dysphagic and dysphonic clients, respectively. Theoretical developments in linguistics and psychology have also transformed our understanding and management of communication disorders. The greater prominence of pragmatics within linguistics, for example, has encouraged clinicians to reconsider how language disorders are assessed and treated – how aphasic adults manage the demands of different conversational contexts and communicative partners is now as likely (and, perhaps, even more likely) to be addressed in assessment and intervention as is the comprehension and production of certain syntactic structures. Psychologists have radically influenced our understanding of the communicative impairments in autism through their proposal of theories of the core cognitive deficit in this developmental psychopathology. The theory of mind proposals of Simon Baron-Cohen and co-workers hold particular resonance for any speech and language therapist who has witnessed the severe pragmatic deficits of many children and adults with an autistic spectrum disorder.

Clearly, developments which have implications for the study of clinical linguistics have been proceeding apace. In this book, the reader is introduced to these developments in the context of discussion of specific communication and swallowing disorders. The latest research findings on these disorders are presented and discussed at length. The structure of the text is intended to make the treatment of each disorder accessible to even the most introductory reader. I begin the discussion of each disorder with an examination of its epidemiology and aetiology. The speech, language, hearing, voice and swallowing features of these disorders receive extended discussion, which will be informative even to advanced readers. Techniques and issues in the assessment and treatment of communication and swallowing disorders are addressed in dedicated sections. The recent emphasis in healthcare on evidence-based practice is never far from sections on intervention with the results of efficacy studies presented, when these are available.

It will be obvious from my comments thus far that I have had a diverse readership in mind in my writing of this book. Clearly, my primary readership is students, researchers and practitioners in speech and language therapy. As anyone who has a professional or academic interest in speech-language pathology will be aware, the field is a multidisciplinary one that draws on developments in and insights from medicine, linguistics, psychology and special education, to name but a few areas. For this reason, I have tried to make the reader aware of those multidisciplinary influences. For example, speech and language therapists are actively involved in research projects that are examining the genetic bases of communication disorders and, accordingly, I examine the findings of this research in the chapters that follow. Although speech and language therapists form the primary readership of this book, they are by no means the only readers who are likely to find the discussion in subsequent chapters relevant to their fields of study and practice. Students of and practitioners in medicine and nursing must understand the pathologies and injuries that can lead to communication and swallowing disorders, as well as the presentation of these disorders. Educationalists encounter children in mainstream and special education settings who have significant communication disorders. A working knowledge of these disorders is thus an essential attribute of these professionals. Social workers and psychologists work with children and adults who have autistic spectrum disorders, mental health problems and learning disabilities. The communication problems that attend these disorders are discussed at length in this book. Finally, parents and carers of children and adults with communication and swallowing disorders rightly expect to be informed about the causes, nature and likely course of these disorders. Many have acquired a considerable level of expertise in the particular communication impairments that affect their child or spouse. It is hoped that this book will contribute to the knowledge base of these individuals as well.

I

The Scope of Clinical Linguistics

1.1 A New Definition of an Established Practice

In this book, I want to give new prominence to the somewhat neglected expression 'clinical linguistics'. I say 'expression' rather than 'field of study' because, of course, clinical linguistics has been a thriving area of enquiry amongst researchers and practitioners in speech and language therapy for many years now.[1] However, while the practice of clinical linguistics in academic and clinical contexts has expanded considerably, the term 'clinical linguistics' has lost out to competitor expressions, such as 'clinical communication studies'. Although the reasons for this shift towards these other expressions are clear enough – for example, the need to have a broader term that can cover the full range of disorders that are encountered by clinicians – I believe the term 'clinical linguistics' gives due emphasis to the role of language in communication and highlights the essentially scientific character of linguistics itself. In this book, I adopt the following definition of clinical linguistics:

> Clinical linguistics is the study of the numerous ways in which the unique human capacity for language can be disordered. This includes 'language disorders', as standardly conceived. However, it also includes disorders that result from disruption to the wider processes of language transmission and reception and disorders of the vegetative functions that are an evolutionary precursor to language. Most notably, it includes all the disorders that are encountered by speech and language therapists[2] across a range of clinical contexts.

This definition emphasises the fact that when we are studying clinical linguistics, we are engaging not simply with an academic discipline, but also with an area of clinical practice. By placing language at the centre of the above definition, I am seeking to re-establish language as the foundation of all human communication. Quite apart from being unrelated to language, speech, voice and fluency disorders on this definition represent various types of breakdown in the mechanics of language transmission. Indeed, it is their capacity to reduce the effectiveness with which language meaning is transmitted that makes these disorders distressing and frustrating for the individuals whom they affect. (To see that this is the case, one need only think about the common complaints of the severe stutterer, apraxic adult or dysarthric child: 'People don't *understand* what I'm saying,' 'It's a struggle to get across to people exactly what I *mean*,' 'I have the *words* in my mind, but I just can't get them out.'). We will return to this issue at numerous points in the following chapters.

A further important dimension of the above definition – one that is frequently overlooked in summaries of this clinical area – is the recognition that language is largely dependent on earlier evolutionary developments in humans, specifically those that have given rise to the neuromuscular mechanisms that make feeding, swallowing and breathing possible. These vegetative functions are frequently disordered as a result of trauma and disease. It will be seen in the chapters to follow that the assessment and treatment of these functions, particularly swallowing, constitute a significant and growing aspect of the work of speech and language therapy.

In conclusion, the above definition seeks to emphasise the place of practice in clinical linguistics, to re-establish the foundational role of language in all human communication and to recognise the important, but frequently overlooked, work on feeding and swallowing disorders in speech and language therapy. In its consideration of all three of these features, this definition moves beyond previous accounts of clinical linguistics.[3] Yet, in doing so, it is not entirely without precedent. An examination of recent issues of the journal *Clinical Linguistics and Phonetics* reveals articles that address swallowing ability after intra-oral cancer (emphasis on vegetative function), the education of speech-language pathologists (emphasis on clinical practice) and a range of language functions in disorders as diverse as stuttering, right hemisphere damage and hearing impairment (emphasis on language). However, having completed this initial examination of clinical linguistics, we are still some way off giving a full account of the scope of its domain. In order to obtain such an account, we must first consider the many different ways in which communication can be disordered in humans.

1.2 Human Communication: Processes

The Royal College of Speech and Language Therapists estimates that 2.5 million people in the UK have a communication disorder.[4] Of this number, some 800,000 people have a disorder that is so severe that it is hard for anyone outside their immediate families to understand them. In this section, I begin an examination of the wide range of communication impairments that make up these large and significant figures. To begin with, however, a few words are in order about the processes of normal communication.

Before we can utter a single word, we have to be capable of forming thoughts that are appropriate for communication. The qualification 'appropriate' is important in this context, as we all entertain thoughts that violate social and moral codes and are rarely, if ever, communicated. Moreover, many other thoughts are below the level of our conscious awareness and, as such, are not communicated. In short, we each entertain many more thoughts than are ever actually communicated. Those thoughts that are to be communicated give rise to a communicative intention. Pragmaticists argue that it is only when a hearer has established a speaker's communicative intention in speaking that a speaker can be said to have communicated anything at all.[5] In order that the hearer may identify the speaker's intention, the speaker must first encode it using a conventional symbol system (one that is recognised and understood by other communicators) that can be readily transmitted. Language is such a symbol system. Language encoding is a complex process that involves many interrelated stages. These stages involve a combination of lexical, semantic, syntactic and phonological processes. Their combined effect is to transform an abstract, nonlinguistic intention into a still abstract, but now linguistic representation. This representation is still not of a form where it can be uttered by a speaker. Various neuromuscular selections must be made during motor programming, before the speaker is finally able to translate these selections into movements of the articulators during speech production (a stage called motor execution).

Thus far, we have outlined the four main processes of communication that are essential to the production (expression) of an utterance. To recap, these processes are: (1) thought genesis, (2) language encoding, (3) motor programming and (4) motor execution. However, even if a communicator is able to fulfil the requirements of these processes, he or she still has not communicated anything at all. As we discussed above, communication can only be said to occur when a hearer is able to retrieve the intention that motivated the speaker's utterance. Our four productive processes must now be matched to four receptive processes, the combined function of which will be to determine this intention on the basis of an input linguistic utterance. In the first of these receptive processes – sensory processing – sound waves are converted into mechanical vibrations via the actions of the tympanic membrane (ear drum) and ossicles. These vibrations trigger a series of neurochemical reactions within the cochlea of the inner ear. From here, nerve impulses make their way along auditory nerves to the auditory cortices of the brain. These cortices, both of which are located in the temporal lobes, are integral to our second main receptive process,

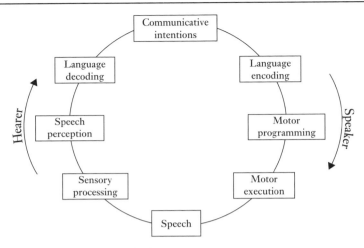

Figure 1.1: The process of communication

speech perception. Although the exact mechanism by means of which hearers perceive speech sounds is still uncertain, it seems clear that top–down processes and contextual influences play a significant role (Massaro 2001). Speech perception is vital to the eventual recovery of a speaker's communicative intention.[6] However, it is by no means the only form of perception that plays a role in this process. One need only consider how often visual information serves to disambiguate a speaker's utterance to appreciate the significance of visual perception in this process too. Before complete disambiguation can occur, the product of perception must undergo a third receptive process, language decoding. In decoding, structural (syntactic) relations within sentences are determined alongside the semantic features of constituent lexemes. Decoding arrives at a propositional meaning of the sentence which is not yet the full intended meaning of the speaker's utterance. This latter meaning can only be obtained by establishing the speaker's communicative intention in producing the utterance, a process that leads us back to the domain of thoughts. It can be seen that in an effort to describe communication between a speaker and a hearer, we have effectively come full circle, a fact that is aptly demonstrated by Figure 1.1.

1.3 Human Communication: Disorders

The communication model that I outlined in the previous section is limited in a number of ways. It assumes an oral–auditory mode of communication when, in fact, other modes of communication are possible (e.g. written–visual communication). At every point in this model, I make claims about communication which appear to be unproblematic, but which are, in reality, deeply contentious (e.g. claims about speech perception, which depend on the psychological reality of the phoneme[7]). The model makes no mention of the role of context in communication and is almost entirely 'mentalistic' in character. But as every student of communication knows, context pervades communication – from deciding what thoughts it is appropriate to express in a certain situation (social context) to speaking more loudly than normal in a busy train station (physical context), it is inconceivable that any form of communication could proceed in the absence of context. However, despite these drawbacks – and no doubt others besides – the above model can be used to demonstrate the loci of communication breakdown and the disorders that result when such a breakdown occurs. In this section, I present an overview of these disorders and indicate to the reader something of their treatment in subsequent chapters.

Many communication disorders have their origin at the level of thoughts and, specifically, in an inability to formulate appropriate intentions for communication. These disorders have a diverse aetiology which includes psychotic conditions like schizophrenia, mental retardation (as occurs, for example, in Down's syndrome) and the early-onset condition of autism. Individuals with advanced dementia lack all communicative intent and are essentially mute. Although Alzheimer's disease is the most common cause of dementia, other causes include human immunodeficiency virus (HIV) infection and Creutzfeldt–Jakob disease (CJD). These conditions and their associated communication disorders present numerous management challenges not just for speech and language therapists, but for other healthcare professionals and carers as well. They will be discussed at various points in subsequent chapters, but primarily in chapters 3 and 5.

Disorders of language encoding and decoding are frequently encountered by both paediatric and adult clinicians. These disorders include aphasia in adults (known as 'acquired aphasia'). Aphasia has been the focus of extensive research and classification for some years. Its linguistic characteristics and impact on communication will be examined in detail in chapter 5. Childhood ('developmental') language disorders are no less diverse than their adult counterparts. These include cases of phonological disorder, children with specific language impairment who present with morphosyntactic deficits and children for whom the pragmatics of language poses considerable barriers to effective communication. These latter children have been variously described as having semantic-pragmatic disorder (Bishop and Rosenbloom 1987) or semantic-pragmatic deficit syndrome (Rapin and Allen 1983), although the validity of this diagnostic category is now strongly disputed in some quarters (Gagnon et al. 1997). In chapter 4, we examine these common language disorders in children. We will also discuss other, not so common language disorders in children, such as Landau–Kleffner syndrome (also known as acquired epileptic aphasia).

In chapters 4 and 5, we examine the motor programming disorder, apraxia. This disorder can affect a range of volitional movements, although automatic movements are unaffected. When the disorder involves movements that are necessary for speech production, the resulting condition is called verbal apraxia or apraxia of speech. (Contrast with limb apraxia, when movements of the arms and legs are compromised.) The disorder has both developmental and acquired forms and can occur in isolation or in conjunction with other communication impairments (e.g. phonological disorder). When the latter situation pertains, a differential diagnosis is both necessary and difficult. In chapter 4, we examine the criteria that guide such a diagnosis. A large number of disorders can disrupt the motor execution of speech. Neurological damage can cause dysarthria, in which impoverished movements of the articulators give rise to varying levels of unintelligibility. The same nerves and muscles that are impaired in dysarthria can also cause disorders of feeding and swallowing (dysphagia), as well as problems such as drooling. Even when nerve and muscle function is normal, the structure and function of the articulators can be compromised through disease and subsequent surgery (e.g. glossectomy) or as a result of defective embryological development (e.g. cleft lip and palate). Benign and malignant lesions of the tissues of the larynx, particularly the vocal folds (cords), can produce disorders of voice; similar lesions in the nasal cavities (e.g. nasal polyps) or dysfunction of the velopharyngeal port (velopharyngeal incompetence) distort normal resonance. Finally, speech production can be severely disrupted in stuttering (stammering). Although the exact causal mechanism at work in this disorder of fluency is unknown, it is unlikely to be simply an organic aetiology, such as occurs in many other motor execution disorders. Cleft lip and palate, fluency disorders and voice disorders will be examined in detail in chapters 2, 6 and 7, respectively. Developmental and acquired dysarthria will be discussed in chapters 4 and 5.

Sensory processing disorders both cause and contribute to communication breakdown in a number of ways. The most obvious way is through complete or partial loss of hearing. At various points in the following chapters, we examine conductive and sensorineural deafness and describe the different forms of audiometry that are used to assess and diagnose hearing disorders. We consider the role of the speech and language therapist in the clinical audiology team. Hearing disorders are not the only sensory processing problems of concern to the speech and language practitioner. Reduced sensation in the oral cavity can result from cranial nerve damage, which may be caused by a cerebrovascular accident (CVA). These and other sensory impairments exacerbate existing communication and swallowing problems and pose a considerable treatment challenge to clinicians. Finally, some individuals who have intact sensory receptors (i.e. normal hearing, vision, etc.) can nonetheless struggle to recognise the sensory information that is the output of those receptors. This disorder, called

Table 1.1 Communication processes and disorders

Communication processes	Communication disorders
Communicative intentions	Problems formulating and establishing communicative intentions. Associated with psychotic disorders (e.g. schizophrenia), mental retardation (e.g. Down's syndrome), autism and dementia (e.g. Alzheimer's disease)
Language encoding and decoding	Problems formulating and understanding various levels of language. Disorders include acquired aphasia and phonological disorder, specific language impairment and pragmatic language impairment in children. Also includes a rare disorder in children, Landau-Kleffner syndrome
Motor programming	Apraxia (developmental and acquired)
Motor execution	Disorders of speech production. Includes dysarthria (developmental and acquired), disorders related to articulation (e.g. cleft lip and palate), phonation (e.g. vocal nodules), resonation (e.g. velopharyngeal incompetence) and fluency (e.g. stuttering). Also includes related disorders of swallowing (dysphagia) and drooling
Sensory processing	Hearing disorders (e.g. conductive and sensorineural deafness) and oral sensory dysfunction
Perception	Agnosia. Affects different sensory modalities, resulting in auditory agnosia, visual agnosia, etc.

agnosia, can affect one or more sensory modalities, resulting in auditory agnosia, visual agnosia and so on. Due to their common neurological aetiologies, agnosia is often found alongside disorders like aphasia. For this reason, it will be examined in chapter 5. However, we will have occasion to discuss agnosia, particularly auditory agnosia, in other contexts as well – for example, in chapter 4, when we will examine auditory agnosia in Landau–Kleffner syndrome.

Communication processes and disorders are shown in Table 1.1.

1.4 The Contribution of Linguistic Science

In the previous section, we described a number of disorders of receptive and expressive language. In order to characterise these disorders, we must draw upon the terminology of different branches of linguistic science. Language can be impaired in any one – and usually it is impaired in more than one – of the following areas: phonetics, phonology, graphology, morphology, syntax, lexicology, semantics and pragmatics. In this section, I describe these linguistic areas and examine the types of deficit that result when these areas are disordered.

Phonetics is the study of speech sounds. This includes the study of the articulatory movements that are required to produce speech sounds (articulatory phonetics) and the measurement of the physical dimensions of speech sounds, such as amplitude and frequency (acoustic phonetics). By contrast, phonology is the study of the sound system of a language. Phonologists examine how speech sounds function to signify meaning: for example, how the difference of one distinctive feature (voice) between 'pin' /pɪn/ and 'bin' /bɪn/ conveys two unrelated meanings. This symbolic dimension of phonology – and the lack of such a dimension to phonetics – is the basis of the long-standing clinical distinction between speech and language disorders. In this way, the dysarthric adult, who cannot perform the articulatory movements that are required in order to produce speech sounds, has a speech disorder. The young child, who cannot signal a difference in meaning between 'sip' and 'zip' (both of which are pronounced [sɪp]), has a phonological (language) disorder. Speech (phonetic) and language (phonological) disorders often coexist; indeed, a speech disorder may contribute to the development of a phonological disorder. For example, the child with a cleft palate may present with severe velopharyngeal incompetence. This inability to achieve full velopharyngeal closure makes it difficult or impossible for the child to articulate oral plosives (the resulting productions are heavily nasalised). The child may substitute all oral plosives with glottal stops, as the glottis is the only point in the vocal tract where the requisite build-up of air pressure can be achieved. No longer able to produce the sound contrasts that would enable a listener to distinguish 'pin' /pɪn/ from 'kin' /kɪn/, or 'bin' /bɪn/ from 'din' /dɪn/ – all of which are realised as [ʔĩn] – this child has a phonological disorder. To the extent that this disorder has its origin in a failure of normal velopharyngeal valving (a speech defect), a phonological and a phonetic disorder are intimately connected in this case.

Graphology is the study of the system of symbols that is used to communicate a language in its written form. Written language has seldom received the extensive treatment that is given to spoken language in books on linguistics in general and on clinical linguistics in particular. Speech and language therapy courses include as routine modules on phonology and phonological disorders. (Phonology is the spoken language counterpart of graphology.) However, these same courses do little more than mention graphology, while disorders of graphology are only briefly addressed, usually in relation to conditions like aphasia. To some extent, this more limited treatment of written language is merely a reflection of the fact that speech is our primary mode of linguistic communication. It is also indicative, however, of the lack of clinical research that has been conducted into written language processes and disorders. Two disorders of written language are acquired dyslexia and acquired dysgraphia. As the term 'acquired' suggests, these disorders occur in individuals who have intact written language skills prior to the onset of a CVA or other neurological event (e.g. traumatic brain injury). Dyslexia and dysgraphia also occur as developmental disorders in children. Given the educational implications of these disorders, they are assessed by educational psychologists and managed by specialist teachers. In their acquired forms, dyslexia and dysgraphia usually exist as part of the central language disorder aphasia. However, even when language is intact, a client may struggle to produce and perceive the letters (graphs) that are used in writing. On some occasions, this is the result of a visual impairment. On other occasions, the client has normal vision, but is unable to recognise letters. On still other occasions, a client is unable to write letters on account of weakness or paralysis of the arm and hand. (This is commonly seen, for example, in right-sided hemiplegia following a left-hemisphere CVA.) In these cases, the disorder is the result of deficits, respectively, in the sensory processing, visual perception and motor execution of the written symbols of language.

For most linguists, grammar consists of two main areas of study: morphology and syntax. Morphology is the study of the internal structure of words. This structure may be simple and consist of a single morpheme. Such monomorphemic words include 'neighbour' and 'crocodile'. (The reader will note that monomorphemic is not the same as monosyllabic.) It is frequently the case, however, that words consist of two or more morphemes. These polymorphemic words – examples include 'cats' and 'navigator' – contain bound and free morphemes. A free morpheme can stand independently of other morphemes as a word of the language. (In the example 'cats', *cat* is a free morpheme.) Bound morphemes, as their name suggests, have no independent existence as words of the language. (In the example *-s* and *-or* are bound morphemes.) These morphemes can inflect to express grammatical contrasts. The *-s* suffix of 'cats' is an inflectional morpheme, as it signals a grammatical distinction between singular and plural. Other bound morphemes are involved in the construction of new words and do not express grammatical contrasts. The *-or* suffix of 'navigator' is such a derivational morpheme.

In chapter 4, we review the findings of studies that have investigated inflectional morphology and other aspects of grammatical morphology (e.g. use of pronouns) in children with specific language impairment (SLI). In general, these studies have revealed that SLI children use significantly fewer inflectional and grammatical morphemes and use significantly more incorrect inflectional and grammatical morphemes than MLU controls (controls matched to SLI subjects on mean length of utterance). Morphemic deficits are also evident in other clinical populations. In chapter 5, we examine a number of these deficits in the language of schizophrenic speakers.

Syntax is the study of the internal structure of sentences. At its most basic, this structure consists of words that are nouns ('man'), verbs ('sing'), adjectives ('blue'), adverbs ('quickly'), prepositions ('beside'), articles ('the') and so on.

These words come together to form phrases, some of which exhibit extensive pre- and postmodification. For example, *the patient* and *the difficult patient in the waiting room* are both noun phrases. However, the complexity of the second noun phrase derives from the presence of a premodifying adjective ('difficult') and a postmodifying prepositional phrase ('in the waiting room'). Phrases combine to form sentences or clauses within sentences. The combination of the noun phrase *the man* and the verb phrase *walks in the park* results in the simple sentence *The man walks in the park*. However, this latter construction may exist as a clause within a larger sentence (*Although the man walks in the park, he is still very overweight*), the parts of which are linked by a conjunction (in this case, the subordinating conjunction 'although').

There are many children and adults for whom the above syntactic levels pose considerable difficulties. Phrase structure is effectively absent in the autistic child who produces only single-word utterances. (More often than not, even single-word utterances are absent.) The agrammatic aphasic omits function words (e.g. articles) and inflectional morphemes. These omissions generate an incomplete, simplified phrase structure that is telegrammatic in appearance (hence, the use of the term 'agrammatism' to describe this type of aphasia). Many clients who fail to produce adequate phrase structure may also be unable to comprehend phrases such as 'the tall man' and 'on the table'. Receptive problems at the level of phrase structure are often most apparent during formal testing, when the client is unable to use contextual cues to facilitate comprehension. Clauses and sentences are often severely compromised in the schizophrenic patient. In addition to impairments at each of these syntactic levels, the language-disordered client may fail to invert subject pronouns and auxiliary verbs (such as occurs, for example, in the asking of questions), may fail to form the negatives of verbs and may be unable to decode the structural relation between subject and object nouns in a passive sentence. We will examine these syntactic deficits, and many others besides, in the following chapters.

Lexicology is the study of the vocabulary of a language. Like graphology before it, lexicology has been largely overlooked by clinical linguists. This neglect is understandable in part; by and large, academic linguists have tended to pursue historical treatments of lexicology, which are of limited relevance to the clinician who must assess and treat language and communication disorders. Yet, there are clear reasons why greater integration of lexicology with clinical linguistics should be encouraged. First, through studies of vocabulary development in children, we have gained considerable insight, not simply into language learning, but also into cognitive developmental processes more generally. The potential exists to expand our knowledge of these processes further. However, that potential will only be realised by embracing the expertise of disciplines like lexicology more fully. Second, for some time studies have indicated that early vocabulary development is a reasonably strong predictor both of the extent of later language development and of the severity of language impairment. Closer integration of lexicology with clinical linguistics will make it possible to articulate more explicitly the nature of this predictive relationship. Third, with the lexicon playing a central role in recent cognitive neuropsychological explanations of disorders such as aphasia and dyslexia, it seems only reasonable that we should attempt to integrate lexicology more closely with clinical linguistics. Having established the need for and possible shape of closer integration of lexicology with clinical linguistics, the challenge for researchers and therapists alike will be to achieve its implementation.

Related to lexicology is semantics, the study of language meaning. Semanticists study lexical meaning (hence, the connection to lexicology). However, they also develop theoretical accounts of sentence meaning, as well as discuss a range of conceptual and applied issues that relate to language meaning. Some of these accounts and issues (e.g. truth-conditional semantics) are not directly relevant to the work of clinical linguistics. However, other semantic theories are contributing in useful ways to our understanding of language disorders. For example, by using the descriptive terminology of semantic components (primitives) in componential theory, it is possible to capture at least some of the semantic errors that occur in aphasia and acquired dyslexia. One such component is [±CONCRETE]. Patients with deep dyslexia can read words with concrete meanings more easily than they can read words with abstract meanings. Similarly, the aphasic patient with lexical retrieval problems may be able to say words with concrete meanings, but may struggle to retrieve words with abstract meanings. As well as providing terminology for the description of semantic errors, componential theory itself receives some validation from these errors. The presence and consistency of a concrete/abstract distinction in the spoken language and reading performance of these patients lend support to the psychological reality of the semantic primitive [±CONCRETE]. Componential theory aside, our increased knowledge of semantics has been a crucial factor in the recent development of cognitive neuropsychological models of language processing in aphasia. Also, semantics has a large, unexplored potential to explain other aspects of language disorder. Many semantic problems occur in the presence of wider cognitive deficits. One effect of these deficits in children, for example, is the failure to develop key concepts. Thus, children with Down's syndrome may fail to use and comprehend locative prepositions like 'in' and 'on', because their concept of space is disordered. Through its investigation of conceptual structures, cognitive semantics may increase our understanding of conceptually based semantic disorders, as well as provide an effective means of remediation of these disorders.

Pragmatics is the study of how speakers and hearers use language in context to communicate nonpropositional meaning (i.e. meaning beyond that encoded in language). In its relatively short intellectual history, pragmatics has included the study of diverse phenomena, not all of which have exhibited conceptual coherence. It is hardly surprising, therefore, that many clinical investigations of pragmatics have lacked both focus and rationale (see chapter 9 in Cummings 2005). More recently, however, clinical studies of pragmatics have been reshaping our views of certain disorders. In Cummings (2005), for example, I argue that the theory of mind hypothesis of autism is none other than a pragmatic explanation of this disorder – autistic children's failure to treat other people as intentional agents is, in the final analysis, not an explanation of their pragmatic deficits, but is itself a pragmatic deficit. Better techniques of description and analysis are revealing previously unrecognised pragmatic impairments in disorders such as acquired aphasia and specific language impairment. An examination of a client's ability to use a range of speech acts or recover the implicature of an utterance is now as much a part of the protocol for assessment as is an analysis of receptive and expressive syntax. Greater understanding of and attention to pragmatics have enabled clinicians to develop more realistic goals of therapy and to achieve these goals through more appropriate means. The pragmatic emphasis on communication of meaning has allowed clinicians legitimately to develop nonverbal methods of communication as the very aim of intervention (and, importantly, not to have this aim treated as an indication of therapeutic failure by the client and family members alike). Also, the pragmatic emphasis on the context of communication has seen the spouse of the client, and indeed other family members and friends, assume an altogether more proactive role in the therapeutic process. We will examine these clinical developments at numerous points in the following chapters. In the meantime, it should be clear to the reader that this 'newest' branch of linguistic enquiry has had by far the most profound impact on clinical linguistic practice.

1.5 The Contribution of Medical Science and its Practitioners

It will not have escaped the reader's attention that, in order to explain the processes of communication, we have had to make use of anatomical and physiological description (the anatomy and physiology of hearing, for example). Moreover, we have appealed directly and indirectly to branches of medicine – neurology, otolaryngology, embryology and so on – in order to understand how communication can be disordered. In short, we cannot go far in the study of clinical linguistics without seriously engaging with various medical specialisms. In this section, I outline these specialisms. Also, I examine the ways in which speech and language therapists must interact with medical professionals from each of these specialisms in the management of specific communication disorders.

Anatomy and physiology form the cornerstone of medical science. Anatomy is the study of the structure of the human body. In earlier centuries, this study largely involved structures that were visible to the human eye through dissection. The brilliantly executed manuscripts of early anatomists contained numerous detailed drawings of large muscles, bones and organs such as the brain, for example. As our techniques for viewing the structure of the body have developed (e.g. electron microscopy and magnetic resonance imaging), so previously unseen structures of the body are now open to examination. We will see in subsequent chapters how magnetic resonance imaging in particular is making possible investigations of the brain that may eventually explain disorders like autism. In the meantime, the reader should be aware that no study of communication disorders can be seriously pursued in the absence of a thorough knowledge of speech- and hearing-related anatomy.

However, simply knowing the anatomical structures of the oral cavity and larynx will not assist us in the study of communication disorders if we do not understand how these structures function to produce speech and voice, respectively. The study of function is the domain of physiology. Throughout this book, we will have occasion to examine communication disorders in which normal anatomical structures fail to function correctly, often as a result of neurological damage. For example, the adult who sustains cranial nerve damage as a result of a CVA may be unable to achieve complete elevation of the velum (soft palate), even though this structure is anatomically sound. The resulting disorder of resonance – hypernasality – is linked to a physiological defect: that is, degraded nerve impulse transmission. In still other communication disorders, abnormal physiological function can cause damage to anatomical structures. For example, the teacher who forcefully adducts her vocal folds when shouting in class risks the development of vocal lesions, such as nodules and polyps. In an effort to compensate for the vocal hoarseness that attends these lesions, this teacher may exacerbate the physiological dysfunction by adducting her vocal folds even more forcibly than normal. This hyperadduction has predictable results – yet more vocal fold damage. As well as demonstrating the vicious circle that is characteristic of vocal abuse and misuse, this scenario is testimony to the functional integrity of anatomy and physiology.

Neurology is the study of the structure and function of the nervous system. This includes the central nervous system (brain and spinal cord) and peripheral nervous system (cranial and spinal nerves), both of which are of interest to the speech and language therapist. The brain contains central speech and language areas, normally in its left hemisphere. These areas can be damaged through trauma, infection or vascular disturbances (e.g. CVA), leading to disorders like dysarthria and aphasia. They are also susceptible to the degenerative effects of Alzheimer's disease and may be adversely affected by conditions which compromise neurodevelopment (e.g. maternal rubella infection). The brain gives rise to nerves that course their way through its structures to the brainstem. These nerves, called cranial nerves, exit the brainstem through foramina (small holes) in the base of the skull and deliver innervation to almost all the muscles involved in speech production. (One notable exception is the phrenic nerves (spinal nerves) that innervate the muscles of respiration.) These nerves are particularly vulnerable to damage through CVAs and progressive neurological disorders like motor neurone disease (MND). The results of this damage are not just speech disturbances (dysarthria and eventually anarthria in MND), but also feeding and swallowing problems (dysphagia). The implications of these neurological conditions for communication and swallowing will be examined in chapter 5, when we will also discuss a number of other neurological diseases (e.g. myasthenia gravis, Parkinson's disease and multiple sclerosis). However, on the basis of this brief discussion of neurology, it should be obvious to the reader that no study of clinical linguistics can afford to ignore this most important medical specialism.

Otolaryngology (or otorhinolaryngology) is the medical study of the ears, nose and throat, from which it takes its common name, ENT medicine. The integrity of all three of these structures is vital for normal communication. It is hardly surprising, therefore, that the otolaryngologist and speech and language therapist liaise closely during the assessment, diagnosis and treatment of a range of disorders. Children can be particularly prone to middle ear disease, which is due largely to inadequate ventilation of the middle ear by the Eustachian tube. (We will see in chapter 2 that this is one of the medical sequelae of cleft palate.) Called otitis media, this disease can significantly impair hearing, a scenario that can have detrimental effects on the young child who is developing speech and language. For this reason, otitis media should be closely monitored by the child's speech and language therapist and doctor, both of whom may refer the child to an otolaryngologist should the condition not respond well to antibiotic medications. The otolaryngologist may prescribe other medications (e.g. more specific antibiotics) and perform a surgical procedure that involves pressure-equalising tubes being inserted into the tympanic membrane. These tubes allow fluid to drain out of the middle ear and enable normal ventilation of the ear to be re-established. The otolaryngologist and speech and language therapist also work closely in the management of voice disorders in children and adults. These will be examined in chapter 7 and include, to name but a few, cases of vocal abuse and misuse, laryngeal carcinoma and psychogenic voice disorders (where the otolaryngologist's role is to eliminate an organic aetiology). Otolaryngology is clearly integral to the work of speech and language therapy. As such, we will have need to discuss otolaryngological methods of assessment and treatment at various points in the chapters to follow.

Psychiatry is the branch of medicine that is concerned with the diagnosis and treatment of mental illness. Many forms of mental illness are not of concern to the speech and language therapist, because they have no direct implications for communication. However, we will examine two conditions – schizophrenia and gender dysphoria – which fall very much within the remit of speech and language therapy. Schizophrenia is a severe mental illness which affects approximately one in every hundred people. Although the disorder affects men and women in roughly equal numbers, it has an earlier onset in men (teenage years and early twenties, compared to thirties in women). Psychiatrists perform a differential diagnosis of schizophrenia based on the identification of positive and negative symptoms. At least some of these symptoms (e.g. thought disorder) have been deemed to play a role in the bizarre language and communication deficits that accompany schizophrenia. We discuss these deficits in chapter 5. Gender dysphoria is a severe and persistent experience of dissonance between one's phenotypic sex and sense of gender identity. Although a diagnosis of gender dysphoria is made by psychiatrists, speech and language therapists are now routinely part of the multidisciplinary team that assesses and treats this condition. The specific role of the therapist is to instruct the pre- and postoperative patient on the use of safe voice modification techniques, to advise the patient and other members of the team of the vocal improvements that can reasonably be expected to be achieved through therapy and voice surgery (if the latter is being contemplated), and to guide the patient in making other communicative adjustments entailed by his or her 'new' sex. The lesson to emerge from this brief discussion of psychiatry is that speech and language therapy has a close clinical affiliation with a number of medical specialisms.

In the same way that the speech and language therapist must have a sound knowledge of speech- and hearing-related anatomy and physiology, he or she must also have an understanding of embryology and of the basic tenets of genetics. Many of the communication disorders that are encountered by therapists exist, not in isolation, but as part of the wide complex of physical and cognitive problems that frequently attend syndromes. The therapist must appreciate, for example, the chromosomal basis of Down's syndrome: namely, the presence of an extra chromosome 21 in body cells (hence, the use of the term 'trisomy 21' to refer to this syndrome). He or she must be aware that phenylketonuria (PKU) – a metabolic disorder, the neurotoxic effects of which can lead to mental retardation – has a genetic aetiology. (A single pair of defective genes is responsible for this disorder.) Chromosomal and other genetic disorders frequently result in abnormalities of embryological development. In fragile X syndrome, mutation of the FMR-1 gene on the X chromosome adversely affects early neurodevelopment, the result of which is mental retardation. Similarly, in velocardiofacial syndrome a genetic defect on chromosome 22 compromises early development of the tissues that form the palate, resulting in cleft palate (usually of the soft palate). Although the speech and language therapist does not need to have a detailed knowledge of the complex biochemical effects of genes on embryological development, some acquaintance with the genetic and chromosomal basis of the disorders that the therapist encounters and with the embryological malformations that cause conditions like cleft lip and palate, is necessary if the therapist is to be an informed, competent clinician.

Speech and language therapists must liaise with a number of other medical professionals. Many child clients of therapists are under the supervision of a paediatrician on account of physical and/or cognitive problems in addition to a communication disorder. The paediatrician will set in motion a range of investigations and therapeutic activities that involve the child and will base all major management decisions on the results of these interventions. The elderly constitute a large and steadily growing number of the clients that are treated by speech and language therapists.[8] Conditions such as dementia are often particularly common in this age group[9] and raise issues such as appropriate short- and long-term care of affected individuals. These decisions are taken by a geriatrician who will consider the views of a range of professionals in the multidisciplinary team (e.g. occupational therapists, psychologists, etc.). During this decision-making process, the speech and language therapist can be a valuable advocate for the communication-impaired patient.

Normal dentition and jaw structure and function are vital for good speech production – witness the reduced intelligibility of the elderly person who is speaking without dentures. Often, however, teeth and jaw abnormalities impact detrimentally on a speaker's communicative effectiveness. Even more importantly, such problems have the potential to disrupt speech development in children. If either situation occurs, it is important that the speech and language therapist liaise closely with an orthodontist, who will decide what surgical procedures, if any, should be undertaken in a particular case. In chapter 2, we will see an example of this professional collaboration, when we come to examine cleft lip and palate. (Children with this congenital defect are at risk of teeth erupting in the area of the cleft.) In the same chapter, we will examine the work of the oro-facial surgeon, who liaises with the speech and language therapist in the treatment of a number of disorders that have implications for communication and feeding (e.g. cleft lip and palate, glossectomy). Oro-facial and dental specialists make frequent use of prosthetics in their work. (For example, a prosthodontist is a dentist who specialises in providing prosthetic appliances like a palatal lift.) The speech and language therapist must be familiar with these devices and be able to assess their impact on communication and feeding. (We will see in chapter 2, for example, that a palatal lift can be used to reduce nasal resonance in cases of velopharyngeal incompetence in cleft palate children.)

In most developed healthcare systems, the patient's first medical contact is with the primary care team. Normally, this team consists of a general practitioner (primary care physician), nurses and health visitors. It is particularly important that the speech and language therapist spends time educating these individuals about communication disorders, as it is these professionals who are often best placed to make referrals to speech and language therapy services. The health visitor is usually first to detect a parent's concern that a child is not making many speech sounds or is not responding normally to environmental noises. An assessment of the child's delayed speech development and otherwise poor auditory response must include information about the child's hearing status. To this end, the speech and language therapist must liaise closely with an audiologist, who will perform a number of audiometric tests. The nurse is normally the primary care professional who implements communication and feeding strategies with patients in both hospital and residential contexts. (Of course, spouses/partners and other family members also have a key role to play in the implementation of these strategies.) Finally, a general practitioner with a high level of awareness of communication disorder can accurately identify a number of conditions that are frequently undiagnosed or misdiagnosed (e.g. spasmodic dysphonia[10]), as well as recognise the early symptoms of serious disease (e.g. laryngeal carcinoma).

In this section, we have described a number of medical disciplines that are an integral part of the knowledge base of a well-informed speech and language therapist (e.g. neurology). We have also described a range of medical professionals with whom the speech and language therapist must work in close collaboration (e.g. the otolaryngologist). In neither of these accounts have our descriptive efforts been entirely exhaustive. We did not discuss, for example, how the speech and language therapist must have at least a rudimentary knowledge of pharmacology, if he or she is to understand how antihistamines and other medications can bring about the dehydration of vocal fold mucosa or how aspirin may result in a vocal fold haemorrhage. Nor did we mention a number of other important professionals with whom the speech and language therapist must liaise – teachers and educational psychologists in school settings, social workers and psychologists in mental health teams, and physiotherapists and occupational therapists in rehabilitation centres. However, none of these areas constitutes a true omission, as we will have occasion to address these topics at various points in the following chapters. But what we have succeeded in demonstrating by way of this discussion is the essentially multidisciplinary nature of clinical linguistics, and the diverse professional roles and collaborations into which speech and language therapists must enter in different clinical contexts.

1.6 The Purpose of Structure

In the remaining chapters of this book, I base my examination of communication disorders on the following three-part structure: (1) epidemiology and aetiology, (2) clinical assessment and (3) clinical intervention. This structure has been motivated by a number of factors, which will be discussed subsequently.

Its effect will be to organise the discussion of complex clinical issues in a manner that is most accessible to the reader.

1.6.1 Epidemology and Aetiology

It is an indication of the regrettable lack of scientific rigour in many books in this area that few of them attempt any serious treatment of the epidemiology and aetiology of communication disorders. (One notable exception is a text by Gerber (1998).) Epidemiology is the study of the prevalence, incidence and distribution of disease and other health-related conditions in a specified population. It is the branch of medical science, for example, that gives us cancer rates for men and women of different ages in different parts of a country or regions of the world. However, it is also the branch of medical science that tells us that autism affects boys and girls in a ratio of 4:1, that schizophrenia affects 1 in every 100 people and that 250,000 people in the UK have aphasia. These figures are relevant to speech and language therapy in all sorts of ways. They indicate which speech and language therapy services should be a priority for funding. They are the basis upon which we can decide if there is an adequate number of training places available to meet the demand for qualified therapists. Most importantly, epidemiological findings often give us clues as to the cause – or aetiology – of a condition. The fact, for example, that autistic spectrum disorder and specific language impairment tend to aggregate in certain families[11] has led researchers to examine the genetic basis of these disorders.[12]

Putting epidemiology to one side, it is even more important that the speech and language therapist has a thorough understanding of the aetiologies of communication disorders. Knowledge of the pathological processes that cause communication disorders is a necessary first step in deciding upon an appropriate form of management of the patient. Patients with rapidly progressive motor neurone disease[13] will derive no benefit from articulation exercises. They will, however, require ongoing assessment of the safety of swallowing, as well as the institution of an alternative communication system. Similarly, the speech and language therapist must pursue very different types of management for the client who has a voice disorder of functional aetiology and the client whose voice disorder has a clear organic aetiology. The duration of speech and language therapy intervention is also largely determined by the underlying aetiologies of communication disorders. Intervention can span years, especially when neurological impairment is extensive and stable (e.g. in cerebral palsy) or is steadily progressive (e.g. motor neurone disease). Alternatively, intervention may last only a few weeks. The client with vocal nodules, for example, will normally have a number of pre- and postoperative sessions with a speech and language therapist in order to establish techniques of safe voice use. In each of these cases, duration refers to the period of time from initial contact to the termination of treatment. However, the duration of individual sessions and the type of activity that is pursued within those sessions are also often determined by the aetiology of a communication disorder. The head-injured patient, who has cognitive deficits, may have limited attention span and be highly distractable. In such a case, short therapeutic sessions are advisable. Finally, the timing of intervention is also related to the aetiology of a communication disorder. Aphasia therapy is usually pursued most intensively in the months immediately following a CVA, as it is during this time that neurological recovery occurs most rapidly. With aetiological considerations informing clinical decisions as diverse as the duration and timing of treatment sessions and the type of activity that is pursued within those sessions, it is clear that no study of communication disorder can afford to neglect aetiology.

1.6.2 Clinical Assessment

Before a speech and language therapist can proceed to treat a client, he or she must be able to describe the client's presenting symptoms. This description is normally undertaken as part of a wider assessment of the client's communication or swallowing disorder. Assessment can be a difficult process, both practically and clinically. Some consideration of those difficulties at this stage will facilitate our discussions of assessment in subsequent chapters.

Paediatric therapists are both familiar with, and ingenious at overcoming, the practical difficulties that can attend assessment. It is not unusual for a reticent child to engage in no verbal communication during an initial clinical contact. However, even in the absence of verbal communication, a wealth of information can be gleaned about the child from an accompanying parent. This information includes details about the child's medical and developmental history, hearing status and communicative behaviour in other contexts. Other information can be obtained through observation of the child's nonverbal communication skills and play skills. Even at this early stage, the therapist will have gathered sufficient information upon which to base a selection of formal assessments. If children are still not ready to engage with the structured tasks in a formal assessment, they may happily talk to their mother about the pictures in a book or tell dolly how to feed teddy during play. All of these activities present the therapist with valuable data upon which to base an assessment of the child's speech and language.

Compared with other cases, however, the reticent child presents therapists with a relatively minor assessment challenge. A number of the children who attend speech and language therapy clinics for assessment exhibit significant emotional and behavioural problems. Some autistic children, for example, are so resistant to interaction that a full assessment of their communication abilities may not be possible. Other children present with considerable sensory and motor deficits which must be overcome in the assessment process; the visually impaired child and the child with athetoid cerebral palsy may both struggle to select pictures in response to verbal stimuli, but this inability may not be indicative of a deficit in receptive language. Still other children have cognitive problems and perform poorly in assessments for reasons related to memory deficits and lack of attention control. None of these assessment difficulties, moreover, is confined to children. The schizophrenic client may pose a behavioural challenge for the therapist who is undertaking assessment. The adult who has sustained a CVA may exhibit sensory and motor deficits; hemianopia and hemiplegia, for example, are relatively common sequelae of CVA. Finally, the patient with traumatic brain injury often exhibits extensive cognitive deficits, including problems in memory, attention and concentration, speed of information processing, executive functioning (planning, organising and problem-solving) and visuo-spatial perception. Limiting the impact of any one of these factors on the assessment process is no small achievement. Managing a number of them simultaneously – as well as controlling the numerous distractions that attend assessment in a busy hospital ward, for example – places considerable demands on even the most experienced of clinicians.

Overcoming the difficulties described above is certainly an essential first step in performing any assessment. However, problems do not end there and continue with the choice of assessement method. Speech and language therapy clinics are now replete with formal assessments that can be used to test language and other communication skills in children and/or adults. These assessments are typically standardised and permit the therapist to compare the client's performance with that of a controlled population. They are seldom the only type of assessment that a therapist will use and are more often employed in conjunction with various informal assessments. These assessments include activities such as recording spontaneous conversation with the adult or older child, observing the client's use of communication skills with nurses and family members, and encouraging the child or adult to tell a story based on a series of pictures. These activities enable the therapist to assess a range of language and communication skills – expressive and receptive syntax, nonverbal communication, discourse coherence and cohesion and so on. At the same time, they permit the therapist to exercise control by determining the skills that should be assessed. ('Informal', in other words, does not mean 'lacking in structure' or 'without clinical rationale'.) For example, the therapist can test a client's reception of syntax by posing certain questions in conversation. Also, he or she can examine the child's expressive vocabulary by introducing pictures of the target lexemes into the story-telling activity. By the time the assessment process is complete, the therapist will have extensive data upon which to base a diagnosis of the client's communication disorder. However, diagnosis is also beset with difficulties of its own, as we will now see.

In most cases, the speech and language therapist will have little difficulty basing a diagnosis of the client's disorder on the results of assessment. However, when clinical opinion about the nature and characteristics of a communication disorder is divided, the process of diagnosis is itself uncertain and contentious. In section 1.3, we saw something of this contention when we described the current clinical controversy that surrounds the diagnostic status of semantic–pragmatic disorder. This disorder has elicited at least four different opinions amongst clinicians regarding its nature and status – it is a subtype of SLI, it is a separate disorder that is unrelated to SLI, it describes pragmatic impairments in autistic spectrum disorder and it does not exist in any capacity. This lack of clinical agreement has even extended as far as the role of organic factors in a diagnosis of semantic–pragmatic disorder. Where Rapin and Allen (1983) applied 'semantic pragmatic deficit syndrome' to children with known organic aetiologies, Bishop and Rosenbloom (1987) excluded such aetiologies from their diagnostic category 'semantic–pragmatic disorder'. (Children whose language impairment is caused by hearing loss or retardation, for example, were not included in the semantic–pragmatic deficit category[14].) Nor are these problems of diagnosis confined to communication disorders in children. For many years, aphasiologists have debated the use of the term 'aphasia'. (Should this term be applied to the adult who has language disorder in the presence of right hemisphere damage or a psychotic condition like schizophrenia, for example?) The reader should be aware that, in the diagnosis of certain communication disorders, there is much that divides clinicians.

1.6.3 Clinical Intervention

In the clinical intervention sections of the following chapters, we examine the activities that are undertaken by the speech and language therapist from the point of assessment and diagnosis to the eventual discharge of the client. Although these activities are too diverse and numerous to discuss in the present context, a few general comments about intervention are in order. More than ever before, speech and language therapy is being required to demonstrate the efficacy of its interventions. Our economic reality is such that, if speech and language therapy cannot demonstrate significant benefits to clients, then it will lose out to other health services in bids for funding. Studies that examine the efficacy of treatment are now as much a part of the work of speech and language therapists as are studies that examine communication disorders themselves. This emphasis on the efficacy of intervention has been a largely positive development for the profession. It has forced us to reflect – in some cases for the first time – on what we do well and to highlight those areas in which we must make improvements. It has encouraged us to be transparent to the purchasers of our services (e.g. schools, hospitals, clients, etc.) about what it is that we do and to establish realistic goals of treatment. On an altogether less positive note, the constant demand for demonstrations of efficacy has placed many therapists under intolerable pressure in their respective work environments. The result has been the loss of many able and experienced therapists from the profession[15] and the listing of speech and language therapy as one of the government's shortage professions, in the UK at least.[16] Clearly, we have not yet succeeded in achieving a satisfactory balance between the need to demonstrate the efficacy of our work and the need actually to do our work.

I described above how the impetus to establish the efficacy of speech and language therapy had forced us, amongst other things, to be transparent about what we do in our work. Speech and language therapists, it has emerged, perform a number of diverse roles. First and foremost, we are the practitioners of a process of therapy. This role involves a large number of activities, ranging from articulation therapy in children to the instruction of the laryngectomy patient on the development of oesophageal voice. The speech and language therapist is also an educator of clients, their families and other health professionals. We discussed in section 1.5, for example, how the speech and language therapist could effect early identification of communication disorders by educating members of the primary care team. Many of our clients and their families are confronting terminal illness (e.g. the patient with motor neurone disease, the client with metastatic cancer); many others are experiencing severe psychological distress, either as a primary disorder (e.g. schizophrenia) or as a result of a communication disorder (e.g. stuttering). For these clients and their families, the speech and language therapist must assume the role of a counsellor and be prepared to examine and discuss issues as diverse as premature death and psychological adjustment following a CVA. We also described in section 1.5 how the speech and language therapist could act as a valuable advocate for the communication-impaired client during discussions regarding options for care. Given my comments in the previous paragraph, it can be seen that the therapist must also act as an advocate for the profession in making the case for sustained funding for speech and language therapy services to managers and government agencies alike. Finally, the speech and language therapist is not simply a practising clinician, but also has a professional duty to contribute to research in the area of communication disorders.[17] As a researcher, the therapist is contributing to the knowledge base that informs all aspects of clinical practice.

We will have occasion to discuss each of these roles further in subsequent chapters. However, before leaving the topic of clinical intervention, I want to expand upon a further comment that I made at the beginning of this section. That was the claim that as part of the drive to prove the efficacy of our work, we have been forced to establish realistic goals of treatment. We must be open with clients and employers alike about the likely outcomes of our work. We must be clear about what we can realistically expect to achieve in therapy and, importantly, about what we definitely cannot achieve. The attainment of normal verbal communication is not a realistic goal for many of the clients that we see in our clinics. Often functional communication – communication that is sufficient to convey basic needs and desires – is the most that therapy can achieve. It is often difficult for the speech and language therapist to encourage the patient with a poor communication prognosis to adjust their expectations of therapy. However, this adjustment can be facilitated by clear explanations of the aims of different therapeutic activities, regular feedback on performance and progress and, in some cases, the signing of a contract by the therapist and client about the goals that might reasonably be achieved by the end of a period of treatment. Contracts are also a valuable way of making explicit the client's role and obligations in the therapeutic process. All too often, therapy is not successful because the client is not performing tasks and practising exercises at home, or the patient is pursuing a behaviour that he or she has been advised to discontinue: for example, the voice patient who refuses to stop smoking. Even when the patient is motivated and engaged in the therapeutic process, progress may be slow or nonexistent and such gains as are made may be very rapidly lost. In all these cases, we must be prepared to examine our techniques critically, and reject or modify them accordingly.

Notes

1. The Royal College of Speech and Language Therapists is the professional body that represents speech and language therapists in the UK. The College was founded in 1945 and gained royal status in 1995. The American Speech-Language-Hearing Association (ASHA) represents 114,035 speech-language pathologists, audiologists and speech, language and hearing scientists in the US. ASHA was founded in 1925. The long-standing existence of both organisations attests to the fact that clinical linguistics has been an active area of enquiry for some years.

2. Terminological distinctions between the US and the UK include differences in the names of the profession (speech and language therapy in the UK, speech–language pathology in the US) and in the names of certain disorders (the genitive form is used in the UK – Down's syndrome and Parkinson's disease – but not in the US, e.g. Down syndrome). These terminological and other variations do not convey differences of meaning, but the reader should none the less be aware of them.

3. One such account is advanced by David Crystal. He defines clinical linguistics as 'the application of linguistic theories and methods to the analysis of disorders of spoken, written, or signed language' (1997:418).

4. The National Institute on Deafness and Other Communication Disorders

(NIDCD) estimates that approximately 14 million Americans have a speech, voice or language disorder. A further figure cited by the Institute is that 1 in 6 Americans has a communication disability.

5. Grice's emphasis on intentions in communication is reflected in his account of non-natural meaning (meaning NN). For Grice, 'A meant NN something by X' is equivalent to saying 'A intended the utterance of X to produce some effect in an audience by means of the recognition of this intention' (1957:385). According to this definition, it is not enough that the speaker intends to cause through his or her use of an utterance a certain effect in the hearer; rather, this effect is only properly achieved when the intention to produce it is recognised by the hearer.

6. I am referring here to typical or normal cases. Of course, deaf communicators are able to ascertain the communicative intentions of others in the absence of speech perception. However, even deaf individuals depend on a form of perception – visual perception of manual signs – in order to establish communicators' intentions. This is another example of the more general point that is made about perception in the main text – forms of perception other than auditory perception have a role to play in the recovery of communicative intentions.

7. The following remarks of Miller convey something of this contention. In his criticism of linear hierarchical models of speech production, Miller remarks that 'the fate of the phoneme as a unit of control has not fared well . . . Arguments for the psychological reality of the phoneme as a perceptual unit must be mustered. However, evidence for its existence as a unit of planning or execution is slim' (2000:176). Clearly, Miller believes that there is little evidence to support the psychological reality of the phoneme in speech perception.

8. This steady increase in the number of elderly clients being treated by speech and language therapists is demonstrated by the following Department of Health statistics for speech and language therapy services in England. If we compare figures for the youngest and oldest age groups on record, we find that for every year between 1998 and 2002, there were 20 new episodes of care (measured by initial contacts) per 1,000 in the age group 0–2 years. (The only exception to this figure occurred in 1999/2000, when 19 per 1,000 new episodes of care were recorded.) While this figure has remained constant over a four-year period, the number of new episodes of care in the age category 85 years and over has steadily increased over the same period: 25 per 1,000 in 1998/99, 27 per 1,000 in 1999/2000, 29 per 1,000 in 2000/01 and 31 per 1,000 in 2001/02.

9. The Alzheimer's Association in the US and Mind in the UK estimate that Alzheimer's disease – the leading cause of dementia – affects as many as 10 per cent of people over 65 years of age and 50 per cent of people over 85 years of age.

10. In a survey conducted by the National Spasmodic Dysphonia Association in 1992, 71 per cent of patients with spasmodic dysphonia had difficulty in obtaining a correct diagnosis, while 70 per cent reported that the physicians they had consulted were unaware of the disorder. General practitioners were consulted by 75 per cent

of the respondents, but only 4 per cent of the respondents were correctly diagnosed by general practitioners. Patients had to consult an average of four (and as many as 25) different doctors over an average of five (and as many as ten) years before receiving a correct diagnosis.

11. We will return to this point in chapters 3 and 4, when we come to examine the epidemiology of autistic spectrum disorder and specific language impairment, respectively. In the meantime, it is worth mentioning another epidemiological finding with clear implications for research into the aetiologies of these disorders: their increased incidence amongst twins.

12. A number of research projects into the genetic basis of autism and specific language impairment are currently active. Two of the most prominent projects are being undertaken by Anthony Monaco of the Wellcome Trust Centre for Human Genetics at the University of Oxford and by researchers in the Developmental Disabilities Clinic at the Yale Child Study Center. Monaco and his team are investigating the genetic basis of developmental disorders in children, including autism, specific language impairment and reading disability. The Yale researchers are examining the molecular genetics of multiple incidence families (families with one autistic child and another child with autism or related pervasive developmental disorder).

13. Of the three types of motor neurone disease (see chapter 5), progressive bulbar palsy is the most rapidly progressive. (Average survival time is between six months and three years.)

14. It wasn't until 1992 that Rapin and Allen excluded similar organic aetiologies from their diagnostic category, semantic–pragmatic deficit syndrome. These aetiologies included severe mental deficiency, hearing loss and cerebral palsy.

15. One method of establishing the extent of this loss is to examine the number of therapists who allow their membership of a professional association to lapse. Such a study was performed in 1999 by the Royal College of Speech and Language Therapists. The College sent a questionnaire to 1,000 lapsed members. Of the 281 returned questionnaires, 161 respondents (57 per cent) had left the profession altogether. A much smaller number – 55 respondents (20 per cent) – had retired. Even amongst respondents who had qualified as recently as 1985–9, respondents who had left the profession outnumbered those who had left the College but were still working in the profession. On average, therapists worked for 11 years before leaving the profession, while 25 per cent had worked for five years or less before leaving. These figures are discussed further by Rossiter (2000).

16. In 2001, speech and language therapy was recognised as a shortage profession by the UK's Department of Health. The decision to so classify speech and language therapy was motivated by two studies of the profession in 1997/8 and 1999/2000, both of which had highlighted increasing recruitment problems (Rossiter 1998, 2000). A follow-up investigation to these studies has revealed yet further deterioration in recruitment levels, with the proportion of filled posts falling from 50 per

cent in 1999/2000 to only 41 per cent in the three-month period from October to December 2001 (Rossiter 2002).

17. This duty is made explicit in *Communicating Quality 2*, a handbook of professional standards compiled by the Royal College of Speech and Language Therapists. This document states that 'if the profession is to continue to develop its expertise and apply this expertise to new and challenging areas of service delivery, research aimed specifically at informing clinical practice must be undertaken' (1996:252).

2

Disorders of the Pre- and Perinatal Period

2.1 Introduction

Many communication, feeding and swallowing disorders encountered by speech and language therapists are the result of events that occur at the time of conception, early in the prenatal period, or before, during and after birth (the perinatal period). The gametes (sperm and egg) that fuse during conception may have an abnormal complement of chromosomes or contain mutated genes. Genetic mutations can also occur during the rapid cell divisions that take place following conception. These genetic and chromosomal abnormalities are just two of the causes of the many hundreds of syndromes that are known to exist.[1] Other prenatal events include exposure of the developing embryo and foetus to infections (e.g. maternal rubella), environmental toxins and agents (e.g. radiation) and noxious substances. Some of these substances are administered by the pregnant woman herself (e.g. alcohol, nicotine and illegal drugs), while others are administered unwittingly by medical personnel in the form of prescribed medications. The effect of these events is the disruption of the various embryological processes that are occurring rapidly in the early prenatal period. Even when these processes have proceeded normally, considerable neurological damage can occur as a result of oxygen deprivation during birth (birth anoxia or hypoxia). Any baby whose pre- and perinatal course has been compromised by one or more of these factors has a significantly increased risk of developing communication, feeding and swallowing problems. These problems and the aetiological mechanisms that bring them about are the subject of the present chapter.

It is important to be clear about the scope of this chapter from the outset. We will not examine syndromes in which there is a significant hearing loss (e.g. Apert's syndrome) here. Nor will we discuss speech and language disorders in children which, by definition, exclude a neurological aetiology (e.g. specific language impairment) or which lack a clear neurological aetiology (e.g. apraxia). These disorders will be examined in chapter 4. We will also omit from this chapter any discussion of autism. Despite growing recognition of the aetiological role of genetic and neuroanatomical factors in autism, this disorder is still characterised by its severe behavioural deficits. Cognitive explanations of these deficits have gained prominence in recent years. For this reason, we will examine autism and the other autistic spectrum disorders in chapter 3. With these various exclusions in place, what remains is a group of communication, feeding and swallowing disorders in which there is a clear neurological or other organic aetiology that is definitive of the disorders themselves (unlike in autism) and that is operative in the pre- or perinatal period.

2.2 Cleft Lip and Palate

A structural defect involving the articulators, cleft lip and palate can have serious implications for speech, language, hearing and feeding in the babies and children that it affects. In the following subsections, we examine the epidemiology and aetiology of this disorder. We also discuss how speech and language therapists assess and treat babies and young children with cleft lip and palate.

2.2.1 Epidemiology and Aetiology

Across sources, there is some minor variation in the estimated rates of occurrence of cleft lip and palate. The American Society of Plastic Surgeons estimates that about 1 in every 800 babies has a cleft lip and/or palate. The American Cleft Palate–Craniofacial Association states that this birth defect affects approximately 1 in 750 newborns each year. Sargent (1999) claims that clefts of the lip and palate occur once in every 700 births (14), a figure that is also advanced by the UK's Cleft Lip and Palate Association. Sargent also states that clefts can occur in infants of all races, although the incidence is highest in the Asian population and lowest in African Americans (14). In general, clefts affect males and females in a ratio of 2:1 (Sargent 1999:14). However, an isolated cleft of the palate is the only form of cleft that occurs more commonly in females (Stengelhofen 1993:3).

Other figures exist for this disorder, some of which have implications for the aetiology of cleft lip and palate. First, 21 per cent of all orofacial clefts have a cleft lip only (unilateral and bilateral), 46 per cent have a cleft lip and palate, and 33 per cent have a cleft palate alone (Sargent 1999:14). Second, cleft lip and palate occur in conjunction with other disorders. There are over 150 syndromes that have cleft lip and palate as part of their differential diagnosis

(Sargent 1999:15). The syndrome most commonly associated with a cleft palate is velocardiofacial syndrome (VCFS),[2] and approximately 50 per cent of children with Pierre Robin syndrome[3] can present with an incomplete cleft of the palate (Sargent 1999:21). The Cleft Palate Foundation in the US estimates that syndromes account for approximately 15 per cent of the total number of cases of cleft lip and/or palate and for almost 50 per cent of cases of cleft palate in isolation.

The precise aetiological mechanism at work in cleft lip and palate is still largely unknown. Notwithstanding this uncertainty, what can be said is that a complex, multifactorial aetiology appears to underlie the disorder. Its association with numerous syndromes (only two of which are mentioned above) and aggregation within families[4] point strongly to a genetic aetiology. Although investigation of the genetic basis of cleft lip and palate is still ongoing, researchers have established that at least one form of cleft palate – a sex-linked form of the defect – results from mutations in a gene called T-box 22. Genetic factors aside, it is thought that various medications play a role in the development of cleft lip and palate. These include anticonvulsive drugs (e.g. phenytoin and sodium valproate), which are used to treat epilepsy. Other drugs that have been implicated in the development of cleft lip and palate are corticosteroids and benzodiazepines (e.g. diazepam), which are used to treat insomnia and anxiety. In some cases, it may be decided that the benefits of taking these drugs (e.g. corticosteroids can help reduce the risk of premature birth) outweigh the risk of a foetus developing cleft abnormalities. Heavy alcohol consumption and smoking have also been linked to clefting, but there is little firm evidence to suggest that nonprescribed medications, trauma or illness during pregnancy contribute in any significant way to the development of this disorder (Cleft Palate Foundation).

Regardless of the specific aetiological factors at work in the development of cleft lip and palate, what is clear is that these factors disrupt the embryological processes that normally occur in the first trimester of pregnancy. For the purpose of understanding how cleft lip and palate arises, we intervene on embryological development at the point at which medial and lateral nasal processes emerge. (I draw on Watson (2001) in the following account.) Scanning electron micrographs (SEMs) are used to demonstrate each of the developments discussed. When available, these SEMs are of human embryos. When SEMs of human embryos are unavailable, SEMs of mouse embryos are used. Given the similarities between human and mouse embryogenesis, the use of SEMs of mouse embryos is unproblematic.

The olfactory placodes and frontal prominence form the upper edge of the stomatodeum, a surface depression in the developing face (see Figure 2.1A). During the fifth and sixth weeks of development, the epithelium of the placodes invaginates (see Figure 2.1B). This process of invagination drives the

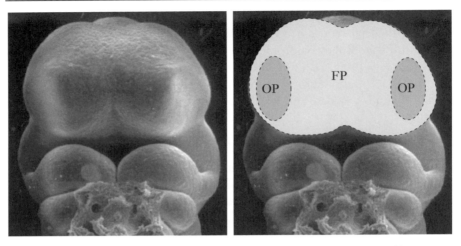

Figure 2.1(A): Frontal view of mouse embryo on day 10 of gestation (fifth week of human gestation) showing two **olfactory placodes** [OP] located on the lateral aspects of the **frontal prominence** [FP]. (Figure 2.1(A) to Figure 2.1(G) are reproduced with the kind permission of Professor Kathy Sulik, Department of Cell and Developmental Biology and Bowles Center for Alcohol Studies, University of North Carolina)

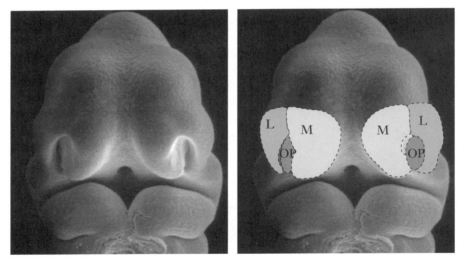

Figure 2.1(B): In the fifth week of human gestation, the **olfactory placodes** [OP] line the nasal pits. **Medial** [M] and **lateral** [L] nasal processes form around the nasal pits

placodes to the bottom of two nasal or olfactory pits. Elevations develop around the sites of invagination. The lateral halves of these elevations give rise to the lateral nasal processes, while the medial halves are known as the medial nasal processes (see Figure 2.1C). The frontonasal process is the area between and

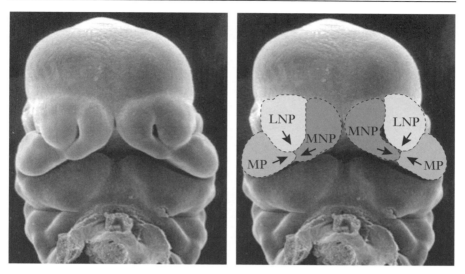

Figure 2.1(C): Frontal view of mouse embryo on day 11 of gestation (sixth week of human gestation) showing union of the **medial nasal processes** [MNP] with the **lateral nasal processes** [LNP] and **maxillary processes** [MP], which is required for normal development of the upper lip to occur

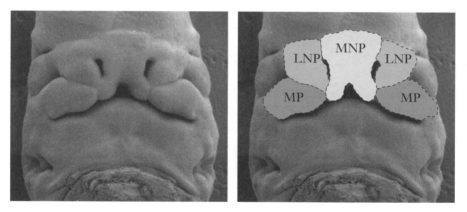

Figure 2.1(D): Frontal view of human embryo (sixth week of gestation) showing how the **medial nasal processes** [MNP] have merged in the midline to smooth the median furrow

including the medial nasal processes. The medial nasal processes grow more rapidly than the lateral nasal processes and converge in the midline (see Figure 2.1D).

Meanwhile, paired mandibular arches at the lower edge of the stomatodeum enlarge and coalesce in the midline. The upper margin of these arches gives rise to the maxillary processes (see Figures 2.1D and E). These processes grow

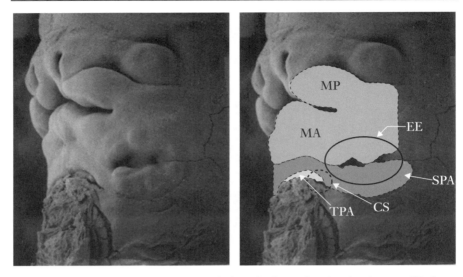

Figure 2.1(E): Human embryo during the sixth week of gestation showing the **mandibular arch** [MA] and the **maxillary process** [MP] of the first pharyngeal arch that contribute the upper and lower jaw. The **external ear** [EE] forms from tissues of the first and **second pharyngeal arches** [SPA]. The **third** [TPA] and fourth pharyngeal arches form very little of the external surface of the neck, their tissues lying deep in the **cervical sinus** [CS]

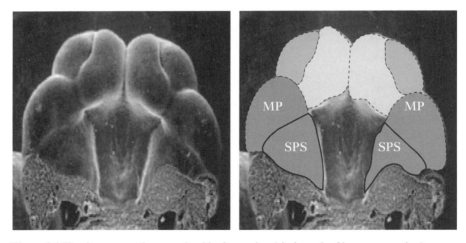

Figure 2.1(F): A mouse embryo on day 11 of gestation (sixth week of human gestation) showing the **secondary palatal shelves** [SPS], which are considered to be part of the **maxillary processes** [MP]

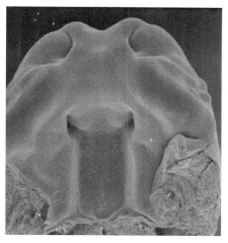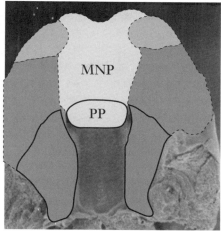

Figure 2.1(G): A mouse embryo on day 12 of gestation (seventh week of human gestation) showing how the **medial nasal processes** [MNP] contribute the tissues that will form the anterior part of the palate, the **primary palate** [PP]

forwards from the superolateral margins of the developing oral cavity towards the midline, eventually fusing with each other in front of the medial nasal processes. Their fusion achieves the formation of the upper lip. The frontonasal process gives rise to the primary palate – that part of the palate that lies in front of the incisive foramen, including the alveolus between the canine teeth (see Figures 2.1F and G). The frontonasal process also gives rise to the primary nasal septum – that part of the nasal septum that is attached to the primary palate. Delayed or inadequate mesenchymal migration will result in clefting of various types. If mesenchymal migration is only minimally disrupted, then a minor defect – notching of the vermilion (see Figure 2.2) of the upper lip – will occur. (The vermilion is last to receive mesenchyme.) If there is a more serious disruption of mesenchymal migration, the cleft may involve the upper lip, alveolus and palate as far back as the incisive foramen. The secondary nasal septum is formed when mesenchyme from the inner aspect of the maxillary process – the tecto-septal process – migrates upwards across the roof of the nasal cavity, merges with mesenchyme from the other side, and moves downwards, fusing with the posterior margin of the primary nasal septum as it goes. The columella and nasal bridge arise from the mesoderm between the medial nasal processes. The nasal alae (see Figure 2.2) develop from the lateral nasal processes.

As its name suggests, the secondary palate develops after the anterior part of the palate (primary palate). Palatal shelves are formed from the inner aspect of the maxillary process below the tecto-septal process. Initially, these shelves hang vertically downwards along the side of the tongue (see Figure 2.3A).

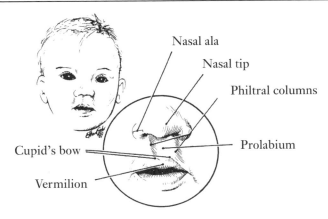

Figure 2.2: The normal lip and nose (Reprinted with the kind permission of the Cleft Palate Foundation, 1–800–24–CLEFT, www.cleftline.org)

During the eighth to ninth week of pregnancy, the neck begins to extend and the tongue moves downwards. The downward movement of the tongue creates space in the developing oral cavity, into which the palatal shelves move (see Figure 2.3B). At this stage of development, the head is not increasing in width and the palatal shelves will be able to fuse in the midline. However, if elevation of the shelves is delayed, fusion may not be achieved and the result will be a cleft of the secondary palate. Palatal elevation occurs approximately seven days later in female embryos than in male embryos and may explain the higher incidence of isolated cleft palate in girls. If the palatal shelves do make contact, they

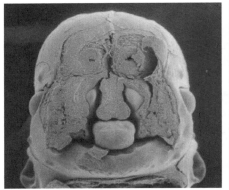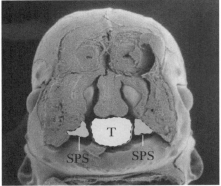

Figure 2.3(A): Frontal view of a mouse embryo on day 14 of gestation (eighth week of human gestation) showing how the **tongue** [T] is initially interposed between the **secondary palatal shelves** [SPS]. (Figures 2.3(A) to Figure 2.3(C) are reproduced with the kind permission of Professor Kathy Sulik, Department of Cell and Developmental Biology and Bowles Center for Alcohol Studies, University of North Carolina)

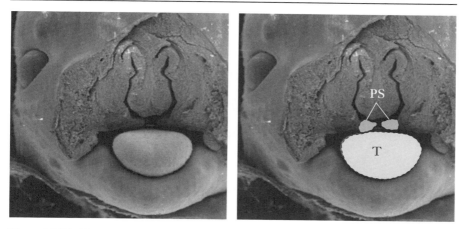

Figure 2.3(B): Frontal view of mouse embryo on day 14 of gestation (ninth week of human gestation) showing how the **palatal shelves** [PS] become positioned above the **tongue** [T] to allow for fusion in the midline

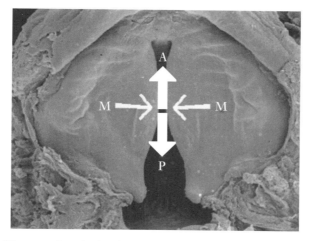

Figure 2.3(C): Human embryo in the ninth week of gestation. The secondary palatal shelves change their contours such that they initially approximate each other close to the **midpoint** [M] and fuse **anteriorly** [A] and **posteriorly** [P] from that point

fuse not only with each other but also with the primary palate anteriorly. Fusion of the palatal shelves proceeds as indicated in Figure 2.3C. Meanwhile, the secondary nasal septum grows downwards and fuses with the shelves in the midline. During fusion of the palatal shelves, the epithelium fuses to make an epithelial seam. Through cell death and migration of cells, this seam disrupts and differentiates subsequently into squamous epithelium on the oral side and ciliated columnar epithelium on the nasal side.

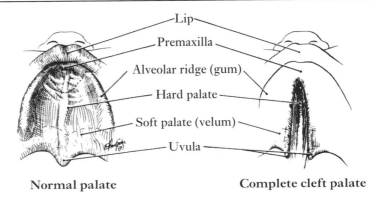

Normal palate   Complete cleft palate

Figure 2.4: The normal and cleft palate (Reprinted with the kind permission of the Cleft Palate Foundation, 1-800-24-CLEFT, www.cleftline.org)

The timing and sequence of these embryological processes explain certain features of clefting. First, these processes are completed within the first three months of pregnancy. Should a foetus be exposed to an environmental agent that is known to cause clefting at some point after this period, this exposure will not lead to the development of cleft lip and/or palate. Second, different embryological processes lead to the development of the upper lip, primary palate and secondary palate. It is possible for these processes to be individually disrupted so that, for example, a cleft lip can occur in the absence of a cleft of either the primary or the secondary palate. Third, depending on which particular embryological processes fail to occur, clefts can vary considerably in severity or extent. A minor cleft might involve only a slight notching of the vermilion border of the upper lip (see Figure 2.2). In a serious defect, the cleft may involve the lip and alveolus (gum ridge) on one side (unilateral) or both sides (bilateral) – see Figures 2.4 and 2.5 – and extend backwards to include the hard and soft palates (see Figure 2.6). In this latter case, the cleft is described as total or complete. When the cleft is limited to the lip, alveolus, hard palate or soft palate, or some combination of these structures, it is described as incomplete, partial or subtotal. Finally, the mucous membrane covering the palate may be intact and conceal an absence of muscle and bone beneath it. Such a defect is described as a submucous or occult cleft palate. Unlike other types of cleft, which are readily identified, a submucous cleft may remain undetected in infancy. An oral examination may reveal a bony notch at the posterior border of the hard palate (this is felt rather than seen), an opaque line medially in the soft palate (zona pellucida) which results from the lack of muscles below the mucous membrane, and a bifid uvula which occurs in almost all cases (Stengelhofen 1993:4). Kono et al. (1981) report an increased prevalence of submucous cleft palate in patients with clefting of the primary palate. McWilliams (1991) found that 44 per cent of a group of 130 patients with

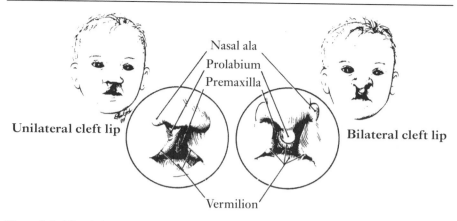

Figure 2.5: The cleft lip and nose (Reprinted with the kind permission of the Cleft Palate Foundation, 1–800–24–CLEFT, www.cleftline.org)

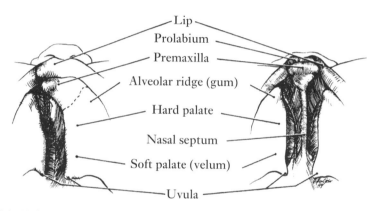

Figure 2.6: Unilateral and bilateral cleft lip and palate (Reprinted with the kind permission of the Cleft Palate Foundation, 1–800–24–CLEFT, www.cleftline.org)

submucous clefts remained asymptomatic into adulthood and that none of these 130 patients required surgical intervention for this clefting condition.

The embryological processes that have been outlined in this section are the basis of a system of classification of cleft lip and palate that was advanced by Kernahan and Stark (1958) and which is now in extensive use (for example, by the American Cleft Palate Association (ACPA)). This classification makes use of an embryologically significant structure – the incisive foramen – to distinguish between clefts of the prepalate (ACPA term) or primary palate (i.e. clefts of the lip and premaxilla), and clefts of the palate or secondary palate (i.e. clefts of the hard and soft palates). The embryological significance of the incisive foramen lies in the fact that it occupies the junction between the embryological processes that give rise to the primary and secondary palates. Located

Table 2.1 Kernahan and Stark's (1958) classification of cleft lip and palate

Clefts of primary palate (lip and premaxilla) only	Unilateral (right or left)	→ Total
		→ Subtotal
	Median	→ Total (premaxilla absent)
		→ Subtotal (premaxilla rudimentary)
	Bilateral	→ Total
		→ Subtotal
Clefts of secondary palate only	Total	
	Subtotal	
	Submucous	
Clefts of primary and secondary palates	Unilateral (right or left)	→ Total
		→ Subtotal
	Median	→ Total
		→ Subtotal
	Bilateral	→ Total
		→ Subtotal

behind the central incisors (see Figure 2.7), from which it derives its name, the incisive foramen is a small aperture through which an artery and nerve supplying the palate pass. The Kernahan and Stark classification is presented in Table 2.1.

2.2.2 Clinical Assessment

The structural malformations associated with cleft lip and palate can have a significant and deleterious effect on feeding in the newborn. Even after extensive surgical intervention, these same malformations can lead to problems in hearing and to disorders of speech and language development in the infant and child with a cleft lip and palate. Assessment of the impact of clefting on each of these domains begins at birth and can continue well into adolescence and adulthood, or until an appropriate functional outcome has been achieved. In this section, we examine the role of the speech and language therapist in this

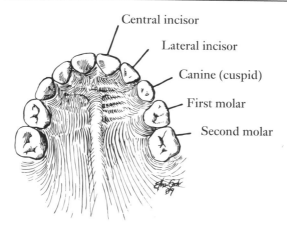

Central incisor

Lateral incisor

Canine (cuspid)

First molar

Second molar

Figure 2.7: Primary teeth (Reprinted with the kind permission of the Cleft Palate Foundation, 1–800–24–CLEFT, www.cleftline.org)

process of assessment. This is not a role that the therapist executes in isolation, but rather as part of a multidisciplinary team. Therefore, we will also need to consider the skills and knowledge that other members of the clinical team contribute to the assessment process.

2.2.2.1 Feeding

In the newborn with cleft lip and palate, there is a clinical imperative to establish a safe and efficient method of feeding. In general, this means instituting a specially adapted method of bottle feeding, as breast feeding a newborn with a cleft of the hard palate is often unsuccessful. (Babies with clefts of the lip or of the soft palate can normally be breast or bottle fed.) A range of soft, squeezable bottles (e.g. Mead Johnson) and orthodontic teats (e.g. the Nuk cleft palate teat) exist for this purpose. Carers can be instructed on how to gently massage the bottle in time with the infant's sucking. Cross-cut teats impede the flow of milk much less than standard teats. The combined effect of feeding technique and special equipment is to reduce the amount of energy that the cleft newborn must expend in order to transfer milk from bottle to mouth. This is an important consideration if the newborn is to avoid the downward cycle of increased energy expenditure and feeding time,[5] fatigue and decreased intake that leads inevitably to malnutrition (Pinder and Faherty 1999:286). The newborn with additional structural or other complications – for example, micrognathia in the infant with Pierre Robin syndrome, and cardiac defects in the newborn with VCFS – is at particular risk from this cycle of events and requires close monitoring of intake and expenditure of calories. In the absence of further complications, dietitians and nurses, who work in close partnership with parents, can overcome many early feeding difficulties. However, if it is decided that some alternative form of feeding is required – newborns with Pierre Robin syndrome may be unable to feed orally and may require gavage (nasal tube) feeding (Lewis and Pashayan 1980) – then a wider range of medical professionals will be involved with the case.

The speech and language therapist's role in the assessment of early feeding problems in the cleft infant is threefold. First, it is to determine the type and extent of any feeding disorder that is related to the cleft infant's structural anomalies. This part of the assessment should take in more than simply the obvious problems that are related to these anomalies – the failure to achieve an adequate lip seal for sucking, the frequency and amount of nasal reflux and so on. It should also include, for example, an assessment of the infant's risk of aspiration due to the presence of nasal residue after a swallow has been completed; liquid that enters the nasal cavities due to inadequate closure of the velopharyngeal port may leak after a swallow into the airway. Ideally, the cleft infant with no neurological involvement would respond to such aspiration with a protective cough, the presence or absence of which should be noted during assessment. The therapist should also take note of any behaviours that the infant employs during feeding to compensate for the problems posed by structural anomalies. Pinder and Faherty (1999) remark that children with isolated cleft lips and palates 'do a remarkable job compensating for the structural abnormalities and eventually can safely eat orally' (290). Maladaptive feeding behaviours should also be recorded, as these may have implications for subsequent speech production. For example, the cleft infant who responds to the sensation of liquid in the nasal cavities with nasal grimaces may later use the same behaviour to reduce nasal air escape during speech.

Second, the speech and language therapist must also assess the impact on feeding of any coexisting disorders. These disorders may take the form of additional structural defects (e.g. micrognathia in the infant with Pierre Robin syndrome). They may also include neurological impairments that result from damage to the central nervous system or cranial nerves. The infant with Pierre Robin syndrome who has severe micrognathia and glossoptosis (retraction of the tongue) is at risk of airway obstruction during feeding. (Protection of the airway may necessitate a tracheostomy.) The resulting breathing difficulties exacerbate a feeding situation that is already difficult on account of clefting of key anatomical structures. The infant with neurological involvement will experience problems with the full range of movements that are required for normal feeding. The child may be unable to coordinate sucking, swallowing and breathing. A flaccid soft palate may obstruct the flow of liquid during the oral phase of swallowing (in addition to causing problems associated with nasal reflux). The swallow reflex may be severely compromised by neurological damage. When this is combined with an ineffective or absent cough reflex, the risk of silent aspiration is considerable. The speech and language therapist must examine each of these dimensions in order to assess the contribution to the feeding disorder of any co-occurring condition. Particularly in cases where there is neurological involvement, it may be decided that oral feeding cannot be safely pursued. In such situations, a range of alternative feeding methods may have to be implemented, such as nasogastric tube feeding and feeding via a gastrostomy tube. The speech and language therapist will be a key member of the paediatric diagnostic team that assesses the viability and potential risks of oral feeding and determines the necessity of alternative feeding methods.

Third, the speech and language therapist's knowledge of feeding anatomy and physiology means that he or she is qualified to advise parents and other team members on the use of prosthetic feeding devices in particular cases. A palatal lift, for example, may achieve sufficient elevation of the soft palate to eliminate nasal reflux during feeding. This is especially likely to be true when velopharyngeal insufficiency is caused by neurological impairment (e.g. cranial nerve damage) or a defect involving the muscles of palatal elevation (e.g. aberrant insertion of the levator palatini muscle in cleft palate). However, if velopharyngeal insufficiency is the result of a short soft palate or an excessively large pharynx, no amount of additional palatal elevation will eliminate nasal reflux. In order to determine the cause of velopharyngeal insufficiency, the speech and language therapist uses techniques such as videofluoroscopic examination. Through the use of these diagnostic instruments, the speech and language therapist is able to recommend the adoption of a palatal lift to treat some cases of velopharyngeal insufficiency, and to identify where the use of this device is contraindicated.

In this section, we have outlined three main ways in which the speech and language therapist contributes to the assessment of feeding disorders in cleft lip and palate. However, the combination of these ways is by no means exhaustive of the therapist's role in assessment of cleft lip and palate. We described in section 2.2 how many babies and infants with clefts present subsequently with problems involving speech, language and hearing. Indeed, these difficulties remain long after feeding problems have resolved, either spontaneously or through medical and therapeutic intervention. At least one of these areas of deficit, speech, has a still somewhat unexplored relationship to feeding.[6] For this reason, we now turn to an examination of the speech defects that occur in cleft lip and palate.

2.2.2.2 Speech

Despite considerable surgical advances in the treatment of cleft lip and palate, a substantial number of children with this disorder go on to develop speech defects of varying severity. In a study of 212 preschoolers who had undergone palate repair, Hardin-Jones and Jones (2005) found that 68 per cent of the children were enrolled in, or had previously received, speech therapy. (Subjects were aged from 2 years 10 months to 5 years 6 months.) Thirty-seven per cent of these children exhibited moderate to severe hypernasality or had received secondary surgical management for velopharyngeal insufficiency. Sargent (1999:20) reports that approximately 70–80 per cent of cleft palate patients develop velopharyngeal competence after palate closure and that 20–30 per cent require speech therapy and/or an additional surgical procedure (a pharyngeal flap) to rectify speech defects. The Cleft Palate Foundation states that approximately 80 per cent of children with repaired cleft palates develop normal speech. The Foundation also claims that over half of children with cleft palate will require speech therapy at some stage during childhood and that approximately 25 per cent of children with repaired cleft palates still present with velopharyngeal inadequacy. Stengelhofen (1993:3) states an altogether larger figure. Some 40 per cent of children with cleft lip and palate, she claims, have 'long-standing problems leading to deficits in their communication skills.'[7] These figures demonstrate the need for an early and comprehensive assessment of speech in the child with cleft lip and palate. It is to an examination of the details of this assessment that we now turn.

For normal development of speech to occur, the following speech production subsystems must be both structurally sound and functionally integrated: (1) articulation, (2) resonation, (3) phonation and (4) respiration. In the child with cleft lip and palate, articulation and resonation are directly compromised by structural defects of the upper lip, hard and soft palates and teeth. In an attempt to compensate for these structural defects, the cleft child may engage in maladaptive vocal patterns that lead eventually to secondary disorders of phonation (e.g. dysphonia related to vocal abuse and misuse). We have already seen how cleft lip and palate may occur in the presence of other structural defects, some of which compromise breathing in a cleft infant (e.g. micrognathia). The child with cleft lip and palate is thus also likely to present with a disorder of respiration. With all four speech production subsystems compromised, either directly or indirectly, in cleft lip and palate, it is unremarkable indeed that speech should fail to develop along normal lines in the cleft infant. The speech and language therapist's aims in assessment are to establish the respective contributions to this development and to any resulting speech disorder of impaired performance in each of these subsystems.

The upper lip is an important articulator in the production of certain speech sounds in English. These sounds are the voiceless and voiced plosive consonants /p/ and /b/, and the voiced nasal consonant /m/, all of which involve a bilabial place of articulation. The upper lip is also an essential structure for sucking, which is a baby's primary method of food intake in the first months of life. Although recommendations about the timing of cleft lip repair vary, there is general consensus that this surgery should be undertaken as early as possible.[8] There are clear functional benefits of early surgery both for feeding and for later speech development. For the first time, a cleft infant will be able to form a complete lip seal during feeding – a requisite skill not just for early bottle feeding but also for later spoon feeding. The cleft infant with a repaired lip and palate is also able to engage in babbling. It is now generally accepted that babbling is an important precursor to later speech development in children. This is no less the case in the cleft palate population where

> evidence of the link between the phonetic repertoire of babbling and the basic sound system of a child's language . . . highlights the need for speech and language therapists to monitor babbling development and to implement intervention if there are indications of delay or deviance. (Russell and Harding 2001:195–6)

Early surgical intervention (palate repair at six months) may permit a normal babble to develop. Where this is not the case, babbling is characterised by a lack of labial and lingual articulations and a dominance of glottal and pharyngeal articulations (Russell and Harding 2001).

However, these early gains in feeding and speech development belie the fact that in a significant number of cases, cleft surgery can restore anatomical structures somewhat more successfully than it can establish normal function in these structures. A repaired cleft lip may exhibit reduced mobility, which can impact negatively on the cleft child's ability to round and spread the lips during speech production. The speech and language therapist can assess the likely effect of this functional impairment on speech production by calculating the cleft child's diadochokinetic rate for the repetition of bilabial plosives (Huskie 1993:68). A functional speech defect related to lip repair may be compounded by a severe nasal defect, particularly in the case of bilateral cleft lip.[9] Here, a shortened columella and the flaring or collapse of both nostrils (nares) may serve to obstruct the nasal airway. Hyponasal speech and an open mouth posture – the latter to facilitate mouth breathing – confirm the presence of an obstructed nasal airway. A secondary surgical procedure, known as an Abbe flap, may be used to correct a shortened columella and severely tightened upper lip in the patient with a bilateral cleft (Sargent 1999:20).[10]

Surgical repair of the hard and soft palates typically occurs some months after lip repair, although the exact timing of this surgery may vary.[11] Of all the primary surgical interventions that are used in the treatment of cleft lip and palate, palate repair is the procedure that achieves the greatest functional gains in speech and feeding. However, even after palate repair, structural defects and functional impairments of the palate can impact negatively on speech production and, for this reason, should be included in the speech and language therapist's assessment of the cleft child. The original surgical repair of the palate can break down. The resulting oro–nasal fistulae vary in size and occur most commonly in the area of the incisive foramen (Stengelhofen 1993:3). Some smaller fistulae are asymptomatic; that is, they have no effect on speech or feeding. These fistulae require no further intervention. The speech and language therapist must decide if a particular fistula is an impediment to normal speech and feeding. In an effort to prevent air passing through the fistula into the nose, the cleft child may engage in maladaptive tongue function during speech production, a finding that is supported by palatographic studies (Stengelhofen 1993:14). The child may shift the place of articulation of consonants further back in the vocal tract, a feature that is also observed in the speech of children who have undergone a delayed repair of the hard palate (Stengelhofen 1993:14). Speech production may be accompanied by audible nasal emission, which can be so severe that it masks friction produced in the oral cavity (Stengelhofen 1993:14). These speech defects – and possible nasal regurgitation of food – may be judged to be sufficiently severe to warrant surgical or prosthetic closure of the fistula. In any event, they must be noted in assessment.

Even in the absence of oro–nasal fistulae, a repaired cleft palate can pose further problems for the production of speech. The height and width of the repaired hard palate may be reduced. Within a reduced palatal space, a tongue of even normal size may be restricted in its movements. Postsurgical scar tissue can reduce sensation in the hard palate. The normally developing child uses sensory information gleaned from the articulators to alter the motor movements that are required to achieve the auditory targets of acceptable speech. If sensory feedback from the oral cavity is impaired, as is frequently the case in cleft palate, it may be particularly difficult for the affected child to achieve the level of motor refinement that is necessary to produce speech sounds. Reduced sensation in the hard palate should be noted during assessment, as it will have an adverse effect on the progress that can be achieved during later articulation therapy. Finally, as part of the oral examination, the speech and language therapist should record the presence of a bony notch at the posterior edge of the hard palate. A bony notch is indicative of a submucous cleft palate, particularly if it is accompanied by a bifid uvula. Such a defect may explain speech problems, persistent otologic (ear) disease and/or swallowing difficulties in a child who has no apparent clefting.

The figures for postsurgical velopharyngeal incompetence at the start of this section clearly indicate that palate repair carries no intrinsic guarantee of normal speech. A range of structural and functional problems affecting the soft palate (velum) can result in inadequate closure of the velopharyngeal port. The repaired velum may lack full mobility, making complete elevation and contact with the posterior pharyngeal wall impossible. Even if complete velar elevation is possible, the soft palate may still not be able to make contact with the posterior pharyngeal wall if the oropharynx is excessively capacious. Shrinkage of adenoid tissue is a common cause of velopharyngeal incompetence during adolescence. In the cleft child with a short or immobile soft palate, the adenoids can provide much-needed bulk in the area of the velopharynx. When the child's adenoids begin to shrink – generally between 10 and 14 years of age – a problem with velopharyngeal incompetence may emerge for the first time.[12] Velopharyngeal incompetence in the cleft child may also be caused by an associated neurological condition. The speech and language therapist's assessment of velopharyngeal incompetence must move beyond a description of its effect on speech – hypernasality of varying degrees – to establish the cause of velopharyngeal malfunction. This is because the aetiology of the disorder determines its prosthetic and surgical management. For example, if velopharyngeal incompetence is related to the immobility of the velum but the velum is a normal length, then a palatal lift will secure the extra velar elevation that is needed to achieve velopharyngeal closure. If a fully mobile velum is too short to make contact with the posterior pharyngeal wall, then an obturator (speech bulb) – a prosthetic device with a plastic extension on its end – will seal off the velopharyngeal port and prevent nasal air escape. However, if velopharyngeal incompetence is permanent (e.g. in the case of neurological damage), severe, unresponsive to speech and language therapy, or likely to deteriorate (e.g. as a result of adenoid reduction or growth changes), or the child cannot tolerate or use a prosthetic device (e.g. because of oral hypersensitivity as a result of early medical interventions), then a surgical procedure such as a pharyngeal flap[13] may be required. Using knowledge of the cause of velopharyngeal incompetence in a particular case, the speech and language therapist is able to advise other team members of the likely functional gains in speech production of prosthetic and surgical methods of intervention.[14]

Of course, any assessment of velopharyngeal function requires observation of a part of the vocal tract that is essentially hidden from view. Moreover, it is not adequate to base an assessment of the causes of velopharyngeal incompetence on the perceived consequences of this incompetence; a range of quite different aetiologies may all present as hypernasal speech. With the development of ever more sophisticated speech technology, the speech and language therapist now has access to an extensive range of instruments and techniques which make it possible to assess objectively the function of the velopharyngeal port. In section 2.2.2.1, we mentioned one of those techniques, videofluoroscopy. In recent years, videofluoroscopy has significantly advanced the assessment and diagnosis of a range of disorders. It is now used routinely in any comprehensive assessment of feeding and swallowing. In the present context, videofluoroscopy permits the speech and language therapist and surgeon to determine if a cleft child has sufficient structural and functional capacity in the area of the velopharyngeal port to support normal resonance during speech. As such, videofluoroscopy can help the cleft team decide if a child with velopharyngeal incompetence will benefit from a particular surgical procedure (e.g. pharyngoplasty).[15] Equally, videofluoroscopy can be used some 6–9 months after surgery has been performed in order to assess its effectiveness.

A videofluoroscopic examination is conducted jointly by the speech and language therapist and radiographer. As one of the health professionals who are most closely involved with the cleft child and his or her family, the therapist will normally explain the purpose of the examination to the child's parent or carer. The older cleft child will also benefit from receiving such an explanation. The therapist is also responsible for devising speech stimuli that will assess the child's ability to maintain and contrast oral and nasal resonance during speech. Videofluoroscopy is an X-ray procedure and, as such, the child undergoing examination must be able to satisfy certain requirements. He or she must be able to tolerate nasal instillation of barium contrast. To reduce exposure to radiation, the child must be cooperative during assessment and must be able to maintain a still head posture. (To facilitate this, the child is asked to look through a viewmaster at pictures while he or she is talking.) Equally importantly, the child must be capable of repeating speech stimuli. (This rules out, for example, the child with mental retardation who may not understand verbal instructions or who may not have the linguistic skills that are required for repetition.) For these reasons, videofluoroscopy is rarely performed in children under three years of age.

After videofluoroscopy has been performed, the speech and language therapist and surgeon can jointly review the videotape. Lateral videofluoroscopy enables the review team to assess the full range of intra-oral movements, not simply those of the velopharyngeal mechanism. This is important, as it has long been recognised that speech intelligibility is a function of the combined operation of all the articulators, rather than of any single articulator. Moreover, as we have already mentioned and as we will discuss subsequently, the cleft child may develop deviant articulations in an attempt to compensate for velopharyngeal malfunction or the presence of oro-nasal fistulae. These deviant articulations can be assessed in lateral videofluoroscopy, but they cannot be observed during another investigative procedure, nasendoscopy. In this procedure, a flexible tube (scope), which is attached to a video camera, is inserted into one of the child's nostrils. As this procedure can be uncomfortable for the child, particularly if the nasal passages are narrow, the nostril that will receive the scope is given a local anaesthetic. This can be through a nasal spray or in liquid form on a cotton wool bud. The whole procedure lasts some 15 minutes and can be performed on children as young as four years of age. Again, speech stimuli are selected that enable the therapist to assess the child's use of oral and nasal resonance during speech. Although this procedure makes it possible to view the velopharyngeal valve directly, and is easier to interpret than the images produced by videofluoroscopy, nasendoscopy is a more invasive technique than other assessments of velopharyngeal function. It is thus not suitable for use with many children and is often the last method of assessment to be used to investigate velopharyngeal incompetence.

Nasendoscopy and videofluoroscopy permit direct and indirect visualisation of the velopharyngeal port, respectively. As such, they are the assessment methods of choice for the surgeon who is planning corrective surgery for velopharyngeal dysfunction. However, the results of these investigations can be supplemented by acoustic and other objective measures of the perceptual consequences of velopharyngeal dysfunction. (A recent perceptual assessment of cleft palate speech – the Great Ormond Street Speech Assessment – will be examined briefly later in this section.) These measures can be obtained through the use of techniques such as spectrography, accelerometry and nasometry. Nasometry records nasal and oral sound pressures and uses these pressures to calculate nasalance scores. (These scores are arrived at by calculating a numeric ratio of nasal to nasal-plus-oral acoustic energy.) Sell and Grunwell (2001) cite their earlier work, which shows that nasalance scores correlate well with perceptual judgements of nasality (Sweeney et al. 1999a). Where nasometry produces acoustic measures, other techniques provide the assessing clinician with aerodynamic measures. (The former measures concern the movement of vibrational energy through the vocal tract, while the latter measures involve airflows and air pressures in the vocal tract (Sell and Grunwell 2001).) Aerodynamic techniques include manometers and combinations of pressure transducers and airflow meters. Sell and Grunwell (2001) draw upon one of their earlier studies to demonstrate that there is a moderate to good relationship between the perceptual judgement of nasal emission and pressure flow measurements during the production of /p/ in 'hamper' (Sweeney et al. 1999b). Clearly, these measures are not adequate by themselves for a diagnosis of velopharyngeal dysfunction to be made. However, when combined with the findings of other assessment techniques, particularly nasendoscopy and videofluoroscopy, they provide the clinical team with additional information about the nature and extent of this disorder.

Velopharyngeal incompetence can have a significant and negative impact on the developing phonetic repertoire of a cleft child. The child with velopharyngeal incompetence cannot achieve the build-up of intra-oral air pressure that is required for plosion. (The child with oro-nasal fistulae experiences a similar articulatory difficulty.) Oral plosives may be substituted by glottal stops, as the glottis is the only point in the vocal tract where the child can achieve an increase in air pressure. (When fully adducted, the vocal cords present a barrier to the pulmonary airstream.) The substitution of oral plosives by glottal stops can bring about a significant reduction in speech intelligibility. In this case, however, only the place of articulation is affected by the substitution – bilabial, alveolar and velar stops are replaced by glottal stops. Speech intelligibility is compromised yet further if glottal stops replace fricatives and affricates as well as plosives. In this situation, manner and place of articulation are both affected by glottal substitution.

Glottal substitutions are part of a general backward shift in place of articulation in cleft palate speech. Weak intra-oral air pressure leads the cleft child to substitute the palato-alveolar fricatives [ʃʒ] with palatal [çj], velar [xɣ] or pharyngeal fricatives [ħʕ]. Secondary articulations (e.g. pharyngealisation, velarisation and nasalisation) and double articulations (e.g. alveolar and glottal contacts) are common. The loss of air through the velopharyngeal port – and oro-nasal fistulae, if present – may lead to weakened fricatives, plosives and affricates. In an attempt to compensate for this loss of air, the cleft child may accommodate to a new speaking volume or strain the voice in other ways. D'Antonio and Scherer (1995) remark that

> the most recent theory for the cooccurrence of velopharyngeal and laryngeal symptoms is that speakers with velopharyngeal dysfunction may attempt to compensate for the inability to achieve complete closure and maintain adequate speech pressures by compensatory activity at the level of the larynx. (190)

The exit of air from the nasal cavities during speech production creates audible nasal emission, which can mask articulations in the oral cavity.

Dental and occlusal problems are common in cleft palate.[16] However, owing to increasingly sophisticated orthodontic and orthognathic procedures,[17] many of these problems now have little detrimental impact on speech development and intelligibility. In relation to dentition, clefts occur between the cuspid and lateral incisor (see Figure 2.7). In some cases, there is a twinning of the lateral incisor (one on either side of the cleft). In other cases, the lateral incisor may be absent. In either event, the consequences for speech production are usually minimal. If the lateral incisor is absent, for example, tongue protrusion through the space that is created by its absence may cause alveolar plosives and fricatives to have a fronted realisation (Stengelhofen 1993:15). Additional dental problems can also have a number of minor effects on articulation. Less commonly, the central incisor on the side of the cleft may exhibit some of the same problems as the lateral incisor. Precise alveolar contacts may be difficult for the child to achieve in such a case. Tongue movement during speech may be restricted owing to the overcrowding of teeth and the eruption of teeth in abnormal positions. Many cleft children have to wear orthodontic appliances (e.g. palatal expansion device) which reduce the palatal surface area for speech. As well as causing short-term reductions in speech intelligibility, these devices could also lead the child to develop maladaptive articulatory patterns. The impact of all dentition problems on articulation should be noted by the speech and language therapist during assessment.

Alveolar placement during speech may be difficult to achieve in the child who has a protruded premaxilla as a result of an unrepaired bilateral cleft of the alveolus (an unlikely event in developed countries). Even in the repaired alveolus, scarring and poor sensory awareness in the region of the gum ridge may make it difficult for the child to establish precise alveolar contacts during the articulation of plosive and fricative sounds (Stengelhofen 1993:15). Malocclusions occur in several of the syndromes that are associated with cleft palate. For example, in Pierre Robin syndrome and Treacher Collins syndrome, micrognathia causes the mandibular base to be set back in comparison to the maxilla. The resulting Class II malocclusion may not have a marked effect on articulation, although alveolar contacts may be fronted or dentalised (Stengelhofen 1993:17). In repaired cleft cases, the maxilla may lack width or be underdeveloped. In the Class III malocclusion that results, the maxillary base is set too far back and the maxillary teeth rest within the mandibular teeth. The normally sized tongue has a restricted maxillary space within which to move during speech and, as a result, consonants may undergo fronting and lateralisation (Stengelhofen 1993:17). As the tongue tip is too far forward in a Class III malocclusion to achieve contact with the alveolar ridge, it adopts a passive posture behind the lower incisors and the tongue blade assumes its role in articulation. However, the blade is less sensitive and flexible than the tip and it can achieve only imprecise articulations. Finally, because the maxillary teeth rest within the mandibular teeth in a Class III malocclusion, it may be difficult for the cleft child to achieve the labio–dental placement that is necessary to articulate /f/ and /v/. The bilabial fricatives [ɸ] and [β] may be substituted in their place (Stengelhofen 1993:17). The effects of malocclusion on the phonetic repertoire of the cleft child should be recorded during assessment and monitored over time.[18]

In the preceding paragraphs, we have described a range of factors that must be considered by the speech and language therapist who is undertaking an assessment of cleft palate speech. Some of these factors are properly part of the comprehensive oral examination that must be undertaken in order to assess the structure and function of the speech articulators. Other factors describe the phonetic sequelae of the various structural and functional defects that are typical of cleft palate. Previously, speech and language therapists, who had to evaluate the speech of cleft palate children, used a range of general speech assessments (e.g. formal standardised tests of articulation that are not specific to the cleft palate population). In recent years, assessment profiles that are specific to the unique characteristics of cleft palate speech have been developed. One such profile is the Great Ormond Street Speech Assessment (Sell et al.

1994, 1998, 1999), which is known by the acronym GOS.SP.ASS. This profile enables the therapist to assess resonance, nasal emission, nasal turbulence, grimace, articulation features (consonant production and cleft-type characteristics) and phonation, as well as evaluate the visual appearance of speech and perform a thorough oral examination. The therapist must also indicate the role of various aetiologies in the speech disorder, as well as discuss a management plan. The cleft-type characteristics include many of the speech categories that were described earlier – for example, lateralisation and glottal articulation. They also enable the assessing clinician to distinguish between nasal realisations of fricatives that are the result of an active compensatory strategy on the part of the child (and which can be resolved through speech therapy) and those that are due to an anatomical or functional defect (and, hence, require surgical intervention). Noseholding will facilitate the production of [s] in the latter case (passive nasal fricative), but will have no impact on [s] production in the former case (active nasal fricative) (Sell and Grunwell 2001).

In this section, we have examined the impact of cleft lip and palate on speech production by examining how the structural and functional anomalies associated with this disorder compromise articulation, resonation, phonation and respiration in cleft children. We have discussed the full range of factors that must be considered by the speech and language therapist who is undertaking a comprehensive assessment of speech in the cleft child. However, given the recognised link between hearing loss and speech and language impairment, any assessment of cleft speech that does not include audiological findings is at best incomplete. In the next section, we examine the type of hearing problems that are typical of cleft lip and palate. Many of these problems are chronic in nature and, as such, they put speech and language development at risk in the cleft child. In order to assess that risk, the speech and language therapist must be aware of the nature and extent of any hearing disorder in the cleft child. We examine how audiometric assessment of hearing in the cleft child proceeds. We also discuss how the speech and language therapist might usefully liase with other medical and health professionals – most notably, the otolaryngologist and audiologist – in an assessment of a cleft child's hearing.

2.2.2.3 Hearing

Cleft lip and palate aside, hearing loss is the most common defect in newborns. The National Institute on Deafness and Other Communication Disorders estimates that between 2 and 3 out of every 1,000 children born in the US are deaf or have some degree of hearing loss. Otological disease is also one of the most common forms of childhood illness. For example, 3 out of 4 children experience middle ear infection (otitis media) by the time they are 3 years old (National Institute on Deafness and Other Communication Disorders). These

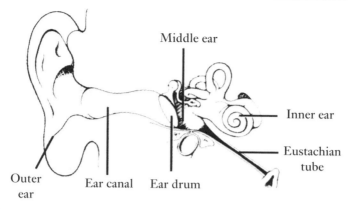

Figure 2.8: Gross structure of the ear (Reprinted with the kind permission of Dr Karlind T. Moller (Chair), Cleft Palate and Hearing Loss (2002), Cleft Palate Foundation)

already high figures are higher still in children with cleft palate. (Children with cleft lip only have the same rate of ear disease as children without clefts.) The Cleft Palate Foundation claims that over 90 per cent of children with cleft palate have recurrent or persistent ear infections or fluid build-up. Moreover, about 15 per cent of children and adults with cleft palate have a sensorineural hearing loss (Cleft Palate Foundation). In this section, we describe why children with cleft palate are particularly vulnerable to ear disease and hearing loss. We examine the audiometric tests that are used to assess hearing in the cleft palate child. Finally, we discuss how the speech and language therapist can integrate audiological results into an assessment of speech and language in the cleft palate child.

Hearing problems in cleft palate stem from anomalies of the palatal muscles. The Eustachian tube connects the middle ear to the nasopharynx (see Figure 2.8). Normally, the contraction of the tensor veli palatini muscle causes the Eustachian tube to open, which in turn achieves the ventilation of the middle ear (see Figure 2.9). In cleft palate, this pair of palatal muscles is abnormal and fails to open the Eustachian tube to the extent that is required for ventilation of the middle ear to occur. In the absence of adequate ventilation, fluid accumulates in the middle ear, resulting in a condition that is commonly known as glue ear (otitis media). This fluid may become infected and pus may form (suppurative otitis media). With no other point of exit, pus may rupture the tympanic membrane and leave the ear through the canal. (Van Cauwenberge et al. (1998) report that over 50 per cent of children with cleft palate have recurrent episodes of acute suppurative otitis media.) To avoid this sequence of events in cleft palate children, otolaryngologists perform a minor surgical procedure called a myringotomy, usually during lip and/or palate repair. By making a small incision in the tympanic membrane, the otolaryngologist is able to drain

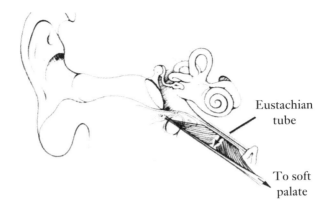

Eustachian
tube

To soft
palate

Figure 2.9: Opening of the Eustachian tube (Reprinted with the kind permission of
Dr Karlind T. Moller (Chair), Cleft Palate and Hearing Loss (2002), Cleft Palate Foundation)

fluid out of the middle ear. This incision normally seals naturally, but by inserting a pressure-equalising (PE) or ventilating tube into it, the otolaryngologist
can establish a temporary aperture in the ear drum (see Figure 2.10). This tube
takes over the task of ventilating the middle ear, thus preventing fluid from
reforming.[19] In order to maintain good otological health and function, some
two-thirds of children with cleft palate have PE tubes inserted (Cleft Palate
Foundation).

Of course, in order to treat hearing loss in cleft palate children, the otolaryngologist must first establish what is causing the loss. Using a range of
increasingly sophisticated audiometric tests, the audiologist and otolaryngologist can determine the type and severity of any hearing loss, as well as assess the
function of the hearing mechanism. One such test of ear function is tympanometry. The accumulation of fluid in the middle ear that is typical of otitis
media impedes the normal vibratory movements of the tympanic membrane
and ear ossicles (malleus, incus and stapes). The resulting conductive hearing
loss is so called on account of the failure of sound waves to reach the cochlea in
the inner ear through air conduction in the outer and middle ear. The role of
middle ear pathology in that loss is established by means of tympanometry. By
measuring sound reflection from the tympanic membrane while varying air
pressure in the ear canal, the audiologist can use tympanometry to assess
middle ear pressure and Eustachian tube function. Otoacoustic emission measurement can be used to test for the presence of sensorineural hearing loss in
cleft palate babies and other newborns. This technique is based on the observation that the cochlea in the inner ear can actually generate sounds (techni-
cally, emissions) either spontaneously (spontaneous otoacoustic emissions) or
in response to acoustic stimulation (evoked otoacoustic emissions). These
emissions are absent in mild inner ear deafness. The sensorineural component

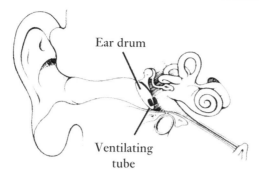

Figure 2.10: Ventilating tube in the ear drum (Reprinted with the kind permission of Dr Karlind T. Moller (Chair), Cleft Palate and Hearing Loss (2002), Cleft Palate Foundation)

of hearing can also be assessed through auditory brainstem response (ABR). In this test, brief sounds are used to evoke electrical activity in the VIII cranial nerve (acoustic nerve) and brainstem. Through the use of this test, it is possible to locate the lesion that is responsible for sensorineural hearing loss in the cochlea, acoustic nerve or brainstem. Finally, behavioural observation audiometry (BOA) can be used to test hearing in infants from 0 to 6 months of age. BOA makes use of a range of behavioural responses to sound in babies, including head turning (head turn technique) and the infant's startle reflex (startle technique). A combination of these procedures will be used to assess hearing in the newborn and child with cleft palate.

Audiological assessment of the cleft palate child should be ongoing.[20] Normal audiological results on one occasion of testing is not an indication that a cleft child has no hearing loss; the child who experiences recurrent episodes of otitis media may present with hearing in the normal range[21] on some occasions, but have depressed hearing on other occasions. Lennox (2001) states that the hearing impairment is 'variable and unpredictable' and that it may be as little as 10dB or as much as 40dB (213). This hearing loss has significant implications for the child's reception of speech sounds and development of language. The child with a hearing loss of 40dB misses most conversational speech sounds. (The intensity of speech sounds varies between 20 and 60 dB HL, with an average of approximately 40dB HL.) At this level of hearing loss, vowels are better heard than consonants. (Vowels are usually more intense and relatively longer than consonants.) The voiceless consonants /s,p,t,k,θ,f,ʃ/ will not be heard by these children in most speaking situations. (Indeed, these sounds contain so little speech energy that they are often not heard by people with normal hearing during average rapid conversation.) Alternatively, when these sounds are heard, it is with a considerable degree of distortion of the speech signal.

Clearly, an assessing clinician must be aware of hearing loss. Depending on the duration and timing of such a loss, the speech and language sequelae are variable. The cleft child with recurrent otitis media during critical periods of speech and language development will be more at risk of impaired speech and language than the child who has an isolated episode of otitis media during less sensitive periods of development.[22] The cleft child who cannot hear certain consonant sounds will omit and distort consonants in his or her own speech. (This is in addition to the other phonetic defects that are related to abnormalities in the structure and function of the speech mechanism.) The cleft child with depressed hearing will have poor auditory discrimination of speech sounds. Such a child may be unable to discriminate consonant sounds according to voicing (e.g. /p/ and /b/) and place of articulation (e.g. /t/ and /k/). In the absence of such discrimination, this child will be unable to produce sound contrasts in his or her own speech. So as well as having a phonetic disorder, a cleft child who cannot realise the phonetic differences between /pɪn/ and /bɪn/ or between /tɪn/ and /kɪn/ in his or her own speech also has a phonological (language) disorder. The child with moderate hearing loss also has difficulty hearing short, unstressed words (e.g. prepositions) and word endings (e.g. -s, -ed). These are important linguistic cues of grammatical and semantic categories and relations. It is unsurprising, therefore, that the child with moderate hearing loss should have limited vocabulary, difficulty with multiple meanings of words, difficulty in developing object classes, confusion of grammatical rules, errors in word placement in sentences, and omission of articles, conjunctions and prepositions (Northern and Downs 2002:22). As well as requiring ongoing audiological assessment, it is clear that the hearing–impaired cleft child also requires ongoing assessment of his or her speech and language. It is to this issue that we turn in conclusion.

Before conducting any assessment of a child's speech and language, it is vital that the assessing clinician have access to the results of a recent audiological examination of the child. The findings of such an examination can explain certain types of speech and language impairment. Also, it is often important to exclude hearing as a cause of speech and language impairment (e.g. in a diagnosis of specific language impairment in children). Given the incidence and severity of otological disease in the cleft palate population, it is even more important that the speech and language therapist have access to recent audiological results before completing an assessment of a cleft child's speech and language. However, speech and language screening of this clinical group raises a number of special considerations in relation to audiology. As with audiological examination, speech and language assessment must be an ongoing process. Even in the prelinguistic child, the speech and language therapist must be able to assess the implications of subnormal hearing for the child's later development of speech and language.[23] Through early involvement with the cleft baby on matters of feeding, the therapist is ideally placed to provide parents with information about speech and language stimulation in the young child. Like audiological assessment, speech and language assessment should be timed to coincide with key events in the child's otological management. In this way, the clinician can assess the effectiveness of procedures such as myringotomy and the placement of grommets by performing pre- and postoperative assessments of speech and language.[24] Moreover, speech and language assessment that is undertaken regularly may reveal a regression in the cleft child's skills. If such regression is detected, further surgical intervention may be required (e.g. repetition of myringotomy and insertion of grommets). So as well as assessing the impact of various otological procedures on speech and language development, regular assessment can reveal problems that act as an impetus to repeat these procedures or perform additional procedures. If amplification is in use (e.g. hearing aids), regular assessment can help the therapist determine if the chosen method of amplification is adequate to support the development of speech and language.

Although many otological problems in cleft palate resolve by the end of the first decade, speech and language assessment should continue to track audiological evaluation into adolescence.[25] The reasons for continuing speech and language monitoring of the cleft child into adolescence are threefold. First, ongoing otological problems, including middle ear infections, may continue to pose a risk to hearing and further threaten the cleft teenager's speech and language. (Persistent middle ear infection should be medically monitored because of its potential to cause complications.[26]) Second, new otological problems may emerge during adolescence, which can put hearing, speech and language at risk. Also, old otological problems may re-emerge, but with different aetiologies. Middle ear infections, once caused by inadequate Eustachian tube opening and ventilation of the middle ear, may be caused by infection via the Eustachian tube when there is chronic infection in the nasopharynx, palatine tonsils or sinuses. Third, the social communication aspects of language undergo considerable development during adolescence and beyond.[27] The context of this development – social interaction with peers – may be denied to the cleft teenager who has hearing loss. For all these reasons, assessment of speech and language in cleft palate should be viewed as an ongoing process that may extend over many years and that must intersect with assessment in other areas, most notably audiology[28] and otolaryngology.

2.2.2.4 Language

In the last section, we described how cleft children are at risk of language delay on account of otological problems, the most significant of which is otitis media. This middle ear infection, which is ubiquitous in the cleft palate population,[29] can cause fluctuating hearing loss during the first decade and beyond. In reality, however, hearing loss is only one of many factors that are believed to play a causative role in language delay in cleft palate. Other factors that contribute to this language delay include mental retardation,[30] a lack of language stimulation (particularly pertinent in the case of the cleft child who has undergone extensive periods of hospitalisation), defective anatomical structures and psychosocial problems. Along with hearing loss, these factors form a complex, multifactorial aetiology for the language delay that is present in cleft palate. And while some of these factors assume greater significance than others in particular cases, none of them can be said to operate truly independently of the others. (For example, the child with mental retardation will require above-normal levels of language stimulation in order to develop even basic language skills.) In this final section under clinical assessment, we examine the nature and extent of language delay in the cleft palate population. We discuss a number of important factors that must be considered by the speech and language therapist who is performing an assessment of the cleft child's language skills. Having completed this section, we will then be in a position to address the treatment issues that apply to this clinical group.

Russell and Harding (2001) state that 'cleft speech development is a combination of normal simplification processes and cleft type strategies' (198). Normal phonological immaturities resolve spontaneously and require no direct intervention from the speech and language therapist.[31] However, in addition to these normal processes, the cleft child must also cope with certain phonological consequences of his or her disordered articulation. One such consequence involves the backing of certain consonant sounds. In an attempt to establish intra-oral pressure during articulation, the cleft child with oro-nasal fistulae may engage in backing of alveolar and post-alveolar consonants. In this way, the consonant sounds /d,t,z,ʃ,tʃ,dʒ/ may all be realised as [g]. This backing process can become so well established in the child's phonological system that when the alveolar fricatives /s,z/ emerge, they undergo backing to the velar fricatives [xɣ]. The process of backing develops in the first instance in response to 'articulatory constraints' that are imposed on the speech mechanism by structural anomalies. (Oro-nasal fistulae are one of the conditions which impose these constraints (Russell and Harding 2001).) However, to the extent that backing becomes an organising principle within the child's sound system, its significance is ultimately more phonological than articulatory.

The child who substitutes alveolar fricatives with velar fricatives may still be able 'to signal meaning differences, even though phonetic realisation is abnormal' (Stengelhofen 1993:41). Certainly, Stengelhofen believes that the child who uses the palatal fricatives [çj] in place of the alveolar fricatives /s,z/ 'is able to communicate effectively and intelligibly, although he is not using the adult pronunciation of the intended target phoneme' (41). For Stengelhofen, such a case demonstrates that 'phonetic deviance may occur without a phonological consequence' (41). It is clear, however, that the often restricted range of a cleft child's phonetic realisations can considerably reduce the extent to which a cleft child can 'signal meaning differences'. For example, the cleft child who has a phonetic inventory that consists only of the nasals /m,n,ŋ/, the velar plosive /k/ and the glottal stop /ʔ/ has a much-reduced system of sound contrasts and a correspondingly severe phonological impairment.

Babbling presents the speech and language therapist with an early opportunity to record the consonant-like sounds that the cleft child is able to use. Features gleaned from these recordings can be compared with those that are known to typify normal babbling and, if necessary, intervention can be initiated. This early analysis may reveal, for example, a lack of labial and front of tongue plosives, which may lead to the backing pattern described above.[32] Later, when the child is using recognisable speech, the therapist can perform a detailed phonological analysis as well as a phonetic analysis.[33] It is important to establish if the child is able to use sounds contrastively, as an inability to do so will considerably reduce the intelligibility of his or her speech. We have already seen that a number of possibilities exist here. The child may have a phonetic deviance that does not impact on his or her ability to signal meaning differences. (Recall the child who uses palatal fricatives in place of alveolar fricatives.) More typically, however, the cleft child's difficulties at the phonetic level have consequences for his or her developing phonology. (Recall the child whose phonology is structured in part by a process of backing that has its origin in an articulatory disorder, the inability to achieve intra-oral air pressure in the presence of oro-nasal fistulae.) Superimposed on these possibilities are a host of normal phonological immaturities, some of which resolve normally (as in noncleft children), but many of which will display speech cleft-type characteristics on their way to phonological maturity. While a range of assessments are available to the clinician who wishes to screen phonology in the cleft palate child, Russell and Harding (2001) state that PACS TOYS (Grunwell and Harding 1995) can be particularly useful for this purpose.

Studies have also revealed delays in lexical development in cleft palate children (Broen et al. 1998). In a study of 30 cleft children and 30 noncleft children aged between 16 and 30 months, Scherer and D'Antonio (1995) report significantly lower frequencies for both the total number of words (a measure of vocabulary use) and the number of different words (a measure of vocabulary diversity) used by the cleft group. While no definitive explanation of these delays exists, the findings of a number of investigations point strongly to an aetiology in the speech production skills of cleft palate children. One such investigation was undertaken by Chapman et al. (2003). These researchers demonstrated that at 21 months, the expressive vocabulary of cleft palate children – measured using the expressive vocabulary checklist of the MacArthur Communicative Developmental Inventories (Fenson et al. 1993) and a 10-minute sample of caregiver-child interaction – correlated positively with the percentage of true stops produced postsurgery (at 13 months). No such positive correlation was observed in noncleft children. Also, lexical development was delayed in the cleft palate group when number of words in a 10-minute sample of caregiver-child interaction was the metric. Of particular interest in this context is a study by Estrem and Broen (1989), which found that cleft palate children targeted more words with word-initial nasals, approximants and vowels and fewer words with word-initial stops, fricatives and affricates. Moreover, a preference for sounds with a labial, velar or glottal place of articulation was shown by these children at least until the end of the 50-word stage. Clearly, the reduced expressive vocabulary of cleft palate children is related to their limited phonetic inventory – these children tend not to use words that their compromised speech mechanism cannot produce. However, the cleft palate child who does not use certain words more often than not will understand these words. In this way, the child's receptive vocabulary performance will exceed his or her performance in expressive vocabulary. This disparity in expressive and receptive performance extends beyond vocabulary. For example, Scherer and D'Antonio (1995) found that there were no differences between cleft and noncleft subjects on the receptive language subtest of the Preschool Language Scale – 3 (Zimmerman et al. 1992). However, cleft subjects had a lower mean length of utterance (MLU)[34] and used fewer bound morphemes – both aspects of expressive syntax – than noncleft subjects.

In addition to delayed lexical development, cleft palate children also exhibit delayed development of syntax. In a recent study, Chapman (2004) calculated the MLU in 15 children with unilateral or bilateral cleft lip and palate. (MLU was only one of several speech and language measures that were included in this study.) Although Chapman made no explicit comparison in this study between the MLU of her cleft subjects and the MLU of noncleft subjects, it is clear that an average MLU of 2.80 morphemes in cleft subjects of 39 months represents a considerable delay when compared with an MLU of approximately 3.5 morphemes in noncleft children of the same age.[35] Some account of this delay is to be found in a number of correlations that formed the focus of Chapman's investigation. Significant correlations were found between speech measures at presurgery (9 months) and postsurgery (13 months) and language measures at 39 months of age. (One other language measure, number of different words (NDW), was used in addition to MLU.) This was the case even in the absence of significant correlations between pre- and postsurgery speech variables and speech measures at 39 months of age. On the basis of this study at least, it would appear that language is more at risk from the early articulatory performance of cleft children than speech itself. However, as Chapman points out, the exact nature of the relationship between speech problems and language delay in cleft children is still unclear. This study does not establish, for example, if cleft children are purposefully reducing the length of their verbal output in an attempt to maintain intelligibility, as is suggested by

Scherer and D'Antonio (1995). Some support for this latter explanation derives from the fact that while expressive syntax is delayed according to MLU measures, all cleft subjects in this study scored within normal limits on the receptive language component of the Preschool Language Scale – 3 (Zimmerman et al. 1992). So cleft subjects clearly understood syntactic categories and relations, even though they were constrained – possibly on account of articulatory problems – not to use these categories and relations within their own speech. Whatever is ultimately shown to be responsible for delays in expressive syntax in children with cleft lip and palate, the speech and language therapist must be alert to the presence of these delays and establish their nature and extent during language assessment.

There are many ways in which speech and language therapists can proceed to assess receptive and expressive language in cleft children. Formal language assessments are now available in abundance. Many of these assessments contain normative data, which permit the therapist to compare the scores of cleft children with those of noncleft children of the same age. The Preschool Language Scale – 3 used by Chapman (2004) is such an assessment. Formal assessments can be more or less specific, with some examining a single dimension of language (e.g. the Peabody Picture Vocabulary Test – III (Dunn and Dunn 1997) measures receptive vocabulary only) and others assessing language on a number of levels (e.g. the Clinical Evaluation of Language Fundamentals (Semel et al. 2003) assesses language skills in a number of areas, including phonology, syntax and semantics). Formal assessments have other advantages over informal methods of assessment (i.e. those assessment methods that are devised and implemented by the individual therapist). These assessments are often described as 'standardised', which means that there is strict control of the language stimuli that are used and of the order in which these stimuli are presented. With the same stimuli being presented on each occasion of testing, the therapist may use these tests to assess the language progress of the cleft child over time (progress being indicated by improvement in test score between testing on one occasion and then again at a subsequent point in time). Standardised assessments are also vital for the purposes of conducting research and performing clinical audit. Until recently, the lack of a standardised speech assessment for use with cleft children had seriously hindered progress in both of these areas.[36] On a more practical level, all speech and language therapists are trained in how to administer formal assessments and interpret their results. So, on the not infrequent occasions when caseloads transfer between therapists, the results of all previously conducted formal assessments are immediately meaningful to a new therapist. Quite simply, formal assessments have a level of objectivity and universality that is lacking in most informal procedures.

This said, informal procedures have an important role in the assessment of language in cleft palate children. By assessing language subsystems in isolation from each other, formal assessments often miss the interactions that occur between language levels. It is particularly important to examine these interactions in the case of cleft children, given what we now know about the relationship between phonetic and phonological levels in these children on the one hand and lexical and syntactic levels on the other hand. Recordings of spontaneous conversation and story-telling activities enable the therapist to determine if the child is using lexical and syntactic strategies to increase intelligibility in the presence of articulatory problems. (For example, is the child limiting both the amount and type of verbal output – using words that contain easily articulated sounds – in an attempt to improve intelligibility?) Informal assessments are also more versatile than formal procedures. They can be used with young and/or uncooperative cleft children who cannot undergo formal assessment. Because informal methods can be built into play and everyday activities, the therapist can obtain a better understanding of how cleft children are using their language skills to communicate in a range of natural contexts than is possible using formal assessments. It is often only in these contexts that the true intelligibility (or, rather, lack of intelligibility) of the child's speech is revealed. (In formal procedures, where the target response is known, the therapist may judge the child to be more intelligible than is actually the case.) The skilled clinician will be able to integrate formal and informal methods in an assessment of language (and of its interaction with speech) in cleft children.

2.2.3 Clinical Intervention

Having completed a comprehensive assessment of the cleft palate child, the speech and language therapist must proceed to implement an appropriate programme of therapy. However, what constitutes 'appropriate' is likely to differ in each case. This is because cleft palate children do not form a homogeneous clinical group to which a single model of, or approach to, therapy can be applied. Accordingly, we will examine in this section a number of general considerations that apply to the treatment of cleft palate children. Before examining general principles of speech and language intervention in cleft palate children, we discuss aspects of the surgical management of these children. Surgical decisions concerning, for example, the timing of palate repair have implications for speech development in cleft children. To this extent, some discussion of the issues that motivate these discussions is warranted in the current section.

2.2.3.1 Surgical Intervention

Surgery to achieve palatal closure (palatoplasty) can affect maxillofacial growth and speech development. Specifically, the timing of palatoplasty presents the following dilemma for surgeons: early palatoplasty can achieve a good speech outcome but can disrupt maxillofacial growth. The decision about when to conduct palatoplasty can be influenced by variables other than speech development and maxillofacial growth – a cleft child with severe medical complications, for example, will normally warrant later surgery. However, to the extent that in medically uncomplicated cases, speech development and maxillofacial growth are key factors in a decision about the timing of palatal surgery, we restrict discussion in this section to a review of clinical investigations into these two variables.

Schweckendiek (1978) reported the long-term results of a timing protocol, in which the soft palate was repaired between six and eight months, but the hard palate was not repaired until between 12 and 14 years of age. While this protocol produced favourable facial growth results – Schweckendiek states that 'the results after primary veloplasty for some hundred adult patients show normal maxillary and cranial growth both clinically and radiologically' (1978:268) – only 40 per cent of subjects had normal speech at 15 years of age and above (i.e. after the time when the residual cleft of the hard palate is repaired). However, acceptable facial growth has also been found in subjects who undergo palate repair well before one year of age. Enemark et al. (1990) report normal and acceptable profiles in 50 out of 57 subjects who underwent hard palate repair at ten weeks. With good growth results being reported in early and late palatoplasty, maxillofacial growth appears to be less susceptible to the timing of palatal surgery than speech. Since Schweckendiek's (1978) study, subsequent investigations have consistently shown that late palatal repair produces a poor speech outcome. Dorf and Curtin (1982) examined the effect of the timing of palate repair on speech production. They compared the speech performance of children who underwent palate repair before one year with the speech performance of children who underwent palate repair after one year. Only 10 per cent of the subjects who underwent repair before one year of age developed compensatory articulations, compared with 86 per cent of subjects who had palatoplasty after one year. Trost-Cardamone (1990) states that the speech pathologist should monitor babbling development in order that palate repair can be performed prior to the stages of late (reduplicated and variegated) babbling: 'Palatoplasty that is physiologically successful and timed to precede and facilitate these stages might avert the development of compensatory and other related backed articulations in cleft palate individuals' (211). Dalston (1992) claims that a child's speech and language development is not 'ill-served' by early palate repair, but that there are few clinical data which indicate that surgeons who perform palatoplasty after one year 'should make a concerted effort to change their surgical protocol' (37). In a study of 212 preschoolers who underwent palate repair, Hardin-Jones and Jones (2005) conclude that 'an optimal treatment regimen for these children is one that includes primary palatal surgery no later than 13 months of age' (7).

The timing of palatal repair also has implications for Eustachian tube function. We described in section 2.2.2.3 how tube dysfunction can lead to otitis media with associated hearing loss in cleft palate children. Hearing loss can both delay and disrupt normal speech development. Any surgical intervention that has a positive impact on Eustachian tube function must thus be assessed for the benefits that it can confer on speech development. Bluestone et al. (1972) report that, following palate repair, there is an improvement in prograde clearance of radiopaque fluid media from the Eustachian tube and middle ear into the nasopharynx. Prograde clearance reflects the drainage function of the Eustachian tube. Bluestone et al. also recorded that the retrograde flow of fluid media from the nasopharynx into the Eustachian tube – a measure of the protective function of the tube – appeared normal after palate repair in over half the ears tested. The ventilatory function of the Eustachian tube was shown to be abnormal, even after palate repair. In a study of Eustachian tube function in 24 children, all of whom had tympanostomy tubes inserted between 3 and 6 months and had undergone palate repair between 14 and 18 months, Doyle et al. (1986) report an improvement in passive tubal function following palate repair[37] (though results for active tubal function are less convincing). These researchers attributed this improvement to the realignment of the levator veli palatini muscle during palatoplasty. Also, surgical intervention to correct velopharyngeal dysfunction can result in significant improvements in speech resonance. In a study of 100 patients who underwent pharyngoplasty for velopharyngeal incompetence, Albery et al. (1982) found that 97 per cent of subjects had been cured of unacceptable nasal escape (63 per cent had no audible escape, 19 per cent had intermittent audible escape and 15 per cent had slight audible escape), while 93 per cent no longer exhibited unacceptable nasal resonance. Sometimes, however, velopharyngeal surgery can result in undesirable speech consequences (e.g. hyponasality) or other complications (e.g. respiratory obstruction), as well as effecting little improvement in hypernasality and nasal escape. For example, in a group of subjects who received sphincter pharyngoplasty, Witt et al. (1994) observed that in only 18 per cent of subjects were hypernasality and nasal emission corrected, while 30 per cent of subjects exhibited hyponasal speech after surgery. Peat et al. (1994) found that in patients who had been assigned to undergo one of four different pharyngoplasty procedures, acceptable nasal resonance was obtained in 78 per cent of patients, while 9 per cent of subjects (12 patients out of 132) required some reversal of their procedure in order to alleviate obstructive symptoms.

Unlike palate repair, speech outcome appears to be less strongly correlated with the timing of velopharyngeal surgery. Hall et al. (1991) remark that 'when well designed, [pharyngeal flap] is quite as effective in adults as it is in children' (182). However, although hypernasality was completely eliminated in 90 per cent of Hall et al.'s adult subjects – a figure that is similar to those obtained in studies of child subjects – the 15 per cent of adults who developed hyponasal speech still presented with hyponasality 4 years or more later. (Hyponasality is normally a temporary complication of this procedure in child subjects.) The question of whether articulation therapy should precede or follow velopharyngeal surgery has exercised many researchers. Van Demark and Hardin (1990) advise against the use of articulation therapy to eliminate nasalisation in the presence of an incompetent velopharyngeal mechanism; however, therapy may be used to promote correct articulatory placement:

> The speech pathologist must recognize . . . that attempts to establish correct sound production in the presence of an incompetent velopharyngeal mechanism may lead a child to develop aberrant posterior patterns of articulation if emphasis is placed on elimination of nasalization rather than on placement alone. (804)

The emphasis for these theorists is clearly on prior surgical management of VPI. According to Sell and Grunwell (2001), however, a period of presurgery articulation therapy may reduce the extent of any planned surgery and, in some cases, even remove the need for surgery altogether. A similar debate surrounds the timing of articulation therapy in relation to orthodontic treatment. If therapy is delayed until orthodontic treatment is complete, the cleft child will have entered puberty and will have missed the critical period during which it is easier to learn speech (Sell and Grunwell 2001). However, performing therapy before necessary orthodontic work has been undertaken can be difficult and unsuccessful. Fistulae are normally repaired at the time of alveolar bone grafting, which is generally performed between 8.5 and 10.5 years (Mars 2001). However, fistula repair may be conducted earlier if the fistula is symptomatic: that is, causing resonance and articulation disorders. If earlier surgery is contraindicated, the fistula may be temporarily obturated through the use of a small plate until alveolar bone grafting is performed (Sell and Grunwell 2001). Finally, maxillary advancement (maxillary osteotomy) has produced varied speech results. While some studies have demonstrated spontaneous improvement in consonant sounds following surgery (Kummer et al. (1989) report improvement in articulation of sibilant sounds in 7 of 11 patients who underwent Le Fort 1 maxillary advancement), Sell and Grunwell remark that 'there would appear . . . to be a growing body of more recent evidence to substantiate the adverse effects of standard osteotomy on speech production' (2001:249).

2.2.3.2 Speech and Language Intervention

In this section, we describe a number of techniques and principles of speech and language intervention in cleft palate children. The reader should not regard the following discussion as a practical guide to therapy with cleft palate children. Such guides already exist (e.g. Stengelhofen 1999; Albery and Russell 1994) and will not be replicated in this context. Nor should the reader view each technique as effective in all cases. Indeed, for many techniques it is difficult to say just how effective they are – few efficacy studies have been conducted in this area. This said, we will neglect to discuss techniques that have failed to demonstrate even a minimal standard of effectiveness (e.g. behavioural management of hypernasality). With these provisos in mind, we begin by examining treatment techniques and principles that could be said to apply to several paediatric clinical groups in addition to cleft palate (e.g. the role of parental participation). We then turn to examine other techniques and principles that are specific to the particular characteristics of cleft palate (e.g. techniques used to treat maladaptive articulation patterns).

Parental participation is one of the key components in any paediatric therapy programme. Where the speech and language sequelae of a particular disorder are likely to persist for some years – as in cleft palate – securing parental motivation, cooperation and participation is crucial if therapy is to achieve certain goals. During the initial contact with the parents – which can be early in the neonatal period, if the therapist has been involved in feeding, or some weeks later – the therapist should seek to explain to the parents the role of speech and language therapy within the child's overall management. At a minimum, this explanation should include a description of the structural anomalies in cleft lip and palate and an account of how these anomalies affect speech production. To this end, the therapist can use diagrams and a range of other, excellent information resources that are now available from support organisations such as the Cleft Lip and Palate Association in the UK and the Cleft Palate Foundation in the US. This information session is necessary for three reasons. First, earlier explanations of the disorder are usually given by medical staff at a time when parents are distressed and are unable to take in information and ask pertinent questions. Indeed, it may only be some weeks or months later before parents even feel sufficiently empowered to ask questions of medical and health professionals or are able to become more proactive in the decision-making processes that surround the management of their child. Second, we have already seen that the cleft lip and palate population is not a homogeneous group. Information resources that are designed for clinical populations as a whole cannot address specific issues that are raised by individual cases. For example, simply reading that clefts are associated with many different syndromes is unlikely to address parental concerns about the potential for speech and language acquisition in the case of a child with a particular syndrome. During the first meeting with the parents, the speech and language therapist can usefully tailor general information about the condition to the particular situation of the individual child. Third, this initial meeting provides the therapist with an opportunity to outline how he or she will be involved with the child over the coming months and years. This involvement may be minimal, taking the form of speech and language monitoring at regular intervals but with little direct intervention. (It is important to point out to parents that not all cleft children will have ongoing problems with speech and language.) Where speech and language therapy involvement is likely to be considerable, the therapist should give the parents some indication of its nature and frequency.

Even before palate repair takes place, the therapist should encourage parents to engage their infant in vocal play and stimulation. These vocal interactions 'establish early patterns of turn taking and vocal response' (Russell and Harding 2001:200). Rather than viewing these early vocal behaviours within a wider process of emerging communication, parents who are misguided about the abilities of an infant with an unrepaired cleft may both devalue and disregard them. After palate repair has been performed, the child's vocalisations should begin to change to reflect his or her new oral structures. The child should begin to produce sounds that he or she was not previously able to produce. Accordingly, glottal and back articulations should become less prominent during babbling, while there should be a corresponding increase in labial and lingual articulations (e.g. [p,m,l]) and oral plosives (Russell and Harding 2001). If these articulatory patterns fail to develop, parents can be instructed on how to model target consonants during babbling with the child. Cleft infants who are repeatedly exposed to new consonant sounds are more likely to adopt these sounds and respond with recognition when they are used by others. To achieve this level of exposure, the therapist must rely on the involvement of parents, who have numerous opportunities each day during which they can model sounds naturally and reinforce their child's productions. The therapist who devotes considerable time and effort to the instruction and support of parents in these activities is thus making a most valuable contribution to the cleft child's developing communication skills.

Parental participation is again important when children begin to receive structured articulation and phonological therapy. The maladaptive articulation patterns of cleft children are often well entrenched. Eliminating these patterns and establishing new motor programmes requires maximum exposure to the new articulations involved and repeated practice in producing them. It is a simple clinical reality in many healthcare systems that clinicians are not able to work with cleft children with either the frequency or the intensity that is required in order to effect changes in articulation behaviour. Parental input serves to augment the amount of stimulation that the child receives in clinic. While increased stimulation certainly brings about gains in specific aspects of articulation, it is not adequate in itself to achieve long-term changes in articulatory behaviour. For the latter to occur, there must be generalisation and carryover of new patterns of articulation to situations beyond the clinic. It is only when the child is using recently acquired sounds consistently in new contexts that these sounds can be said to be an established part of his or her phonetic inventory. Parents who have been properly instructed in how to model, facilitate and reinforce new patterns of articulation are not only achieving a much-needed increase in the amount of sound stimulation that the child receives; they are also extending the therapy programme to the home environment, which will be an important test case of the child's ability to achieve generalisation of these new articulation skills.

Phonological therapy can also be facilitated by the participation of parents. Everyday situations provide parents with numerous opportunities in which to develop the child's awareness of how sounds are used to convey different meanings. For example, if the cleft child uses [keɪk] for 'cake', 'Kate', 'gate' and 'take', it is relatively easy for parents to provide a model of the target word 'Kate' before handing the child her favourite doll. To facilitate the child's production of target phonemes, it is quite easy for parents to engineer situations in which the child is required to request certain objects. (For example, the child should ask for Kate when going to bed, rather than simply being handed the doll.) It is also important for the child to experience something of the communication failure that results from using the incorrect form (e.g. that a request for [keɪk] will result in the child being given something to eat rather than receiving her doll). As well as providing the cleft child with opportunities to produce problematic sound structures in words, activities such as looking at picture books together and telling stories based on pictures can be used by parents to stimulate lexical and syntactic development in language-delayed children. These simple yet effective activities will be undertaken relatively effortlessly by some parents; indeed, many parents implement variations on these activities as part of their routine interactions with young children. Other parents will require more explicit direction from the speech and language therapist in order to achieve maximum benefit from these activities for their children. In all cases, the therapist should provide parents with ongoing support and guidance; parental participation is not a substitute for therapy, but will be viewed as such by parents who feel neglected by the therapeutic process. The therapist who is transparent about the aims of therapy and about the contribution of parents to therapy is best placed to secure parental cooperation and, ultimately, optimal speech and language outcomes.

Clearly, much speech and language intervention with cleft children is mediated through parents. This type of indirect intervention, we have already seen, is ultimately clinically motivated – it is necessary in order to achieve the generalisation of new skills and so on. However, to be truly effective, indirect intervention must exist alongside a range of direct techniques that are administered by the speech and language therapist. The choice of these techniques varies in accordance with factors such as the clinical needs and characteristics of the child, the preferences of the individual therapist and the use of particular treatment programmes within cleft lip and palate centres. At a minimum, they all involve some form of phonological therapy and articulation therapy, with the latter making more or less extensive use of instrumental techniques such as electropalatography. In the remainder of this section, we review these direct methods of intervention. It should be pointed out from the outset that these methods are not unique to the cleft palate population, but are also employed in the treatment of other clinical groups.

Before attempting articulation therapy, the clinician must establish if the child has adequate auditory discrimination of speech sounds. Poor auditory discrimination may be an indication that the child has a previously undetected hearing loss, which requires investigation. Even when the child's hearing is within the normal range, he or she may still exhibit poor auditory discrimination of speech sounds for other reasons (e.g. an attention deficit). The child who cannot discriminate between different speech sounds lacks an essential skill for articulation therapy. The therapist may need to spend time developing the child's discrimination and self-monitoring skills before embarking on therapy itself. The issue of the order in which to treat sounds in articulation therapy is by no means uncontroversial. Albery (1993) supports treating sounds in cleft children in the order in which they occur in normal phonetic/phonological development. Accordingly, plosive sounds would be targeted in therapy before fricative and affricate sounds. However, Russell and Harding (2001) state that 'it is common to follow an idiosyncratic sequence of consonant acquisition when working with cleft palate children' (204). They go on to suggest that 'it may be appropriate to target fricatives before plosives.' Other theorists advocate working on sounds that are most easily elicited in isolation or are stimulable or that contribute most to the child's reduced intelligibility. It is generally accepted that voiceless sounds are more readily elicited than voiced sounds and should be attempted first in therapy (Albery 1993). Therapy may target a number of consonant sounds or, less frequently, only one consonant sound (Russell and Harding 2001). It is often necessary to adopt a combined phonetic and phonological approach to therapy (Sell and Grunwell 2001). For example, it is not infrequently the case that a group of sounds is similarly affected by a cleft-type process (e.g. a backing process). And while therapy may favourably influence a group of sounds simultaneously, Sell and Grunwell (2001) remark that 'identification and targeting all errors affected by a process is important in therapy' (239).

Consonant sounds must be produced accurately in isolation before their integration into words and sentences is attempted in therapy. The correct production of consonants in isolation is no minor achievement for cleft children. Albery (1993) remarks that 'this is the level at which most children with cleft palate "fail" if they have a problem' (104). The therapist's spoken model of a target sound is often not sufficient in itself to elicit accurate production of the sound by the cleft child. For the child with a well-established pattern of backed articulation, visual and tactile cues may be necessary to encourage an anterior pattern of articulation. The child may require the additional visual stimulus that is provided by a mirror in order to achieve proper placement of the tongue tip/blade against the alveolar ridge during the production of alveolar sounds. Simple diagrams of the positions assumed by the articulators during the production of target sounds might be helpful in the case of the older child. While visual stimuli obtained through mirror work can be used to encourage correct alveolar placement during articulation, another type of visual stimuli, produced by electropalatography (EPG), can be used to eliminate abnormal lingual-palatal contacts in cleft palate speech. Gibbon (2004)[38] describes EPG as 'a visual feedback facility that provides a real time display of tongue-palate contact patterns that can be used as part of a speech therapy programme' (286). The visual displays produced in EPG help to make subconscious and hidden lingual misarticulations concrete and real for cleft children. Once observed, these abnormal lingual patterns are more readily modified in therapy. Of course, EPG is not suitable for every cleft child. Some cleft children are unable to tolerate the artificial palate that must be worn in this procedure; other cleft children have associated learning problems and will derive little benefit from the use of this technique. However, it is clear that in the cooperative, motivated cleft child, EPG is an effective therapeutic device that can be used to establish new patterns of articulation and modify or eliminate existing patterns of articulation.[39]

Many lingual misarticulations in cleft palate speech develop as compensatory strategies in the presence of structural and other defects (e.g. oro-nasal fistulae). The resistance of compensatory strategies to change is what necessitates the use of EPG both in the case of lingual misarticulations and in the case of another prominent group of compensatory speech behaviours, glottal articulations. Gibbon (2004) remarks that 'glottal and pharyngeal errors are classic compensatory speech errors learned as a strategy to impound air and maintain phonological contrasts, and as a result these speech errors are prime targets for therapy with EPG if other techniques have failed to resolve the difficulty' (301). Some of these other techniques involve modified whispering and sighing and are described in detail by Golding-Kushner (1995). They include the use of sustained /h/, over-aspiration and gentle whispering to keep the vocal folds apart. Noseholding can be used to help the child with VPI achieve intra-oral air pressure. Through the use of visual and other cues, the child can then be encouraged to attempt bilabial and alveolar placements, where previously only glottal articulations were used. (Van Demark and Hardin (1990) claim that therapy can be used to promote correct articulatory placement prior to surgical correction of velopharyngeal incompetence.) Correct placement must be accompanied by proper management of the airstream if glottal coarticulations are to be avoided. (Golding–Kushner (1995) reports that these can occur in patients who have been instructed in therapy on how to achieve correct bilabial and alveolar placement, but who have not been taught techniques in airstream management.) To encourage appropriate use of the airstream, Albery (1993) suggests holding a paper tissue in front of the child's mouth during the production of /p/ – the paper tissue will only move if an oral airstream and release of air are used. Other sounds can be facilitated through the use of additional techniques – Russell and Harding (2001) suggest that the use of blowing with subsequent production of a voiceless bilabial fricative can be effective in eliciting /f/. Whatever sounds are targeted in therapy, they must be used accurately in isolation before further progress can be made.

The newly acquired consonant sounds can be integrated into meaningful units of language – words, phrases and eventually sentences – in a staged approach. The first step is to include the target sounds in simple CV and VCV combinations (e.g. 'ta, ta, ta' and 'ata, ata, ata'). These combinations enable the child to develop articulatory proficiency in producing the target sound in a range of positions (such as occurs in words). When words are introduced, it may be necessary initially to separate the target sound from the rest of the word. Albery (1993) states that it is easier to practise the target sound first in word final position and then in word initial position. The therapist should adopt words and sentence structures for sound training that are appropriate to the child's level of language development. This is because there is often a trade-off observed between the child's linguistic level and articulation performance – as the child is pushed beyond his or her level of linguistic competence, articulation performance tends to deteriorate. Once targeted sounds are well established across all language levels, the therapist can begin to tackle the child's delayed language, particularly expressive language, in an equally systematic fashion. The therapist should begin to incorporate target sounds within increasingly complex syntactic structures, whilst all the time striving to maintain the level of articulation performance and intelligibility attained by the child. Initially at least, articulation performance may deteriorate, necessitating some linguistic simplification of the sentences being used in therapy. However, using appropriate facilitation techniques, the experienced clinician will be able to guide the cleft child through these problematic speech–language interactions and through other difficulties as well.

Phonological therapy must underpin any attempt to integrate newly acquired sounds into language. The therapist must actively develop in the child a sense of how sounds function contrastively and meaningfully in language. A cleft child may understand the need to effect phonological contrasts within his or her speech but, on account of structural or other defects, he or she may be unable to do so (e.g. the child with velopharyngeal incompetence who uses glottal articulations for all pressure consonants). On other occasions, the child may develop compensatory articulations in an attempt to effect phonological contrasts. Some of these articulations will be effective in signalling phonological contrasts; others will be unsuccessful. On still other occasions, the child may not express phonological contrasts within speech, not because of any structural defects of his or her speech mechanism – although such defects will undoubtedly restrict the child's ability to signal contrasts – but because he or she lacks basic phonological awareness of the contrastive function of sounds. The therapist must attempt to establish which of these scenarios best captures the child's difficulties, as each will necessitate a slightly different approach in therapy. However, even in the case where phonological disorder is related to a child's articulation problems, articulation therapy must be underpinned by phonological therapy if the new articulations achieved in therapy are to be successfully generalised. A range of phonological therapy activities can be used for this purpose. For example, the therapist can encourage the child to sort words according to contrasting consonants – e.g. [t] versus [k] – and to produce the correct word from a minimal pair, which must then be incorporated in a meaningful way into sentences and stories (Russell and Harding 2001). Of course, none of these therapeutic activities – articulatory or phonological – will be successful if the cleft child is lacking essential motivation. And renewed motivation some years later, when critical periods for learning speech and language have passed, is less easily converted into success in therapy. Accordingly, the therapist who is working with children must develop an appropriate reward system, which should be applied in a consistent and proportionate manner.

2.3 Cerebral Palsy

The pre- and perinatal period is also a time of considerable neurodevelopment. This is reflected in the fact that while the newborn has a body weight that is only 5 per cent of its adult value, its nervous system is one-fourth of its adult weight (Perkins and Kent 1986). Moreover, neurodevelopment is still an active process long after birth. For example, the brain gains weight dramatically up until about five years of age and the myelination of axons continues into middle and even late childhood (Perkins and Kent 1986). However, there are a significant number of babies and children who present with disorders when neurodevelopment does not proceed along normal lines. Known by the term cerebral palsy, these disorders involve aberrant control of movement and posture that appears early in life. This abnormality of control is secondary to a lesion of the central nervous system or other dysfunction that is not the result of a degenerative brain disease. The events that cause brain damage in cerebral palsy occur during the pre- and perinatal period or early postnatal period. Amongst other motor control problems, children and adults with cerebral palsy present with the speech disorder dysarthria. The neurological damage that occurs in cerebral palsy is also responsible for feeding and swallowing problems in this clinical population. If mental retardation accompanies cerebral palsy, the child or adult will also exhibit a language disorder. For all these reasons, the speech and language therapist is a key member of the multidisciplinary team that assesses and treats individuals with cerebral palsy.

2.3.1 Epidemiology and Aetiology

The United Cerebral Palsy Research and Educational Foundation reported in 2003 that there are between 550,000 and 764,000 persons in the USA with cerebral palsy. Recent studies have shown that cerebral palsy affects approximately 2.0–2.5 people in every 1,000 in the population. This figure is confirmed in a report that produced an overview of medical literature published between 1966 and 1978 on the epidemiology of cerebral palsy.[40] It has also been confirmed in a major study of cerebral palsy across 14 centres in eight countries in Europe (Surveillance of Cerebral Palsy in Europe 2002).[41] Parkes et al. (2001) report that rates of cerebral palsy among normal birth weight groups have remained relatively constant over time (about 1 per 1,000 live births). However, these authors also report that rates among low birth weight and very low birth weight groups increased by about threefold during the period from the 1960s to the late 1970s and that rates among babies weighing less than 1000g are also increasing. These increased rates among low birth weight babies reflect the rising survival rates of these babies during this period, which can be attributed to significant improvements in neonatal services at this time.[42] Since the late 1980s, rates of cerebral palsy appear to have stabilised (Parkes et al. 2001).

In many cases of congenital cerebral palsy[43] it is difficult to say with certainty what the cause of the disorder is. However, a number of events that occur in the pre- and perinatal period are known to damage the motor centres in the brain. These include infections during pregnancy (e.g. rubella, cytomegalovirus and toxoplasmosis), rhesus (Rh) incompatibility leading to jaundice,[44] and severe oxygen shortage in the brain or trauma to the head during labour and delivery. (The National Institute of Neurological Disorders and Stroke reports that about 6 per cent of congenital cerebral palsy cases are caused by birth complications, including asphyxia.) Strokes can also occur in the foetus and newborn baby. A number of other factors are responsible for cases of acquired cerebral palsy. In the first few months of life, for example, brain damage can be caused by infections such as bacterial meningitis or viral encephalitis or by trauma resulting from a motor vehicle accident, a fall or child abuse. In addition to events that are known to cause brain damage in the foetus and neonate, research studies are increasingly revealing a range of risk factors that are associated with cerebral palsy. Some of these factors describe attributes of one or both parents – for example, maternal hyperthyroidism, mental retardation, seizures, maternal race and maternal and paternal age have all been linked to an increased risk of cerebral palsy.[45] Other factors concern features of the pregnancy and labour. In this way, various studies have established multiple births,[46] breech presentation, a complicated labour and delivery, maternal bleeding during the sixth to ninth months of pregnancy and severe proteinuria (the presence of protein in the urine) late in pregnancy as risk factors for cerebral palsy. Still other risk factors describe features of the neonate. These factors include a low Apgar score,[47] prematurity (less than 37 weeks), low birth weight,[48] nervous system malformations[49] and seizures in the newborn. Ongoing research is revealing yet further risk factors.[50] It is worth emphasising that while each of these factors has been associated with an increased risk of cerebral palsy, a normal baby may emerge from a pregnancy that exhibits a number of these factors and a pregnancy displaying none of these factors may result in a newborn with cerebral palsy.

Cerebral palsy is most commonly classified according to its most obvious external characteristic, movement disorder. In this way, children and adults with spastic cerebral palsy[51] display slow, restricted movement and increased muscle tone (hypertonia). This is caused by one or more lesions in the motor cortex and corticospinal tract (also called the pyramidal system). The child with athetoid cerebral palsy[52] produces slow, writhing involuntary movements that block volitional attempts at movement. The lesion(s) responsible for the disorder in this case are located in the extrapyramidal motor system and/or pyramidal system and basal ganglia. In ataxic cerebral palsy, movement is poorly coordinated and may be accompanied by an intention tremor. In this form of cerebral palsy, the cerebellum is the site of lesion. Finally, a number of mixed forms of cerebral palsy also exist. In the most common mixed form – spastic-athetoid cerebral palsy – spasticity is combined with athetoid movements. In this case, lesions occur in both pyramidal and extrapyramidal systems.

A classification of the movement disorder is commonly accompanied by a description of the parts of the body that are affected by cerebral palsy. Thus, it is commonplace to find terms such as 'hemiplegia' and 'quadriplegia' used alongside 'spastic' and 'athetoid' (i.e. spastic hemiplegia, athetoid quadriplegia). In hemiplegia,[53] one side of the body is affected, although the arm and leg may be affected to varying degrees.[54] In diplegia, both legs are affected more than the arms. All four limbs are involved in quadriplegia.[55] Less commonly in cerebral palsy, only one limb is involved (monoplegia) or three limbs are affected (triplegia), usually both legs and one arm. Finally, cerebral palsy may also be classified according to the severity of the functional limitations that attend the disorder. This form of classification divides individuals with cerebral palsy into mild, moderate and severe types.[56]

The brain damage that causes motor dysfunction in cerebral palsy is often accompanied by damage to other areas of the brain.[57] These damaged areas cause a number of additional physical and cognitive problems for the child with cerebral palsy. These problems include epilepsy, visual and hearing impairments, mental retardation, abnormal sensation, and perception and growth deficits. In a study of 204 children with cerebral palsy, Murphy et al. (1993) found that approximately 75 per cent had either mental retardation, visual impairment, hearing impairment or epilepsy. Among these children, 65 per cent were mentally retarded, 46 per cent had epilepsy and 15 per cent had a sensory impairment. Many of these additional problems have negative implications for communication in the child and adult with cerebral palsy (e.g. hearing loss). Others are consequences of feeding and swallowing problems in this clinical population (e.g. growth deficits). For these reasons, we discuss some of them briefly in the present context.

Impairments of hearing and vision are commonly found in cerebral palsy. Using data from four UK-based case registers of cerebral palsy, Parkes et al. (2001) report that 1 in 10 children with cerebral palsy has no useful vision and 1–2 in every 100 children has no useful hearing. In a recent review of literature, Ashwal et al. (2004) report that visual impairments and disorders of ocular motility are common, occurring in 28 per cent of children with cerebral palsy, while hearing impairment occurs in approximately 12 per cent of cerebral palsied (CP) children. We will see in later sections that visual defects can compromise communication in the child with cerebral palsy. Visual problems include acuity loss (either myopia (short-sightedness) or hyperopia (long-sightedness)), field loss (such as hemianopia, when either the right or left, upper or lower half of the visual field is missing), oculomotor problems (such as strabismus, in which there is eye misalignment due to muscle imbalance), and visual processing problems that are caused by cortical visual impairment. Hearing loss has serious implications for speech and language development in the child with cerebral palsy. On account of the presence of one or more central nervous system lesion(s) in cerebral palsy, it is to be expected that hearing loss in this clinical population is predominantly sensorineural in nature.[58] It is also to be expected that many of the same factors that cause lesions to develop in the central nervous system will be linked to hearing impairment in cerebral palsy. In this way, Ashwal et al. (2004) report that hearing impairment occurs more commonly if the aetiology of cerebral palsy is related to very low birth weight, kernicterus (encephalopathy that results from bilirubin deposits in the brain), neonatal meningitis or severe hypoxic-ischaemic insults.

In addition to visual and hearing problems, the child and adult with cerebral palsy can have deficits affecting other sensory modalities. Reduced tactile sensation, particularly when this affects the articulators, can have adverse implications for oromotor therapy with this clinical group. The perception or recognition of tactile sensation may also be impaired. The individual with cerebral palsy may be unable to recognise even everyday objects through tactile sensation (a disorder called stereognosia). For example, the CP child may have to look at his or her hand in order to identify correctly the ball or comb that is held within it. Sensory and perceptual deficits, particularly across a number of modalities, compound an already difficult set of clinical considerations in cerebral palsy. We will see subsequently that the speech and language therapist must be aware of the nature and extent of these deficits and of their effect upon assessment and treatment.

Many children and adults with cerebral palsy also have cognitive impairments. The National Institute of Neurological Disorders and Stroke state that one-third of children with cerebral palsy are mildly impaired intellectually, a third are moderately or severely impaired and a third are intellectually normal. Ashwal et al. (2004) report that the incidence of mental retardation in their study of 886 children with cerebral palsy is 52 per cent. Parkes et al. (2001) states that 1 in 4 children with cerebral palsy has severe learning disability. Researchers in the SCPE found that 1 in 5 children with cerebral palsy (20.2 per cent) had a severe intellectual deficit. In general, the severity of cognitive impairment is related to the type of cerebral palsy. Spastic quadriplegic children have greater degrees of mental impairment than children with spastic hemiplegia (Ashwal et al. 2004). Cognitive impairment serves to limit language acquisition in the child with cerebral palsy. It is also a key consideration in the planning of communication intervention in this clinical population – many forms of augmentative and alternative communication (AAC) require functional language skills and some capacity for learning on the part of the child or adult with cerebral palsy. For these reasons, we will return to consider cognitive impairment at various points in the following discussion.

Growth problems also attend cerebral palsy. The National Institute of Neurological Disorders and Stroke states that failure to thrive is common in children with moderate to severe cerebral palsy, particularly those with spastic quadriparesis. Undoubtedly, poor nutrition has a major role to play in growth failure. The evidence of malnutrition in the CP population is undeniable.[59] This is still the case, even though the nutritional status of individuals with cerebral palsy has improved considerably in recent years, largely as a result of gastrostomy feeding and the use of commercially prepared formulas. However, it is also likely that failure to thrive is caused by damage to brain centres that control growth and development.[60] Gastrostomy feeding requires an initial surgical procedure and can result in complications of varying severity.[61] As such, its use is normally only recommended when investigation reveals oral feeding to be unsafe or incapable of meeting the CP child's nutritional needs. The speech and language therapist is a key member of the multidisciplinary team that makes an assessment of the suitability of oral feeding in a particular case.

The details of that assessment and of the speech and language therapist's contribution to it will be examined further in the next section.

2.3.2 Clinical Assessment

The child with cerebral palsy presents the speech and language therapist with a number of unique assessment challenges. These challenges stem in large part from the complex neurological basis of this disorder. It will be recalled that the trauma or insult that causes cerebral palsy occurs at a time when the central nervous system is immature and still has to undergo considerable neurodevelopment. As the central nervous system matures, the clinical expression of cerebral palsy changes, even though the encephalopathy is essentially static in this disorder. Within this evolving clinical profile, the severity and type of communication impairment and feeding and swallowing problems can also be expected to vary. Assessment that is performed infrequently and in isolation from ongoing treatment is an inadequate basis upon which to monitor these clinical changes and to adjust intervention, where this becomes necessary.

The brain injury in cerebral palsy also poses challenges for assessment. When the injury is widely distributed (such as occurs in kernicterus[62]) or multifocal in nature (as a result, for example, of trauma in the postnatal period), a mixed neurological picture will emerge. The child may exhibit signs of pyramidal and extrapyramidal damage – for example, slow, writhing athetoid movements combined with a positive Babinski sign.[63] This mixed neurological picture is reflected in an equally mixed set of speech features, with the child exhibiting characteristics of both spastic and athetoid dysarthrias. Establishing the respective contributions of spastic and athetoid speech features to the overall unintelligibility of a child's speech is a difficult, yet necessary, component of assessment. Also, widely distributed and multifocal brain injury can cause a number of other impairments that occur alongside the motor dysfunction of cerebral palsy. Some of these associated impairments contribute to the speech and language disorder (e.g. hearing loss and cognitive impairment) and it is the task of the assessing clinician to determine the extent of that contribution. Other associated impairments can make assessment of the CP child more difficult in practical terms. For example, the child with severe physical disabilities may struggle to point to pictures during language comprehension tasks. Where oculomotor problems also occur, eye gaze cannot be reliably used to indicate responses during assessment. Finally, many children with cerebral palsy require pharmacotherapy, not only to relieve the distressing symptoms of the motor disorder (e.g. spasticity and athetoid movements), but also to control seizure activity and to reduce drooling. A number of the drugs used for these purposes can cause drowsiness[64] and irritability,[65] both of which will adversely affect the child's attention and cooperation during assessment. We will return to each of these factors in the following paragraphs, as we come to examine how feeding, speech, hearing and language are assessed in the CP population.

2.3.2.1 Feeding

Feeding and swallowing problems are amongst the most common and distressing consequences of motor dysfunction in cerebral palsy. A recent study of the parents of children with oromotor dysfunction on the Oxford Register of Early Childhood Impairments confirms the severity and extent of feeding problems in the CP population (93 per cent of the children included in this study having cerebral palsy). In this way, Sullivan et al. (2000) report that 89 per cent of children needed help with feeding, 28 per cent of parents described prolonged feeding times (three hours a day) and 20 per cent of parents found feeding to be stressful and unenjoyable. These researchers also found that 56 per cent of children choked with food, 31 per cent had suffered at least one chest infection in the previous six months (an indication that aspiration is occurring), and 28 per cent had continuous drooling of saliva. It is undoubtedly a sad reflection of the state of paediatric dysphagia services in the UK that, although 38 per cent of respondents considered their child to be underweight, 64 per cent of children had never had their feeding and nutrition assessed. This lack of assessment may also explain why only 8 per cent of children were receiving caloric supplements and only 8 per cent of children were fed nonorally via a gastrostomy tube, when the high rate of chest infection indicates that there was a significant risk of aspiration of food among the subjects in this study. Clearly, there is still considerable room for improvement in the delivery of dysphagia services to children with oromotor dysfunction.[66] For our present purposes, we are concerned to examine a key component of these services, assessment.

The central question that must be addressed by the multidisciplinary team during assessment is whether oral feeding is a safe and effective method of feeding. Using knowledge of oral and pharyngeal musculature and of the neural pathways that innervate this musculature, the speech and language therapist is ideally placed to address questions about the safety of oral feeding. The question of the effectiveness of oral feeding is addressed both by the team's dietitian, who has knowledge of the CP child's nutritional needs and can determine if those needs are adequately met through oral feeding, and by the occupational therapist, who can establish if a better sitting position and the use of special equipment can improve the effectiveness of oral feeding. Beyond the important task of establishing the safety of oral feeding, the involvement of the speech and language therapist in an assessment of feeding is justified on other grounds. It has been argued that early feeding skills may have some predictive value in relation to later speech development. The exact nature of the relationship between feeding skills and articulatory proficiency is unclear – indeed, some clinicians argue that there is little or no relationship between these functions.[67] However, it remains the case that an early feeding assessment provides the speech and language therapist with an opportunity to examine part of the neuromuscular mechanism that will be used in speech production and to do so in children who are too immature to participate in more formal neurological testing (e.g. cranial nerve testing).

Six cranial nerves (V, VII, IX, X, XI and XII) innervate the oral and pharyngeal muscles of feeding. The motor nuclei of each of these nerves are located in the brainstem (cranial nerve XI also has motor nuclei in the spinal cord). Any one of these nuclei – and usually several of them – may be damaged in cerebral palsy. The result is an impairment of both oral and pharyngeal stages of feeding. In order to determine the nature and extent of this impairment, speech and language therapists routinely include an examination of oral-pharyngeal reflexes within an assessment of feeding.[68] Each of these reflexes is mediated through the brainstem at the level of the pons, medulla and/or midbrain. (The rooting reflex is also mediated through the cervical spinal cord.) As such, reflexes that are absent or exaggerated or that persist beyond an expected time may be taken to indicate underlying central nervous system pathology.[69] For discussion of each of these reflexes, the reader is referred to Love and Webb (2001). We examine how the function of cranial nerves in feeding can be assessed by means of a technique called modified feeding.

The assessment of oral-pharyngeal reflexes in isolation gives clinicians early insight into the function of certain cranial nerves and the brainstem levels through which these reflexes are mediated. Ultimately, however, it is necessary to examine how these same neural mechanisms subserve the altogether more complex motor patterns of feeding. This can be achieved through a technique called modified feeding, in which small pieces of food are placed in different locations within the oral cavity and the child's responses to them are noted. Modified feeding may be used with healthy children from birth to 36 months and in motor-impaired children with oromotor dysfunction well beyond three years of age (Love and Webb 2001). As well as examining feeding skills, the therapist should use this assessment as an opportunity to note all clinical signs of neurological impairment apparent in the structures of feeding.

The first component of feeding to be examined is the neuromuscular mechanism by means of which food is transported to the oral cavity. The lips and tongue are actively involved in retrieving food from a spoon and in mopping up food debris around the mouth. This transportation stage of feeding can be assessed by placing a small bolus of food in the midline of the lower lip. The therapist can establish if tongue protrusion is sufficient to retrieve food from the lip. Purposeful protrusion of the tongue may be accompanied by a powerful and excessive tongue thrust,[70] particularly in athetoid cerebral palsy. Also in athetoid cerebal palsy, the tongue may exhibit writhing movements similar to those that affect the trunk and limbs. The child with spastic cerebral palsy may fail to achieve adequate tongue protrusion and elevation for food retrieval purposes. The therapist should also determine the presence and extent (unilateral or bilateral) of atrophy of the tongue, as this is a sign of lower motor neurone damage. The tonicity of the lips should be assessed and the therapist should establish if the child can form a lip seal. Drooling and the spillage of food from the mouth occur when the lip seal is weak or absent. Impoverished or exaggerated lip and tongue movements compromise the child's ability to transport food into the oral cavity and are caused by impairment of cranial nerves VII and XII, respectively.

Having assessed the transportation stage,[71] the therapist then begins an examination of the oral phases of feeding.[72] The actions of the tongue and jaw are integral to mastication (the oral preparatory phase of feeding) and should be thoroughly assessed by the therapist. The tongue must deliver food between the molars, where it can be crushed. It must also be able to elevate and crush food against the hard palate. The tongue is also responsible for moulding food particles into a bolus. If either lateral tongue movement or tongue elevation is compromised, the effectiveness of the mastication stage of feeding will be considerably diminished. Evidence that such compromise is occurring includes a small, poorly formed bolus and deposits of food around the teeth and on the floor of the oral cavity. A poorly formed bolus which contains large food particles that are inadequately held together is also likely to be unstable. (Impoverished tongue movements are unable to achieve the necessary mixing of food with saliva to produce a cohesive bolus.) An unstable bolus can disintegrate during swallowing, which places the child at an increased risk of aspiration. After mastication has occurred, the tongue propels the bolus backwards in the direction of the oropharynx. This is achieved by the elevation of the tongue, which sequentially makes contact with the hard palate as it moves backwards. For the CP child with motor involvement of cranial nerve V, this sequence of tongue movements may not be possible or such movements as do occur may be ineffective in propelling the bolus towards the oropharynx.

Mandibular muscles are also active during mastication. Like the tongue muscles just described, mandibular muscles are innervated by the motor fibres of the mandibular branch of cranial nerve V. Under normal circumstances, the mandible is necessary for biting to occur and it can move in an anterior-posterior direction as well as laterally (the latter movement being the essence of the grinding action that takes place during mastication). Abnormal jaw movements and reflexes are evident in the child with motor dysfunction and should be noted by the clinician during an assessment of feeding. A bite that is exaggerated and too powerful indicates an abnormal jaw reflex and the presence of an upper motor neurone lesion above the level of the pons. The clinician can test for a hyperactive jaw reflex by tapping the lower jaw and observing if a clonus occurs. Deviation of the mandible during opening and mastication suggests weakness of the pterygoid muscle on the side of the deviation. Finally, the jaw may be used in athetoid cerebral palsy to achieve tongue elevation during feeding (Love and Webb 2001).

Unlike the oral phases of swallowing, the pharyngeal phase is involuntary and totally reflexive. This phase begins with the closure of the nasopharynx, which is brought about by the actions of the soft palate (velum) and pharyngeal constrictors. The hyoid bone and larynx move upwards and forwards. The vocal cords move to the midline and the epiglottis protects the airway by folding backwards. The tongue helps propel the bolus through the pharynx by pushing downwards and backwards. Further propulsion of the bolus is achieved by contractions of the pharyngeal walls. The oesophagus is ready to receive the descending bolus. Its upper sphincter is pulled open by the forward movement of the hyoid bone and larynx. When the bolus passes into the oesophagus, the sphincter closes and the pharyngeal structures return to reference position. The entire swallowing reflex lasts approximately 1 second and is under the control of the sensory and motor tracts of cranial nerves IX and X.

Impairment of the pharyngeal phase of swallowing can lead to aspiration, which has serious and life-threatening consequences for the child and adult with cerebral palsy.[73] It is often not possible to assess an individual's risk of aspiration from clinical examination alone. Although coughing with swallowing, postprandial wheezing, laryngeal gurgling[74] and recurrent pneumonia are strong clinical indicators of aspiration (Arvedson and Brodsky 2002), there are many patients in whom aspiration may occur in the absence of signs or symptoms (i.e. silent aspiration[75]). For this reason, a reliable diagnosis of aspiration usually awaits the results of one or more of the following techniques: chest X-ray, computerised tomographic (CT) scan of the chest, flexible fibreoptic nasopharyngolaryngoscopy (FFNL), flexible endoscopic examination of swallowing (FEES), videofluoroscopic swallow study (VFSS), and rigid airway endoscopy including evaluation of bronchial secretions (Arvedson and Brodsky 2002). Videofluoroscopy is the most important instrumental technique in the assessment of aspiration and forms the 'gold standard' against which other techniques are measured (Arvedson and Brodsky 2002). In permitting a full examination of swallowing from oral to oesophageal stages, VFSS allows clinicians to ascertain an exact aetiology of aspiration as well as the timing of aspiration. It is possible to establish, for example, if aspiration occurs because of a delay in swallow initiation (aspiration before a swallow), if aspiration is the result of ineffective laryngeal closure (aspiration during a swallow) or if aspiration is due to residue in the larynx and hypopharynx being drawn through the larynx during the next inhalation (aspiration after a swallow). VFSS also allows clinicians to assess the effect of body posture and sitting position on swallowing, as well as to establish the relationship between the textures of different foods and aspiration.

During the final stage of swallowing – the oesophageal phase – the bolus is propelled along the oesophagus by means of peristalsis. The bolus may take some 8–20 seconds to move along the oesophagus before being deposited in the stomach through the cardiac sphincter (lower oesophageal sphincter). If closure of this sphincter is weak, ingested food, acid, bacteria and enzymes from the stomach will pass back into the oesophagus. This gastro-oesophageal reflux is a threat to the airway of the CP child and adult and can cause indirect aspiration.[76] For this reason, clinicians must consider reflux as a possible cause of aspiration during an assessment of dysphagia in cerebral palsy.[77] Although a diagnosis of gastro-oesophageal reflux is not made by the speech and language therapist,[78] the therapist should nonetheless be alert to the signs of reflux during history-taking. These signs include irritability, inability to tolerate large feeds, early satiation and frequent vomiting.[79] In addition to the significant risk of aspiration that gastro-oesophageal reflux poses for the child and adult with cerebral palsy, reflux has also been linked to a number of laryngeal and voice disorders (see chapter 7). These disorders are no less the concern of the speech and language therapist than dysphagia itself. Clearly, there are clinical grounds beyond aspiration that can be used to justify an assessment of oesophageal phase swallowing and reflux status in cerebral palsy.

By necessity, a systematic evaluation of feeding in cerebral palsy must include assessment of specific neuromuscular mechanisms at different stages or phases of swallowing. However, concentration on the details of such an assessment should not entail neglect of the social interaction that attends feeding. This interaction can provide the speech and language therapist with a valuable opportunity to observe how the CP child and adult communicate choices about food and a variety of needs to family members and carers. On the basis of this observation, the speech and language therapist can establish the extent to which various modes of communication – vocalisations, speech, eye gaze, gesture and systems of augmentative and alternative communication – are used by the CP child or adult and can determine the effectiveness of each of these modes. The therapist can also use this opportunity for informal observation to gauge the presence and extent of verbal comprehension impairment and to establish the impact of sensory deficits (e.g. hearing loss) on communication. Other responses can be assessed in terms of what they can tell the therapist about the child's or adult's oromotor dysfunction. In this way, a weak or asymmetrical smile should be recorded, as an asymmetrical smile and flattening of the nasal fold on one side of the face may indicate unilateral paresis. The therapist should also take note of the child who fails to smile altogether and in whom there is an evident lack of facial expression. The absence of these normal interpersonal responses from the child may be clinically significant and may indicate bilateral corticobulbar damage in which the facial nerves (cranial nerve VII) are involved. Even the uncooperative child can provide the clinician with an opportunity to assess oromotor dysfunction. The failure of the tongue to cup during crying, for example, suggests problems with the innervation of the tongue musculature by cranial nerve XII. These examples could be multiplied. However, the point that is demonstrated by them is nonetheless clear – a feeding assessment should examine the CP child's oromotor dysfunction in considerable detail, but not at the expense of understanding how this dysfunction operates as part of a wider pattern of communication.[80]

2.3.2.2 Speech

Speech disorder is common in cerebral palsy. Sullivan et al. (2000) report that 78 per cent of children with oromotor dysfunction in their study had speech difficulty. Love and Webb (2001) state that 75–85 per cent of children with cerebral palsy show obvious speech problems. The speech disorder most often found in cerebral palsy is developmental dysarthria.[81] Dysarthria can affect all four speech production subsystems (articulation, resonation, phonation and respiration) and can vary considerably in severity. In some cases, speech is intelligible to all but the unfamiliar listener. In other cases, speech may be completely unintelligible and the CP child or adult may communicate by means of an alternative communication system.[82] We will discuss a number of these systems in section 2.3.3. (Technological developments have brought about a rapid proliferation of these systems in recent years.) In this section, we outline the main components of a speech assessment in cerebral palsy.

A few introductory comments are necessary to explain the disordered speech patterns that are likely to be revealed during assessment. Speech development in cerebral palsy occurs against the background of considerable physiological limitations. We will see in section 2.3.3 that these limitations have implications for the setting of treatment goals in therapy. However, they also account for features of the prelinguistic period and for features of speech development in cerebral palsy. One such feature is the lack of early babbling in CP children.[83] The sensory and motor experiences that the normal child derives from early babbling are a necessary first step on the road to developing the complex, coordinated neuromuscular mechanisms that are involved in mature speech production. The CP child who is deprived of these experiences on account of physiological limitations may fail to attain oromotor control for speech. Moreover, he or she may develop maladaptive articulation patterns in an attempt to produce speech sounds from within a physiologically compromised speech mechanism. These maladaptive articulations, which may include sound distortions and speech sounds not normally found in the child's native language, reveal problems at the phonetic level of speech production. When these various distortions become organised into a system of contrasts that is itself deviant, the child may present with a phonological disorder as well as a phonetic disorder. The problems imposed on speech development by physiological limitations may be compounded by additional difficulties such as hearing loss, perception problems and learning disability. Moreover, caregivers may not engage in early vocal play with the CP infant in an attempt to avoid extensor spasms that may accompany the child's vocal productions (Milloy and Morgan–Barry 1990). The combination of these factors in the CP child threatens speech development and places the child at risk of phonetic and phonological disorders.

Dysarthria in cerebral palsy is the result of disturbances in tone, strength, endurance and coordination of the speech musculature. Some of these disturbances are particularly prominent in certain types of cerebral palsy. For example, the child with spastic cerebral palsy exhibits increased tone (hypertonia) of the speech musculature, while the child with ataxic cerebral palsy has difficulty coordinating the muscles of speech. A typical clinical picture, however, is one in which a combination of these disturbances characterises the speech of the CP child. For this reason, the speech and language therapist must assess the speed, force, steadiness, range and timing of speech movements in all CP children and adults. When disturbances of the speech musculature affect both temporal and spatial dimensions of speech production, the CP child's intelligibility will be considerably compromised. In such a case, assessment will reveal a preponderance of phonetic and phonological processes that are related to problems of temporal coordination and spatial configuration. One process that is related to temporal incoordination is the devoicing of initial consonants. Devoicing occurs when delays in the initiation of phonation mean that voicing fails to coincide with the placement of articulators. Other processes are related to a failure of the articulators to attain particular spatial configurations. For example, persistent hypernasalisation of speech is an indication that the child cannot achieve elevation of the soft palate and closure of the velopharyngeal port. During assessment, the speech and language therapist must not only establish the phonetic and phonological processes that are contributing to the unintelligibility of the CP child's speech; he or she must also be aware of what these processes reveal about the role of temporal and spatial factors in the child's disordered speech.

Clearly, a speech assessment in cerebral palsy must include a description of the phonetic and phonological processes that are responsible for sound errors in the CP child's speech. This part of the assessment can be completed by using a formal test of articulation and phonology, the choice of which will be determined by factors such as the age of the subject.[84] A speech assessment must also include an account of how the child's sound errors relate to temporal and spatial dimensions of the underlying motor disorder. In order that therapy may be effective, it is as important for the therapist to know how the articulators move through space and time on the way to their articulatory destinations as it is for him or her to know the positions of the articulators at those destinations. (Speaking is, after all, a dynamic activity that takes place in real time.) Finally, a speech assessment in cerebral palsy must also include a description of the prosodic features of pitch, loudness and duration. Prosody can be seriously disrupted in dysarthria and prosodic disturbances reduce quite substantially the intelligibility of the CP child's speech. Having outlined the key features that should be addressed during a speech assessment in cerebral palsy, we can now proceed to elaborate on these features according to the speech production subsystems of articulation, resonation, phonation and respiration.

During an assessment of articulation, the therapist should observe the precision, speed, range and diversity of movement of the oral articulators. Articulators often lack the precision of movement that is required to produce consonant sounds. This lack of precision is sometimes particularly evident in one specific articulator and may affect sounds produced by that articulator – for example, liquids, affricates and lingual fricatives reflecting tongue impairment. Other articulators (e.g. lips) may produce asymmetrical movements. Articulators may be slow to initiate and execute movement. The range of movement of an articulator may be considerably reduced (e.g. marked impairment of tongue elevation). There may also be limited diversity of movement of one or more articulators. For example, the tongue may not be able to elevate, retract, arch and so on, but may only be able to protrude forcefully and reflexively. The tongue and jaw may lack independence of movement and the jaw may compensate for the lack of tongue elevation.

Restricted, slowed and mistimed movement of the lips, tongue and jaw can lead to significant problems of articulation in the CP child. These problems are more evident during the articulation of consonants. However, vowels may also be distorted and simplified (e.g. diphthong reduction) and the child's vowel space may be considerably reduced. Simplification errors involving consonants are common and include stopping and cluster reduction. In a study of a nine-year-old girl with mild spastic quadriplegia, Milloy and Morgan–Barry (1990) observed stopping of affricates in syllable initial word initial position (e.g. 'chimney' [tʰɪmːɪ]) as well as stopping of approximants (a phonological deviance). This subject had a limited consonant cluster inventory with most target clusters being reduced to one element. Milloy and Morgan–Barry noted that /s+/ clusters were reduced to the fricative element, which was routinely lateralised in their subject's speech (e.g. 'stamps' [ɬæmpɬ]; 'spoon' [ɬun]).[85] In plosive-approximant clusters, the plosive was usually preserved and was often devoiced (e.g. 'glove' [kʰʌ f]; 'great' [kʰeɪʔt]). These examples of devoicing reflect a more general problem of coordinating voicing with articulation in dysarthria. The subject in Milloy and Morgan–Barry's study found it more difficult to initiate a voiced consonant when combined with the [(+) continuant, (+) friction, (+) sibilance] features. Articulation errors may be inconsistent, for example, voicing. (In addition to [kʰeɪʔt], 'great' was also realised as [geɪf] by Milloy and Morgan-Barry's CP subject.) Prosodic disturbances are evident in the prolongation of speech sounds.

The muscles that regulate valving of the velopharyngeal port – muscles of the soft palate and lateral and posterior pharyngeal walls – can be individually weak and poorly coordinated during speech production in dysarthria. Velar elevation may not be adequate to achieve closure of the velopharyngeal port. The result may be marked hypernasality of speech and nasal air emission during speech production. The child's inability to generate intra-oral air pressure has consequences for articulation. Oral obstruents are often weak – the subject in Milloy and Morgan-Barry's study produced weak, lax plosives. Phonetic and phonological processes include nasal addition and substitution errors. An examination of the speech of Milloy and Morgan-Barry's subject reveals nasalisation of approximants (/wrʌl/ → [n]) and some nasalisation of the voiced dental fricative (/ð/→[n] or [m]).

The loss of air pressure through the velopharyngeal port also has implications for respiration. In the presence of velopharyngeal insufficiency, there is a marked reduction in the number of syllables that can be produced on a single breath (the breath group). To counteract this reduction, the dysarthric child may increase his or her respiration rate during speech. Along with this increase in rate, the CP child may develop abnormal patterns of breathing for speech. To compensate further for this loss of air, the CP child may also make various phonatory adjustments. These adjustments may include an increase in speaking volume and/or the use of a more attacking pattern of vocal fold adduction (a possible source of some voicing errors). Both of these compensations may result in a hyperfunctional voice disorder and must be considered by the therapist who is assessing a CP child with significant velopharyngeal insufficiency.

Even in the CP child with velopharyngeal insufficiency, the resonance pattern is not invariably one of hypernasality. An immobile soft palate that cannot achieve elevation for velopharyngeal closure may also obstruct the velopharyngeal port during the production of speech. In such a case, resonance can fluctuate between hypernasal and hyponasal patterns. Not only is the range of palatal movement reduced in dysarthria, but the speed and timing of movement can also be disrupted. The disruption of these dimensions of palatal movement can make it almost impossible for the CP child to effect a transition from nasal to oral resonance in the word 'nap' /nap/, for example. Slow or mistimed palatal movement will cause the nasal resonance of /n/ to persist during the articulation of the subsequent oral sounds. The vowel sound /a/ in particular will assimilate the nasality of the preceding nasal consonant /n/. The presence of assimilative nasality in vowels should be noted by the therapist during assessment, as it is a further important indicator of velopharyngeal function in the dysarthric CP child.

We discussed above how phonatory disturbances can result from the CP child's attempt to compensate for failings of the velopharyngeal mechanism during speech production. However, phonation can also be impaired as a result of the motor disorder in cerebral palsy. This impairment can affect the pitch, loudness and quality of the voice to a greater or lesser degree.[86] Pitch may be poorly regulated with frequent pitch breaks and tremor. It may also be inappropriately high or low and the pitch range may be reduced. The spastic CP child can display a lack of vocal inflection. The dysarthric CP child may have poor regulation of the loudness of the voice – uncontrolled volume is a common feature of spastic cerebral palsy. He or she may speak too loudly or too softly and may have a reduced loudness range. Abnormal voice qualities can occur in cerebral palsy. The voice may be breathy, hoarse or strain-strangled. The athetoid CP child may produce whispered, hoarse or ventricular phonation, while the spastic CP child's voice may have a gutteral or breathy quality. The dysarthric child may present with intermittent dysphonia.

In addition to abnormalities of the pitch, loudness and quality of the voice, the dysarthric CP child may display other phonatory disturbances. He or she may be unable to initiate phonation or may have difficulty initiating phonation. Adventitious, involuntary phonations may be in evidence. In the presence of continuous voicing, the dysarthric child may be unable to distinguish voiced from voiceless consonants. Poor coordination of phonation with respiration may find the CP child producing audible airflow prior to the start of voicing, for a spoken breath group. Insufficient laryngeal valving of the pulmonary airstream can result in short breath groups, as fewer syllables are produced on each exhalatory breath. Clearly, phonation is at considerable risk of impairment in dysarthria and must be comprehensively examined during a speech assessment.

The function of the respiratory muscles – muscles of the diaphragm and intercostal and abdominal muscles – must also be examined during a speech assessment in cerebral palsy. Problems with the motor control of respiration[87] may result in disturbances in the depth, rate and timing of breathing for speech. The CP child who cannot regulate the timing of respiration may take linguistically inappropriate inspirations within words. As well as having difficulties with the timing of respiration in relation to speech, the CP child may also produce long inspiratory pauses between utterances. In the child with a shallow breathing pattern, airflow may be insufficient to support phonation, with reductions observed in both the intensity (loudness) of the voice and the length of breath groups. In other cases, the airflow may be sufficient for phonation to occur, but it may be poorly controlled. This lack of respiratory control may manifest itself in disturbances of vocal intensity. For example, the dysarthric CP child may experience excessive alterations in vocal loudness and the fading of loudness towards the end of a breath group. The child with poor respiratory control may also be unable to vary the length of breath groups. Respiratory inefficiency may cause the CP child to inspire at all pauses in an effort to maintain a sufficient airflow for phonation. There may be poor coordination of phonation with respiration, such that the CP child may initiate speech at an inappropriate point in the respiratory cycle – for example, near the end of expiration with no preparatory inhalation prior to speaking.

The dysarthric CP child, whose respiratory mechanism is severely compromised during speech production, faces a considerable problem of fatigue when speaking. There are two related sources of fatigue in the CP child's speech. First, the speech muscles (including the muscles of respiration) are typically weak in dysarthria. The movement of these muscles demands an increased level of energy expenditure on the part of the CP child.[88] Second, to counteract the functional limitations of the respiratory muscles, the CP child may spontaneously develop compensatory patterns of breathing – for example, the CP child may institute clavicular breathing, in which the shoulder girdle and upper portion of the chest are elevated through the actions of the external intercostal muscles and the accessory muscles with evident tension and effort in the infrahyoid muscles of the neck. Many of these compensatory behaviours involve an inefficient use of energy, with maximal energy expenditure producing minimal gains in speech function. When this additional energy expenditure is incurred over a period of time – such as occurs during extended speaking – the CP child will experience fatigue. Fatigue can lead to yet further deterioration in speech production. A vicious cycle ensues as the child expends more energy and sustains more fatigue in an effort to maintain intelligibility. Cumulative fatigue can be avoided by instituting rest periods during and between treatment sessions. (These sessions can be very numerous when the CP child is receiving physiotherapy and occupational therapy in addition to speech and language therapy.) For the purposes of assessment, however, the clinician can establish the extent to which the CP child's intelligibility fluctuates with fatigue (and with emotional states such as anger and excitement) by interviewing the child's parents and/or carers.[89] A common parental observation is that intelligibility decreases as the child tires towards the end of the day.

In section 2.2.2.2, we examined a number of radiological and instrumental techniques that can be used by the therapist to assess articulation and resonation. (Of course, videofluoroscopy may also be used to assess swallowing.) Other instrumental devices may be used to assess phonation and respiration. Many of these techniques have been made possible through recent technological developments (e.g. the Kay Computerised Speech Lab). The objective nature of the acoustic and aerodynamic measurements produced by techniques such as VisiSpeech and spirometry serves to validate a perceptual assessment of features such as vocal pitch and loudness. However, the clinical utility of these techniques extends beyond assessment, with many of these devices also able to provide the child or adult with biofeedback during treatment. The reader should be aware that instrumental techniques are a useful adjunct to assessment in the case of the dysarthric child with specific phonatory and respiratory disturbances.

2.3.2.3 Hearing

Hearing problems affect between 25 and 30 per cent of people with cerebral palsy (Turkington and Sussman 2004). These problems are largely sensorineural in nature. This is because many of the same pre-, peri- and postnatal events and illnesses that cause cerebral palsy also cause sensorineural hearing loss. Each of these events and illnesses should alert medical personnel, audiologists and speech and language therapists to the possibility of hearing loss in the CP infant and child. It is particularly important that these children are identified early so that appropriate methods of intervention can be commenced as soon as possible. This can only be effectively achieved through universal neonatal hearing screening. The two audiometric techniques that are used during screening are transient evoked otoacoustic emissions (TEOAEs) and automated auditory brainstem response (AABR). We describe how these techniques are being used to make a diagnosis of hearing impairment in newborns, including those with cerebral palsy.

Hearing impairment in cerebral palsy can be the result of breakdown at a number of different levels in the overall auditory mechanism. The organ of Corti may be destroyed as a result of bacterial meningitis, causing cochlear deafness. The cochlear nuclei in the brainstem may be damaged in kernicterus. The developing auditory centres in the cortex may be damaged as a result of cerebral infarction, leading to cortical or central deafness. It is important to establish the exact point(s) of hearing breakdown, as these different levels of impairment will necessitate quite different forms of audiological intervention. For example, the CP child with cortical deafness may hear speech sounds but have difficulty recognising them, so that amplification alone may not be appropriate in this case. TEOAEs enable clinicians to assess the cochlea's response to sound. In this technique, a stimulus emitter produces a small click and the resulting emission is recorded by a microphone and displayed on a computer screen. By using a broadband click, it is possible to obtain information between 500 and 5000Hz, which covers the frequencies of most speech sounds. Emissions are detectable in nearly 100 per cent of normal ears and are not measurable in ears with a hearing loss greater than 25–30dB (Ramsden and Axon 2001). This test is an effective means of screening neonatal hearing, with the main drawback of this technique being a lack of response in middle ear disease (e.g. otitis media).

The presence of TEOAEs only establishes that there is a normal preneural response to sound. However, hearing may still be impaired if any part of the neural pathway from the cochlea to the auditory cortex of the brain is damaged. AABR is used to test the part of that pathway from the auditory nerve (a branch of the acoustic nerve) to the brainstem. During this technique, surface electrodes are placed high on the forehead, on the mastoid and on the nape of the neck. The click stimulus, which is usually set at 35dBHL, is delivered to the infant's ear through earphones that are designed to attenuate background noise. To determine if the test has been passed or failed, the resulting waveform is compared with a template that is based on normative data. AABR cannot provide information on the degree or nature of hearing loss. Nevertheless, it is an effective method of detecting infants who require further audiological assessment.

On the basis of these two screening techniques, it is possible to identify those infants who have a normal preneural response to sound, but an absent neural response, as indicated by AABR. Such auditory neuropathies have been reported in babies who require special care (Watkin 2001), a significant proportion of whom will also have cerebral palsy. A diagnosis of hearing impairment has serious implications for the development of communication skills in the CP infant and child. Hearing impairment compounds a most difficult communication situation for the CP child. Speech development, which must already occur against the background of motor disability, is compromised further by the fact that one's incoming speech signal is attenuated and/or distorted. There is clear evidence of a detrimental effect of sensorineural hearing loss on a range of phonological skills in children. Briscoe et al. (2001) found that mean scores on tests of phonological short-term memory, phonological discrimination and phonological awareness were significantly lower in children with mild-to-moderate sensorineural hearing loss than in age-matched controls. This study found no clinically significant deficits in the wider language and literacy skills of children with sensorineural hearing loss. However, amongst hearing-impaired subjects with two or more indicators of phonological impairment, language and literacy skills tended to be poorer than those of hearing-impaired subjects in a phonologically unimpaired subgroup.

A similar pattern of findings emerges in a study by Norbury et al. (2001). In this case, children with sensorineural hearing impairment did not differ significantly from age- and language-matched control groups on measures of tense marking. However, 22 per cent of the hearing-impaired group met criteria for language impairment (the prevalence of language impairment in the normal hearing population is estimated to be 7.4 per cent (Tomblin et al. 1997)), and all of the hearing-impaired children had problems with finite verb morphology. In the absence of an adequately developed language base, the hearing-impaired CP child may lack the requisite structural language skills with which to take turns in conversation and perform a range of pragmatic functions. The speech and language therapist must be aware not only of the effect of hearing impairment on the CP child's developing communication skills, but also of the implications of this impairment for communication assessment and intervention. For example, the CP child's conversational partners may need to be trained to supplement their own speech with manual or graphic signs when hearing impairment is a consideration.

2.3.2.4 Language

As the discussion of section 2.3.2.3 demonstrates, there is some initial support for the claim that sensorineural hearing impairment predisposes affected children to language deficits. In addition to the morphosyntactic problems addressed in that section, Gilbertson and Kamhi (1995) found that 50 per cent of their child subjects with sensorineural hearing loss also had language impairments. However, hearing impairment is only one of a number of factors that places the CP child at risk of language disorder. The child's motor disability limits his or her participation in many of the early childhood experiences that are so integral to language development. The CP child with severe motor impairment is unable to explore his or her environment or participate easily in play activities with other children and adults. These prelinguistic experiences are vital if the child is to develop cognitive skills and early knowledge that will be central to communication interaction. Of course, the same neurological injury that causes motor disability may also result in intellectual deficits. These deficits limit the extent to which learning based on these prelinguistic experiences is even possible. Individually, hearing impairment, motor disability and intellectual deficits are significant factors in the development of language disorder in any child. The combination of these factors in cerebral palsy – as well as other factors, such as a less interactive parenting style, early and prolonged periods of hospitalisation, missed education through illness – poses a considerable and serious threat to language development in the CP child. In this section, we describe language impairment in cerebral palsy and discuss how language may be assessed in this clinical population.

Where learning disability is not a consideration, language comprehension abilities often surpass expressive language skills in cerebral palsy. Poor expressive language skills may account for the dominant use of single-sign utterances by alternative communication users (see section 2.3.3.2). An expressive language deficit may also explain the reduced language output of CP subjects. For example, in a study of seven CP children, Falkman et al. (2002) found that the amount of linguistic communication that was used (12 per cent) was considerably less than could be expected given the age of the subjects (5–7 years of age) and the fact that they were of normal intelligence. One explanation advanced for this finding is motor impairment which, these authors contend, limits the child's interactions with the environment and, in doing so, restricts the development of linguistic skills. Establishing the nature and extent of language impairment in cerebral palsy is not an easy task. Reduced language output makes any assessment of expressive syntax all but impossible. The CP child or adult with severe motor impairment may be unable to signal understanding of language, even with the use of an alternative communication system. In what follows, I discuss research findings that reveal the presence of phonological processing problems in cerebral palsy. Related to these problems are associated deficits in vocabulary and literacy. Meanwhile, there is evidence to indicate that the understanding of grammatical structures appears to be intact in CP subjects with these various impairments.

We described in section 2.2.2.4 how structural anomalies of the speech production mechanism have adverse consequences for the development of phonology in the cleft palate child. It emerges that dysarthric speech impairments in cerebral palsy can also disrupt developing phonological skills in affected children. In this way, Bishop et al. (1990) found that dysarthric or anarthric CP subjects performed less well than control subjects with normal speech on a phoneme discrimination task that required them to judge whether pairs of nonwords were the same or different. When tested a year later, speech-impaired subjects still performed less well than control subjects on the same-different task. However, there was no difference in performance on a word judgement task, in which subjects were asked to judge if a word was spoken correctly or if one sound had been altered. Bishop et al. conclude that these CP subjects can discriminate phoneme contrasts adequately (as indicated by their performance on the word judgement task), but that they have weak memory for novel phonological strings (same–different task). Other phonological deficits in cerebral palsy are revealed by a study of 32 CP subjects who had no intelligible speech and who were AAC users. Vandervelden and Siegel (1999) examined three areas of phonological processing in these subjects: retrieval of whole-word phonology, phoneme awareness and phonological recoding. Compared with a group of reading level-matched controls, the AAC users and a group of 32 speech-impaired but intelligible subjects scored significantly lower in all areas of phonological processing.

Phonological deficits such as those described above have consequences for the development of wider language and literacy skills in cerebral palsy. Bishop et al. (1990) argue that CP subjects' weaker memory for novel phonological strings is responsible for impaired receptive vocabulary amongst these subjects – anarthric and dysarthric CP subjects were impaired relative to their matched controls (also CP subjects, but with normal speech) on the British Picture Vocabulary Scale (a British version of the Peabody Picture Vocabulary Test). For unfamiliar words to be retained, such as occurs in vocabulary acquisition, novel phonological strings must be converted into an articulatory code (see Foley and Pollatsek (1999), who challenge the necessity of articulatory coding). Bishop et al. contend that this process is facilitated by the ability to repeat novel strings and is either impossible or severely disrupted in anarthric or dysarthric CP subjects. Moreover, this vocabulary deficit occurs in the absence of any impairment of the understanding of grammatical structure – there was no significant difference between test and control CP subjects on the Test for Reception of Grammar (Bishop 1983). Phonological problems are also identified as playing a key role in the poor literacy skills that are found among nonspeaking CP children. For example, the CP subjects in Vandervelden and Siegel's (1999) study showed low skill in using sound–letter correspondences to spell. Moreover, the effect of phonological problems on the development of literacy skills is altogether greater than any effect produced by the child's home literacy experiences. In this way, Sandberg (1998) found that the home literacy experiences of 35 children with cerebral palsy had at best a marginal influence on reading development. The speech and language abilities of these children were much more likely to explain their poor literacy skills.

Clearly, the speech and language therapist must include a comprehensive examination of language and literacy skills as part of an overall assessment of communication in the CP child and adult. Even in cases where speech is unlikely to provide an effective means of communication for the CP individual, language development must be monitored and facilitated in order that the CP child may have the requisite language skills for the use of an alternative communication system. It is worth remarking that while norms for language development in speaking children are well documented, norms for alternative language development are lacking (von Tetzchner and Martinsen 2000). Literacy skills should also be examined during an assessment of communication in cerebral palsy. Moreover, where there is potential for improvement, these skills should be developed during a programme of intervention. For example, the graphic sign user may proceed to learn orthographic writing. However, many motor-impaired individuals never achieve functional reading skills, or learn to read quite late and may need to use graphic signs until seven or eight years of age (von Tetzchner and Martinsen 2000).

Motor disability presents the clinician with a number of unique challenges during language assessment. Many language comprehension tests require subjects to point at pictures or manipulate objects. For example, in the Reynell Developmental Language Scales (Reynell 1985), children are asked to 'Put the doll on the chair' and 'Put all the pigs behind the brown horse.' These test items will be difficult or impossible for the motor-impaired child to execute. Computer-based language comprehension tests are now available and can be used to overcome many of the problems posed by motor impairment. In Bishop et al.'s (1990) study, CP subjects who were unable to speak or point indicated their responses on the British Picture Vocabulary Scale and the Test for Reception of Grammar by selecting numbers on a computer.

Formal language assessments should be supplemented by observations and parental reports of language use and comprehension in a range of contexts. Such observations and reports are likely to indicate a greater level of linguistic competence than that which is revealed through formal language testing. This discrepancy occurs because many of the natural cues that facilitate comprehension of language in everyday situations are not available to the CP child and adult during formal testing. For example, the CP child who fails to comprehend the instruction 'Give me the cup' during language testing may have no difficulty in complying with this command when it is uttered during dinner by a parent whose hand is outstretched towards the child. The combination of formal testing and informal observation enables the therapist to assess the extent to which the CP child is using contextual cues to augment poor receptive language skills. By combining the results of formal testing with parental reports, the therapist can make a number of other important determinations about the child's language skills. For example, parents are often best placed to comment on the particular strategies the child uses to indicate comprehension of spoken language. These strategies can be unusual and difficult for other people to identify. This is no less true of the speech and language therapist, who often has limited time in assessment with which to become acquainted with the child's particular communicative strategies. However, parents can also engage in over-interpretation of their child's communicative and other responses. In this way, the child who gives over a cup in response to a parent's outstretched hand may understand little or nothing of the verbal instruction 'Give me the cup.' Yet, parents may take the successful execution of the task to indicate complete comprehension of the verbal command. By assessing all parental reports of language skills in the context of the findings of formal language testing, the therapist is able to minimise this over-interpretation effect and to arrive at an accurate estimation of the child's language abilities in everyday communication.

2.3.3 Clinical Intervention

Having assessed the CP child and adult, the speech and language therapist can then make a number of recommendations for treatment. In relation to feeding, recommendations may include specific guidance about positioning and food textures or the advice to avoid oral feeding in the case where aspiration is clearly demonstrated. An equally diverse range of interventions may be recommended for the treatment of dysarthria in cerebral palsy. Where there is adequate physiological support for speech, the emphasis of therapy will be on developing aspects of motor speech function with a view to improving the child's or adult's overall intelligibility. In the case of severe motor impairment, the CP child may never develop intelligible speech and treatment may focus instead on establishing an effective means of augmentative or alternative communication. In this section, we examine a number of techniques that may be used by the speech and language therapist to treat oral motor feeding dysfunction in the CP child and adult. Later, we discuss different approaches that may be used by the speech and language therapist to enhance communication skills in individuals with cerebral palsy.

2.3.3.1 Feeding Intervention

Growth failure, undernutrition and aspiration pneumonia are just some of the problems that attend feeding disorder in cerebral palsy. Given the severity of these medical sequelae, there is clearly a clinical imperative to treat dysphagia as aggressively as possible in this clinical population.[90] Where oral feeding is possible, such treatment may consist in advice to parents and carers on matters such as safe food textures and positioning techniques. It may also involve extensive work on improving the child's sensory awareness of foods and/or decreasing sensory defensiveness in the child who is hypersensitive in and around the oral cavity. The therapist will also concentrate on developing independent and socially acceptable feeding practices in the CP child and adult. To this end, treatment will focus on encouraging the child to use utensils appropriately during feeding and on the control of drooling. Many of these techniques can be used with gastrostomy-fed children and adults who are also oral feeders and who are receiving tube feeding in the short or long term as a supplement to oral feeding (e.g. to increase nutritional intake during a period of illness). We begin by describing positioning techniques.

The importance of correct positioning for feeding cannot be overstated. The motor-impaired child and adult are unable to make the various neuromuscular adjustments that are required to maintain safe and effective feeding in a range of suboptimal positions. In general, the aim of positioning is to obtain a central postural alignment. This requires neutral head flexion with a balance between flexion and extension, neck elongation, stable and depressed shoulder girdle, trunk elongation, a stable and symmetrical pelvis in neutral position, hips at 90° and feet in neutral position with slight dorsiflexion and never plantar-flexed (Arvedson 1998). Variations in this position may be required, depending on which stage of swallowing contributes most to the CP child's feeding problems. If the child has major oral phase swallowing problems, feeding is best undertaken in the reclined position, in which the whole of the child's wheelchair is tipped back to approximately 30° to the vertical and the neck and hips are in a flexed position. In the CP child with more difficulties in the pharyngeal phase of swallowing, the erect position with flexed neck and hips is recommended (Morton et al. 1993). The child's position can often be improved by simple changes in seating (e.g. altering the position of the chair's head support and support for feet and using a foam insert in the seat to improve stability at the hips). Whatever positioning techniques are adopted, they should not be so restrictive that the child is unable to participate actively in feeding. In this way, the child's trunk and arms should be as free as possible in order that he or she may lean forward to reach a spoon or pick up food.

Oral hypersensitivity may make the CP child reluctant to have food in his or her mouth or even touching the lips and cheeks. This hypersensitivity may also involve the child's hands. In such a case, the child may refuse to touch food, which is an obstruction to attempts to encourage the child to pick up food and feed independently. Many of these hypersensitivity problems are compounded by a sense of invasiveness when parents use forceful and unexpected actions to wash their child's face and brush his or her teeth. Food presents an array of sensory input that may be too intense for the hypersensitive child. For this reason, the therapist should spend time prior to the introduction of food developing a more graded set of responses in the child to sensory stimuli. This can be achieved through simple modifications of the everyday activities of face wiping and tooth brushing. Using a small square of cloth, which the child should be encouraged to hold, the therapist can wipe each of the child's cheeks in turn. Firm pats should be used rather than fine strokes, as the deep pressure that is exerted by the former action is more easily tolerated by the child in the initial stages of sensory work. A clear midline focus is achieved by patting in the direction of the mouth. Deep pressure is also applied above and below the lips, with the lower lip pressed up and the upper lip pressed down towards the centre position. As the child's ability to tolerate the sensory input from these activities increases, the pressure that is applied to the cheeks and lips can be gradually reduced. Tooth brushing presents the hypersensitive child with a greater amount of sensory input. The teeth are brushed in four quadrants in the same order, with each brush stroke beginning and ending in the midline. (The four quadrants arise from the artificial division of the upper and lower teeth along the midline.) Teeth should be brushed first on the outside and then on the inside. It may be necessary initially to avoid the use of toothpaste, which will present the child with additional sensory input and will stimulate the production of saliva. By encouraging the child to spit or swallow between each quadrant, brushing can assist the child in developing control of drooling. Finally, play with different food textures and other materials can help the hypersensitive child develop a tolerance for touching and picking up food. Progression in sensory play is achieved by moving from dry textures (e.g. lentils and beans) through to damp textures (e.g. play dough) and lastly wet textures, as in pudding and finger paint (Pinder and Faherty 1999).

The previous sensory work is undertaken with a view to preparing the child for the intense sensory stimulation that is produced by food. When introducing food into an oral motor feeding programme, consideration must be given to its texture, temperature and taste. I will focus on food texture in my comments below. Food texture is important because different textures require different oral skills in the child. For example, crisp foods such as raw apple require extensive chewing, while foods with more than one texture (e.g. vegetable soup) involve the gathering and swallowing of liquid while chunks are retained and then chewed. Food textures present the following dilemma for the clinician. Some food textures can be eaten relatively easily and safely by the motor-impaired child. However, unless the child is exposed to more difficult (and potentially unsafe) food textures, he or she will not be able to develop better oral skills for feeding. The paediatric dysphagia therapist must therefore chart a difficult course between safe food textures on the one hand and food textures that can trigger further development of oral feeding skills on the other hand. The therapist is guided in all aspects of treatment planning, including issues relating to food texture, by clinical guidelines[91] and by techniques such as videofluoroscopy, which can be used to monitor the safety of various foods (and of feeding positions). In what follows, I provide only an overview of general principles that underpin feeding guidance.

In general, thin liquids are less easily managed by the CP child than thickened liquids. Thin liquids travel quickly through the oral-pharyngeal cavities and cannot be controlled by the motor-impaired child. Water is a particularly difficult thin liquid for the motor-impaired child – its lack of taste makes it difficult for the child to sense its location and movement in the oral cavity. The use of starch-based thickeners is recommended for thickening thin liquids (Tilton et al. 1998). Thickened liquids provide the child with tactile input and they have an increased oral-pharyngeal transit time which is beneficial for the child whose swallowing reflex is delayed. Gisel (1988) observed a strong effect of food texture on chewing efficacy in cerebral palsy. She found that CP children with spastic quadriparesis were able to eat solid foods more efficiently than either viscous or pureed foods. Foods with multiple textures are more problematic for the feeding-impaired child than foods that have a single, consistent texture. The introduction of differently textured foods follows the developmental progression that occurs in the child's oral motor skills. The foods which place least demand on these skills – smooth foods which range from being semi-solid (easiest) to slightly lumpy (most difficult) – are first to be introduced. The therapist will then introduce foods with a granular texture (e.g. mashed potato), foods that are lumpy and require some chewing (e.g. steamed vegetables) and foods that are firm and chewy (e.g. moist chicken) in that order. Foods requiring more complex oral motor skills – crisp foods and firm foods that demand good chewing skills – are last to be introduced (Pinder and Faherty 1999).

Bolus consistency and size must also be considered by the therapist. Inadequate chewing skills can result in a poorly formed bolus that lacks cohesiveness. Food particles may break away from the bolus, drift backwards in the mouth and cause choking, gagging, coughing or airway obstruction. Small bites are generally recommended. However, a large bolus can increase sensory awareness in the oral cavity, which can assist the formation and transit of the bolus (Arvedson 1998). The therapist should also be aware of the effects of certain foods on the child's secretions and should avoid these foods where appropriate. Sugar and citrus acids can cause increased saliva production. The therapist may decide to avoid sweet tastes during oral stimulation taste trials when a child is known to have difficulty controlling his or her own secretions. Milk products can cause mucus and saliva to thicken. Thickened mucus may pool in the pharynx and present an aspiration risk to children who may already have weakened respiratory systems (Pinder and Faherty 1999).

The introduction of utensils into a feeding programme is significant in at least two respects. It marks an important opportunity for the child to exert control and develop independence during feeding. The child is now an active participant in the feeding process rather than a passive recipient of food from others. This sense of involvement and control on the part of the child is likely to diminish feelings of frustration and powerlessness during feeding, feelings which can all too often manifest themselves in temper tantrums and a refusal to eat. The use of utensils is also an additional load on the child's limited motor skills. This extra burden may serve to increase the child's tone and trigger abnormal reflexes such as the asymmetrical tonic neck reflex. Even oral reflexes (e.g. jaw and tongue thrusting) that had decreased during feeding therapy, may become evident again under the pressure of self-feeding (Pinder and Faherty 1999). These physical problems can be resolved through careful attention to positioning during feeding – positioning should emphasise the midline and discourage excessive extension or flexion. They can also be lessened or eliminated by using simpler food textures at first, so that the child may focus on the gross and fine motor skills that are required to manipulate the utensils. The child's enthusiasm for greater participation in feeding may also have to be balanced against other considerations. Mealtimes are likely to take longer, which may detract from other activities at home and at school. The child who is involved in feeding may fatigue rapidly. Fatigue may increase the child's risk of aspiration. It may also lead to a reduction in the amount of food consumed and to a decrease in the child's nutritional intake. Where this decrease is judged to be significant, some adjustment of the feeding programme may be required. The therapist will undertake all such adjustments in consultation with the team's dietician.

With these general considerations about the use of utensils in mind, the therapist can turn his or her attention towards establishing safe, effective use of specific utensils. The primary therapeutic aims during spoon feeding are to encourage tongue stability and lip and jaw closure. In order to maintain a safe and effective position for feeding, the spoon should approach the child from the midline and below eye level. If the child must extend his head and neck to receive the food, swallowing is more difficult and the risk of aspiration increases.[92] To encourage participation, the child's hand can be placed on the therapist's hand as the spoon moves to and from the mouth. Once in the mouth, spoon pressure on the tongue can serve to stabilise its position in the jaw. Previous feeding experiences may have encouraged passivity on the part of the child. The passive child may not respond to the presence of the spoon by raising the lower jaw and forming lip closure around the spoon. The therapist must actively discourage the child's expectation that food will be deposited in the mouth through the feeder scraping the contents of the spoon against the upper lip and teeth. With sustained practice and encouragement, the passive child can learn to form an effective lip seal around the spoon and remove food from it, where previously an open mouth posture was adopted.

Drinking from a cup makes different demands of a child's oral motor skills. The rim of the cup should be placed between the lips and not between the teeth or on the tongue, which can elicit a bite reflex and forward tongue posture, respectively. At first, the child may gain stability by biting on the cup. Also, the child with wide jaw excursions during drinking may need the stability of a hand placed below the jaw. This assistive hand placement can be lessened as the jaw develops internal stability. With the lower lip supporting the rim of the cup, the cup can be tipped slightly so that the (thickened) liquid touches the upper lip. The upper lip can then control the amount of liquid that enters the oral cavity. Sipping actions are followed by swallowing before further liquid is taken into the mouth. Liquid should not be poured from the cup into the child's mouth. Pouring removes the need for the child to draw liquid actively into the mouth and, thus, encourages passivity on the part of the child. Poured liquid is also more likely to cause coughing, choking and aspiration, as the child is unable to control when liquid enters the oral cavity or, indeed, how much liquid enters. For the child who is learning to drink, an open cup is recommended over a spout cup, which tends to encourage suckling (Arvedson 1998). Modified utensils (e.g. spoons and forks with built-up handles, plate guards and scoop bowls) can facilitate feeding in the motor-impaired child. The speech and language therapist should discuss with the occupational therapist how these different utensils can best be employed in a particular case.

Chewing is integral to bolus preparation and must also receive attention during feeding therapy. The motor-impaired child is unable to use lateral tongue movements to move food between the teeth for chewing. The therapist can begin to establish a more effective pattern of chewing by holding food between the teeth as the child repeatedly raises and lowers his or her jaw against it. When the chewed food is swallowed, the same procedure is repeated on the opposite side of the mouth. Lateral tongue movement can be encouraged by stimulation to the lateral edge of the tongue. When food is placed in the middle of the tongue, a suck-swallow response is stimulated, with the tongue moving in an unproductive forwards–backwards direction (Pinder and Faherty 1999).

Drooling is a significant obstacle to social integration and vocational opportunity, particularly in the motor-impaired adult.[93] Although saliva control is routinely addressed in feeding therapy, drooling is less of a problem during feeding than it is between mealtimes – saliva is regularly removed from the oral cavity during feeding by the swallow reflex. There are three main approaches to the management of drooling: (1) oral motor therapy, (2) medication and (3) surgery. No single approach is totally effective and treatment usually involves some combination of these techniques.[94] Also, less invasive methods – namely, oral motor therapy and medication – are usually implemented before surgery is undertaken. In the remainder of this section, we describe each of these techniques and briefly discuss their efficacy in the treatment of drooling.

Oral motor therapy is an integral part of drooling management.[95] Not only is it the first treatment technique to be adopted by clinicians, but it continues to play an important role in saliva control when intervention includes pharmacotherapy or surgery. Oral motor therapy focuses on many of the same areas that we have already discussed in relation to feeding. Attention to positioning is a key component in the management of drooling. Oral structures that are poorly supported by the head, shoulders and trunk cannot control the flow of saliva from the mouth. The drooling child and adult often have oral sensory deficits that contribute to a lack of saliva control. Oral motor therapy must also address these sensory deficits. Key aspects of this work include increasing the child's sensory awareness of lip closure, helping the child to distinguish between a wet and a dry face, and developing the child's sensation of saliva overflow at the lips. Finally, as the strength of lip, tongue and jaw movements increases, so too will the child's control of saliva. Oral motor therapy must, therefore, also focus on developing the strength of these oral movements.

In cases where drooling is severe and oral motor therapy has been minimally effective, it may be necessary to institute pharmacotherapy. A range of drugs exists for the treatment of drooling.[96] Antihistamines and anticholinergic agents are the most commonly used. Some of these drugs are more effective than others, but all of them produce various side effects. The anticholinergic drug, glycopyrrolate, 'remains theoretically the drug of first choice' (Blasco 2002:780). Studies have shown this drug to produce response rates of between 70 and 90 per cent. However, between one-third to two-thirds of patients develop side effects that include an excessively dry mouth (xerostomia), constipation, urinary retention, decreased sweating and skin flushing, and irritability or other behavioural changes (Blasco 2002). However, not all side effects produced by these drugs are undesirable. For example, trihexyphenidyl has tone reduction as a side effect and has been used to reduce drooling in children with rigid or dystonic cerebral palsy.[97] The therapist must be aware of the effect of drugs on the viscosity of saliva. Blasco (2002) urges caution in the use of drugs to control drooling in children who choke on their own secretions. He warns that changes in the viscosity of saliva threaten to undermine yet further the already poor respiratory status of these children.

Surgery is normally only undertaken when oral motor therapy and medication have failed to lessen drooling. This is because surgery can result in complications that do not attend other forms of treatment. For example, several of O'Dwyer and Conlon's (1997) subjects who underwent submandibular duct relocation developed postoperative pneumonia secondary to salivary aspiration, submandibular gland swelling and a ranula (retention cyst). Moreover, surgical procedures are irreversible, so if the surgery does not ameliorate drooling, the patient may be left with undesirable long-term problems. Several surgical techniques are available. One of the more effective techniques is submandibular excision with parotid duct ligation (a modification of the earlier Wilkie procedure). The submandibular glands are responsible for a large percentage of resting salivary production. Their excision, along with the ligation of the ducts of the parotid glands, can serve to decrease the volume of saliva that is produced. In submandibular duct relocation, the ducts of the submandibular glands are dissected and re-routed to the posterior tonsillar pillar. This enables saliva to flow backwards towards the throat rather than forwards and out of the mouth. In transtympanic neurectomy, the otolaryngologist interrupts the parasympathetic nerve supply to the parotid, submandibular and sublingual glands as the nerves traverse the middle ear along the medial wall. These surgical techniques produce varied results. In a study of 52 patients who underwent different surgical procedures for the treatment of sialorrhoea (increased saliva flow), Shott et al. (1989) state that 'bilateral submandibular gland excision with parotid duct ligation is the only procedure in which consistent control of sialorrhoea can be expected' (47). In a study of 53 patients who underwent submandibular duct relocation, O'Dwyer and Conlon (1997) report that 94 per cent of parents stated that their child had benefited from the procedure and over half of the parents reported complete cessation of all drooling within three months of the operation. In transtympanic neurectomy, an initial success rate of between 50 and 80 per cent can be expected, with later failures related to the regeneration of the nerve fibres (Vaughn and Brown 2003).

2.3.3.2 Communication Intervention

Normal speech is not a realistic goal of treatment for CP children and adults with dysarthria. Rather, the focus of intervention in this clinical population is on establishing functional communication skills, whereby the child is able to fulfil his or her communication needs through a range of verbal and nonverbal means. Where the child's physiological limitations do not preclude improvements in speech, this may involve the therapist working directly on articulation and other aspects of speech production (e.g. breathing) with a view to increasing the intelligibility of speech. In the severely motor-impaired child who has little prospect of developing verbal communication, the priority of intervention is to establish a suitable system of augmentative and alternative communication. In a condition like cerebral palsy, where associated cognitive, visual and hearing impairments not only disrupt the development of normal communication skills, but also restrict the type of AAC system that an individual can use, it is clear that this particular priority of intervention is not always achieved with ease. The focus on functional communication over normal speech has other implications for intervention. The therapist must consider the wider context in which communication occurs. We will see subsequently that context is a very broad notion indeed and includes not only the physical setting in which interaction occurs, but also the conversational partners of the CP child and adult. Considerable effort in therapy is directed towards training parents and carers in the use of strategies that can facilitate communication with the CP child and adult. Later in this section, we will examine these strategies and discuss their efficacy. In the meantime, we consider the place of techniques that are aimed at improving speech production within a wider programme of communication intervention.

In section 2.3.2.2, we described how articulation, resonation, phonation, respiration and prosody could be impaired to varying degrees in dysarthria. Treatment of the speech disorder in cerebral palsy must, therefore, give due consideration to each of these components of speech production. Treatment techniques are diverse in nature but tend, in general, to fall under one of the following therapeutic approaches: (1) traditional therapy, (2) instrumental therapy, (3) prosthetics, (4) surgery and (5) pharmacotherapy. With the possible exception of (4) and (5), each of these approaches aims to maximise speech function within physiological limitations that are imposed on the speech musculature through neurological impairment. (Approaches (4) and (5) improve speech function by reducing the physiological limitations on the speech production mechanism.) Traditional therapy subsumes the large range of behavioural techniques that use repeated practice of speech and nonspeech behaviours as a means of improving speaker intelligibility. Instrumental therapy includes the growing number of biofeedback techniques that make the physiological processes of speech production accessible to the dysarthric client through auditory, visual and tactile sensory modalities. Prosthetics aims to augment the function of the speech musculature through the use of artificial devices. We will discuss these five therapeutic approaches in turn and assess their contribution to attempts to improve speech production in cerebral palsy.

The decision to treat dysarthria using behavioural techniques is based on an assessment of the CP child's stimulability. The child who can improve his or her speech performance by exaggerating articulatory movements or by changing speaking rate exhibits some capacity to compensate for the various speech impairments associated with dysarthria. The behavioural techniques that are used to treat the stimulable child range from those that treat particular components of speech production (e.g. articulation) to those that target nonspeech movements. The former techniques typically involve some modification of the pattern of speaking – increasing effort, slowing rate and over-articulating speech (clear speech) are three such modifications. The latter techniques use nonspeech exercises to improve the speed, range, strength and timing of muscle movements for speech. In this way, blowing and sucking exercises are used to strengthen the muscles of the velopharyngeal port and achieve a reduction in the hypernasality of speech.

The problem with behavioural techniques that are used to increase muscle strength, or rectify other pathokinesiologies of dysarthria, relates largely to the efficacy of these techniques. In many cases, it is doubtful that these techniques are serving any useful speech purpose. For example, it is now widely recognised that behavioural techniques such as blowing exercises are not an effective means of reducing hypernasality during speech production.[98] Moreover, it is not even clear that behavioural techniques can increase muscle strength or improve other pathokinesiologies associated with dysarthria. As Hodge and Wellman remark 'the efficacy of behavioural treatments that attempt to normalize pathokinesiologies underlying dysarthric speech in children is by and large unknown' (1999:222). This lack of knowledge is attributable in part, if not in whole, to the problem of measuring the effect of behavioural techniques on speech production.[99] The need to address this problem has been one of the major impetuses for the emergence of an instrumental approach to the treatment of dysarthria.

Instrumental techniques provide objective, measurable data on different aspects of speech production. For example, electropalatography (EPG) enables the clinician to quantify and describe objectively lingual–palatal contacts during articulation. Using these techniques, clinicians are now able to record and quantify speech along a range of dimensions that were previously either inaccessible to study or accessible only to perceptual analysis. Clearly, instrumental techniques make a significant contribution to efficacy studies, where the data that is provided by instrumentation is used to demonstrate treatment outcomes. However, these techniques also play a key role in therapy, where they facilitate speech motor learning by providing biofeedback to the speaker. In this way, the visual feedback that is provided by EPG can help the dysarthric child attain alveolar placement of the tongue for the articulation of the consonants /t,d/, for example. Indeed, instrumental techniques are so effective in establishing new speech behaviours that they have often succeeded where traditional therapy techniques for dysarthria have failed. Gibbon and Wood (2003) describe the case of an 8-year-old boy with cerebral palsy who consistently fronted velar targets and who did not respond to conventional speech therapy techniques. EPG analysis revealed two features of diagnostic significance – an unusually asymmetrical pattern of tongue–palate contact and unusually long stop closure durations. After 15 sessions of EPG therapy over a period of four months, there was a significant improvement in the boy's ability to produce velar sounds. Following Gibbon and Wood, this result suggests a clear role for EPG in the diagnosis and treatment of articulation disorders in individuals with mild cerebral palsy.

Instrumental techniques have undoubtedly transformed therapy for motor speech disorders in a number of clinical groups, including cerebral palsy. When sensory problems are known to be a factor in a child's speech disorder (as is the case in cerebral palsy), the provision of biofeedback can be an important catalyst in speech motor learning. Also, motivation is a key factor in learning and children tend to be more motivated by a therapeutic process that involves instrumentation and computer displays of speech activity than by a process that is based on traditional techniques. Yet, it should not be overlooked that there are CP children and adults who are not suitable candidates for instrumental therapy or who are unlikely to benefit from this particular therapeutic approach to their speech disorder. Despite efforts to reduce oral hypersensitivity, for some CP children and adults hypersensitivity remains a persistent problem. These individuals are unlikely to tolerate instrumental techniques that use invasive oral appliances, such as the artificial palate that must be worn during EPG training. Moreover, many CP children and adults have visual and hearing impairments that restrict the type of instrumental technique that can be employed during therapy. For example, a child with a severe visual defect will not be able to monitor computerised displays of lingual–palatal contacts in EPG. Finally, the successful use of any instrumental technique requires that the CP child and adult possess certain cognitive and intellectual skills. For example, in the case of EPG, the CP child and adult must understand how two-dimensional configurations on a computer screen relate to lingual–palatal contacts in the oral cavity. The CP child and adult, in whom these cognitive and intellectual skills are either lacking or seriously impaired, will not be able to participate to any effective extent in a therapeutic programme that uses instrumental techniques.

On account of their invasive nature, prosthetic devices tend to be employed only when traditional and instrumental approaches to therapy have failed to bring about significant improvements in speech function. These devices effect speech improvements by one of two means. They can augment the function of certain muscle groups. For example, palatal lifts can improve the function of the velopharyngeal port and, through doing so, reduce the hypernasality of speech. Prosthetic devices can also be used to eliminate muscle movements that interfere with speech production. In this way, bite blocks can be used to inhibit or limit involuntary jaw movements. Few studies have directly examined the use of prosthetic devices to treat dysarthria in cerebral palsy.[100] When studies have been undertaken, results tend to indicate that these devices are not effective in the treatment of specific speech problems. For example, Lotz and Netsell (1989) used a palatal lift to improve velopharyngeal closure for oral plosive consonants in a CP boy with severe dysarthria. These researchers concluded that the palatal lift was unsuccessful in the case of this boy, who eventually underwent pharyngeal flap surgery in order to correct his velopharyngeal incompetence. For this CP child at least, speech movements appeared to be more difficult and laboured with the lift in place. Hardy et al. (1969) implemented prosthetic management of velopharyngeal incompetence in five children with cerebral palsy. Four of these children were fitted with palatal lifts, while the fifth child used a bulb–type obturator. (This child had a bifid uvula and short soft palate.) Prosthetic intervention was initiated for these children either because behavioural therapy had proved to be ineffective or because progress had plateaued. Hardy et al. judged prosthetic intervention to be of minimal assistance to the child with severe neurological involvement, in whom there are severe restrictions of mobility affecting the tongue, lips and jaw.

In general, prosthetic management of velopharyngeal incompetence is attempted before surgical management. This is because surgery can produce complications that are not encountered during prosthetic intervention (e.g. surgical risks, new resonance problems). Moreover, surgical procedures are permanent, so the patient may be left with long-term problems if surgery does not have a successful outcome. For all these reasons, surgery to correct velopharyngeal incompetence is normally only undertaken after behavioural and prosthetic management have been tried, but have been found to fail. There are few reports in the literature of the use of surgery to correct velopharyngeal incompetence in cerebral palsy. When studies have been conducted, findings have been variable. Early favourable results from pharyngeal flap surgery (Hardy et al. 1961) have given way to less positive outcomes (Hardy et al. 1969). Other surgical techniques are used to alleviate spasticity in cerebral palsy. However, these techniques do not target spastic speech muscles and, hence, lack an application in the treatment of dysarthria – selective dorsal root rhizotomy, for example, aims to reduce spasticity in the legs by selectively severing sensory nerves entering the lower spinal cord.

Pharmacotherapy is being used increasingly to provide the CP child and adult with relief from the various movement difficulties associated with cerebral palsy. Antiparkinsonian drugs (e.g. anticholinergic and dopaminergic drugs), antispasticity agents (e.g. baclofen) and, to a lesser degree, anticonvulsants, antidopaminergic drugs and antidepressants have been used in the management of dystonia. Spasticity can be managed through the use of benzodiazepines and baclofen. Benzodiazepines, neuroleptics and antiparkinsonian drugs (e.g. levodopa) are used to manage chorea and athetosis. Anticonvulsants (including benzodiazepines such as diazepam, valproic acid, barbiturates) are useful in the management of myoclonus. Despite the proven value of these drugs in controlling movement difficulties in some cases, no studies have been conducted to date of their effect on dysarthric speech in cerebral palsy.

When physiological limitations are so great that they preclude any prospect of an improvement in speech, the speech and language therapist should consider the introduction of an alternative communication system. Such a system may also be required to support or augment speech in the case where some limited speech is possible, but is not readily intelligible. The choice of system is dependent on a range of factors, including the particular competencies and deficits that the CP child or adult brings to communication, the communication purposes for which the system is used and the settings in which communication occurs (e.g. in school, at home). Cost is also a consideration, particularly in the case of recent aids that are based on advanced computer technology. Many forms of alternative communication require the active participation of a communication partner – for example, the partner must be relied upon to interpret the meaning of graphic signs that are selected by the CP child and adult. Clearly, the therapist must also consider the role of the communication partners of the CP individual during AAC intervention. We examine a number of these factors in more detail below.

The motor disability in cerebral palsy is one of the most important factors that influence the choice of alternative communication system. The motor-impaired CP child or adult, who has poor control of arm and hand movements, may be unable to point with an extended forefinger at Rebus signs[101] on a communication board or to give signs to a communication partner, such as occurs in the Picture Exchange Communication System (Bondy and Frost 1998). For the CP individual with good head and body control, head sticks can be used to provide an effective, alternative form of pointing. In the absence of such control, eye gaze can be used to point to signs on a communication board. For eye-pointing to be successful, the communication partner must be situated where he or she can follow the user's gaze. The difficulty in identifying the target of eye gaze and the fact that the eyes are used for a number of functions other than pointing make it preferable that another form of pointing is developed. It is important that the therapist, parents, carers and other professionals build upon whatever form of pointing the CP child and adult can most easily manage. In this way, von Tetzchner and Martinsen (2000) describe the case of a 30-year-old disabled man whose language acquisition was hindered because staff at his school refused to accept his use of the innermost joint of his thumb to point at his communication board. Even when motor problems do not preclude the CP child or adult reaching towards signs on a communication board, poor movement control may reduce the accuracy of sign selection. In this case, the graphic signs or letters on a communication board must be large. Also, when switches are used to control the aid, a low degree of accuracy will require that they have large fields and considerable space between them.

A number of other impairments must also be considered when introducing a system of alternative communication. Problems of visual acuity may determine the size of graphic signs and make it difficult for the CP child and adult to distinguish graphic signs that are similar to one another. The CP individual with visual field deficits may only be able to see and point to signs in part of the communication board. Oculomotor problems may make it difficult to scan signs on a communication board or computer screen. These problems will also preclude the use of eye gaze as a form of pointing. Cortical visual impairment may disrupt the perception of graphic signs. For example, it is not uncommon for brain-damaged children and adults to identify objects using only one or a few of the available cues. If such stimulus over-selectivity is suspected, it may be necessary to introduce signs that do not have many features in common (von Tetzchner and Martinsen 2000).

Many CP individuals are also learning-disabled. Learning disability places various limitations on the type of alternative communication system that can be employed. For example, efforts to teach Blissymbols[102] to learning-disabled subjects have been largely unsuccessful, owing to the complex graphic formation and similarity in form of many of these signs (von Tetzchner and Martinsen 2000). Pictogram Ideogram Communication[103] has largely replaced the use of Blissymbolics among individuals with learning disability. Communication boards often contain photographs and pictures from magazines. However, it is a common misconception that pictures are more readily recognised and understood than graphic signs. Many learning-disabled individuals find it difficult to understand what pictures represent. This difficulty is compounded when photographs of familiar people, objects and animals are used to represent classes – for example, a photograph of the family dog that is used as a generic term for 'dog'. For learning-disabled children and adults, a graphic sign system may be more easily understood and acquired than a system which makes use of drawings and photographs. Some learning-disabled individuals may struggle to understand the communicative purpose of a manual communication board. These children and adults may benefit from hearing a word spoken at the same time as a graphic sign is selected; this scenario simulates spoken communication and, as such, is more comprehensible to the individual with learning disability. In such a case, the learning-disabled child and adult may benefit from the use of a communication device with artificial speech output.

Many CP individuals have good language comprehension and delays in expressive language. The consistent use of single signs should lead during language intervention to the establishment of multiple sign utterances. These utterances require a vocabulary that not only is capable of expressing the needs and interests of the CP child and adult,[104] but will also promote multi–sign use. In this way, signs that can be combined with more than one activity sign (e.g. FINISHED as in FINISHED WORK, FINISHED JUMP) or more than one object sign (e.g. CARRY as in CARRY MILK, CARRY SACK) permit a natural developmental progression to occur from single signs to two–sign utterances. These so-called pivots are always used in the same position by the individual child and, as such, they have syntactic significance. (Pivots such as 'gone' in 'gone milk' and 'gone dog' have been taken by child language researchers to represent the emergence of syntax in speaking children.) Other signs that achieve an expansion in sign use include commands such as FETCH in FETCH CUP and FETCH MINERAL WATER. These signs can be readily built into expressive language activities – for example, the child producing commands which are then carried out by the therapist or teacher. Verb signs are an effective means of facilitating multi–sign use and syntactic development. Verbs take a number of other elements. For example, the verb 'carry' implies that someone is doing the carrying ('Mummy') and that something is being carried ('milk'). The verb sign CARRY thus leads to the construction MUMMY CARRY MILK. It also creates the possibility of further syntactic expansion through the introduction of other elements, e.g. MUMMY CARRY MILK IN JUG.

These expansions increase the size of the child's sign vocabulary. However, they also extend the vocabulary beyond action and object signs to include signs from other categories. For example, MUMMY CARRY MILK IN JUG introduces a new category of spatial locatives through the use of the sign IN. These multi–sign utterances also represent an important opportunity to build upon the child's developing knowledge of semantic roles, such as agent, action and location in the signed utterance MUMMY SLEEP IN BED. These roles will often require direct attention during language intervention. This is because the implied agent is more often than not the sign user and children may not understand that other people can also act as agents. It is not until children accept and use photographs of other people in the role of agent that these photographs can be said to function as semantic agents. Also, photographs in which the child is present make it difficult for a sign user to distinguish the agent semantic role from other semantic information in the picture. Different semantic roles can be established by using a separate photograph of the sign user, which can then be combined with photographs or graphic signs of roles such as action and location. Fill–in strategies are an effective technique for developing the use of semantic roles. Signs are selected by the therapist or teacher while the child is watching (e.g. ROBERT EAT?). The child must then complete the informa-tion by selecting an appropriate graphic sign from his or her total vocabulary (or from a smaller number of graphic signs, if this proves to be too difficult).

Despite efforts to encourage the use of multi-sign utterances, it remains the case that children with good comprehension of spoken language tend to use a high proportion of single-sign utterances (von Tetzchner and Martinsen 2000). A number of factors have been advanced to explain this lack of multi-sign use, including the additional cognitive resources (particularly working memory) that sign selection requires and the specific forms of interaction that are adopted by the communication partners of the CP child and adult. Interaction training for the conversational partners of CP individuals is now a routine part of communication intervention with this clinical population. Although the effectiveness of this training has yet to be clearly established,[105] its widespread inclusion within therapeutic programmes warrants its exam-ination in the rest of this section.

It is frequently remarked that CP children and adults adopt a passive com-municative style. The main feature of this communicative style is a lack of initiative in conversation, with CP individuals preferring to respond to the con-versational turns of others rather than initiate turns of their own. Moreover, the passivity of CP children and adults during communication is dispropor-tionate to their motor impairment, with many otherwise competent communi-cators in speech and sign also failing to initiate turns in conversation.[106] In explanation of this behaviour, researchers have argued that conversational partners are largely responsible for the passive communication style of CP indi-viduals. The conversational dependency on others of CP speakers and alter-native communicators is fostered by these partners, many of whom are parents and carers who have been used to performing other activities for the motor-impaired child or adult.

Typically, conversations follow a restricted pattern in which there are high levels of partner control and children's responsivity (Pennington et al. 2004). Conversational partners select the topics to be discussed, complete the con-versational turns of CP subjects and constrain subjects' contributions to con-versation through their use of questions. When a CP subject is using alternative communication, partner control can be even more evident. Conversational partners often fail to give alternative communicators time to respond.[107] They tend to guess responses (often incorrectly) after the subject has selected only one sign. This encourages single-sign use and can cause considerable confu-sion when errors are made. Partners ask alternative communicators a dispro-portionately large number of yes-no questions, even when their access to a sign vocabulary indicates that they are capable of a more extensive response.[108] Moreover, the very semblance of sincere communication is removed when partners follow a question with a series of subquestions, and fail to wait for a response to any of them, or ask questions to which they already know the answer. By insisting on the use of a communication aid when simple pointing to an object will suffice, the conversational partner can create considerable frustration in the alternative communication user. The effect of these communicative behaviours on the CP child or adult is, at best, to limit the CP subject to making responses to the topics, questions, comments and directives of others. At worst, these behaviours can cause the CP subject's total disengagement from communication.

During interaction training, the therapist seeks to educate partners in how they can best facilitate conversational exchanges with the CP child or adult. This training can involve a range of instructional methods. Initially, the therapist should observe interaction between the CP subject and one or more conversational partners, who are usually parents or carers. If sufficient time and appropriate facilities are available, it is helpful to make a video recording of these conversational exchanges. This recording can be used by the therapist to raise partners' awareness of the behaviours that facilitate and hinder effective communication with the CP subject. When post-training recordings are also made, this allows partners to examine the transition within their own communicative behaviours and makes it possible for the therapist to assess the efficacy of interaction training. Some techniques are easily implemented by partners and require little more than verbal instruction from the therapist – for example, advice on increasing face-to-face contact with the CP subject. Other techniques are less readily implemented and may require demonstrations as well as verbal instruction before they can be successfully executed – for example techniques to increase the CP subject's responsiveness. In the rest of this section, we examine a number of strategies that may be used to increase the CP subject's participation in and initiation of conversation.

Interaction training aims to modify those communicative behaviours that enable partners to exert control in conversation and that reduce the role of the CP subject to a passive responder. These behaviours are varied and include the extensive use of questions by partners and the failure to allocate turns to the CP subject. Importantly, they include the rights to initiate and terminate conversation, rights that are assumed almost exclusively by conversational partners. By initiating conversation, the conversational partner determines the topic of conversation. He or she also determines the duration of conversation and the point at which conversation will be terminated, neither of which may satisfy the conversational needs of the CP subject. Conversational partners must learn to recognise the often indistinct signs that a CP subject is attempting to initiate conversation. This is less of an imperative for the partners of CP subjects who use communication aids with artificial speech output – in such a case, a ready-made opening phrase is adequate to indicate a desire to communicate. However, for other CP speakers and alternative communicators, vocalisation, gesture or other body movements may be the only indication that the CP subject wishes to initiate conversation. Involuntary vocalisations and movements are common in cerebral palsy, so these communication-oriented behaviours may simply be overlooked by a potential conversational partner. The extent of this problem is demonstrated by Calculator and Dollaghan (1982), who found that teachers responded to only 39 per cent of the communicative initiatives produced by nonambulatory students in a residential classroom setting. These problems are more evident at the beginning of conversation, when the CP speaker or alternative communicator must first attract the attention of a conversational partner, than they are at the end of a conversation, when the CP subject can simply use speech or signs to indicate that he or she wishes to finish the exchange.

The issue of who initiates conversation also has implications for how the internal structure of a conversation will develop. As we discussed above, the conversational partner more often than not opens exchanges with the CP subject. To the extent that a question forms the first conversational turn, the roles of questioner and responder are assigned from the outset to the partner and CP subject, respectively. Moreover, the nature of the partner's questions limits the CP subject's ability to reverse these conversational roles. Closed questions constrain the content of the CP subject's responses and preclude his or her development of new topics of conversation. If the CP subject is unable to introduce new topics of conversation, he or she may not feel motivated to ask questions about the conversational partner's chosen topic. Yes-no questions are even more limiting in this regard. And while these questions may be conversationally expedient in some respects – they reduce the CP subject's response times and remove the partner's need to use unreliable guessing strategies – yes-no questions deny the CP subject many valuable opportunities in which to make extended responses and develop cognitive and expressive language skills.

Clearly, any effort to reduce partner control during conversation must include an examination of the number and type of questions that are employed by the conversational partner. Wherever possible, questions should be replaced by other speech acts that permit the CP subject to make an extended contribution to conversation (e.g. 'I'd like to hear about your holiday' as opposed to 'Where did you go on holiday?'). When questions are used, they should be open and not yes-no questions (e.g. 'What did you do on holiday?' rather than 'Did you swim on holiday?'). The aim should be to encourage the CP child or adult to develop extended responses within boundaries that are set by the CP subject rather than by the conversational partner's questions.

Although questions dominate conversational exchanges with CP subjects, they conceal the fact that little genuine turn-taking occurs within these exchanges. Questions place an obligation on the CP subject to produce a response (an obligatory turn) in conversation. However, conversational partners often do not give CP individuals time to respond to questions in conversation. This problem is even more acute for users of communication aids, who lose their turns in conversation because they are slow to initiate communication. Voluntary turns are more difficult still for alternative communicators.[109] This difficulty is largely the result of the CP subject's inability to use facial expression and intonation to indicate an intention to take turns in conversation. Motor-impaired individuals struggle to produce these nonverbal signals. Moreover, they are often misinterpreted by conversational partners as expressions of hostility or of a lack of interest in conversation. (For example, the CP individual who cannot raise his or her head may routinely find that conversations are terminated.) Clearly, the accurate identification and interpretation of the CP subject's turn-taking cues must form a central part of any interaction training with conversational partners.

Notes

1. A syndrome consists of multiple defects or impairments, all of which have a single aetiology. Although genetic abnormalities are a major cause of syndromes, other causes are infections (e.g. rubella) and intoxication (e.g. excessive consumption of alcohol). In this way, the deafness, cataracts, mental retardation, neuromotor dysfunction and cardiac problems that result from prenatal exposure to rubella constitute a syndrome. Similarly, cardiovascular, craniofacial and limb defects, along with prenatal growth deficiency and developmental delay, are symptoms of foetal alcohol syndrome.

2. VCFS is also known as Shprintzen's syndrome, DiGeorge's syndrome, craniofacial syndrome or conotruncal anomaly unusual face syndrome. The most common defects associated with this syndrome are cleft palate, heart defects, a characteristic facial appearance, minor learning problems and speech and feeding problems. VCFS is a genetic disorder in which part of chromosome 22 is missing. In 10–15 per cent of cases, the syndrome is inherited. (The type of inheritance is autosomal dominant.) Over 130,000 people in the US have this syndrome, which accounts for some 5–8 per cent of children who are born with a cleft palate (National Institute on Deafness and Other Communication Disorders).

3. This syndrome is characterised by micrognathia (severe underdevelopment of the mandible) and glossoptosis (falling back of the tongue) that causes airway obstruction and respiratory distress. It is often called Robin sequence, because one defect leads to the development of another defect. Initially, micrognathia (usually caused by a single gene) results in the tongue remaining high in the oropharyngeal space during development. This prevents closure of the palatal shelves. The result is a cleft palate. Affected children experience the same speech impairments that accompany cleft palate in the absence of a syndrome (i.e. velopharyngeal insufficiency and hypernasal speech).

4. Studies of multiple incidence families have enabled geneticists to establish recurrence rates for cleft conditions. These rates form the basis of genetic counselling of parents who are considered to be at risk of having a child with cleft lip and/or palate. These rates are described by the Cleft Palate Foundation and are summarised in the present context. Every parent has a 1 in 700 risk of having a child with a cleft disorder. A parent who has a child with a cleft condition runs an increased risk of between 2 and 5 per cent (2–5 chances in 100) that the next child, and any subsequent child, will be affected. The risk increases yet again, to between 10 and 12 per cent, if there is more than one affected person in the immediate family. When no other member of the family is affected, an individual with a cleft has a 2–5 per cent chance of having a child with a cleft disorder. If a close relative is affected, an individual with a cleft has a 10–12 per cent chance of having a child with a cleft disorder. Unaffected siblings of a child with a cleft have a 1 per cent risk of having a child with a cleft disorder. When more than one family member has a cleft, an unaffected sibling has a 5–6 per cent risk of having a child with a cleft condition. Finally, when a syndrome is involved in the cleft disorder, the familial recurrence risk can be as high as 50 per cent.

5. Newborns can normally be fed within 20–30 minutes. When feeding time exceeds 45 minutes, the newborn is expending calories on feeding that are necessary for early weight gain (Sargent 1999:15).

6. On the basis of several 'clinically observed parallels' between feeding and speech, Pinder and Faherty (1999) remark on this relationship as follows: 'Although the causal, or at least contributory, connection between the oral motor skills of feeding and of speech requires further research, these clinically observed parallels are intriguing and may ultimately serve to augment or enhance treatment with these children' (282).

7. This larger figure is likely to reflect the full gamut of problems that affect communication (hearing, language, etc., as opposed to just velopharyngeal incompetence). It is also probably related to the fact that Stengelhofen is a speech and language therapist and, as such, is better placed to detect and diagnose speech deficits than medical professionals. Stengelhofen makes this very point in relation to velopharyngeal incompetence:

> Many cases of velopharyngeal incompetence remain undiagnosed until well on into speech development. The author has seen cases at referral from 3 years to 42 years; the appropriate differential diagnosis had not been reached in the adults although several medical specialists had already been consulted. (1993:6)

8. The American Society of Plastic Surgeons states that cleft lip surgery is generally undertaken when the child is about 10 weeks old. Sargent (1999:18) claims that a bilateral cleft lip is usually repaired in one surgical procedure that is performed at three months of age. The American Cleft Palate–Craniofacial

Association recommends that surgical repair of the cleft lip should usually be undertaken in the first six months or as early as is considered to be safe for the child. Stengelhofen (1993:10) remarks that lips are repaired at a few hours in some centres, but it is usually the case that lip repair occurs between three and six months.

9. In the child with bilateral cleft of the lip, separation of the upper lip along the philtral columns (see Figure 2.2) causes isolation of the prolabium (see Figure 2.5). A bilateral cleft of the lip accounts for 15 per cent of all lip clefts (Sargent 1999:18).

10. Many secondary surgical procedures are undertaken when facial development is complete – normally between 16 and 18 years of age in men, and between 14 and 16 years of age in women. However, certain factors may necessitate earlier surgery. For example, the American Cleft Palate–Craniofacial Association recommends that secondary surgical procedures involving the nose (e.g. rhinoplasty and nasal septal surgery) should be performed only after completion of nasal growth, or earlier if there are airway problems or nasal tip deformities.

11. The American Cleft Palate–Craniofacial Association recommends that the palate should be repaired by the age of 18 months in a normally developing child, and earlier if possible. Sargent (1999:19) states that surgical repair of the palate is best achieved in one procedure before 12–14 months of age. The American Society of Plastic Surgeons claims that palate repair is usually performed when the child is 9–18 months old. Stengelhofen (1993) states that 'the repair of the palate will more usually be undertaken between 6 and 18 months' (10) and that 'the best time for palate surgery appears to be around 12 months' (8).

12. A less common cause of the emergence of velopharyngeal incompetence in adolescence is growth processes. Facial growth during childhood and adolescence occurs in a downward and forward direction. This carries the hard and soft palates away from the posterior pharyngeal wall, thus creating a larger space to be bridged during elevation of the velum. If the velum is short or immobile, it may not be able to bridge this gap. So some children with previously normal function of the velopharynx may develop velopharyngeal insufficiency as they mature.

13. In this procedure, a flap of tissue is raised from the posterior pharyngeal wall and inserted into the soft palate. Lateral ports or holes remain, so that the nose is not obstructed (Sargent 1999:20). It is most suitable for patients who have good lateral pharyngeal wall motion but poor palatal motion.

14. As well as indicating when surgical intervention is warranted, the speech and language therapist is also able to indicate when a particular surgical procedure is not appropriate. In many cleft children, surgical removal of the adenoids (adenoidectomy) and/or tonsils (tonsillectomy) may exacerbate an existing problem of velopharyngeal incompetence, or create a problem of velopharyngeal incompetence where none had previously existed. Donnelly (1994) reports that VPI-related hypernasality occurs in approximately 1 in 1,500 adenotonsillectomy procedures and that up to 50 per cent of patients so affected will require surgical

intervention for the correction of this resonance problem. Of course, this is not to overlook other circumstances in which adenoidectomy and/or tonsillectomy are necessary – these surgical procedures may be indicated to permit safe performance of a pharyngeal flap or other type of pharyngoplasty. When a cleft child is being considered for adenoidectomy and/or tonsillectomy, the speech and language therapist and otolaryngologist must discuss the possible impact of these procedures on speech, amongst other factors.

15. Like pharyngeal flap (see note 13), pharyngoplasty is a surgical procedure for the correction of velopharyngeal incompetence. It is most suitable for patients who have inadequate lateral pharyngeal wall motion. A further type of surgical proce- dure – posterior wall augmentation – is used to correct velopharyngeal incompe- tence that is caused by a gap in the central velopharyngeal port that measures at most 1–3mm. It is also indicated when velopharyngeal closure is not tight enough to prevent air escape during high oral pressure and when there is persistent velopharyngeal incompetence following adenoidectomy. Both the patient's own tissues (e.g. fat or dermis) and foreign implants (e.g. Teflon) may be used to augment the posterior pharyngeal wall.

16. Semb and Shaw (2001) obtain the following figures for lateral incisor anomalies from a number of sources: the lateral incisor is congenitally missing in the primary dentition in 12–14 per cent of cases and is missing in the permanent den- tition in about 50 per cent of cases. Semb and Schwartz (1997) cite several authors who report that canine impaction occurs 10 times more often in patients with clefts than in noncleft individuals. Ranta (1990) reports that the prevalence of congenital absence of permanent teeth (excluding the cleft-side maxillary lateral incisor and third molars) in Finnish children with unilateral cleft lip and palate is approximately 50 per cent. As for occlusal problems, Semb and Shaw (2001) report that crossbite of one or more teeth on the cleft side is the commonest devi- ation from normal dental arch form in the primary dentition in unilateral cleft lip and palate. On account of shorter dental arches, particularly in unilateral cleft lip and palate, it is common for crowding in the posterior dentition when all teeth are present (Semb and Shaw 2001). In one cross-centre study, Mars et al. (1992) found that between 10 per cent and nearly 50 per cent of unilateral cleft lip and palate subjects aged 8–10 years had Goslon scores in groups 4 and 5 and, as such, required surgical maxillary advancement to correct poor dental arch relation- ships. (The Goslon Yardstick is an accurate and effective means of determining the quality of dental arch relationships in comparative cross-centre studies.)

17. These procedures begin early in life. Before lip repair is performed, an ortho- dontic appliance may be fitted in an effort to rotate the maxillary alveolar seg- ments into position for repair of the alveolus (gingivoperiosteoplasty). The alveolus may be repaired during lip repair in infancy. If gingivoperiosteoplasty is not performed at this stage, a bone graft may be performed some years later (5–10 years of age). This involves taking a small section of bone from the patient's hip,

head, ribs or leg and inserting it into the cleft near the teeth. This procedure provides support for unerupted teeth and teeth next to the cleft, as well as the lip and nose. Also, it stabilises the alveolus and premaxilla, particularly when a bilateral cleft is present. Ideally, bone grafting should be performed before the eruption of the permanent maxillary teeth in the area of the cleft. In a patient who presents late for treatment, bone grafting may necessarily occur after the permanent teeth have erupted. Once the bone graft is in place, the orthodontist can replace missing teeth in the area of the graft by moving adjacent teeth into the graft, using a prosthetic replacement (dental bridge) or by using dental metallic bone implants. The cleft child may also undergo orthognathic surgery to correct malocclusion (an abnormal relationship between the upper and lower jaws, such that the mandibular teeth protrude and overlap the maxillary teeth (underbite) or the maxillary teeth extend beyond the normal line of occlusion (overbite)). In the child with Pierre Robin syndrome and severe micrognathia (underdevelopment of the mandible), for example, expansion of the mandible can be achieved through a technique called distraction osteogenesis (Sargent 1999:22). The mandible is cut and secured to the expansion device with pins. The device is turned daily for a period of 4–5 weeks. It is then kept in place until new bone growth bridges the gap in the mandible, a process that takes 8 weeks.

18. Unlike repair of the lip and palate, which occurs early in the child's life, orthognathic surgery is normally not undertaken until physical maturation is complete. An obvious exception would be early orthognathic surgery to correct severe micrognathia which is compromising the child's airway. The detrimental impact of malocclusion on speech development may also be judged to be sufficiently severe to warrant earlier orthognatic surgery. The speech and language therapist is thus a vital member of the team that decides the timing of this surgery.

19. The commonest type of ventilating tubes are Shepherd or Shah grommets. These remain in the tympanic membrane for nine months and a year, respectively, and are then extruded. Where more than three grommet insertions are required, a more permanent ventilation tube may be necessary (e.g. Goode T tube or Permavent tube). However, these carry an increased risk of persistent perforation. A persistent perforation in the pars flaccida region of the membrane may lead to the growth of skin (keratin) in the middle ear. This condition is called cholesteatoma.

20. The American Cleft Palate–Craniofacial Association has established a number of recommendations for the audiological care of this clinical population. The Association recommends that all children with craniofacial anomalies – cleft palate included – should undergo an assessment of hearing sensitivity for each ear before the age of one year; that follow-up examinations should continue through adolescence; and that audiological assessment should take place yearly for the first six years of the child's life, even in the absence of a positive history of otological disease or hearing loss.

21. Hearing in the range 0–25dB HL is considered to be normal for adults. However, Northern and Downs (2002) argue that 15dB HL should be considered the lower limit of normal hearing for children – children, they argue, lack adult strategies for understanding speech in context, and must therefore be able to hear all speech sounds in order to establish perceptions of these sounds.

22. In their discussion of the speech and language sequelae of otitis media, Northern and Downs remark that 'the important factors seem to be the onset of the recurrent problem in the first few months of life and the duration of time the child has MEE (and thus conductive hearing loss) during the initial 2 years' (2002:80). MEE stands for middle ear effusion and is a description of the fluid (effusion) that attends otitis media.

23. On account of the recognised link between otitis media and speech and language delays, Northern and Downs (2002) recommend that all children should undergo language screening tests at six months and every six months thereafter until three years of age (84). They recommend also that 'if MEE exists for 3 months despite vigorous medical or surgical treatment or if the hearing impairment persists after 3 months, a language screening test should be applied' (85).

24. The American Cleft Palate–Craniofacial Association recommends that all children undergoing myringotomies and placement of ventilating tubes should be seen pre- and postoperatively for audiological assessment.

25. Even if speech and language development has been appropriate, the American Cleft Palate–Craniofacial Association recommends that screening of speech and language should take place on a regular basis (preferably annually) until after adenoid involution, and at least every three years thereafter until dental and skeletal maturity are reached.

26. One such complication is mastoiditis. This is the inflammation of the air cell system of the mastoid process, a bony protuberance that lies behind and below the external ear. It can exist in both acute and chronic forms. Chronic mastoiditis is associated with a history of otitis media. The resulting hearing loss often has a sensorineural component. The middle ear infections which cause mastoiditis are treated with antibiotics. Moreover, antibiotic treatment is usually very successful, as the reduced rates of mastoid surgery since the introduction of antibiotics indicate. For example, Nadol and Eavey (1995) report a 1954 study that showed that between 9.3 per cent and 69.5 per cent of patients with acute otitis media before the introduction of antibiotics eventually required mastoid surgery, compared to 1.5–28 per cent of patients in the period thereafter. Where surgery is required, a mastoidectomy is performed. This procedure can be more or less extensive – the middle ear structures may be preserved (modified radical mastoidectomy) or moved along with the tympanic membrane (radical mastoidectomy).

27. 'Conceptual and social-communicative aspects of language do not appear to be constrained in similar ways by biological time factors. Development may continue

in these aspects for years beyond puberty, at least in some ways' (Rondal and Comblain 1996:9).

28. In the same way that the speech and language therapist must develop a sound working knowledge of audiological assessment, the audiologist must also have an understanding of speech and language development and of language assessment procedures:

> Because language delay can be a significant factor in the identification of young children with mild to moderate hearing impairment or history of otitis media with effusion, it behoves the audiologist to develop competency in the observation of normal speech-language milestones as well as skill in administering language screening tests. (Northern and Downs 2002:85)

29. Robinson et al. (1992) state that the prevalence of otitis media with effusion in children between 2 and 18 months of age is 92 per cent. (Grant et al. (1988) cite the higher figure of 97 per cent for children between 2 and 20 months of age.) In children aged two years without a cleft palate the prevalence of otitis media with effusion is 20 per cent (Zielhuis et al. 1990).

30. Mental retardation is found not infrequently alongside cleft palate. This is because substantial numbers of clefts occur with other disorders as part of a syndrome. (Shprintzen et al. (1985) found that 31 per cent of 1,000 cleft patients studied had a recognisable syndrome, sequence or association.) Mental retardation is one of these other disorders. Three syndromes/associations in which clefting and mental retardation often occur together are foetal alcohol syndrome, G syndrome (Opitz-Frias syndrome) and the CHARGE association.

31. Even in the transition from normal phonological immaturities to a mature phonological system, cleft-type characteristics are evident in the speech of cleft palate children. For example, in the transition from stopping to the production of fricatives, the cleft child may use velar or uvular fricatives or nonoral pharyngeal or nasal fricatives. So, the cleft child who is using the developmentally normal process of stopping may first use [p] to realise the initial consonant sound in 'four'. However, he or she may then progress to use the nasal fricative [m̃] for /f/. An expansion of the child's phonological system may thus convey the impression that the child's speech is deteriorating (Russell and Harding 2001).

32. This is one of a number of features that Albery and Russell (1994) use to arrive at a decision about the need for early intervention. Other features necessitating early intervention include a predominant pattern of glottal and pharyngeal articulations (4).

33. Russell and Harding (2001) provide explicit guidance about the timing of the cleft child's first phonological assessment. They state that 'it is recommended that all children who have cleft palate should receive routine screening of speech and language development at 18 months' (196). They advocate the use of systematic

phonological screening 'at subsequent assessments, when children are producing more language' (202).

34. Measuring MLU is a commonly used index of grammatical development. MLU is normally determined by counting the number of morphemes per utterance and dividing by the number of utterances.

35. The best-known MLU measure was devised by Roger Brown in the 1960s. This measure consists of five stages, each of which corresponds to a specific age range (in months). According to Brown's system, children in the age range 35–40 months (recall that Chapman's cleft subjects were 39 months of age) should occupy stage IV, which covers an MLU between 3.0 and 3.5 morphemes. At only 2.8 morphemes, Chapman's cleft subjects occupy the middle of the MLU range of stage III (2.5–3.0 morphemes), the age range for which is 31–34 months. Chapman's subjects are operating at a MLU level that is approximately six months below their chronological age. In most contexts, a delay of six months is taken to be clinically significant. (For example, in a study of 30 cleft children, Scherer and D'Antonio (1995) use a delay of six months below the child's chronological age as a criterion for referral for a more thorough speech-language evaluation.)

36. A national audit protocol is now available in the form of the Cleft Audit Protocol for Speech (Harding et al. 1997). This protocol is based on the more detailed Great Ormond Street Speech Assessment (see section 2.2.2.2 in the main text for a brief description). These clinical tools have done much to address the lack of standardised assessments in both research and clinical audit.

37. Passive tubal function describes the mechanical properties of the Eustachian tube in terms of compliance, resistance and closing forces; active tubal function describes the ability of the paratubal musculature to dilate the Eustachian tube during activities such as swallowing. Even though palatoplasty resulted in improvements in passive tubal function, Doyle et al. (1986) found that this procedure failed to bring about direct improvement in Eustachian tube function:

> these data imply that the effect of palatoplasty on Eustachian tube function is minimal and can be accounted for solely on the basis of the changes in the relative position of the levator veli palatini muscle. There is little to no evidence that the efficiency of the tensor veli palatini muscle, recognized as the sole tubal dilator, is much improved by palate repair. (67–8)

38. In a review of 23 articles published over 20 years, Gibbon (2004) discusses eight abnormal patterns of tongue–palate contact that have been identified using EPG data. These patterns are: (1) increased tongue–palate contact, (2) retraction of anterior consonants to palatal or velar placement, (3) fronted placement of velar targets, (4) complete closure across the palate, (5) minimal tongue–palate contact ('open pattern'), (6) double articulations, (7) variability in EPG patterns and (8) abnormal timing.

39. As well as being an effective therapeutic tool, electropalatography is also a valuable diagnostic technique. For example, Gibbon (2004) describes how we are able to distinguish through EPG the phonological process of placement contrast neutralisation (such as occurs in the backing of alveolar targets to velar placement) from the phonetic process of reduced placement separation (the result of a combination of retracted placement for alveolar targets and fronted placement for velar targets). Using EPG, the clinician is able to detect an articulatory distinction in the latter process (a distinction that is being used by the speaker to signal phonemic contrasts) that is absent in the former process.

40. This report was commissioned by Scope (a UK-based support and information service for people with cerebral palsy) and carried out by researchers at Queen's University Belfast.

41. In this study, the overall prevalence rate for the period 1980–90 was 2.08 cases per 1,000 live births. This study is part of a collaborative project called Surveillance of Cerebral Palsy in Europe (SCPE).

42. Mortality rates among low birth weight and very low birth weight (VLBW) babies have continued to decrease since this time. Gould et al. (2000) report that between 1987 and 1993 in California, VLBW infant mortality rate decreased by 28.4 per cent, VLBW neonatal mortality rate decreased by 30.3 per cent and VLBW postneonatal mortality rate decreased by 25.3 per cent.

43. In congenital cerebral palsy, the developing brain sustains damage before or during birth or within the first 28 days of life. In acquired (or postneonatal) cerebral palsy, damage occurs after the 28th day of life but before the child's fifth birthday. United Cerebral Palsy states that 70 per cent of people with cerebral palsy have congenital cerebral palsy due to prenatal brain damage, 20 per cent have congenital cerebral palsy due to brain damage sustained during birth and 10 per cent have acquired cerebral palsy.

44. Rhesus (Rh) incompatibility occurs when a rhesus negative mother develops antibodies against a rhesus positive foetus. The mother is sensitised to rhesus positive blood during an earlier mismatched blood transfusion or as a result of foetal blood entering her circulation. Her immune system develops antibodies which cross the placenta during pregnancy and cause haemolysis of foetal red blood cells. This results in mild jaundice and anaemia or, in more severe cases, hydrops foetalis in utero. The latter is usually fatal.

45. Cummins et al. (1993) found an increased risk of cerebral palsy in mothers under 20 years or 40 years or older and in fathers under 20 years. This study also revealed an increased prevalence of cerebral palsy among children born to black women.

46. Twinning has been described as a risk factor for cerebral palsy in a number of studies. Grether et al. (1993) report that a twin pregnancy results in a child with cerebral palsy 12 times more often than does a singleton pregnancy. However, this increased risk cannot be fully explained by the greater tendency of twins in this

study to have a low birth weight – ten times more twins than singletons weighed less than 1500g at birth – as it was also found that a twin of normal birth weight has a higher probability of developing cerebral palsy than does a singleton of normal birth weight. Grether et al. also report that in children who survive foetal death of a co-twin, cerebral palsy is 108 times more prevalent than in singletons and 13 times more prevalent than in twins whose co-twin is born alive.

47. Developed in 1949 by the anaesthesiologist Virginia Apgar, the Apgar score is a measure of the neonate's condition in the minutes immediately following birth. The score (rated from 0 to 10) is based on four factors – heart rate, respiratory effort, reflex irritability and colour – and is an accurate predictor of infant survival.

48. Numerous studies have linked low birth weight (less than 5.5lb) and very low birth weight (less than 3.3lb) to an increased risk of cerebral palsy. SCPE (2002) found that among babies weighing less than 1500g (3.3lb) at birth, the occurrence of cerebral palsy was more than 70 times higher than in babies who weighed 2500g (5.5lb) or more at birth. In a large, population-based American cohort study, Cummins et al. (1993) found that children with birth weights less than 2500g contributed 47.4 per cent of the cerebral palsy in the population, children weighing less than 1000g contributed 7.8 per cent and children with birth weights of 4000–4500g were at lowest risk of developing cerebral palsy.

49. One such malformation is microcephaly (small head). The presence of nervous system malformations like microcephaly is indicative of a problematic course for neurodevelopment during the prenatal period. As part of this problematic course, the motor centres of the brain may not have developed along normal lines, which may lead to congenital cerebral palsy.

50. The role of genetic factors and maternal infection and inflammation in the development of cerebral palsy are two areas of ongoing research. Although cerebral palsy has always been described as a nongenetic disorder, the findings of some studies are suggestive of a role for genetics in the disorder. One such study was conducted by Sinha et al. (1997), who studied the prevalence of cerebral palsy in an Asian and non-Asian population in Bradford, England. The prevalence rate of cerebral palsy in the Asian population varied between 5.48 cases per 1,000 persons (assuming that none of five unexamined children had cerebral palsy) and 6.42 cases per 1,000 persons (assuming all five unexamined children had cerebral palsy). The prevalence rate of cerebral palsy in the non-Asian population was 3.18 cases per 1,000 persons. The researchers attributed the significantly higher prevalence rate among the Asian subjects to genetic factors. One-half of the Asian families in Bradford who had a child with cerebral palsy had at least one first-cousin marriage. Also, almost one-third of the children with cerebral palsy in the Asian group had a sibling, cousin or aunt with the same type of cerebral palsy. These researchers conclude that 'consanguinity appears to play a major part in the pathogenesis of CP in the Pakistani population living in Bradford' (Sinha et al. 1997:260–1). Notwithstanding ongoing research, the link between cerebral

palsy and maternal infection and inflammation is still unclear. It is claimed that nonsymptomatic vaginal infection in pregnant women is an important risk factor for premature birth, which is known to be associated with an increased risk of cerebral palsy. However, Klebanoff et al. (1995) treated bacterial vaginal infection (group B streptococci) in pregnant women with no symptoms of illness and found that treatment did not prevent premature delivery. Grether et al. (2003) found that intrauterine infection approximately doubled the risk of cerebral palsy among the premature, low birth weight infants of white women, but not among the premature, low birth weight infants of Hispanic, black or Asian women. Yoon et al. (1997) found evidence in their study to support the hypothesis that inflammatory cytokines, produced as a result of microbial invasion of the amniotic cavity, lead to brain white matter lesions and cerebral palsy.

51. The National Institute of Neurological Disorders and Stroke in the US estimates that spastic cerebral palsy affects between 70 per cent and 80 per cent of the cerebral palsy population. Athetoid cerebral palsy is less common, accounting for between 10 per cent and 20 per cent of cerebral palsy cases. Ataxic cerebral palsy is the least common form, affecting between 5 per cent and 10 per cent of cases.

52. This form of the disorder is also known as dyskinetic cerebral palsy. The label 'athetoid cerebral palsy' reflects only one of several movement problems that result from extrapyramidal damage. In addition to athetosis, children and adults with extrapyramidal damage may display chorea (abrupt, irregular, jerky movements), choreoathetosis (a combination of athetosis and choreiform movements) and dystonia (slow, rhythmic movements with muscle tone abnormalities and abnormal postures).

53. In a Swedish population-based study of cerebral palsy, in which 241 children born between 1991 and 1994 were examined, Hagberg et al. (2001) found that diplegic (spastic/ataxic) and hemiplegic subtypes accounted for the vast majority of CP cases, 44 per cent and 33 per cent, respectively. Spastic tetraplegia was present in 6 per cent of cases. Diplegic and hemiplegic subtypes had converse patterns of distribution according to prematurity. In this way, diplegia was present in 83 per cent of the extremely preterm group, 76 per cent of the very preterm group, 56 per cent of the moderately perterm group and 25 per cent of the term group. By contrast, hemiplegia was present in 9 per cent of the extremely preterm group, 10 per cent of the very preterm group, 32 per cent of the moderately preterm group and 44 per cent of the term group.

54. In spastic hemiplegia, the affected side of the body is opposite to the side of the brain in which the lesion occurs. This is because the brain has contralateral control of the body, with the right and left cerebral hemispheres controlling the left and right sides of the body, respectively. This is possible because at the point where the medulla becomes the cervical spinal cord, the large majority of nerve fibres forming the pyramids cross over to the opposite side of the brainstem. (Between 15 per cent and 20 per cent of the nerve fibres forming the corticospinal

tract do not cross over and give rise to the anterior corticospinal tract.) This cross-ing is called the decussation of the pyramids.

55. Tetraplegia is another term for quadriplegia. In spastic quadriplegia, legs are gen-erally affected as much as or more than arms. However, if arms are more involved than legs, the disorder is classified as double hemiplegia.

56. In a study of 170 children with spastic cerebral palsy, Grether et al. (2003) found that 32 per cent had a mild form of the disorder, 36 per cent had moderate cere-bral palsy, 30 per cent had severe cerebral palsy and severity was unknown in 2 per cent of subjects. The criteria that Grether et al. used to classify the severity of cerebral palsy cases were no functional impairment (mild), some functional ability in the most-affected limb, although assistive devices may be used (moder-ate), and no functional ability in the most-affected limb (severe).

57. A report produced in 2002 by the United Cerebral Palsy Research and Educational Foundation states that an estimated 50–75 per cent of people with cerebral palsy have an associated injury to other areas of the brain. Boyle et al. (1996) report that some 66 per cent of individuals with cerebral palsy have other disabilities, primarily mental retardation and vision impairment.

58. Sensorineural hearing loss can be caused by disorders of the inner ear, cochlea, cranial nerve VIII, central nervous system pathways, nuclei or cerebral process-ing of sound. However, the very definition of cerebral palsy – that CP is caused by central nervous system damage – means that the inner ear, cochlea and cranial nerve VIII (part of the peripheral nervous system) are less likely to be involved in the sensorineural hearing loss in cerebral palsy than the part of the auditory pathway that is mediated through the central nervous system (i.e. from the cochlear nucleus in the lower part of the brainstem to the auditory processing of sound in the cerebral cortex).

59. Samson-Fang et al. (2003) report that 27 per cent of children with moderate to severe cerebral palsy were found to be malnourished in a study conducted under the auspices of the North American Growth in Cerebral Palsy Project.

60. Poor nutrition alone cannot explain the type of growth disturbances that occur in cerebral palsy. For example, in spastic hemiplegia, limbs (particularly the hand and foot) on the affected side of the body may not grow as quickly or as large as limbs on the unaffected side. (If poor nutrition alone was responsible for growth problems, we would expect limbs on both sides of the body to be equally under-developed, and so on). Moreover, this disparity in growth cannot be explained by lack-of-use atrophy of the limb, particularly the foot, on the affected side of the body, as it is also observed in spastic hemiplegic patients who can walk (National Institute of Neurological Disorders and Stroke).

61. Major complications include bowel obstructions, gastrointestinal bleeds, ulcera-tion, peritonitis and ostomy infection. Some minor complications were related to the devices that were used and include leakage through or around the tube, dis-lodgement, disconnection, blockage, site irritation, infection and granulation

tissue. Other minor complications involved gastrointestinal problems such as constipation, diarrhoea, cramping and vomiting.

62. The encaphalopathy caused by hyperbilirubinaemia (known as kernicterus) is usually widespread and involves the basal ganglia (particularly the globus pallidus and subthalamic nucleus), hippocampus, substantia nigra, cranial nerve nuclei (particularly oculomotor, vestibular, cochlear and facial nerve nuclei), brainstem nuclei such as the reticular formation of the pons, the inferior olivary nucleus, cerebellar nuclei such as the dentate and the anterior horn cells of the spinal cord.

63. The Babinski sign (or extensor plantar sign) is an abnormal reflex that is indicative of corticospinal (pyramidal) damage. Normally, when the sole of the foot is scratched, there is a slight retraction of the foot and curling of the toes. In a neurological patient who displays a Babinski sign, the large toe extends upwards and the other toes fan outwards as the foot withdraws. The Babinski sign usually reaches stability by the age of two years (Love and Webb 2001). Until this age, the sign is highly variable, even in normal infants, as the nervous system is still in an immature state. (The immature and the damaged nervous system both exhibit reflex behaviours that are normally inhibited by higher centres.)

64. The three drugs that are used most often to control spasticity are diazepam, baclofen and dantrolene. Drowsiness is a significant side effect of these drugs.

65. A range of drugs can be used to treat severe drooling in cerebral palsy. As well as providing varying degrees of relief from drooling, these drugs can have undesirable side effects. Benzhexol hydrochloride (Artane) can cause restlessness and overactivity, while atropine has been found to cause irritability and restlessness.

66. In the UK, at least, there is considerable variability in the provision of paediatric dysphagia services. Suzanne Fox (Head Speech and Language Therapist in the Special Needs Service of City Hospitals Sunderland, NHS Foundation Trust) remarks that 'there are considerable differences in levels of services (from highly organised regional centres of excellence to limited services) provided in paediatric dysphagia in terms of caseloads, expertise, time available, availability of multi-professional teams and interest, access to specialist clinics and assessment, training and education' (personal communication, 18 November 2004).

67. This argument emphasises that feeding is mediated by the brainstem while speech production falls under the control of higher centres in the brain:

> Evidence indicates that the feeding reflexes are mediated at the brainstem level and that voluntary speech is controlled at the cortical, subcortical, and cerebellar levels, with the prime voluntary pathways for speech being the corticobulbar fibers ... Therefore, early motor speech gestures probably are not directly related to the development of motor reactions in feeding during infancy and childhood, even though some of the motor coordinations and refinements in speech acquisition are analogous to some of the biting and chewing gestures in feeding. (Love and Webb 2001:299)

68. These reflexes include rooting, suckling, swallowing, tongue, bite and gag reflexes. Laryngeal reflexes may also be examined during an assessment of feeding. With the recent development of sensory testing as an adjunct to flexible endoscopic evaluation of swallowing (FEES), it is now possible to test the laryngeal adductor reflex (LAR). This reflex is triggered by delivering a calibrated puff of air to the aryepiglottic fold region of the larynx. In the subject with normal laryngopharyngeal sensory capacity, this stimulation will produce a brief closure of the vocal cords with or without a swallow. Link et al. (2000) found that reduced laryngopharyngeal sensory capacity (as indicated by a LAR that is absent or difficult to elicit) correlates with laryngeal penetration and aspiration during a feeding evaluation in children.

69. Oral-pharyngeal reflexes are not the only reflexes in cerebral palsy that persist beyond the point of normal developmental suppression. The Moro reflex and the asymmetrical tonic neck reflex are two primitive reflexes that may persist in cerebral palsy.

70. In the CP child, the normal developmental suppression of oral-pharyngeal reflexes may not take place. As a result, these reflexes may become a permanent and marked feature of the child's oromotor dysfunction and may be evident during both feeding and speech production.

71. It is a weakness of most accounts of feeding that they fail to describe how food is transported to the oral cavity. The neglect of this transportation stage stems from a rather narrow view of feeding as starting with the process of chewing – the oral preparatory phase. An account of oral feeding that includes a stage before the oral preparatory phase can be justified on at least two grounds: (1) the ability to transport food into the oral cavity can be seriously compromised in the presence of oromotor dysfunction and (2) the same neuromuscular mechanisms that are responsible for later stages of feeding also innervate this initial transportation stage.

72. There are two oral stages or phases of feeding – the oral preparatory phase and the oral phase (Logemann 1983). During the oral preparatory phase, food is transformed into a bolus. The bolus is produced by means of chewing (mastication) – the combined actions of the lips, cheeks, tongue and jaw serve to break food down and mix it with saliva. In the oral phase, the bolus is propelled by the action of the tongue towards the oropharynx. This phase ends with the initiation of the swallowing reflex. While the length of the oral preparatory phase varies in relation to the texture of the food and the age of the child, the oral phase lasts less than 1 second, regardless of factors such as food texture.

73. Aspiration puts the airway at risk of mechanical obstruction, bacterial pneumonia, chemical tracheobronchitis and pneumonitis. Long-term complications of aspiration include tracheal and bronchial granuloma formation, stenosis, recurrent pneumonia, bronchitis, bronchiectasis and lung empyema (Arvedson and Brodsky 2002).

74. Gurgling, wet respiration, laryngeal wheezing and other abnormal laryngeal and respiratory sounds are indicative of aspiration. These sounds may be detected by placing a stethoscope against the neck during swallowing, respiration and phonation in a technique called cervical auscultation.

75. Arvedson and Brodsky (2002) report that in CP children who aspirate, 94 per cent can be shown to do so silently using videofluoroscopic swallow study (VFSS).

76. Indirect (secondary) pulmonary aspiration occurs when the contents of gastro-oesophageal reflux spill into the larynx and the tracheobronchial tree. In direct (primary) pulmonary aspiration, saliva, oral flora, mucous and ingested food enter the tracheobronchial tree.

77. Given the high rate of occurrence of gastro-oesophageal reflux (GOR) in cerebral palsy – Trier and Thomas (1998) report that GOR occurs in up to 75 per cent of children with cerebral palsy – it is clear that reflux should be one of the first factors that clinicians consider during dysphagia assessment in this clinical population.

78. A range of professionals may be involved in a diagnosis of GOR. Using flexible fibreoptic nasopharyngolaryngoscopy (FFNL), an otolaryngologist may detect physical changes in the larynx that are associated with reflux (e.g. true and false vocal fold swelling). Radiologists, gastroenterologists and pulmonologists may be involved in administering radionuclide studies such as the scintiscan. This is used primarily for the evaluation of gastro-oesphageal reflux disease and extra-oesophageal reflux disease. (This latter term describes reflux that emerges from the upper oesophageal sphincter into the pharynx, larynx, mouth and nasal cavities.) When scanning is delayed from 4 up to 24 hours after radioactive material has been ingested, it may reveal radioactivity in the lungs (Arvedson and Brodsky 2002).

79. Sullivan et al. (2000) found that 22 per cent of the children with oromotor dysfunction in their study had significant problems with vomiting.

80. These examples demonstrate the interplay that occurs between micro- and macro-elements during assessment. In this way, assessment must consider how damage to cranial nerves (micro-elements) affects a child's oromotor function and, ultimately, his or her ability to communicate and achieve social interaction (macro-elements). By the same token, however, a number of macro-elements (e.g. the failure to smile and produce other facial expressions during caregiver-child interaction) can shed light on the function of specific cranial nerves (micro-elements).

81. Muscular dystrophy is the most common neurological disorder after cerebral palsy to result in developmental dysarthria (Love and Webb 2001). In muscular dystrophy, all striated muscles, including those of the speech mechanism, atrophy and weaken. Developmental dysarthria may also be caused by cranial nerve impairment. In Möbius syndrome, lesions of a number of the cranial nerves related to speech – trigeminal (V), facial (VII) and hypoglossal (XII) nerves – can produce a marked dysarthria. The muscular defects in muscular dystrophy and

the cranial nerve impairment in Möbius syndrome also cause dysphagia in affected individuals.

82. When there is a complete lack of speech as a result of severe paralysis, weakness and/or incoordination, the term 'anarthria' is used instead of 'dysarthria'.

83. 'Clinical experience has shown that most cerebral palsy children do not babble freely and readily, nor do they vocalize much' (Milloy and Morgan-Barry 1990:113).

84. Milloy and Morgan-Barry (1990) used the Edinburgh Articulation Test (Anthony et al. 1971) and the Phonological Assessment of Child Speech (Grunwell 1985) to examine articulation and phonology in a nine-year-old child with mild spastic quadriplegia.

85. The use of the lateral fricative [ɬ] in place of /s/ is not necessarily an example of phonetic deviance, as many members of the child's family also used the lateral fricative for /s/. For this reason, the lateral fricative was not targeted for correction in therapy.

86. The terms 'pitch', 'loudness' and 'quality' describe perceptual characteristics of the voice. These terms correspond, in turn, to the acoustic features of fundamental frequency (f_0), intensity and the frequency distribution of energy (the aspect of a sound that is independent of pitch and loudness).

87. Unlike the muscles of articulation, resonation and phonation, which are innervated by cranial nerves, the muscles of respiration are innervated by cervical (C) and thoracic (T) spinal nerves. Diaphragmatic, abdominal and intercostal muscles are innervated by spinal nerves C3–C5, T7–T12 and T1–T11, respectively.

88. The author knows of no direct evidence to support this claim. However, it receives considerable indirect support from two types of evidence. (1) Other motor activities in cerebral palsy have been associated with increased energy expenditure. For example, children with cerebral palsy often have reduced mechanical efficiency, resulting in a higher energy cost of walking compared to age-matched peers (Lennon et al. 1996); (2) Abnormal muscular activity in cerebral palsy is associated with increased energy expenditure. Johnson et al. (1995) found that adults with athetoid cerebral palsy had increased energy requirements. This was partially explained by athetotic movements which increased the resting metabolic rate of the subjects in their study by an average of 524kcal/day.

89. By virtue of their extended contact with the CP child, parents and carers are often the best judges of the factors that cause intelligibility to fluctuate. However, parents and carers are seldom the most reliable judges of a child's overall intelligibility. A child that is highly unintelligible to the unfamiliar listener may be judged to be only moderately unintelligible by a familiar parent or carer.

90. This has not always been the approach to feeding and swallowing problems in cerebral palsy. Sullivan et al. (2000) remark that '[g]rowth failure and undernutrition have often been accepted as inevitable and irremediable consequences of CP' (674).

91. The Royal College of Speech and Language Therapists (2005) has produced clinical guidelines that cover all aspects of the assessment and management of dysphagia. Under management, guidelines exist for the timing of intervention, the type of food or liquid given (including food texture), the behavioural strategies that facilitate feeding and the use of intra-oral prosthetics, amongst other things.

92. In a study of 14 children with neurological problems mostly associated with cerebral palsy, Morton et al. (1993) found that aspiration occurred when laryngeal movement was insufficient to push the laryngeal inlet fully against the underside of the epiglottis. This type of aspiration was particularly evident when the neck was extended.

93. O'Dwyer and Conlon (1997) state that an estimated 10 per cent of children with neurological impairment suffer significant interference with everyday living due to excessive drooling.

94. Pharmacotherapy and surgery may be used together in treatment. Blasco (2002) reports from his own clinical experience that medication is considerably more effective following surgery than it had been before surgery.

95. 'I still believe hands-on oral-motor therapy techniques and proper positioning interventions remain the fundamental management modalities' (Blasco 2002:780).

96. These drugs can be delivered orally or transdermally. A commonly used transdermal drug is scopolamine. Applied as a patch that is about 1.8cm in diameter and 0.2mm thick to hair-free skin behind the ear (the absorption rate is best when the patch is applied in this location), this system allows a gradual release of scopolamine through the intact skin into the blood system. The benefits of this drug last up to 72 hours. Side effects include mild sedation and dry eyes.

97. 'The use of trihexyphenidyl has been thought provoking because of the potential beneficial side effect of tone reduction. This particular drug may have a special place in the management of drooling in children with rigid or dystonic CP and is favored by me in that clinical setting' (Blasco 2002:779).

98. The Academy of Neurologic Communication Disorders and Sciences states that there is currently no evidence to support the effectiveness of strengthening exercises, such as blowing and sucking. These techniques fail, it is argued, because nonspeech exercises do not target the neuromuscular mechanisms that are involved in speech production.

99. 'Some of the difficulties with using the behavioral therapy techniques . . . include the lack of sensitivity, calibration, and quantitative nature of the data obtained' (Murdoch et al. 1997).

100. In 1997, the Academy of Neurologic Communication Disorders and Sciences established a committee to develop practice guidelines in dysarthria. As part of the research for these guidelines, searches of the literature in the period from 1966 to July 2000 were undertaken. These searches revealed some 32 articles that addressed the effectiveness of velopharyngeal management, especially palatal lift fitting. Of these 32 articles, six (19 per cent) described subjects with cerebral palsy.

101. The Rebus system consists of 950 graphic signs. These signs are primarily picto-graphic, but the system also includes a smaller number of ideographic signs. All signs are black line drawings on a white background. The system was originally developed in the USA. A British version has been developed and is closely linked with the Makaton project (Von Tetzchner and Martinsen 2000).

102. The Blissymbolics system was originally devised as an international written lan-guage which aimed to promote peace by facilitating communication between states-men (Bliss 1965). The system took Chinese as its model, thus explaining the graphic complexity of its signs. There are 100 basic Blissymbols which are then combined to form words. The first graphic sign system to be used in many countries, Blissymbolics is now in steady decline in Europe and North America. However, there is a risk that by avoiding an advanced sign system such as Blissymbolics, chil-dren who could master such a system may be denied a valuable opportunity to develop their expressive language skills (von Tetzchner and Martinsen 2000).

103. Pictogram Ideogram Communication (PIC) (Maharaj 1980) consists of around 1300 signs, each of which is a stylised drawing that forms a white silhouette on a black background. An English gloss is written in white lettering above the drawing. Although PIC signs are easier to use than Blissymbols, they are more limited than Blissymbols in other respects. For example, PIC signs may be used to form sentences. However, given the relatively small number of these signs, it may be necessary to use signs from other systems for this purpose (von Tetzchner and Martinsen 2000).

104. Although ready-made vocabularies exist, these are often poorly suited to express individual needs and interests. Von Tetzchner and Martinsen (2000) describe the case of a 36-year-old woman with cerebral palsy who chose her own vocabulary in consultation with a team of professionals. When this chosen vocabulary was compared with 11 standard or core vocabularies, it was found that none of the latter vocabularies contained all 240 words chosen by the CP subject. Most of the standard vocabularies covered well below 50 per cent of the subject's words. The total of all these standard vocabularies – 2327 words – did not cover this subject's core vocabulary needs.

105. Pennington et al. (2004) have conducted a recent review of experimental studies of interaction training with the conversational partners of CP individuals. These authors conclude that trends in behaviour change have been suggested by these studies but that further investigations, which address the methodological inade-quacies of the original research, are required in order to establish the effectiveness of this training.

106. In a study of seven nonambulatory users of Blissymbols, Calculator and Dollaghan (1982) found that subjects occupied the respondent role nearly three times as frequently as the initiator role. Similar results were demonstrated by Light (1985), who found that the primary caregivers of four- to six-year old users of Blissymbols took communicative initiative 85 per cent of the time.

107. Conversational partners find the longer waits during alternative communication difficult. Light (1985) found that when pauses of more than 1 second occurred, the primary caregivers of four- to six-year-old children began to speak 92.5 per cent of the time. Children who needed more time to make a response using Blissymbols were only able to respond to yes–no questions, which they did quickly by nodding, vocalising or shaking their heads. When alternative communicators are given more time by conversational partners, they also produce more initiations in communication. The child in Light's study who produced most initiations – 45 initiations in 20 minutes – also had the caregiver who waited the longest (for periods as long as 47 seconds in duration). The average number of initiations produced by the other children was 11.7 in 20 minutes. Glennen and Calculator (1985) found that when conversational partners were instructed to wait, communicative initiatives – specifically, object requests – increased in two children aged five and twelve years.

108. Von Tetzchner and Martinsen (1996) report that even motor-impaired individuals who have good comprehension of spoken language and who have access to a communication board with a reasonable number of signs receive a disproportionate number of yes–no questions.

109. Voluntary turns are not prompted by the conversational partner. Smith (1991) found no voluntary turns in a study of a nine-year-old girl who communicated using Blissymbols.

3

Disorders of Cognitive Development

3.1 Introduction

Cognition includes a diverse range of intellectual skills in the absence of which communication is not possible. Amongst other things, these skills include mental processes such as reasoning and perception and cognitive resources like memory and attention. In recent years, considerable progress has been made in our understanding of how acquired impairments of these cognitive skills come to impact on language and communication in general. However, much less is known about the specific effects of cognitive impairment on the development of language and communication skills in children. There are several reasons for this discrepancy in our current state of knowledge. First, cognitive development is incomplete in the immature brain. When cognitive immaturity exists alongside cognitive impairment, it is difficult for clinicians to derive conclusions about the specific cognitive factors that may be contributing to a child's language and communication problems. Second, many of the disorders that are associated with cognitive impairment in children lack clear neurological correlates. This is not the case in acquired disorders that cause cognitive deficits. One need only compare the still largely uncertain neurobiological basis of autism with the focal neurological damage that occurs in a cerebrovascular accident or brain tumour. Neurological correlates function as an important diagnostic marker of cognitive impairment in adults. (For example, frontal lobe damage is associated with cognitive deficits like rigidity, perseveration and poor planning and problem-solving skills in closed head injury.) The absence of these correlates in many developmental disorders limits efforts to produce models of cognitive impairment in children that can then be applied to the study of language and communication problems. Third, while acquired cognitive deficits may be very specific in nature – closed head-injured subjects may present with a specific deficit in memory or attention – cognitive impairment in a disorder such as Down's syndrome involves a wide range of intellectual skills (e.g. reasoning, memory, attention). Where a number of cognitive skills are compromised by a disorder, it is difficult for clinicians to determine the specific effects of each impaired skill on the child's language and communication abilities.

In this chapter, we examine two disorders in which communication impairments are related to deficits in cognitive development. The first of these disorders – learning disability – includes a wide range of conditions, the most common of which is Down's syndrome. For this reason, our discussion will focus largely on communication in Down's syndrome, although we will also discuss other syndromes and disorders in which learning disability occurs. We will see subsequently that a significant number of autistic individuals are also learning disabled. However, it is also the case that the communicative and other impairments associated with autism are increasingly being linked to an underlying cognitive deficit. We begin our examination of learning disability by describing epidemiological and aetiological features of this disorder.

3.2 Learning Disability

A substantial number of children fail to develop normal communication skills because of significant retardation of cognitive, mental or intellectual development. Historically, various labels have been used to describe these individuals. Changing social attitudes towards affected individuals have seen the label 'learning disability' replace the less acceptable terms 'mental handicap' and 'mental retardation' in many professional and everyday contexts. ('Mental retardation' is still used extensively in medical literature and is a valid diagnostic term.) Definitions of learning disability have also undergone considerable change. While definitions have historically been located within a biomedical paradigm, recent definitions of learning disability have been based on functional descriptors and the level of support that is required by affected individuals. In the following extract from a report produced by the UK's Department of Health, a functional descriptor (social functioning) is emphasised:

> Learning disability includes the presence of:
> - A significantly reduced ability to understand new or complex information, to learn new skills (impaired intelligence), with;
> - A reduced ability to cope independently (impaired social functioning); which started before adulthood, with a lasting effect on development.
> (Department of Health 2001:14)

Traditionally, intelligence quotients (IQs) have been used to indicate the severity of 'impaired intelligence' in learning disability.[1] However, Mencap[2] reports that the practice of relying on IQ ratings in assessments of learning disabilities is no longer as important as it once was. The Department of Health report, from which the above extract is taken, states that 'the presence of a low intelligence quotient, for example an IQ below 70, is not, of itself, a sufficient reason for deciding whether an individual should be provided with additional health and social care support' (2001:14–15).

3.2.1 Epidemiology and Aetiology

In the UK, the Department of Health estimates that around 25 people per 1,000 population have mild/moderate learning disabilities – that is, some 1.2 million people in England alone. The Department estimates that a further 210,000 people have severe/profound learning disabilities. Within this figure, there are 65,000 children and young people, 120,000 adults of working age and 25,000 older people. The Department of Health predicts that the number of people with severe learning disabilities may increase by around 1 per cent per annum for the next 15 years. This predicted increase is the result of several factors – increased life expectancy, particularly amongst Down's syndrome individuals; the growth in numbers of children and young people with complex and multiple disabilities who now survive into adulthood; the rise in the number of school-age children with autistic spectrum disorders, some of whom will have learning disabilities; and the greater prevalence of learning disabilities among some minority ethnic populations that are of South Asian origin.

In the United States, the Centers for Disease Control and Prevention (CDC) have been involved in several studies to determine the prevalence of mental retardation (a term commonly used in the US). As part of the Metropolitan Atlanta Developmental Disabilities Surveillance Program, the CDC is tracking the number of children with mental retardation in a five-county area in metropolitan Atlanta. This study has revealed that between 1991 and 1994, on average about 1 per cent of children between the ages of 3 and 10 years had mental retardation. The CDC also found that mental retardation was more common in older children (6–10 years) than in younger children (3–5 years), in boys than in girls, and in black children than in white children. In 1993, the CDC used data from the Department of Education and the Social Security Administration to determine prevalence rates for mental retardation in children and adults in the US. This study showed that an estimated 1.5 million persons aged 6–64 years in the US had mental retardation and that the overall rate of mental retardation was 7.6 cases per 1,000 population. The mental retardation rate was higher for children (11.4 cases per 1,000) than for adults

(6.6 cases per 1,000). Lower prevalence rates in the US compared to the UK may be explained by the criteria used to admit subjects to the CDC study, such as participation in a public education programme and eligibility for financial assistance through the Social Security Administration.

The learning-disabled population is not a homogeneous group. Rather, this population consists of diverse syndromes and disorders, all of which have learning disability as one of their main clinical features. Chief amongst these syndromes and disorders are cerebral palsy (see section 2.3 in chapter 2), autism (see section 3.3), Down's syndrome and fragile X syndrome. Down's syndrome is the most common cause of learning disability. This syndrome affects about 1 in every 1,000 babies born – the National Association for Down Syndrome in the US reports the higher figure of 1 in every 800 live births. The Down's Syndrome Association states that there are an estimated 60,000 people with this syndrome living in the UK and that some 600 babies with this syndrome are born each year in the UK. It is expected that the number of people with Down's syndrome in the UK will rise from 26,045 in 1981 to 27,459 in 2021 (Prasher and Smith 2002). This increase is due in part to the increasing life expectancy of individuals affected by this syndrome; the average life expectancy of someone with Down's syndrome has increased from 18 years in 1961 to 57 years at the start of the twenty-first century (Prasher and Smith 2002). The incidence of Down's syndrome is known to rise with increasing maternal age. It is nevertheless the case that 80 per cent of children with Down's syndrome are born to women who are under 35 years of age (National Association for Down Syndrome).

Fragile X syndrome is the most common inherited form of learning disability, accounting for some 40 per cent of X-linked learning-disabled cases (CDC). The gene that is responsible for this syndrome – the fragile X mental retardation 1 (FMR1) gene on the X chromosome – can exist in a number of forms. The full mutation form of the gene causes clinical features of the syndrome in males. Such features are less common in full mutation females, presumably because of X-inactivation, and in cases where the premutation form of the gene occurs. (This form can occur in males and females.) Crawford et al. (2001) report that population-based studies suggest that the prevalence of the full mutation form ranges from 1 in 3,717 to 1 in 8,918 Caucasian males in the general population, while prevalence estimates for the premutation form range from 1 in 246 to 1 in 468 Caucasian females in the general population. Other syndromes associated with learning disability have much lower prevalence rates. For example, Prader-Willi syndrome[3] affects 1 in 12,000 to 15,000 individuals (Prader-Willi Syndrome Association, US), while Williams syndrome[4] occurs in 1 in 20,000 live births (Williams Syndrome Association).

Despite improvements in genetic screening and other diagnostic techniques, it remains the case that no cause can be found for learning disability in approximately 30 per cent of severe cases and in 50 per cent of mild cases (Sebastian 2002). Known aetiologies include genetic disorders, infections, trauma, metabolic disorders and toxic agents. Within genetic disorders, learning disability can be caused by an abnormal number of chromosomes (e.g. Down's syndrome[5]), by deletions of parts of chromosomes (e.g. the short arm of chromosome 5 in cri du chat syndrome[6]) or by sub-microscopic deletions (microdeletions) of DNA (e.g. Prader-Willi syndrome and Angelman's syndrome[7]). Some forms of learning disability are inherited. Inheritance can occur through the X chromosome, as in fragile X syndrome. Other disorders involve autosomal dominant inheritance (e.g. tuberous sclerosis[8]). Most of the metabolic disorders that cause learning disability have an autosomal recessive pattern of inheritance. The best known and most common of these disorders is phenylketonuria.[9]

Research into the genetic basis of many of the disorders that are associated with learning disability is still in its early stages. For example, the gene that causes fragile X syndrome (FMR1) was discovered as recently as 1991 and scientists are currently trying to understand the effects of a lack of usable fragile X mental retardation protein (FMRP) on the brain. Even more recently, in October 1999, scientists sponsored by the National Institute of Child Health and Human Development in the US announced that they had discovered that a change in the sequence of a single gene can cause Rett syndrome (a further disorder in which learning disability occurs). The gene in question produces a protein called methyl cytosine binding protein 2 (MECP2). Rett syndrome is generally classified as an autistic spectrum disorder or a pervasive developmental disorder. For this reason, we will examine it again in section 3.3 of this chapter.

Maternal infections can put an unborn baby at risk of mental retardation. Prior to the rubella vaccine being licensed for use in the US in 1969, congenital rubella was a significant cause of mental retardation. In the last rubella epidemic to occur in the US prior to the introduction of the vaccine,[10] there were some 20,000 congenital rubella syndrome cases. Mental retardation occurred in 1,800 of these cases. Deafness and blindness resulted in 11,600 and 3,580 cases, respectively. Rubella presents the greatest risk of damage to the foetus during the first trimester of pregnancy – up to 85 per cent of infants infected during this time will exhibit problems when followed after birth. When rubella infection occurs after the twentieth week of gestation, defects are rare (CDC, National Immunization Program).

Other maternal infections that can have an adverse effect on prenatal neurodevelopment are cytomegalovirus (CMV), toxoplasmosis and human immunodeficiency virus (HIV). CMV is the most common cause of congenital infection in the US, occurring in approximately 1 in 40,000 live-born infants per year (Reddy et al. 2004). The mother's CMV immune status is important in determining if placental infection occurs and if the foetus and newborn develop symptomatic disease – symptomatic CMV congenital disease is less likely to occur in women who have pre-existing immune responses to CMV than in CMV-naive individuals (Goodrich 2004). CMV is the leading cause of sensorineural hearing loss in young children (Reddy et al. 2004). CMV can also cause significant learning disability or mental retardation. Goodrich (2004) reports a study of 12 children with congenital CMV infection. Three of these children were of average intelligence, eight were moderately to severely retarded and one child was mildly retarded.

Toxoplasmosis is an infection caused by the protozoan parasite, *Toxoplasma gondii*. *Toxoplasma* infection can occur through ingesting contaminated food or through exposure to oocysts in cat faeces. Also, a mother can transmit *Toxoplasma* infection to her unborn child. Infection in the prenatal period can cause mental retardation, blindness and epilepsy. Toxoplasmosis is not a nationally reportable disease in the US, so it is difficult to establish the extent of congenital infection. However, three studies that examined *Toxoplasma* infection in pregnant women have led researchers to conclude that there are an estimated 400–4,000 cases of congenital toxoplasmosis each year in the US (Lopez et al. 2000). Another infection that has food-borne transmission, listeriosis, can result in foetal death, premature delivery or severe illness, including mental retardation, in the newborn. Pregnant women have accounted for some 16–90 per cent of patients in many *Listeria* outbreaks (Reddy et al. 2004).

Maternal HIV infection poses a serious health risk to the unborn baby and neonate. Transmission may occur during pregnancy (intrauterine infection), during labour and delivery, and in the postnatal period if an infected mother breast feeds. Up to 25 per cent of infants who are infected with HIV through mother to child transmission progress to serious disease or death by their first birthday (Department of Health 2004). In those children who survive the first year, there can be significant neurodevelopmental problems. Smith et al. (2000) found evidence that early (i.e. intrauterine) HIV-1 infection increases a child's risk for poor neurodevelopmental functioning within the first 30 months of life. These researchers found that early infected infants scored significantly lower than late infected infants by 24 months of age and beyond on both mental and motor measures.

Herpes simplex virus type 2 (HSV-2) accounts for 80–90 per cent of neonatal and almost all congenital infections (Patel 2005). The newborn who is exposed to genital HSV-2 during delivery is at significant risk of encephalitis and neurological impairment. Infected newborns develop symptoms in the first week of life and exhibit one of the following presentations at 10–17 days. The disease may be limited to the skin, mouth and eyes (category 1) or there may be primary central nervous system (CNS) involvement (category 2). In the most severe form – category 3 – there is disseminated disease that involves the CNS, lung, liver, skin and eyes. The prognosis is good for neonates with category 1 disease who receive appropriate drug therapy (an aciclovir dosage of 30mg/kg/d). Ninety eight per cent of infants will show normal development at the age of one year. However, where there is CNS involvement or disseminated disease, 75 per cent of infants die or have permanent neurological impairment (Patel 2005).

Learning disability is one of the sequelae of bacterial meningitis. The bacterial pathogens that are most often responsible for bacterial meningitis in the neonate are *Streptococcus agalactiae* (group B streptococci) and *Escherichia coli*. A newborn may develop meningitis through exposure to group B streptococci in the female genital tract during delivery. The meningococcus is the most common cause of bacterial meningitis in children and adults in the UK. Poor host defences in newborns, particularly in low birth weight babies, leads to bacterial meningitis being fatal in about one-third of neonates. This is higher than the overall fatality rate that occurs in bacterial meningitis.[11] In a study of outcomes of bacterial meningitis in children, Baraff et al. (1993) found that 83.6 per cent of sufferers have no detectable sequelae, 10.5 per cent have sensorineural hearing loss, 4.2 per cent have mental retardation, 3.5 per cent have spasticity and/or paresis and 4.2 per cent develop a seizure disorder.

A number of different substances can have teratogenic effects on the developing embryo. Chief amongst these toxic agents is ethanol (alcohol), which can cause foetal alcohol syndrome (FAS)[12] when consumed by women during pregnancy. The main characteristics of this syndrome are abnormal facial features (flat philtrum, short nose, short palpebral fissures, epicanthal folds), growth deficiencies (low birth weight, small stature) and CNS defects (mental retardation, amongst others). However, the phenotypic expression of this syndrome is highly variable and depends on the amount of alcohol consumed, the duration of exposure to alcohol, the mother's ability to metabolise alcohol before it reaches the placenta, and the stage of pregnancy at which alcohol exposure occurs. (Exposure in the first trimester causes structural anomalies, while exposure in the last trimester has adverse effects on brain development.) It is difficult to estimate prevalence rates for foetal alcohol syndrome as these can vary considerably depending on the location and population investigated. Niccols (1994) states that foetal alcohol syndrome affects between 1 and 3 infants per 1,000 live births. The prevalence is much higher – 23–29 cases per 1,000 births – among babies born to women who are identified as problem drinkers or alcohol abusers (Spiegler et al. 1984).

Lead exposure can have teratogenic effects on the developing foetus as well as serious consequences for a child's physical and cognitive development. In a recent meeting[13] of the Advisory Committee on Childhood Lead Poisoning in the US, Dr Howard Hu of the Harvard School of Public Health summarised the findings of several studies that examined the risks posed by the mobilisation of maternal bone lead stores to the developing foetus. In one study, children who were born to women who had survived lead poisoning were three times more likely to be learning disabled than their control counterparts. In October 1991, the CDC produced a statement entitled 'Preventing Lead Poisoning in Young Children'. In this statement, the CDC acknowledges that blood lead levels as low as 10μg/dL are associated with decreased intelligence and impaired neurobehavioural development. These effects are all the more serious when one considers the number of children who have blood lead levels in excess of 10μg/dL. In 1997, a UNEP-UNICEF report entitled 'Childhood Lead Poisoning: Information for Advocacy and Action' stated that 28 per cent of children between three and five years in the world's most developed countries and 78 per cent of children under two years have average blood lead levels exceeding 10μg/dL.

Events in the perinatal period can put the neonate at risk of brain damage and learning disability. Premature, low birth weight babies are more likely to develop intracranial haemorrhage and periventricular leukomalacia than full-term infants of normal birth weight. Prematurity and low birth weight are linked to multiple births and conditions such as pre-eclampsia. Haemolysis of foetal red blood cells and decreased excretion of bilirubin due to an immaturity of liver function may lead to hyperbilirubinaemia and possible brain damage (kernicterus). The baby's central nervous system may sustain damage during a breech or high forceps delivery. Complicated deliveries present a greater risk of asphyxia, although birth asphyxia is a less common cause of neonatal brain injury than was previously thought to be the case (National Institute of Neurological Disorders and Stroke).

Injury and disease in the postnatal period can also result in brain damage and cognitive impairment. A child may sustain a head injury which can have serious implications for language and cognitive development. Brookes et al. (1990) found that falls were the most common cause (57 per cent) of head injury of all severities in 2118 children who attended Scottish Accident and Emergency departments in 1985. Sharples et al. (1990) examined fatal paediatric head injuries between 1979 and 1986 in Newcastle-upon-Tyne in England and found that of the 255 children who died of their head injury, 195 (76 per cent) were involved in road traffic accidents. Head injuries may involve concussion or, in more serious cases, cerebral laceration and contusion, and subarachnoid, subdural and extradural haemorrhage. In a recent review of literature, Homer and Kleinman (1999) found that the prevalence of intracranial injury in children with mild head trauma varied from 0 to 7 per cent. This same review revealed that in the absence of significant intracranial haemorrhage, the long-term outcomes for children with minimal or mild head injury are generally very good, with only a small increase in risk for subtle deficits in particular cognitive skills. However, even children with mild head injury may be at risk of poor outcomes, with the risk increasing considerably in more severely injured children.[14]

The CNS in children can also be damaged by tumours that originate within it (e.g. posterior fossa tumours) or that infiltrate it, usually during the advanced stage of acute lymphocytic leukaemia (ALL). The United States Cancer Statistics indicate that, in 2001, ALL was the most common form of cancer in the age group 0–19 years and was the second most common cause of cancer death in this age group. (Excluding the figure for combined leukaemia deaths, tumours of the brain and nervous system were the most common cause of cancer death in the 0–19 age group.[15]) ALL is also referred to as acute lymphoblastic leukaemia, because the leukaemic cells which are produced in the bone marrow and which can cause leukaemic infiltration of the CNS, are called lymphoblasts. Posterior fossa tumours are also known as infratentorial brain tumours. This is because they grow below the tentorium, a fold of the dura mater which separates the cerebellum from the cerebrum and encloses a bony process or plate of the skull called the tentorium. The most common posterior fossa tumours are astrocytomas, medulloblastomas and ependymomas, in that order.[16]

Significant improvements in survival rates in these neoplastic conditions are largely attributable to the use of radiotherapy and chemotherapy.[17] However, as more children survive these conditions, it is becoming increasingly clear that radiotherapy and chemotherapy can induce structural and functional changes in the CNS that can lead to long-term negative sequelae. Cranial irradiation has been linked to grey matter damage (particularly basal ganglia calcification), white matter necrosis and calcification, generalised cerebral and cerebellar atrophy and cerebrovascular disease (Murdoch et al. 1999). These structural changes are accompanied by functional deficits in cognitive, motor, sensory and communication abilities. Intellectual impairment has been observed to occur in children who have undergone cranial irradiation, with reported incidences ranging from 25 to 60 per cent (Murdoch et al. 1999).[18] Many children who undergo radiotherapy for the treatment of cancer may also receive chemotherapy.[19] In cases where combined radiochemotherapy is used, it is difficult to say with certainty which structural brain changes and linguistic and cognitive impairments are related to the use of chemotherapy per se. For this reason, researchers have looked to cases of ALL to understand the long-term effects of chemotherapy on neurological and neuropsychological functioning. (As there is no disease mass (tumour) present in ALL, chemotherapy may be the only form of therapy used in the treatment of this leukaemia.) These cases have revealed three main groups of effect of CNS prophylaxis in ALL patients – structural changes in the brain[20] and other nervous system anomalies, endocrine disturbances and cognitive deficits. Reports of cognitive deficits are numerous and include accounts of intellectual impairment (reduced IQ), poor attention and concentration (which has resulted in parallels being drawn between the symptoms exhibited by ALL children and attention deficit disorder in children) and memory deficits (Murdoch et al. 1999).

3.2.2 Clinical Presentation

It can be seen from section 3.2.1 above that many diseases and injuries can cause cognitive impairment in children. The time of onset of these causal events has implications for the nature of any resulting cognitive impairment. For example, the 10-year-old child who develops ALL and who exhibits specific cognitive deficits subsequent to CNS prophylaxis will have a very different cognitive impairment from the 10-year-old Down's syndrome child who has never acquired age-appropriate cognitive abilities. Given that cognition is fundamental to the development of communication skills, it is to be expected that different patterns of cognitive impairment will give rise to different communication disorders. The heterogeneity of these disorders makes any general characterisation of childhood communication disorder in the presence of cognitive impairment all but impossible. Accordingly, we will describe communication disorders across a range of clinical populations in which cognition is impaired or fails to develop normally. The child who presents with impaired cognitive functioning and concomitant disorders of communication will also often experience feeding and swallowing difficulties that can extend well beyond the postnatal period. It is to an examination of these difficulties that we now turn.

3.2.2.1 Feeding

Feeding problems are common amongst infants, children and adults with cognitive impairment and learning disability. The severity and course of these problems are related to their underlying aetiology, and also to the child's level of linguistic and cognitive functioning – the child who can follow commands and learn new behaviours has a more favourable feeding prognosis than the child who has poor linguistic and cognitive skills. We describe below the feeding problems that occur in several of the disorders introduced in section 3.2.1. At relevant points, we discuss the implications of these problems for a feeding assessment. For a fuller discussion of this assessment, the reader is referred to sections 2.2.2.1 and 2.3.2.1 in chapter 2. The disorders that we will now revisit from section 3.2.1 include Down's syndrome, traumatic brain injury, brain tumours, HIV/AIDS, foetal alcohol syndrome and Rett's syndrome. Each of these disorders places the affected neonate, infant and child at significant risk of feeding and swallowing problems.

Genetic syndromes that cause learning disability or mental retardation can also cause neurogenic dysphagia. Feeding and swallowing problems occur commonly in Down's syndrome. Early feeding is compromised by hypotonia and cardiovascular anomalies. Oral structural defects include a large tongue (macroglossia) which can protrude, a small oral cavity and fissures of the tongue. However, the role of these structural anomalies in feeding is likely to be minimal. Arvedson and Brodsky (2002) state that 'the more common feeding difficulty with Down syndrome relates to oral sensorimotor coordination rather than a structural problem' (36). Drooling may also be evident and can be caused by a number of factors that require evaluation by an interdisciplinary team. Arvedson and Brodsky describe the case of a four-year-old boy with Down's syndrome who had a six-month history of chronic profuse drooling and facial chapping that resolved after tonsillectomy. Examination of this child by an otolaryngologist had revealed massively enlarged tonsils with an open month posture, anterior tongue placement and severe posterior pharyngeal cobblestoning. A further factor contributing to this child's drooling problem was extra-oesophageal reflux disease, for which treatment in the past year had involved dietary control, head elevation at night and a maximally dosed medical regimen. Interdisciplinary evaluation was also integral to the diagnosis of another case reported by Arvedson and Brodsky, that of a 12-year-old Down's syndrome boy who presented with progressive dysphagia. This boy had C1-C2 vertebral instability and the compression of his medulla by the floor of his skull had resulted in dysphagia and chronic aspiration.

Down's syndrome is only one of many syndromes that cause learning disability or mental retardation, and in which significant feeding and swallowing problems can occur. The nature and cause of these problems can vary considerably with each syndrome. In Prader-Willi syndrome, for example, dysphagia is often severe in the neonatal period and nasogastric tube feeding may be required. However, dysphagia is usually transient, and hyperphagia and obesity typically characterise the preschool and school-age years. A quite different course occurs in Rett syndrome, where feeding skills begin to regress after an initial period of normal development. Problems with chewing, swallowing, choking and emesis (vomiting) ensue, with female sufferers being restricted to pureed or soft foods in the later stages of the disease. Nor is every feeding and swallowing problem in genetic syndromes related to neurological impairment. Even in syndromes in which there is learning disability or mental retardation, structural anomalies such as cleft lip and palate and micrognathia, and gastric-oesophageal disorders may be equally significant causes of feeding problems. In this way, cleft palate may compromise feeding in velocardiofacial syndrome, while micrognathia and its subsequent contribution to airway obstruction is a significant factor in the feeding disorder of Dubowitz's syndrome.[21] Also, oesophageal dysmotility has been reported in connection with feeding problems in Opitz-Frias syndrome.[22]

In inflicted and accidental head trauma, the child may be comatose and dependent on a ventilator in the early postinjury period. During this acute phase, the child's nutritional needs are met through nonoral routes. A child may be fed by means of a gastrostomy tube when brain damage is severe. The speech and language therapist is a key member of the interdisciplinary team that assesses the child's readiness to resume oral feeding. Such an assessment must consider the child's level of alertness, sensory and motor function, respiratory status and risk of aspiration, amongst other factors. The therapist must also be aware of the effect of a tracheotomy tube on swallowing efficiency[23] and of tube safety issues – for example, that deflating a cuffed tracheotomy tube can cause secretions and food pooled above the cuff to enter the lower airway. If either oral secretions or refluxate are removed from the tube during suctioning, aspiration is occurring and oral feeding should not be resumed until instrumental investigation using endoscopy and fluoroscopy has taken place. In cases where oral feeding is considered to be unsafe, and provided that the child is medically stable, the therapist can begin a programme of oral-motor stimulation that has a non-nutritive focus (if aspiration is occurring). This will help prepare the child for the later introduction of oral feeding.

Head-injured children are also at risk of behavioural feeding problems. They may refuse food due to confusion and agitation, because of discomfort (related, for example, to reflux[24]) or because they lack sensations of hunger and thirst. During a long period of hospitalisation, a head-injured child may develop problems with feeding because of the distractions in his or her environment, time constraints on feeding and the presence of multiple caregivers. If physical problems have been eliminated as causes of the child's refusal to engage in oral feeding, then a diagnosis of conditioned dysphagia may be advanced to explain this behaviour. The therapist should be alert to behavioural feeding problems during assessment.

HIV-infected children are also at risk of feeding and swallowing problems. These problems can be caused by opportunistic infections and by CNS damage. Oral and oesophageal candidiasis are common sequelae of HIV infection in children. This fungal infection can cause dysphagia and lead to inadequate oral intake. In a study of 448 HIV-infected children followed between 1987 and 1995 for a history of oesophageal candidiasis, Chiou et al. (2000) found 51 episodes of oesophageal candidiasis in 36 patients (a frequency of 8.0 per cent). Oropharyngeal candidiasis was the most common clinical presentation of oesophageal candidiasis (94 per cent of cases). Other feeding and nutritional problems associated with this infection included odynophagia (80 per cent), retrosternal pain (57 per cent), nausea/vomiting (24 per cent), drooling (12 per cent), dehydration (12 per cent), hoarseness (6 per cent) and upper gastrointestinal bleeding (6 per cent). *Candida albicans* was the causative organism in 36 of these 51 episodes.

The CNS in children with HIV is also susceptible to opportunistic infections. Viral infections can be caused by herpes simplex virus, varicella zoster virus and by cytomegalovirus. However, CNS infections are rare in children compared to adults. The most common CNS manifestation of HIV infection in children is encephalopathy, with between 50 and 90 per cent of children having clinical or radiological evidence of HIV encephalopathy at some stage (Jeanes and Owens 2002). Two main patterns of HIV encephalopathy are found in children.[25] In static encephalopathy, there is a nonprogressive developmental delay. Progressive encephalopathy is associated with microcephaly, pyramidal tract signs and spasticity.[26] Feeding and swallowing problems are sequelae of neurological impairment in HIV encephalopathy. Davis-McFarland describes the case of an HIV-infected boy called Andy[27] who was fitted with a gastronomy tube for enteral feedings and medication intake at 5 months. At 15 months, Andy underwent magnetic resonance imaging (MRI), which revealed bilateral enlargement of the sulci and brain atrophy[28] (Zuniga 1999).

Children with brain tumours can develop feeding and swallowing problems. Where there is cranial nerve involvement, children can experience oral sensorimotor deficits and pharyngeal phase swallowing problems that place them at risk of aspiration (Arvedson and Brodsky 2002). Cornwell et al. (2003b) found problems in the oral preparatory, oral and pharyngeal phases of swallowing in a 7.5-year-old child AC, who had been treated for a recurrent posterior fossa tumour. Problems revealed by a videofluoroscopic evaluation of swallowing in AC included a pattern of tongue extension-retraction (oral preparatory phase), premature spillage of the bolus to the level of the valleculae and pyriform sinus (oral phase) and laryngeal penetration with epiglottic undercoating (pharyngeal phase). Many chemotherapy drugs that are used to treat brain tumours – for example, CCNU (Lomustine) – can cause nausea and emesis (vomiting), which adversely affect appetite.

Feeding problems in foetal alcohol syndrome (FAS) can be caused by cleft lip and palate, micrognathia and associated airway obstruction and by hypertonia. Infants with FAS display limited sucking patterns. They are irritable and distractible during feeding and may also fatigue easily. In some children with FAS, nonoral feeding supplements may have to be extended beyond 12 months (Arvedson and Brodsky 2002). Infants with FAS may be at risk of further damage in the postnatal period if mothers, who are lactating and breast feeding, continue to consume alcohol. It has been demonstrated, for example, that alcohol in breast milk – estimated to be less than 2 per cent of the maternal dose[29] – can alter the odour of milk (Mennella and Beauchamp 1991) and cause infants to consume significantly less milk (Mennella and Beauchamp 1993).

3.2.2.2 Speech

Speech disorders are common in the learning-disabled population. As with feeding anomalies, these disorders vary with the syndrome or other medical aetiology that has caused the child's learning disability. A speech disorder may be caused by a structural defect of one or more articulators (e.g. cleft lip and palate, macroglossia and micrognathia). The same neurological insult that caused the child's learning disability may also cause a neurogenic speech disorder. Quite often, the speech disorder has both structural and neurological components. It is the task of any speech evaluation to determine the respective contribution of structural and neurological factors to the child's speech disorder. Such an evaluation must also determine the contribution of cognitive impairment and hearing loss to the child's speech impairment. In order to make an assessment of these factors, the therapist must draw upon information from a range of disciplines during a speech evaluation (e.g. otolaryngology, audiology, psychology). For a full discussion of speech evaluation in children, the reader is referred to sections 2.2.2.2 and 2.3.2.2 in chapter 2. In this section, we describe the speech disorders that occur in learning-disabled individuals. These disorders include neurogenic speech impairments such as dysarthria, as well as structural articulation deficits. We discuss the factors that predispose learning-disabled children to speech disorders, with particular emphasis on the role of cognitive impairment in the development of these disorders.

Dysarthria is a common neurogenic speech disorder in learning-disabled children. Many of the same illnesses and injuries that are known to cause cognitive impairment in children are also responsible for this speech disorder. In a retrospective study of motor speech disorders at the Glenrose Rehabilitation Hospital, Hodge and Wellman (1999) found that, of the children diagnosed with dysarthria, 50 per cent had some type of cerebral palsy, 23 per cent had some other type of congenital condition, 21 per cent had a later-onset condition (e.g. traumatic brain injury), 3 per cent had a neuromuscular disorder (e.g. muscular dystrophy) and 3 per cent did not have a neurological diagnosis in their medical records. In congenital conditions such as cerebral palsy, the speech disorder will typically be one of developmental dysarthria (see section 2.3.2.2 in chapter 2). A somewhat different clinical picture attends acquired childhood dysarthria in later-onset conditions such as traumatic brain injury or where treatment of a posterior fossa tumour has occurred. In this section, we examine the features of dysarthria in several congenital and late-onset conditions. Later, we discuss other speech disorders (e.g. dyspraxia) that occur in these conditions.

Few studies of Down's syndrome have examined the neurogenic basis of speech problems in the clinical population. A notable exception in this regard is a study of three young Down's syndrome adults by Hamilton (1993). Hamilton used electropalatography to identify dysarthric speech features in these subjects. These features included increased tongue-palate contact patterns, the omission of /k,g/ or their production as velar fricatives (undershoot), overshoot for fricatives resulting in complete closure, the absence of any adequate auditory or articulatory difference between /s/ and /ʃ/, the absence of coarticulatory patterns in consonantal clusters and the failure to use the tongue tip for the articulation of the alveolar sounds /t,d,n/. Hamilton relates several of these features – increased tongue-palate contact patterns, undershoot, overshoot and the absence of coarticulatory patterns in consonantal clusters – to dysarthric speech features identified in children and adults by Hardcastle et al. (1985, 1987, 1989). The subjects' hypotonic tongues made it difficult for them to achieve coarticulation in consonant clusters, as they were unable to move the tip/blade (front) of the tongue and the body (back) of the tongue to different places on the palate at the same time. Hamilton also attributes the failure of the tongue tip to be used during articulation to the hypotonic state of the subjects' tongues.

Dysarthric speech errors have also been described in a range of other syndromes. In a study of 13 subjects with Prader-Willi syndrome (PWS), aged from 7;0 to 29;5 years, Defloor et al. (2002) found phonetic difficulties that are consistent with hypotonia in PWS individuals. The subjects exhibited partial devoicing of voiced obstruents, derhotacising of /r/ and the loss of the plosive or fricative character in voiceless plosives and fricatives. Defloor et al. remark that similar errors are present in individuals who present with flaccid dysarthria following a neurological insult. Solot et al. (2000) describe dysarthric speech errors in two children with the 22q11.2 microdeletion syndrome. These children exhibited reduced respiratory support, reduced rate and volume, prosodic abnormalities and imprecise articulation with poor ability to duplicate new speech targets. Solot et al. also report dysarthria in a sample of 31 children with this syndrome who were more than five years of age.

Dysarthria is frequently acknowledged to be an acute sequela of treatment for cerebellar tumours in children. However, this clinical finding has only rarely been the focus of research, with the result that there is still little known about the features and course of later-onset dysarthria in children. In a study of 11 children who underwent treatment for a cerebellar tumour,[30] Cornwell et al. (2003a) address a range of questions relating to the nature and severity of this type of dysarthria. Dysarthria in these subjects was judged to be mild and persistent – subjects were examined six months after the completion of treatment. Although the severity of dysarthria was generally mild, more severe impairments were evident in some cases. For some children, perceptual speech analysis revealed moderate impairment of three speech dimensions: precision of consonant production, ability to vary pitch and audible inspirations. Individual subjects displayed moderate and moderate-severe deficits of tongue function on the Frenchay Dysarthria Assessment (Enderby 1983). These moderate and severe impairments led to a classification of moderate dysarthria in three children. Twenty-one of the 33 speech dimensions examined were present in three children at least. However, only three features – a hoarse vocal quality, imprecision of consonants and decreased pitch variation – occurred with a frequency greater than 50 per cent. Thus, it was not possible to establish a definitive set of deviant speech features that could be taken to characterise the dysarthria in these children.

Cornwell et al.'s study is significant in at least two further aspects. The late onset of the dysarthria of the subjects in this study – the mean age of these children was 10.3 years – raises interesting questions about the contribution of developmental and acquired components to the speech disorder. Cornwell et al. failed to find a significant developmental component in the dysarthria of their child subjects. In fact, only one of the 11 subjects studied exhibited developmental speech characteristics. This study also allows us to examine the pathophysiology of dysarthria in children treated for cerebellar tumour. Hypotonia and ataxia are both present in adults with cerebellar damage and have been linked to dysarthric speech features. These features include deviant speech characteristics in the areas of articulation, prosody and phonation, such as impaired stress patterns (excess and equal stress) and imprecise consonant production. While hypotonia and ataxia were present as generalised motor signs in many of Cornwell et al.'s subjects, and their deviant speech features were prosodic, articulatory and phonatory in nature (typical of ataxic dysarthria in adults), these child subjects lacked the most distinctive feature of ataxic dysarthria in adults, excess and equal stress. Cornwell et al. attribute the absence of this stress pattern to a number of differences between their child subjects and adults with ataxic dysarthria.[31] They conclude that

> the clustering of deviant speech dimensions in the prosodic, articulatory and phonatory aspects of speech production, despite the absence of the most definitive aspect of the ataxic dysarthria in adults, excess and equal stress, could be interpreted to indicate that the dysarthria [of child subjects treated for cerebellar tumour] could be classified as ataxic. (Cornwell et al. 2003a:611)[32]

Late-onset dysarthria can also be a long-term sequela of traumatic brain injury (TBI) in children. Theodoros et al. (1998) used physiological and perceptual techniques to obtain a comprehensive profile of the dysarthria of a 14-year-old boy who had sustained a severe TBI 12 months before the study. For 2.5 months post-injury, this boy was mute and used hand gestures and pictures to communicate. By five months postinjury, he used a word/phrase/letter communication display and a Canon communicator as his primary means of communication. He was able to produce a few single-word approximations. At seven months postinjury, he presented with a moderate dysarthria. The physiological techniques used to assess this boy's speech included clinical spirometry and kinematic assessment of chest wall movements (respiratory function), electroglottography (laryngeal function), a modified version of the nasal accelerometric technique proposed by Horii (1980) (velophayngeal function) and lip and tongue pressure transducers (articulatory function). The boy's speech was assessed perceptually using the Frenchay Dysarthria Assessment (Enderby 1983), a perceptual analysis of a speech sample and the Assessment of Intelligibility of Dysarthric Speech (Yorkston and Beukelman 1981). Overall, these assessments revealed that tongue function was severely reduced and that lip, velopharyngeal and laryngeal function was moderately impaired. There was a mild impairment in respiratory function. The boy's speech was severely impaired in relation to rate, pitch variation and consonant precision. (Reduced pitch variability and consonant imprecision occurred with a frequency greater than 50 per cent in the children with cerebellar tumours in Cornwell et al.'s (2003a) study.)

A slower speaking rate was also observed by Campbell and Dollaghan (1995) in a study of nine children with traumatic brain injury. Five of these nine children were judged by naive listeners to have a slower speaking rate than control subjects. Of the five TBI subjects with slower speaking rates, three had average syllable durations more than 2 standard deviations (SD) above the average duration for the control group. These were the only subjects diagnosed with dysarthria. Four of the five TBI subjects with slower speaking rates also had percentages of pause time more than 2SD above the average for the control group. Where longer average syllable durations were related to the speech motoric deficits of the TBI subjects, increased percentages of pause time were judged by Campbell and Dollaghan (1995) to reflect cognitive-linguistic deficits in these subjects. These authors conclude that articulatory speed and linguistic processing speed may contribute independently to slowed speaking rates more than one year after traumatic brain injury.

Learning-disabled children and adults may also exhibit dyspraxic-type speech errors. Dyspraxia is a disorder of motor programming during speech production. As such, it disrupts voluntary movement sequences for speech in the absence of paralysis or paresis of the speech musculature (see section 4.2 in chapter 4 for a fuller discussion of dyspraxia). In her study of three young Down's syndrome adults, Hamilton (1993) found several speech errors which, she claimed, are typical of dyspraxia. Hamilton's subjects displayed long closure durations and, in one subject at least, slow approach and release phases for closures. Two of her subjects exhibited abnormally long transitions between different elements in consonant clusters. All three subjects experienced difficulty in rapidly repeating polysyllabic consonant-vowel sequences during diadochokinetic (DDK) tests. The production of these sequences was erratic and arrhythmic. Asymmetry and variability were features of fricative articulation, particularly during /s/ and /ʃ/ production, in two of Hamilton's subjects. Becker et al. (1990) observed mild verbal apraxia in three of their eight subjects with FAS. Dyspraxic speech errors demand a quite different therapeutic approach from that used to treat other articulation problems (see section 4.2.4 in chapter 4). The speech and language therapist must therefore be alert to the possibility of a dyspraxic component in the speech production problems of learning-disabled individuals during speech evaluation.

Speech problems in learning-disabled individuals may result from structural defects of the peripheral speech mechanism. These defects are varied and include clefts of the lip and palate, problems with dentition, abnormal jaw relationships, a small buccal cavity, macroglossia, pharyngeal disproportion, hypertrophy of the tonsils and adenoids and laryngeal abnormalities. A number of these structural anomalies occur in Down's syndrome (DS) and are linked to articulation, resonance and phonation problems in this clinical population. DS individuals have a small buccal cavity and a large muscular tongue,[33] which influence the production of lingual consonants (Stoel-Gammon 2001). When accompanied by tongue protrusion, macroglossia may lead to the use of the tongue blade, as opposed to the tip, during alveolar articulation. Enlarged adenoids can cause resonance problems and hyponasal speech. Enlargement of the lingual tonsil in DS individuals can result in narrowing of the lower pharynx and the superior laryngeal aperture (Rondal and Edwards 1997). This can alter the resonatory capacity of the pharynx. The bridge of the nose, bones of the midface and maxilla are relatively small in Down's syndrome (Pilcher 1998). This underdevelopment or hypoplasia of the midfacial region can cause a prognathic Class III occlusal relationship, which may in turn cause articulation errors. Dental abnormalities are common in Down's syndrome and include delayed eruption (possibly by as long as 2–3 years), missing teeth in both the primary and permanent dentitions, microdontia and malformed teeth (Pilcher 1998). Dental anomalies can affect articulation. Dentition problems may also result in defective dental occlusion and alter the size of the oral cavity, which may impair sound resonance (Rondal and Edwards 1997). Further resonance problems may be caused by a short or cleft palate, which can also lead to the use of compensatory substitutions (Shprintzen 2000). Phonatory disturbances occur in Down's syndrome. Voice quality deviations include breathiness, hoarseness and harshness (Rondal and Edwards 1997). Pryce (1994) relates the phonation problems of Down's syndrome individuals less to any structural anomalies of the larynx than to flaccidity of the extrinsic laryngeal muscles and pharyngeal resonator, and to the drying effect of an open mouth posture on the laryngeal mechanism.[34]

Speech production problems are present in many other congenital syndromes with associated learning disability or mental retardation and are related to structural and functional defects of the peripheral speech mechanism. Hyponasal/denasal resonance was identified in all nine children with Apert's syndrome studied by Shipster et al. (2002). This resonance abnormality is consistent with certain structural anomalies present in this syndrome, viz. midface hypoplasia, reduced pharyngeal height, width and depth, choanal atresia or stenosis and a long, thick soft palate. Structural abnormalities of the palate are extremely common in the 22q11.2 microdeletion syndrome and include cleft palate, submucous cleft palate (classical or occult), congenitally absent musculus uvulae and palatopharyngeal disproportion (Solot et al. 2000). Reduced mobility of the palate and/or lateral pharyngeal walls may result in velopharyngeal incompetence. These palatal anomalies have been linked to articulation, resonance and voice problems in 22q11.2 microdeletion syndrome. In a study of 31 children with this syndrome who were more than five years of age, Solot et al. (2000) found that 77 per cent had articulation disorders. The most common articulation errors were compensatory articulations secondary to palatal abnormalities. These errors included glottal stops, nasal substitutions, pharyngeal fricatives, linguapalatal sibilants, reduced pressure on consonant sounds, or a combination of these articulations. Solot et al. found that all children identified with palatal defects were also hypernasal. Hypernasality was mild in 12 of the 40 children with palatal abnormalities who were studied by Solot et al. (2000). A further 12 children (30 per cent) exhibited moderate hypernasality on perceptual rating scales, while 16 children (40 per cent) displayed severe hypernasality. Phonatory disturbances are often seen in this clinical population. Hoarseness and reduced vocal volume are particularly evident and are related to velopharyngeal incompetence.[35] Similar articulation and resonance findings were reported by Persson et al. (2003) in a study of 65 subjects with this syndrome who were aged between 3 and 33 years of age (median age 9 years and 4 months).[36]

Speech disorders in learning-disabled children and adults may be related to problems of phonological development. Kumin et al. (1994) found that the order of phoneme emergence in 60 children with Down's syndrome was unlike that of typically developing children. Moreover, there was considerable age variation amongst the DS subjects in the emergence of specific phonemes. For example, the range of ages for the emergence of the /p/ phoneme was from one year to eight years of age. Also, even when norms for the emergence of certain phonemes were missed by the DS subjects, the DS children nevertheless went on to acquire these phonemes – one DS child was eight years old before he began to produce /b/, a sound typically developed by age three. Phonological processes have been observed to persist in the speech of children and adults with learning disability or mental retardation. In a study of a 10-year-old girl with Wolf-Hirschhorn syndrome,[37] Van Borsel et al. (2004) report the frequencies of 13 phonological processes. Several syllable structure processes were evident in this girl's speech, the most frequent of which were cluster reduction and final consonant deletion. Fronting and gliding were the most frequent substitution processes, while assimilation also occurred with some frequency. All

10 children with Apert's syndrome studied by Shipster et al. (2002) had varying degrees of delayed phonological development. Immature phonological processes exhibited by these subjects included stopping of fricatives and affricates, final consonant deletion, voicing of voiceless consonants, and fronting of velar and palato-alveolar sounds. In a study of eight children with FAS, Becker et al. (1990) found a greater incidence of assimilatory or harmony processes in FAS subjects during single word production than was observed in control subjects. Moreover, a five-year-old boy with FAS displayed an idiosyncratic phonological pattern, the use of a voiced velar stop /g/ in substitution for /tʃ/ and /s/ in the initial position of words. Finally, Defloor et al. (2002) report that, while phonetic problems (namely, distortions) were more evident with increasing age in 13 individuals with Prader-Willi syndrome, errors reflecting a phonological problem (phonotactic errors, phonological process errors, omissions and substitutions) decreased with increasing age.

Problems with speech fluency are also more common in mentally retarded or learning-disabled individuals. Wingate (2002) reports that the average prevalence of stuttering in the mentally retarded population is about 8 per cent. (In the population in general, the prevalence figure most often cited is 1 per cent.) This figure masks the fact that there is considerable variation in the prevalence of fluency problems, both between studies and between the different disorders that constitute the learning-disabled population. In a study of 20 children with FAS, Church et al. (1997) found that two subjects (10 per cent) displayed significant speech dysfluency that included severe stuttering and word cluttering/dysrhythmia. Solot et al. (2000) observed dysfluent speech in two (6.4 per cent) of their 31 school-age children with the 22q11.2 microdeletion syndrome. Van Borsel et al. (1999) report the presence of stuttering in 4 (3.1 per cent) of their 128 subjects with Turner syndrome.[38] We will return to this issue in chapter 6, when we examine disorders of fluency.

It is routinely acknowledged in the clinical communication literature that cognitive impairment can result in significant problems of speech acquisition in children. However, few theorists have attempted to describe the nature of the relationship between cognition and speech development in any detail.[39] Fewer theorists still have attempted to relate speech disorders in learning-disabled individuals to cognitive development in these subjects. Most studies have merely noted the presence and severity of cognitive impairment in children with speech disorders. An example is a retrospective study by Hodge and Wellman (1999) of dysarthric children at the Glenrose Rehabilitation Hospital. Amongst the dysarthric children studied by Hodge and Wellman, 22 per cent fell below the average range of cognitive ability, 11 per cent had low-average cognitive ability and 46 per cent had borderline cognitive ability. A further 8 per cent were mentally retarded and 13 per cent had no record of cognitive abilities.

Studies that have investigated the relationship between cognitive and speech development demonstrate that impaired cognitive functioning can have a significant deleterious effect on prelinguistic vocal development and speech acquisition. Sohner and Mitchell (1991) examined the early babbling patterns of a female subject with cri du chat syndrome through the ages of 8–26 months.[40] Babbling development was greatly slowed and coincident with sensorimotor cognitive levels. Multisyllable (reduplicated) babbling did not occur until 13 months in this subject, when in normal infants this behaviour typically occurs between 9 and 11 months (Sohner and Mitchell 1991). At 25 months, the subject displayed behaviours that were typical of the late Sensorimotor Stage III to Early Stage IV (4–8 and 8–12 months, respectively) on the Uzgiris-Hunt Scales of Infant Psychological Development (Uzgiris and Hunt 1975). At the same time, the subject's babbling behaviour was typical of normal vocal development during the 4–6-month age range. No meaningful words were observed or reported between the ages of 8 and 26 months in this child.

Clearly, the cognitively impaired child in Sohner and Mitchell's study experienced considerable delays in prelinguistic vocal development. However, this study falls short of demonstrating a correlation between cognitive impairment and delays in babbling and other aspects of vocal development. Moreover, Sohner and Mitchell's subject failed to produce speech by 26 months of age. Hence, this subject cannot be used to examine the impact of cognitive impairment on speech development in the learning-disabled child who acquires speech. Defloor et al.'s (2002) study of articulation in Prader-Willi syndrome (PWS) overcomes both these limitations of Sohner and Mitchell's investigation. Thirteen PWS subjects (chronological age 7;0 to 29;5 years) underwent a comprehensive speech evaluation that included a phonetic inventory analysis, a phonotactic analysis, an assessment of error rate, an analysis of sounds affected, an error analysis in terms of the traditional categories of omission, substitution and distortion, an analysis of error patterns and a phonological process analysis. The subjects had a total IQ from 38 to 83. Defloor et al. found a significant inverse correlation between overall error rate on the one hand and total IQ on the other hand. Also, the IQ level of the PWS subjects accounted for the considerable variation that was found in overall error rates. (These ranged from 4.24 to 30.65 per cent.) Variation was particularly evident in phonotactic errors (0.00–31.11 per cent) and phonological process use and frequency. (Frequency for cluster reduction ranged from 1.39 to 42.42 per cent.)

3.2.2.3 Hearing

Hearing disorders are common in the learning-disabled population. These disorders include conductive and sensorineural hearing losses as well as central auditory processing deficits. In a study of 22 subjects with FAS, Church et al.

(1997)[41] found 17 cases (77 per cent) of conductive hearing loss due to recurrent serous otitis media and 6 cases (27 per cent) of mild sensorineural hearing loss[42] which ranged from a low of 15–20 dB in one child to a high of 15–30 dB in two children. Of 12 subjects who were old enough to be evaluated for central auditory processing ability, all produced performances on the Word Recognition with Ipsilateral Noise test and the Competing Sentence Test that were poor enough to be classified as abnormal. Becker et al. (1990) found a positive history of recurrent otitis media in 3 of their 8 children with FAS. One of these 3 children failed pure tone conduction screening that was administered at 25dBHL across the octave frequencies of 250–4000Hz. The 10-year-old girl with Wolf-Hirschhorn syndrome studied by Van Borsel et al. (2004) had a history of otologic disease and hearing loss. At 4;10 years, this child was diagnosed with bilateral secretory otitis media. At 8;9 years, pure tone audiometry revealed a bilateral conductive hearing loss of 30dBHL on average, which was somewhat more severe in the low frequencies. Shipster et al. (2002) found hearing problems in all 10 of their children with Apert's syndrome. Nine of these children had a history of fluctuating mild to moderate conductive hearing loss. This was related to persistent otitis media with effusion (OME) or ossicular chain fixation combined with OME in four cases. A mixed severe loss that was predominantly sensorineural in nature was present in the tenth child.

It can be seen from the brief survey of hearing impairment above that conductive hearing loss (CHL) is particularly common in those syndromes in which there are significant craniofacial anomalies (that is, FAS and Apert's syndrome). Moreover, CHL is typically associated with a history of otitis media with effusion in individuals with these syndromes. Solot et al. (2000) found that CHL and otitis media were similarly prevalent in their subjects with the 22q11.2 microdeletion syndrome (another syndrome in which there are significant craniofacial anomalies). Of 47 children who received audiometric evaluations, 19 children (39 per cent) exhibited hearing loss in one or both ears, 18 of which had conductive hearing loss averaging 25–35 dBHL. Middle ear pathology was observed in 16 of the 19 subjects with hearing loss and included tympanometry-confirmed serous otitis media, retraction of the tympanic membrane or perforation of the tympanic membrane. The high prevalence of otitis proneness and CHL in craniofacial syndromes is explained by Eustachian tube dysfunction in these syndromes. Tube tortuosity and stenosis or deficiencies in the muscles (the tensor veli palatini) surrounding the proximal opening of the Eustachian tube result in poor aeration and drainage of the middle ear cavity and lead to an increased risk of middle ear disease. The association between palatal muscle anomalies and otitis media/CHL is particularly well established. Only four of Solot et al.'s 19 subjects with hearing loss were found to have normal palatal function and three of these subjects had hearing problems that were presumed to be the result of ossicular abnormalities (as opposed to otitis media).

Learning-disabled individuals often present with more than one type of hearing disorder. This is very clearly demonstrated in the case of FAS, where affected individuals can have conductive and sensorineural losses, central auditory processing problems and a developmental delay in the maturation of the auditory system. CHL in FAS subjects and their otitis proneness[43] is related to Eustachian tube dysfunction and immunodeficiency in these subjects[44] (Church et al. 1997; Church and Kaltenbach 1997). Animal models of FAS are helping to clarify the aetiological mechanism that underlies sensorineural hearing loss in FAS subjects. These models indicate that alcohol has embryotoxic effects on the embryological precursors (otic placode and neural crest cells) of certain inner ear structures (viz. cochlear hair cells and the auditory nerve). Animal and human FAS studies provide preliminary evidence that pre-natal alcohol exposure can damage key anatomical structures in the central auditory system, including the cochlear nucleus, inferior colliculus, medial geniculate body, cortex and corpus callosum. Abnormal auditory brainstem responses in humans and animals prenatally exposed to alcohol indicate the presence of developmental delays in auditory maturation.[45] Clearly, structural, functional, immunological and neurological anomalies can cause hearing impairment in learning-disabled subjects. When more than one of these anomalies occurs – as in FAS – clinicians should be aware that several types of hearing disorder may be present.

It has long been recognised that hearing impairment and otitis media can have an adverse effect on speech and language development in children. Petinou et al. (1999) examined the effects of OME on early speech production in two groups of subjects. One group contained infants who had an otitis media history during the first year of life, while the other group consisted of infants who were otitis media-negative. Phonetic transcriptions of recorded babbling samples at 10, 12 and 14 months of age revealed that otitis media- negative infants produced more alveolar stops and nasals than their positive counter-parts. Within the otitis media-positive group, children with better hearing thresholds showed more diversity in their phonetic inventories than children with poorer thresholds. Shriberg et al. (2003b) found that children with positive OME histories had significantly lower intelligibility scores than children with negative OME histories. Friel-Patti and Finitzo (1990) studied language development in children with early experience of OME. The hearing of these children was significantly related to scores on the Sequenced Inventory of Communication Development Scale, beginning with receptive language at 12 months of age. At 18 and 24 months, both receptive and expressive language were significantly related to average hearing loss from 6 to 18 months.

These deleterious effects of hearing loss on early speech and language development can also be expected to operate in learning-disabled children. Indeed, it is likely that these effects may be somewhat more pronounced in individuals with impaired cognitive functioning. The detrimental impact of hearing impairment on the speech and language of learning-disabled individuals is amply demonstrated by Church et al. (1997) in their study of 22 subjects with FAS. Language disorder was present in 15 (88 per cent) of 17 subjects with peripheral hearing disorder (conductive and/or sensorineural hearing loss). All 12 FAS subjects with central hearing disorder also had language disorder. Hearing impairment had an even more deleterious effect on speech in these subjects. Fifteen subjects with peripheral hearing disorder underwent speech assessment. All 15 subjects displayed evidence of speech pathology. Of 12 subjects with central hearing disorder, 11 (92 per cent) were also found to have speech pathology.[46] Persson et al. (2003) found a significant relationship between the hearing variable pure-tone average and speech intelligibility in their study of subjects with the 22q11.2 microdeletion syndrome. In a study of 48 children and adolescents with Down's syndrome, Chapman et al. (2000) found that hearing status contributed 8 per cent of the variance in intelligibility in their subjects. This level of variance was borderline significant.

Several studies report a significant relationship between hearing loss and expressive and receptive language in learning-disabled subjects. In the same study of Down's syndrome children and adults discussed above, Chapman et al. (2000) found that hearing status contributed 8 per cent of variance in lexical performance (number of different words produced). This level of variance indicated a trend of significance. Hearing status also accounted for 7 per cent of the variance in the syntax measure (mean length of utterance) in these DS subjects. Laws (2004) found that hearing thresholds significantly correlated with expressive language in DS subjects with impaired hearing (thresholds above 40dB). Other studies suggest that hearing level does not contribute significantly to receptive and expressive language in DS subjects. Chapman et al. (2002) found that hearing did not contribute significantly to the best-fitting model of longitudinal change in syntax comprehension and production in 31 Down's syndrome subjects aged between 5 and 20 years at the start of the study. Each of these 31 subjects had passed hearing screening at 45 dBHL.

3.2.2.4 Language

Among its most serious consequences for communication, learning disability has a significant deleterious effect on a child's ability to acquire language. Language learning is a complex process that draws upon a diverse array of cognitive skills. For language learning to take place, children must be able to attend to speech stimuli. An input speech signal must be stored in auditory short-term memory before further linguistic processing can take place. Attention and memory are two vital cognitive resources for language learning and are impaired to a greater or lesser extent in most children and adults with learning disability.[47] The effect of memory on language acquisition is demonstrated by Chapman et al. (2002), who investigated longitudinal change in syntax comprehension and production skill in 31 individuals with Down's syndrome. Chapman et al. found that auditory short-term memory, along with age at the start of the study and visual short-term memory, best predicted syntax comprehension in the DS subjects over the six-year period of the study. In a study of 30 children and adolescents with Down's syndrome, Laws (2004) confirmed the much-reported presence of a specific deficit in verbal short-term memory (phonological memory) in DS subjects. Laws also found that nonword repetition contributed about 50 per cent of the variance in MLU and sentence recall scores. This level of variance constituted a significant correlation between phonological memory and expressive language abilities in these Down's syndrome subjects.

The findings of Chapman et al. (2002) and Laws (2004) confirm a close association between auditory or verbal short-term memory on the one hand and language performance on the other hand. However, not all language performance in learning-disabled subjects correlates with memory and other measures of cognitive function. Sometimes, expressive and/or receptive language is not associated with an individual's level of cognitive ability. Shipster et al. (2002) found that the scores of children with Apert's syndrome on two measures of cognitive ability – a general conceptual ability (GCA) measure and a nonverbal composite (NVC) score – were significantly higher than the scores of these children on a combined expressive language measure. In 5 of the 8 children for whom scores were available, the gap between expressive language and the nonverbal composite score surpassed 15 standard points (or more than 1SD). GCA and NVC scores correlated with receptive language scores in these Apert's syndrome subjects. Amongst their cohort of children with the 22q11.2 microdeletion syndrome, Solot et al. (2000) report expressive language delays that went beyond the cognitive levels of these children. Speech was absent in 20 of 29 preschool children in whom there was exact reporting of developmental milestones or observation of language skills. A further two children had just a few words or signs at two years of age. In some children, persistence of limited expressive language at 2.5–3 years of age was noted. At 9;8 years, the language skills of the subject with Wolf-Hirschhorn syndrome studied by Van Borsel et al. (2004) were commensurate with those of a 3- to 4-year-old child. This language performance was unexpected given the typically poor cognitive profile of subjects with this syndrome.[48]

Clearly, not all language performance in learning-disabled subjects can be directly related to the cognitive abilities of these subjects. Indeed, there are cases in which language performance surpasses an individual's cognitive level to such an extent that language is described as exceptional, even though it is still not comparable to the language performances of normal functioning subjects.

Such 'exceptional language', it has been argued, can be found in individuals with Williams syndrome (WS). Amongst the wider phenotype of this syndrome,[49] affected individuals have typically been described as having 'relatively spared language capacities alongside seriously impaired visuo–spatial cognition, number, planning, and problem solving' (Grant et al. 1996:615). Not all language components are equally intact in Williams syndrome, however. It has generally been claimed that intact morphosyntax exists alongside impairments of lexical semantics in WS individuals. Such impairments are particularly evident in WS infants.[50] Paterson (2001) found receptive vocabulary delays in 15 WS infants aged from 24 to 36 months. Using a visual preference paradigm, Paterson observed that WS infants looked longer at stimuli that matched a verbal label than chronological age controls. The performance of these infants was equivalent to mental age controls. The WS infants also had smaller receptive vocabularies than controls, as measured on a standardised parental assessment of vocabulary (MacArthur Communicative Development Inventory, Fenson et al. 1993).[51]

However, there is a growing body of evidence which indicates that syntax may also be impaired in WS subjects. Karmiloff-Smith et al. (1998) used a word monitoring task (on-line) and a sentence–picture matching task (off-line) to investigate syntax in eight WS subjects (mean chronological age 20;7 years). The results of the word monitoring task revealed that WS subjects were sensitive to the violation of auxiliary markers and phrase structure rules like normal controls. However, unlike normal controls, they did not display sensitivity to violations of subcategory constraints.[52] Karmiloff-Smith et al. interpret these results as indicating that dissociations also exist within syntactic processing in Williams syndrome. The performance of the WS subjects on the sentence–picture matching task was poor in general. The order of difficulty of the various syntactic structures examined was similar in the WS subjects as it was for normal, elderly controls – control and WS subjects found sentences (both actives and passives) with nonagentive verbs the most difficult and sentences containing locatives the least difficult. The poorer performance of WS subjects on the sentence–picture matching task is explained, Karmiloff-Smith et al. argue, by the greater cognitive demands of this off-line task. To match a spoken sentence to a picture, a subject must first listen to and decode the sentence, maintain it in memory and compare the sentence to each one of the pictures before finally selecting the picture that is the best match. Cognitively impaired WS subjects may be overwhelmed by the extra cognitive demands of such a task.[53]

That syntactic impairments occur in Williams syndrome is clear from the above study by Karmiloff-Smith et al. (1998). However, what this study does not tell us – and what is required if we are to assess the exceptionality of WS language – is whether or not the syntactic performance of these WS subjects is commensurate with the IQ of these subjects. (Although Karmiloff-Smith et al. (1998) report the verbal and performance IQ of these subjects, no attempt is made to relate the receptive syntax performance of these subjects to these indices of mental function.) Other studies have attempted to relate the syntactic performance of WS subjects to the verbal mental age of these subjects. In an earlier study, Karmiloff-Smith et al. (1997) examined receptive and expressive morphosyntax in WS subjects. The mean test age of 18 WS subjects on the Test for Reception of Grammar (Bishop 1983) was 6;3 years. While this test age turned out to be significantly lower than the mean chronological age of these subjects (18;7 years), it was commensurate with their nonverbal mental age (6;0 years), as measured on the Raven's Progressive Matrices (Raven 1986). Areas in which deficits were particularly evident included comparatives, prepositional phrases and a variety of embedded structures.[54]

In a second study conducted by Karmiloff-Smith et al. (1997), serious deficits were observed in the expressive syntax of WS subjects. Grammatical gender assignment was investigated in 14 monolingual French-speaking WS subjects and 18 monolingual French-speaking controls. Real and nonce terms were used to test generalisation of gender assignment on the basis of either the article (i.e. *un* versus *une*) or the partially regular system of word endings (e.g. *-on* is a typical masculine ending in French, while *-onne* is a typical feminine ending). By hiding her ring under pictures of real or invented objects and animals of different colours and then asking subjects to indicate its location, the experimenter was able to establish if WS subjects and normal controls could assign grammatical gender correctly across all sentence elements (e.g. *un cochon gris*, 'a grey pig') or only some or none of these elements (e.g. *un cochon grise* – incorrect form of adjective). Despite the greater mental age of the WS subjects compared to that of the normal controls, as measured on French tests of vocabulary (7;3 years: WS; 5;9 years: controls) and syntax (6;8 years: WS; 5;5 years: controls), the WS subjects made a significantly larger number of errors of gender agreement compared to the young normal controls. In a recent study of 21 WS subjects, Thomas et al. (2001) found no selective deficit in the production of irregular English past tense forms when controlling for verbal mental age (VMA) in these subjects. (VMA was measured using the Word Definitions and the Verbal Similarities subtests of the British Abilities Scales II (Elliott 1996).) However, even when Thomas et al. controlled for verbal mental age, the WS subjects had an additional deficit in generalising regular past tense formation to novel verbs.

As the above studies demonstrate, there are very real areas of depressed language performance in WS subjects. In areas such as lexical semantics and syntax, the performance of WS subjects is often equivalent to that of verbal mental age controls. However, there is also clear evidence that syntactic performance particularly may fall below that of verbal mental age controls and may even be commensurate with the nonverbal mental age of WS subjects. In the WS subjects studied by Karmiloff-Smith et al. (1997), the subjects' mean mental age on the Test for Reception of Grammar (TROG) was 6;3 years (well below the mean chronological age of the subjects: 18;7 years). This mean TROG mental age was much closer to the mental age of these WS subjects on the Raven's Progressive Matrices (6;0 years), a measure of nonverbal cognitive ability, than it was to their mental age on the British Picture Vocabulary Scale (8;10 years), a test of vocabulary comprehension. Williams syndrome has typically been characterised as a disorder in which relatively spared language abilities exist alongside deficits in nonverbal cognition, particularly visuo-spatial skills. To the extent that studies are now beginning to reveal significant syntactic and other linguistic deficits in the WS population,[55] it seems likely that this standard characterisation of the disorder may have to undergo some revision.

There is no suggestion in the above paragraphs that language performance in WS subjects is anything but superior to the nonverbal cognitive abilities of these subjects. Nevertheless, it remains the case that in areas such as syntax, language performance is more commensurate with the nonverbal mental age of WS subjects than was previously thought to be the case. Mental age-consistent language abilities were also demonstrated by Becker et al. (1990) in a study of language performance in eight children with FAS. The Raven's Coloured Progressive Matrices test was used to obtain a measure of these subjects' nonverbal cognitive ability. Grammatical and semantic abilities were assessed using a battery of standardised tests. On all but one grammatical test – the expressive portion of the Northwestern Syntax Screening Test (NSST, Lee 1969) – the performance of the FAS subjects was similar to that of normal controls who were matched to the FAS children on nonverbal cognitive ability. Even on the expressive portion of the NSST, the little difference that did occur in FAS and control performance – there were a general trend towards lower scores on the part of the FAS subjects – did not achieve statistical significance. On one further grammatical measure – the Grammatical Closure subtest of the Illinois Test of Psycholinguistic Abilities (Kirk et al. 1968) – FAS and control subjects' derived scores did not differ statistically when comparing performance based on either chronological age or mental age. When the performance of FAS and control subjects was compared by mental age, no significant differences were found on any of the four semantic tests used. On two of these tests, there were no significant differences between FAS and control subjects when performance was compared by chronological age. Becker et al. (1990) conclude that 'when matched to MA controls, FAS subjects did not exhibit MA inconsistent language' (119).

Williams syndrome and FAS are noteworthy disorders for clinical linguists in the following respect. Even when language performance in WS and FAS subjects is mental age-consistent, language is significantly impaired in both WS and FAS individuals compared to chronological age peers. However, these impairments are masked to a considerable extent by these subjects' apparently sophisticated social use of language. Abkarian (1992) states that '[b]ecause of a superficial conversational talent, adults may wrongly surmise that children with FAS have better linguistic skills than they actually possess' (227). The advanced, if somewhat unusual, skills in the use of language by WS subjects have led clinicians and theorists to use the term 'cocktail party syndrome' of this disorder. Schultz et al. (2001) remark that

> [u]pon meeting a person with WS for the first time, one might not immediately guess that the person has developmental cognitive delays. They frequently show 'cocktail party' verbal abilities – language abilities that are superficially quite intact, coupled with good adherence to social conventions and mores and a rather intense social interest. (607)

Also, individuals with Williams syndrome often display a strong desire to engage in communication with others: 'they often have good social relationships with adults whom they seek out for linguistic interaction' (Karmiloff-Smith et al. 1995). This desire for communicative interaction is also evident in other learning-disabled children and adults: for example, males with fragile X syndrome. However, the appearance of sophisticated language use and the pursuit of linguistic interaction with others belie the presence of considerable pragmatic deficits in Williams syndrome and in many other learning-disabled populations. We conclude our discussion of language disorder in learning disability by examining pragmatic impairments in some of these populations.

In a recent study of pragmatic skills and social relationships in Williams syndrome, Laws and Bishop (2004) observed significant levels of pragmatic language impairment in 17 of 19 WS subjects examined. Parents of WS individuals were asked to complete the Children's Communication Checklist[56] (Bishop 1998), or an adult form of the checklist where the WS subject was over 18 years of age. The same checklists were completed for 24 Down's syndrome children and adolescents by teachers or classroom assistants, for 17 children with specific language impairment by teachers or speech and language therapists and for 32 typically developing children by parents or teachers. Only the WS subjects achieved a pragmatic composite score below the 132 cut-off indicative of impairment. The WS subjects obtained significantly lower scores than controls on all five subscales of the composite – inappropriate initiation, coherence, stereotyped conversation, use of context and rapport. In two of these subscales – inappropriate initiation of conversation and the use of stereotyped conversation – WS subjects achieved a significantly poorer score than either subjects with Down's syndrome or specific language impairment. WS subjects produced fewer coherent narratives and conversations than normal controls, even though they had similar levels of syntactic ability to these typically developing children. The WS subjects' ratings in these areas were comparable to those of DS and SLI subjects. Depressed performance in these latter subjects was related to poor syntactic skills.

The poor performance of WS subjects on subscale C (inappropriate initiation) is consistent with reports describing the lack of normal inhibition shown by WS individuals with strangers. It is also consistent with responses to one item on the social relationships scale used by Laws and Bishop. Most parents of WS subjects believed that the statement 'talks to anyone and everyone' applied to their son or daughter. However, the typical social phenotype of Williams syndrome is not supported by other findings of Laws and Bishop's study. WS subjects achieved a poorer rating (albeit marginal) than control subjects and a lower, but not significant, rating than DS and SLI subjects for conversational rapport. The finding that WS subjects had poorer ratings for social relationships than both DS and SLI subjects was also unexpected. Many WS subjects displayed a tendency to be babied, bullied or teased by other children, a finding that could not be explained by the attitudes of other children to any observed differences (physical characteristics and learning disabilities) in these subjects – DS subjects, who also exhibited differences, did not display a similar tendency. Finally, WS subjects differed most from controls and DS and SLI individuals on the interests scale in having large stores of factual information and one or more overriding interests. WS subjects also used significantly more unusual words than either DS or SLI individuals.

The above study by Laws and Bishop (2004) is important in at least three respects. First, it demonstrates that individuals with Williams syndrome do indeed experience considerable deficits in pragmatic aspects of language. Fifteen (79 per cent) of the 19 WS subjects studied by Laws and Bishop scored 132 or less on the pragmatic composite, the level at which an individual may be said to have pragmatic difficulties. This compares with only 12 (50 per cent) of the subjects with Down's syndrome and 7 (41 per cent) of the children with SLI. Second, the findings of this study also force us to revise the standard view of the social phenotype in Williams syndrome. Quite apart from being an area of strength in the WS subjects, social relationships were more impaired in these subjects than in any of the other groups examined by Laws and Bishop. Third, this study provides us with a comprehensive analysis of pragmatic and social skills in another learning–disabled population, that of Down's syndrome. It is to an examination of these skills in Down's syndrome that we now turn.

Laws and Bishop's study confirms for the most part the view that social communication is an area of strength in Down's syndrome. DS subjects were the only clinical group to score at the same level as controls on the scale measuring social relationships. Ratings on the interests scale were quite unlike those associated with pervasive developmental disorders and were largely explicable in terms of the language and cognitive skills of DS subjects. In this way, only two DS children were described as using unusual words. (DS children have limited vocabulary and are thus less likely than normal controls even to know words judged to be unusual.) Also, only one DS child was judged to have a large store of factual information. (Memory limitations in Down's syndrome would make it particularly difficult for DS subjects to have such stores.) However, 10 (42 per cent) of the DS subjects were rated as preferring to be with adults or, in the case of adult subjects, were said not to enjoy the company of others of the same age. Twelve (50 per cent) of the subjects with Down's syndrome scored 132 or less on the pragmatic composite, the level at which pragmatic impairments can be said to be present. Examination of individual subscales, however, showed that pragmatic problems were more closely associated with the coherence of narratives and conversations rather than with other scales on the checklist and that coherence was a function of the speech production and syntactic skills of DS subjects.

Other studies have confirmed that pragmatic skills are relatively intact in much younger DS subjects also. (The mean age of the DS subjects studied by Laws and Bishop (2004) was 15;11 years.) Ramruttun and Jenkins (1998) examined a range of communication skills in 10 DS children with a mean age of 35.6 months. These subjects were matched to 10 nondelayed children (mean CA: 19.7 months) and 5 non–Down syndrome children with learning disabilities (mean CA: 70.4 months) on one word comprehension level. Parents were asked to complete the Pragmatics Profile of Early Communication Skills (Dewart and Summers 1988) and to engage in low structured free play with the children in their own homes. Video recordings were made of each mother and child dyad during play sessions. Results revealed that there was no significant difference between DS children and nondelayed infants in the number and range of non-verbal, vocal and gestural communicative behaviours used. Children with Down's syndrome used fewer words than nondelayed infants. The total vocabulary (words and signs together) of DS children was not significantly different from the word vocabulary of nondelayed children, showing that the DS children are able to use signing to compensate for their delay in using words. There was no significant difference in the average number of times children with Down's syndrome and nondelayed infants used the following behaviours: smiling, shaking head, vocalising, looking at objects, looking at mother, reaching and vocalising, showing, giving, vocal imitating, turning away and clapping hands. However, children with Down's syndrome were significantly delayed at using referential looking. Ramruttun and Jenkins (1998) conclude that 'it is remarkable how well children with Down syndrome are shown to match the control group of nondelayed infants in their ability to communicate intentionally' (58).

Clearly, pragmatics is an area of relative strength in the DS population.[57] However, pragmatic skills are much less well developed in other learning-disabled populations. Sarimski (2002) found that the mean number of intentional communicative acts was significantly lower in 13 children with Cornelia de Lange syndrome[58] (CdLS) than in a control group of children with Down's or cri du chat syndrome. All 13 subjects with CdLS had severe cognitive impairments.[59] Subjects with cri du chat syndrome had a similar level of intellectual impairment to CdLS children, while those with Down's syndrome had milder cognitive impairments and expressive language deficits. Video recordings were made of a 40-minute low structured play session between each of the subjects and an educational therapist. Each videotape was coded for child behaviours and intentional communication acts.[60] Analysis revealed significant between-group differences in the mean frequencies of intentional communicative acts – 3.46 communicative acts were used by the CdLS subjects, 12.33 by the DS subjects and 11.17 by the cri du chat syndrome subjects. Children with Down's syndrome and cri du chat syndrome used more preverbal communicative acts for directing other's attention and for maintaining the topic by responding to a previous statement or answering a question. Importantly, there were no significant differences in the use of intentional play behaviours by CdLS subjects and by the total control group, indicating that the lack of intentional acts on the part of CdLS subjects was confined to communication.

In this section, studies by Ramruttun and Jenkins (1998) and Sarimski (2002) have been described at length for the following reason. The early communicative behaviours examined by these studies may form the most effective means of communication in children who have a serious cognitive disability and who are unlikely to develop language. Owing to their subtlety, however, parents and caregivers may fail to recognise the communicative significance of these behaviours. They may also lack effective strategies for facilitating early communicative skills in learning-disabled infants. Awareness and development of these early skills are an integral part of communication intervention in learning-disabled subjects. It is to an examination of this intervention that we now turn.

3.2.3 Clinical Intervention

For many learning-disabled subjects, the clinical picture is a complex one consisting of multiple physical and cognitive impairments. The diverse nature of these impairments necessitates intervention by a range of medical and health professionals, often over many years. The speech and language therapist's contribution to intervention is considerable and begins with early assessment and support of feeding and communication skills. The development of these skills is likely to be significantly delayed in all but the most mildly cognitively impaired children. Indeed, children with serious cognitive disability may never be able to feed orally or acquire verbal communication. The nature of any feeding intervention will reflect the combination of neurological and structural factors that may be the cause of feeding problems in a particular case. However, it is also crucially influenced by the child's cognitive level – the child with cognitive disability may be unable to follow verbal instructions or learn new feeding behaviours. The reader is referred to section 2.3.3.1 in chapter 2 for discussion of some of the techniques that may be used during dysphagia therapy.

In this section, we present an overview of the main approaches to communication intervention in learning-disabled subjects. These approaches include early parental guidance and support in the use of activities that are designed to promote communicative behaviours in the prelinguistic child. They also include more traditional techniques such as those employed in language and articulation therapy, the latter with and without the use of instrumental methods. Finally, intervention must necessarily focus on the use of an alternative communication system in the case of the nonverbal child with learning disabilities. In verbal learning-disabled subjects, a sign system such as Makaton can provide essential support of a child's or adult's developing communication skills. We end this section with a discussion of how augmentative and alternative communication systems may be employed in the learning-disabled population.

3.2.3.1 Early Communication Intervention

Prelinguistic communicative behaviours are increasingly the focus of intervention by clinicians. This focus is justified on the following grounds. First, although these behaviours are nonsymbolic, they allow users to enact their needs and interests and are, thus, genuinely communicative in nature. Second, these behaviours may be the sole or most effective means by which the severely cognitively disabled child is able to communicate to those in his or her environment.[61] Third, there is clear evidence to indicate that the rate of intentional nonverbal communication in prelinguistic infants is a predictor of later language skills in these infants.[62] Fourth, the communicative nature of these prelinguistic behaviours is often not immediately apparent to parents and carers. Yet, with even a minimal amount of guidance and support from clinicians, many parents and carers can be encouraged to recognise and facilitate these behaviours in a range of communicative contexts. In this section, we describe the communicative behaviours that are the focus of intervention in this approach. We also examine the strategies that are used to promote these behaviours in clinical and other contexts. However, we begin with a cautionary note.

A wide range of behaviours characterises the prelinguistic period in the development of communication. Many of these behaviours involve a clear intent to communicate.[63] For example, the infant who can use gestures, vocalisations and/or eye contact to direct an adult's visual attention to a communicative referent is producing an intentional communicative act. Many other behaviours are less clearly intentional, but they can still have a communicative effect upon an adult. The infant who points and gazes at a toy, for example, may be interpreted by the adult as expressing a desire to be given the toy, even though these behaviours occur in the absence of coordinated visual attention to the adult. Intentional communicative behaviours in the prelinguistic period have been linked to language outcomes in both normal and developmentally delayed infants (Calandrella and Wilcox 2000; McCathren et al. 1999). However, the relationship between these prelinguistic behaviours and subsequent language skills is by no means a simple one. This is because other factors have been found to mediate this relationship. For example, Yoder and Warren (1999) found that when maternal verbal responsivity was statistically controlled, intentional communication ceased to be significant as a predictor of language outcomes. Moreover, behaviours that lack communicative intent have also been shown to predict language outcomes. In this way, Calandrella and Wilcox (2000) found that the rate of gestural indicating behaviour was a significant predictor of receptive and expressive language outcomes and was the only predictor of receptive language outcomes in a study of 25 toddlers with developmental delay. Clearly, much is still not known about early communicative behaviours and their relationship to subsequent language development. This is particularly true in the case of developmentally delayed infants. To the extent that these behaviours and their relationship to language are at the centre of the communicative interventions that we are about to examine, the reader should be aware that these interventions are at a formative stage and that much research into their use and efficacy, particularly in clinical groups, still remains to be done.

Several studies have now reported on the use of prelinguistic milieu teaching (PMT) in children with cognitive or intellectual disabilities. In a study of 58 children with developmental disabilities, Yoder and Warren (1998) describe the implementation of PMT as follows. PMT treatment sessions were scheduled four times a week for six months. A primary and secondary trainer, who conducted three and one of these sessions, respectively, worked on a one-to-one basis with each child. During PMT intervention, requests for objects or actions (so-called proto-imperatives) were the first communication forms to be targeted. Trainers attempted to engage in play routines with each of the subjects. These routines involved turn-taking sequences around a central theme (e.g. peek-a-boo, ball rolling). When the child had engaged in at least three turns in a routine, the trainer withheld his or her turn. If the child failed to respond by requesting the continuation of the routine or if he or she used a less mature behaviour than that which was targeted, the trainer prompted the child for the targeted behaviour (e.g. by saying 'Look at me'). Prompts were chosen to be minimally intrusive and were subsequently faded out. If the targeted behaviour was forthcoming, the play routine was continued and the child's behaviour was verbally acknowledged (e.g. by saying 'You looked at me!'). If the child still failed to respond appropriately, the routine was continued in order to maintain a positive affective milieu for teaching. When proto–imperatives began to be used more frequently, proto–declaratives were then targeted during PMT. Proto–declaratives involve drawing a partner's attention to or sharing experience or affect about an interesting object. These communicative acts were elicited by the trainer withdrawing his or her attention occasionally from the child. This behaviour was intended to stimulate the child into drawing the trainer's attention to the child's focus of attention and interest. This technique relied on the child's expectation that the trainer would continuously attend to child-selected objects of interest. This expectation was established at least three months into the treatment period.

In efficacy studies, PMT has been compared to, or supplemented by, other communication interventions. In general, these other interventions involve some type of responsivity education for parents. Yoder and Warren (2002) offered the parents of 39 toddlers with intellectual disabilities up to 12 sessions of responsivity training that was based on the Hanen Method. Through small group and one-to-one sessions, parents were instructed in how to produce optimal responses to children's communication acts. These responses included linguistic mapping, in which the adult puts the child's immediately preceding nonverbal communication act into words; compliance, in which the adult immediately carries out what the child requested in the prior communication act; and vocal imitation, in which the adult imitates the child's vocalisations, either exactly or with slight modifications. Yoder and Warren (2002) used responsivity education alongside PMT in this study. In an earlier study, Yoder and Warren (1998) compared a responsivity treatment to PMT. Described as responsive small group (RSG), this technique was designed to provide children with communicative experiences that do not inhibit development, but that are sufficiently different to permit an assessment to be made of the treatment effect of PMT. The technique required one trainer and three children to engage in parallel play. The trainer was permitted to respond to the children's communication, but he or she could not make communicative demands. Also, the trainer was not allowed to engage in imitation of the children's motor or nonword vocal behaviour, as this was included in PMT. Vocal imitation was one of the 'optimal responses' that Yoder and Warren (2002) included in their responsivity education for parents. Its omission from the responsivity treatment of the current study meant that PMT was not compared to a 'full-blown' responsivity treatment.

The findings of the above studies reveal a complex relationship between interventions based on PMT or PMT combined with responsivity education (RPMT) and language and communication outcomes. Yoder and Warren (1998) found that PMT intervention only resulted in more frequent intentional communication in post-treatment generalisation sessions in those toddlers whose mothers responded to a high percentage of the children's communication acts in the pretreatment period. Where mothers responded to fewer than 39 per cent of their children's communication acts in the pretreatment period, RSG resulted in more frequent intentional communication in post-treatment generalisation sessions than PMT. In explanation of these findings, Yoder and Warren (1998) argue that children of responsive mothers expect adults to respond to their communication attempts. This expectation leads them to persist in their communication attempts longer than children who do not have this same expectation. These children are less likely to change their focus of attention or become unengaged when confronted with a PMT prompt to produce a more mature form. As such, they are more likely to benefit from the information embedded in the prompts and acknowledgements used in PMT. Children who interact with unresponsive mothers may expect to be left alone when in the company of an adult. These children's experience may lead them to initiate communication when they are with an adult who is attentive and responsive, but otherwise undemanding (i.e. the conditions found in the RSG treatment). These children are likely to fare well under the RSG treatment, but they may become passive communicators in the presence of adults who use prompts (i.e. the PMT treatment).

As Yoder and Warren (1998) demonstrate, the extent to which children respond to communication interventions such as prelinguistic milieu teaching is dependent on factors in the pretreatment period – in this study, the degree of maternal responsivity. In a later study, Yoder and Warren (2002) explore further the pretreatment variables that can affect a child's response to prelinguistic communication intervention. Yoder and Warren found that intervention, which consisted of combined responsivity education for parents and prelinguistic milieu teaching for children (RPMT), facilitated parental responsivity in the post-treatment period. Having been instructed in how to produce 'optimal responses to child communication', parents were clearly able to continue using these techniques beyond the treatment period. It was also found that RPMT accelerated growth of productive language (on a measure called lexical density) in children with a low frequency of canonical vocal communication[64] in the pretreatment period. As expected, RPMT accelerated growth of child-initiated comments in children with low frequency comments in the pretreatment period. However, somewhat less expected were the findings that RPMT appeared to decelerate growth in requests in children with Down's syndrome and to decelerate growth in comments and lexical density if children began treatment with relatively frequent comments and canonical vocal communication, respectively. In explanation of the former finding, Yoder and Warren (2002) suggest that DS children may find it difficult to make requests because of hypotonicity and consequent passivity – comments, which required simpler motor skills than forms used to make requests, were produced with greater success by DS children. Also, requests necessitated more prompts than comments and DS subjects, who resist prompts, are unlikely to gain experience in making requests during RPMT intervention. Finally, the deceleration of growth that was observed in comments and lexical density is taken by Yoder and Warren to indicate that a linguistic, rather than a prelinguistic, intervention is more appropriate in children who display relatively frequent commenting and canonical vocal communication in the pretreatment period: 'if the child uses many comments and canonical vocal communication acts, even if the child is not yet speaking, then a linguistic treatment (e.g. Milieu Language Teaching)[65] may be more appropriate than a prelinguistic communication treatment' (2002:1171–2).

3.2.3.2 Speech and Language Intervention

For the substantial number of learning-disabled subjects who develop verbal communication, many of the techniques used in language and articulation therapy also have a role to play in intervention. Where a child's oral–motor skills and level of cognitive functioning do not preclude improvements in intelligibility and development of language, these techniques have been used with considerable success to treat specific speech and language deficits. The methods used in this form of intervention include traditional language and articulation techniques. Also included in this type of intervention are a range of instrumental methods. In this section, we describe both sets of techniques and assess their relative contribution to therapy. We begin, however, by outlining a number of general principles of speech and language intervention in learning-disabled subjects.

In section 3.2.2.2, we described how a number of speech disorders may contribute to reduced intelligibility in learning-disabled subjects. In this way, a child's spoken output may contain articulatory, phonological and dyspraxic components. These different speech disorders require the setting of separate treatment targets. These targets may be worked on simultaneously or in order of priority – it may be decided, for example, that certain phonological processes are contributing most to a child's unintelligibility and that these processes should be addressed first in therapy. Other factors that will affect the choice and order of speech treatment targets include a child's oral–motor skills, hearing status and cognitive level. When devising speech treatment targets for learning-disabled subjects, therapists have been unduly guided by norms in typically developing children. In their study of phoneme acquisition and emergence in 60 children with Down's syndrome, Kumin et al. (1994) caution against this practice and argue that

> [t]he wide range of ages for emergence of individual phonemes indicates that although a child may not have begun to produce a specific phoneme by the timetable suggested in the norms for typically developing children, the child with Down syndrome may still begin to produce the sound at a later age. (300)

As more becomes known about the process of speech sound acquisition in learning-disabled subjects with different aetiologies, it may be possible to devise treatment targets that reflect the particular characteristics of this process in a range of disorders.

Clearly, speech treatment targets must be devised with a number of factors in mind. Several factors must also be considered when devising language treatment targets for learning-disabled subjects. First, therapists should establish separate treatment targets for comprehension and production. This is necessary because language comprehension levels often differ markedly from language production levels in learning-disabled subjects. Buckley and Le Prevost (2002) remark that in children with Down's syndrome 'comprehension in both domains [vocabulary and grammar] is typically significantly ahead of production' (74). Second, intervention should focus on specific structures (grammatical constructions, semantic fields, etc.) in each language level, rather than target several of these structures simultaneously across language levels.[66] However, this is not to neglect the very real interactions that can occur between language levels or between speech and language and that are the basis of various trade-offs that are observed to occur during therapy (e.g. the child who reverts to using phonological immaturities when the syntactic demands of a task push him close to or beyond his level of grammatical competence). Third, in the same way that speech treatment targets are more likely to be effective when these targets reflect features of speech development in particular syndromes, language intervention targets are more likely to be effective when they are based upon the language developmental patterns of syndromes.[67] This treatment principle receives support from the finding that there is considerable variation in language development in learning-disabled subjects with different aetiologies.[68] Fourth, there is plenty of clinical evidence to indicate that language intervention should be extended into adolescence and adulthood. Language intervention in learning-disabled teenagers and adults can facilitate the emergence of late language structures,[69] as well as develop the pragmatic and social skills that are necessary for effective communication.[70] In older learning-disabled subjects, language intervention may serve to minimise the effects of conditions such as Alzheimer's disease.[71] Of course, all treatment targets should be tailored to meet the language needs of individual learning-disabled subjects and should be devised with family members, carers and other professionals at the centre of any intervention.[72]

With more than 95 per cent of children with Down's syndrome using speech as their primary communication system (Kumin 1999), it is clear that any programme of communication intervention in this learning-disabled population should give emphasis to the development and improvement of speech skills. Treatment should aim to improve the overall intelligibility of the child's speech. Articulation therapy can make a direct contribution towards achieving this aim, but it must be supplemented by techniques that address deficits in other aspects of speech production (e.g. phonation, resonation). There is no standard set of techniques for use in articulation therapy. Rather, techniques are chosen that (1) are specific to the particular features of the child's articulation disorder, (2) draw upon areas of strength in different clinical groups and individuals, and (3) can be readily demonstrated to, and implemented by, parents and carers. This last point is particularly significant, as parents and carers are normally integral to generalisation (the process by means of which newly acquired speech skills become established and used consistently in non-clinical communicative contexts). We discuss each of these points in more detail below.

Articulation errors in learning-disabled subjects can have their origin in quite distinct speech disorders. Each of these disorders demands a different emphasis in treatment. Where a child presents with abnormalities of muscle tone (e.g. hypotonicity in Down's syndrome), dysarthric speech errors must be addressed in therapy. In order to develop the range and strength of articulatory movements required for speech production, intervention should contain an oral-motor training component. Rosin and Swift (1999) describe a range of speech and nonspeech tasks that can be used for this purpose. These tasks are designed to encourage oral movements such as tongue protrusion and lateralisation. Tongue protrusion can be achieved, for example, by getting the child to lick peanut butter on a tongue depressor that is held in front of the lips. As soon as an oral movement is achieved on a nonspeech task, it is then integrated into speech tasks of increasing complexity. For example, the child who can demonstrate consistent lip closure on a number of nonspeech tasks (blowing kisses, forming a lip seal around a straw) can progress to producing /p/, first in a single CV sequence and then in sequences in which the vowel is varied. By combining two CV sequences, the child is able to extend his or her articulation of target bilabial sounds to the single-word level: for example, baby. For visible sounds, such as those involving bilabial and alveolar articulation, the use of a mirror may assist the child in achieving accurate placement of the articulators. Depending on the extent of the child's language development, therapy should aim to establish consistent production of the target sound at phrase and sentence levels. Where this is not possible, consistent production of target sounds in a few functional words and phrases can still lead to improvement in the child's intelligibility.

Other articulation errors in learning-disabled subjects are associated with developmental apraxia of speech (DAS). Rosin and Swift (1999) describe speech errors that are consistent with DAS in a 6-year-old boy with Down's syndrome. This boy displayed difficulty in sequencing sounds, prolonged vowels and inconsistency of errors accompanied by groping. Because there is no weakness of the speech musculature in DAS, treatment techniques that are applied to dysarthria are not appropriate for use in DAS. Strand (1995) describes several principles that are deemed to be important to the treatment of DAS. These principles include the use of intensive paired auditory and visual stimuli, production of sound combinations versus isolated phoneme training, focus on movement performance drill, use of repetitive production and intensive systematic drill and careful construction of hierarchies of stimuli. The use of decreased rate with proprioceptive monitoring, the use of carrier phrases, pairing movement sequences with suprasegmental facilitators such as stress, intonation and rhythm, and the establishment of a core vocabulary are also emphasised. What subset of these principles can be most successfully applied to the cognitively impaired child with DAS remains to be seen. Approaches to the treatment of DAS will be discussed in detail in chapter 4.

A phonological disorder may also contribute to the unintelligibility of the learning-disabled child's speech. Rosin and Swift's six-year-old DS subject exhibited the phonological processes of stopping, fronting and final consonant deletion. A range of techniques exists for the remediation of these processes. Two techniques that are mentioned by Rosin and Swift are minimal pair contrasts and the Cycles Remediation Phonological Approach (Hodson and Paden 1991; originally published in 1983). In relation to final consonant deletion, minimal pair contrasts (Fokes 1982) make use of targets that differ only in the presence of a final consonant sound. In this way, boo and boot are contrasted, as are bye-bite, bee-beet and bow-boat. In this approach, the child is encouraged to become aware of how the sound contrast represented by minimal pairs signals a difference of meaning in the language.

In the Cycles approach to phonological process intervention, a variety of processes are targeted for therapy, each for a relatively short period of time (Stoel-Gammon et al. 2002). Phonological processes that occur at least 40 per cent of the time on the Assessment of Phonological Processes-Revised (APP-R) (Hodson 1986) are targeted for elimination during cycles. Within cycles, processes are targeted in phases with progression to subsequent phases and new processes occurring regardless of the level of accuracy attained on a particular phase. The emphasis within cycles is on giving the child experience across the phonological system rather than on achieving mastery of specified targets. At the end of the cycle, the child is assessed again on the APP–R. Any processes that still occur with a frequency of 40 per cent or greater are targeted in the next cycle. Previous processes are also revisited and new advanced processes are targeted in subsequent cycles. Treatment in this approach proceeds by means of (1) auditory bombardment, where the child is provided with slightly amplified auditory stimulation of the new phonological patterns, (2) practice with word exemplars which illustrate new phonological patterns through different phoneme and syllable combinations and (3) brief, but regular, home practice that is carried out by a child's parent (Stoel-Gammon et al. 2002).

Reduced speech intelligibility in learning-disabled subjects may be the result of disorders other than dysarthria, apraxia and phonological impairment. In particular, intelligibility may be compromised by fluency problems, of which there is a higher incidence in Down's syndrome and other learning-disabled subjects (see section 3.2.2.2). Some of these problems are related to deficits in language formulation. However, other fluency problems are consistent with disorders like stuttering and cluttering. Rosin and Swift (1999) identify several features typical of cluttering in the speech of a 11-year-old girl with Down's syndrome. These features include reformulation, a rapid speech rate that increases towards the end of utterances and the use of final consonants that are not well marked and are often imprecise. To address these cluttering features, a rate programme was recommended as part of this girl's intervention. A rate reduction sequence was implemented. This involved (1) modelling slow rate with controlled stimuli, (2) prolonging consonants and vowels, (3) exaggerating mouth movements, (4) stressing each syllable, (5) stressing final consonants, (6) working on appropriate phrasing and pausing and (7) trying unison speaking and fading the clinician's input. Treatment techniques for stuttering and cluttering will be examined in detail in chapter 6.

It was described above how clinicians should aim to use treatment techniques that draw upon known areas of strength in individuals and clinical groups. It is frequently observed that visual processing skills are an area of relative strength in Down's syndrome subjects. Visual memory is particularly notable in this regard, with many authors confirming abilities in this area in individuals with Down's syndrome.[73] Skills in visual processing can be readily adapted for use in articulation therapy. These skills are directly drawn upon when a mirror is used to help a child attain accurate placement of the articulators for the production of sounds. Strengths in visual processing also account for the success in using electropalatography (EPG) to remediate articulation errors in the speech of people with Down's syndrome. We discuss below how EPG is being used in therapy with DS subjects.

EPG therapy provides visual feedback of tongue behaviour that would otherwise not be visible to subjects. This instrumental technique has been successfully used in DS subjects to treat articulation errors that are resistant to traditional methods of intervention. In this way, Gibbon et al. (2003) report the case of a 10-year-old girl with Down's syndrome who underwent EPG training in order to resolve a pattern of velar fronting in which the targets /k,g,ŋ/ had alveolar placement /t,d,n/. At the age of eight years, this subject (known as P) had undergone a six-month period of therapy in which the velar fronting process was specifically targeted. Therapy was unsuccessful and at 10;07 years, P was referred by her speech and language therapist for EPG treatment. P's EPG therapy consisted of 12 weekly sessions, each of which lasted approximately 45 minutes. During these sessions, P used visual feedback of tongue-palate contact patterns to establish velar placement for the targets /k,g/. From four weeks into therapy, P used a portable training unit between clinical sessions. These home sessions were conducted on a daily basis under the supervision of P's mother. Results indicated that while /t/ and /k/ targets had identical alveolar placement before therapy, 87 per cent of /k/ targets had accurate velar placement at the end of therapy. The centre of gravity measure – an indicator of placement on the hard palate – showed no difference in contact patterns for /t/ and /k/ before therapy, but a statistically significant difference midway through and at the end of therapy. Finally, the variability index – a measure of the stability of articulations – showed stable contact patterns before therapy for /t/ and /k/ targets. These contact patterns became unstable midway through therapy, as the new articulation pattern of velar placement began to emerge. By the end of therapy, index values for /t/ had decreased while values for /k/ remained high. Clearly, while the stability of /t/ targets had been restored by the end of therapy, the newly established /k/ targets were still unstable.

Visual skills can also be used to improve speech intelligibility in DS subjects through the use of signing. Many DS children and adults use signing to augment speech. It is observed that improvements occur in the intelligibility of DS adults who use key-word signing[74] to augment speech in 'Total Communication'[75] groups (Powell and Clibbens 1994). To validate this clinical observation and, specifically, to eliminate the possibility that this perceived improvement is related to therapists' knowledge of sign, Powell and Clibbens examined the intelligibility of four DS adults in two signing conditions. In the 'high' signing condition, the person with whom the DS subject conversed always used key-word signing. In the 'low' signing condition, key-word signing was never used by the conversational partner. Three different types of rater assessed the intelligibility of the DS subjects' speech: (1) a 'skilled' listener who knew sign (a speech and language therapist who did not know the subjects), (2) a 'skilled' listener with no knowledge of sign (a speech and language therapist who worked in a different speciality), and (3) two 'naive' listeners who had no knowledge of sign and no prior contact with the subjects or with speech and language therapy. With signs providing nonverbal cues to interpretation, the

DS subjects who used signing may appear more intelligible than they actually are. In order to establish that the intelligibility of the DS speakers is related to speech and not to the nonverbal cues provided by signs, raters were required to assess video segments of speech by listening only ('unseen' condition) and by normal viewing ('seen' condition).

Results indicate that, even when video segments were rated by listening only, subjects were assigned a higher intelligibility rating in the 'high' signing condition than in the 'low' signing condition. For all subjects, an overall mean difference of 12 per cent was found in favour of the key-word signing condition. Speech intelligibility did not vary between the 'seen' and 'unseen' conditions when no signing was used ('low' signing). Clearly, the nonverbal cues that naturally accompany normal spontaneous speech were not adequate in themselves to improve speaker intelligibility. In the 'high' signing condition, however, intelligibility increased by 14 per cent in the 'unseen' condition. These results show that key-word signing has a positive effect on speaker intelligibility. Moreover, this effect goes beyond that explained by nonverbal cues and is achieved in the absence of direct work on articulation and on the phonological system.

As well as improving the intelligibility of speech, signing can also bring about gains in language. We will examine some of those gains later in this section. We will return to signing in section 3.2.3.3, when we come to discuss augmentative and alternative communication in learning disability. In the meantime, a few comments are in order about the role of parents and other caregivers in speech intervention. The aim of any speech intervention is to establish new articulatory patterns and other speech behaviours. There is a widespread clinical consensus that this aim cannot be achieved if parents and other individuals who have contact with the child (family members, professionals, friends, etc.) are not closely involved in the process of therapy. This involvement will vary considerably amongst individual cases, from observation of sessions between the therapist and child to the implementation of therapy techniques at home. At a minimum, however, all parents and caregivers should be aware of the speech goals for the child and of the techniques that are being used by therapists to achieve these goals.

There are a number of reasons why parents and others are so integral to the success of speech remediation. First, aberrant patterns associated with speech disorders are often well entrenched and, as such, are very resistant to change – observe the resistance to change of the velar fronting process in the DS girl studied by Gibbon et al. (2003). Displacing old and establishing new speech patterns requires extensive stimulation and practice. This is particularly true in apraxia of speech, where it has been reported that children require 81 per cent more individual treatment sessions than children with severe phonological disorders (an average of 151 sessions compared to 29 sessions) in order to achieve the same functional outcome (Campbell 1999). Many clinics and therapists are unable to offer this level of treatment and so parents are required to implement speech remediation techniques outside of clinical sessions. Second, even if more treatment sessions were available, additional clinical intervention is not sufficient in itself for speech goals to be achieved. This is because speech behaviours that are newly acquired in clinic must eventually undergo generalisation to nonclinical contexts. The consistent use of new speech patterns in these contexts is the criterion against which the success of therapy is judged. Third, learning-disabled children exhibit poor cognitive skills. Problems in processing information make it difficult for these children to follow instructions during therapy. Memory deficits limit the amount and type of information[76] that can be presented during speech tasks. Also, the child who has memory deficits is less likely to retain knowledge and skills and needs ongoing revision of newly acquired articulatory patterns and speech behaviours. The combined effect of these cognitive impairments is a reduction in the child's capacity to learn new speech behaviours in therapy. This effect can be lessened to some degree by intensive stimulation and practice of new speech behaviours in a home environment that is managed by motivated and informed parents. Fourth, parents and friends are usually best placed to know a child's interests and daily activities. Therapy tasks that are tailored to these interests and activities are more likely to be met with compliance and motivation on the child's part and to result in a successful outcome.

Where a child's cognitive abilities do not preclude improvements in language, intervention may also target language skills. Specific language structures (e.g. grammatical constructions) may be selected for treatment, when it is judged that these structures can best help the learning-disabled subject achieve functional communication. For example, by teaching the learning-disabled individual the syntactic constructions that are needed to form questions and to produce statements, a child or adult can convey greater content and perform more pragmatic functions than is possible through one- or two-word utterances. In addition to direct work on grammatical constructions and other language structures, therapy may also target language skills indirectly. For example, there is now clear evidence that signing, literacy training and work on phonological memory can all improve the expressive language skills of learning-disabled individuals, particularly those with Down's Syndrome. Two of these interventions – signing and literacy training – draw upon visual skills, the relative strength of which in DS subjects was shown above to produce articulatory and intelligibility gains in these subjects. The third intervention – focus on phonological memory – is an attempt to improve language skills by targeting one of the main cognitive deficits (an impairment of verbal short-term memory) that underlie these skills. We will examine each of these interventions in turn in the following paragraphs.

The most pronounced language deficits in Down's syndrome occur in syntax and morphology. Poor syntactic abilities are one of the main reasons why DS children exhibit often severe limitations in expressive language – most children with Down's syndrome do not move beyond the level of simple phrase structure grammar found in normal children younger than three years (Fowler 1990). By targeting syntactic structures in therapy, children can increase their mean length of utterance. DS adults, too, can be encouraged to increase the length of their language output, despite often lacking language intervention at an earlier stage in development.[77] Leddy and Gill (1999) describe a programme of language intervention in which Nicholas, a 43-year-old male with Down's syndrome, was taught to increase the length of his language output. Nicholas's expressive language consisted of two- to four-word phrases such as 'Go eat' and 'Mail go Sue office' – the content of the second utterance reflects the fact that Nicholas was a part-time employee in a county government office, where he delivered mail, amongst other tasks. His comprehension of language was superior to his expressive language (a typical pattern in Down's syndrome) and he could understand multi-step directions and several complex syntactic constructions. Nicholas could also read single words and short sentences with ease.

During an intensive six-week period of individual and group sessions, Nicholas was encouraged to increase the content of his messages by extending the length of his utterances. Group sessions followed individual sessions and gave Nicholas the opportunity to implement in more natural communicative contexts the strategies that were practised with him during individual language therapy. Projects such as cooking and art work provided an overarching structure for the group sessions. Clinicians accompanied members to the group sessions, where they cued them to use their new strategies and created scenarios that would require them to put their communication skills into practice (e.g. remove a cooking utensil, which required the member to request it). A brief conversational exchange between Nicholas and the clinician at the start of each individual session generated the grammatical structures and markers that would be worked on during that session. Nicholas was instructed directly in the use of past tense markers (-ed), past tense irregular verbs and prepositions. This information, along with the utterances from the original conversational exchange, were written on a marker board. After identifying the length of each utterance, Nicholas was encouraged to 'make it longer' or 'say it with more words'. His revised utterance was then written on the board. Once a grammatically improved utterance was obtained – for example, 'I worked on mail' instead of 'I work mail' – Nicholas was encouraged to recount additional information about his work. This information was added to the board. The clinician instructed Nicholas in the use of articles, adjectives and conjunctions, which formed the basis of yet further grammatical expansions (e.g. 'I worked in the mailroom with Lew'). Finally, the clinician rehearsed the conversation with

Nicholas, first using the marker board as a script and then conducting the exchange from memory.

This account of how sentence expansion was achieved in a single subject reflects a number of principles that apply to language intervention in both children and adults with Down's syndrome. First, printed text was integral to intervention and facilitated Nicholas's language learning. By using text, the clinician is encouraging Nicholas to make use of his stronger visual skills during treatment. The expectation is that this area of relative strength in Nicholas's profile of skills will aid his development of language in general and his acquisition of grammatical skills in particular. The use of reading in language intervention can be justified on similar grounds.[78] The pacing board uses a visual and motoric cueing system that can help children with Down's syndrome increase the length of their utterances (Kumin et al. 1995). The board uses circles for each word in an utterance; for example, 'throw ball' would have two circles. The child is encouraged to move from left to right, touching each circle, as he or she says the words in the utterance. (A similar effect is achieved by putting a dot under each word in a book.)

Second, by conducting group sessions after individual sessions, the clinician was able to encourage Nicholas to use his newly acquired syntactic skills in a range of more natural communicative contexts. For language intervention to be successful, language skills must undergo generalisation to nonclinical contexts. It is clear that this was achieved in Nicholas's case. Although Nicholas occasionally had to be reminded to 'use full sentences' during the first few weeks of group therapy, by the end of the period of intervention he was spontaneously producing longer and more complete utterances. There is also evidence that these improvements extended outside of therapy sessions altogether, with co-workers and community support providers reporting significant gains in Nicholas's communication skills.

Third, in the same way that newly acquired language skills must contribute ultimately to improved communication in everyday contexts, the communicative demands of these contexts should in turn inform the clinician's decision to treat certain language skills. The decision to equip Nicholas with strategies that he can use to increase sentence length was motivated by the communicative demands of his work environment. Treatment targets that are developed in isolation from the contexts in which communication takes place are unlikely to result in a successful outcome.

Fourth, group activities such as cooking and art work facilitated Nicholas's use of his new communication skills. These activities draw upon well-known scripts of the events that take place in particular situations and of the people and objects that are present in those situations, e.g. that cooking is likely to involve a range of cooking utensils. Learning-disabled individuals often have reasonably good knowledge of everyday events and routines. This knowledge can be used to facilitate language learning in these individuals. Although in this case scripts were used with an adult, they have also been adopted successfully with children.[79] Rosin and Swift (1999) state that '[s]cript use can be applied with children of all ages. For infants and toddlers, routines, fingerplays, songs, and nursery rhymes are important early scripts' (140).

Fifth, Nicholas's clinician addressed specific grammatical structures during his individual treatment sessions. Nicholas was taught how prepositions, conjunctions and other grammatical elements could be used to achieve an expansion in the length of his utterances. Even though most learning-disabled individuals will never exhibit normal syntax, many children and adults can be taught to use simple syntactic constructions. Moreover, as we understand more about the syntactic errors that learning-disabled children and adults make, we can begin to use this knowledge to develop more specific syntactic interventions.[80]

Thus far, we have discussed an approach to language intervention in which language structures are targeted directly during therapy. However, it is also possible to bring about improvements in language through a number of less direct interventions. One of these interventions is signing. Signing is a particularly effective communication strategy in DS children. This is because signing trades on the strong visual preference of DS children. Also, signing provides DS children with a means of communication at a time when unintelligibility limits the usefulness of speech and receptive language is ahead of expressive language. Signing can thus help to reduce the frustration of many DS children, who know what they want to say, but are unable to say it or make themselves understood. Most importantly, however, signing permits language development to occur during an important developmental period and until such time as DS children are able to produce speech. At this point, signing may either be phased out or continue to be used to support speech as a form of augmentative communication. (We will return to this use of signing in section 3.2.3.3.) Clibbens (2001) reports the findings of several studies which demonstrate that the combined use of signed and spoken input can boost early language development in children with Down's syndrome. Particularly significant gains are made in lexical development[81] as a result of early signing. In a study by Miller (1992), DS children who were exposed to early signing had larger total vocabularies (spoken and signed) from 11 to 17 months (mental age) than typically developing children. Launonen (1996) found that at three years (chronological age), the average vocabulary (spoken and signed) of DS children who received signing intervention was as large as the vocabulary of a control group of DS children at four years of age. (The latter subjects did not receive an intervention package consisting of manual signs, gesture and action from six months to three years.) With these and other studies demonstrating the language gains that can result from the use of signing, it is clear that therapists cannot afford to overlook the most important contribution of signing to language intervention.

In recent years, there has been increasing recognition on the part of clinicians and educationalists that reading can result in wider language gains in DS children. Buckley (1995a) used reading in an intervention programme that was designed to improve the morphosyntax of 12 teenagers with Down's syndrome. At the end of a year's training, all but one of the teenagers were using longer, more complex sentences in conversation, as measured by mean length of utterance. Laws et al. (1995) investigated the language and memory abilities of 14 children with Down's syndrome, half of whom were readers or developed reading during the course of the study. At the start of the study, there were no significant differences between readers and nonreaders on measures of vocabulary and grammar understanding (assessed by the BPVS and TROG, respectively) and auditory and visual memory (assessed by auditory and visual word span tests). However, after nearly four years, readers displayed a significant advantage over nonreaders on all these language and memory measures.

The findings of these studies, and others besides, have convinced practitioners to use reading as a language intervention strategy with DS children. Reading is now successfully integrated into many special education curricula. Buckley (1995b) remarks that the use of reading to teach spoken language 'has been used successfully for more than 25 years in some areas of special education in the United Kingdom' (163). However, some account of the effectiveness of reading in stimulating language development in Down's syndrome is necessary. Many children and adults with Down's syndrome experience conductive hearing loss associated with otitis media. Deficits in verbal short-term memory and auditory processing problems are also reported to occur in this clinical population. These impairments compromise the auditory pathway, albeit at different levels. One consequence of these impairments is that DS children are less able to use auditory stimuli to facilitate language learning than typically developing children. The stronger visual processing skills of DS children, combined with the permanence of the written word, render reading an effective route into language learning in Down's syndrome. Laws et al. (1995) remark that

> for children with Down's syndrome, the visual representation of language offers a way to overcome their auditory processing and memory difficulties. In contrast to spoken language, printed text provides a permanent rather than a transitory signal. This allows more processing time, and gives the child a better chance of learning. (63)

It has long been recognised that reading can improve the language skills of DS children.[82] However, the specific mechanisms through which this is achieved await further research into the visual processing of language in Down's syndrome.

A specific deficit in verbal short-term memory is increasingly being linked to language impairment in Down's syndrome. This deficit is believed to involve the phonological loop component in the model of working memory proposed by Baddeley and his colleagues (Baddeley and Hitch 1974; Baddeley 1986, 2000). In this way, Laws (2004) found a significant correlation between phonological memory (measured by nonword repetition) and expressive language abilities (measured by mean length of utterance and sentence recall) in 30 children and adolescents with Down's syndrome. That this finding reflects a specific deficit in phonological memory and is not caused by the subjects' hearing impairment on the one hand or by mutual output constraints[83] on nonword repetition and spoken language on the other hand is shown by the fact that hearing did not correlate with expressive language measures and that adjusting for word repetition skills did not reduce the above correlation. Laws takes these findings to lend some support to the view that phonological memory stores multi-word utterances, while templates of their syntactic structures are represented in long-term memory. These templates are then used to generate spoken language. If the phonological loop facilitates the process by means of which templates are represented in long-term memory, then intervention, Laws contends, should focus on establishing representations of syntactic structures and not on the serial recall of unrelated words, such as is typically used in programmes that teach a rehearsal strategy. To this end, Laws recommends the use of reading as an intervention strategy: 'Since early reading books tend to be fairly repetitive, reading could provide the opportunity for frequent practice of the syntactic structures and so support children's acquisition of long-term memory representations' (2004:1092).

3.2.3.3 Augmentative and Alternative Communication

Augmentative and alternative systems of communication are now widely used by learning-disabled children and adults. Due to the heterogeneity of the learning-disabled population, these systems must be capable of serving quite diverse communicative needs. Broadly speaking, three main groups of learning-disabled subjects may benefit from the use of augmentative and alternative systems of communication. First, where a subject is unlikely to develop speech, an alternative system may provide the learning-disabled child or adult with an effective means of communication. Depending on the user's motor, sensory and cognitive abilities, such a system may involve pointing to graphic signs mounted on a communication board or the use of a program based on advanced computer technology. Second, where speech does emerge but is unintelligible, an augmentative system may support the child's or adult's spoken output. The

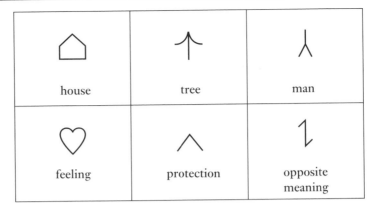

house	tree	man
feeling	protection	opposite meaning

Figure 3.1: Pictographic and ideographic Blissymbols

Makaton vocabulary (Walker 1978) is one such augmentative system that is widely used by learning-disabled individuals in the UK. Third, an AAC system may be used to stimulate speech and language development in the learning-disabled child. In this case, the system may be phased out as the child becomes a proficient oral communicator or it may continue as an alternative to oral communication if speech does not emerge. This third use of AAC systems was discussed in section 3.2.3.2 and will not be examined further in this context.

Several manual and graphic sign systems are currently available. Some systems are more easily acquired than other systems by learning-disabled subjects. Several factors have been proposed to explain these differences in ease of acquisition. Some of these factors relate to features of the systems themselves. In this way, there is a general assumption that iconicity may facilitate the acquisition of both manual and graphic signs. Iconicity describes a similarity between the performance or appearance of a sign and obvious features of the object or action for which the sign is used. Iconicity involves two further notions: transparency (the ease with which people who are unfamiliar with the sign are able to guess its meaning) and translucency (the ease with which people can perceive a relationship between a sign's meaning and its appearance or performance when the gloss of the sign is provided). Generally speaking, pictographic Blissymbols (e.g. HOUSE, TREE, MAN) are transparent, while ideographic Blissymbols (e.g. FEELING, PROTECTION, OPPOSITE) are translucent (see Figure 3.1). Notwithstanding their iconicity for normal subjects, Blissymbols may be anything but iconic for learning-disabled subjects. Von Tetzchner and Martinsen (2000) argue that

> [s]everly learning-disabled individuals are not always able to perceive what a picture is supposed to represent. This may mean that figurative differences that seem great to most people because they convey

meaning are not so clear for individuals who are unable to perceive the content of the picture. (195, 197)

This may account for the observation that Blissymbols are a particularly difficult system for learning-disabled subjects to acquire: 'With the exception of cases in which only the simplest signs have been taught, experiments in teaching Blissymbols to this group have not been very successful' (von Tetzchner and Martinsen 2000:12).[84]

The above discussion is important in the following respect: it demonstrates the relativity of iconicity. Signs that are highly iconic for some subjects may lack iconicity for learning-disabled subjects, who have not developed the necessary pictorial comprehension. Depending on their cognitive abilities and other skills, different users may have a very different learning experience of the same sign system. Attributes of the user constitute the second set of factors that can affect how easily a child acquires a sign system. Many learning-disabled individuals have motor and sensory impairments in addition to their cognitive or intellectual disability. Motor impairments may affect a child's ability to produce manual signs or even point to graphic signs on a communication board. The visually impaired subject may not be able to discriminate between graphic signs of similar form. (Many Blissymbols, for example, have one or more basic signs in common.) Even when an individual's vision is normal, a user may only attend to certain visual stimuli or neglect parts of a sign on account of poor scanning. For example, some learning-disabled individuals may not notice the prongs on the fork and the bristles on the toothbrush in the Picture Communication Symbols FORK and TOOTHBRUSH (see Figure 3.2). As a result, they may be unable to distinguish these signs: 'There is reason to believe that many profoundly learning-disabled individuals have difficulty in perceiving this type of difference, perhaps because of stimulus overselectivity or poor visual scanning strategies' (von Tetzchner and Martinsen 2000:197).

As well as compromising an individual's ability to acquire a sign system, specific attributes of the user may also facilitate acquisition. This can be seen in Down's syndrome, for example. Visual perceptual and motor skills are areas of relative strength in young children with Down's syndrome (Foreman and Crews 1998). Visual short-term memory in particular is consistently reported to be superior to auditory short-term memory in Down's syndrome individuals (Jarrold and Baddeley 2001). Skills in the visual and motor domains are believed to account for the considerable successes of Down's syndrome subjects in acquiring manual signs. Although we do not yet have a precise explanation of why this is the case, it seems likely that any such explanation must include some account of the role of short-term memory. The stronger visual short-term memory of Down's syndrome subjects is able to retain the visual form of a sign longer than auditory short-term memory is able to retain the

fork	toothbrush
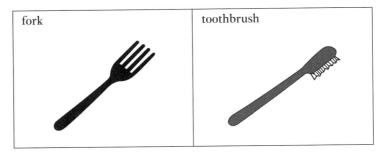	

Figure 3.2: FORK and TOOTHBRUSH Picture Communication Symbols (Picture Communication Symbols © 1981–2006 by Mayer-Johnson LLC. All rights reserved worldwide. Used with permission)

spoken form of a word. This difference in the duration of retention of visual and auditory information is likely to privilege a visual over an auditory route in language learning. As a consequence, it is likely that manual and graphic signs will be more readily acquired than spoken words. At least this much is borne out by the findings of studies. Layton and Savino (1990), for example, report the case of a young Down's syndrome boy called Bobby, who had acquired a manual sign vocabulary of 150 words by the stage his oral-expressive vocabulary contained only about 12 words.

Visual strengths in certain learning-disabled subjects can lead to over-selectivity during the training of expressive signing. Remington and Clarke (1993a) remark that '[s]everal previous studies have shown that when expressive signing is trained using simultaneous communication, in which both visual and spoken cues may function as discriminative stimuli for signing, children with severe mental retardation demonstrate overselectivity, usually to the visual modality' (36). The result of this over-selectivity is that learning-disabled children fail to acquire speech comprehension, notwithstanding their repeated exposure to words and their referents during training. In an effort to overcome over-selectivity, Remington and Clarke (1993a,b) used Extensive Sign Training and Mediated Sign Training. The Extensive condition involved overtraining expressive signing in simultaneous communication, but with a reduced reinforcement schedule. In the Mediated condition, receptive speech functions were trained prior to simultaneous communication training. While the Extensive condition produced faster acquisition of expressive signing than the Mediated condition, it did not overcome over-selectivity and thus did not facilitate speech comprehension. In a second study, Remington and Clarke (1993b) compared Extensive Sign Training and Differential Sign Training. The latter method involved mixing an equal number of simultaneous communication trials and trials in which the cue for manual signing was the referent alone. Once again, the Extensive condition produced the faster acquisition of expressive manual signing. However, only the Differential condition was able to overcome overselective attention and thus facilitate speech comprehension.

It is now widely acknowledged that factors relating to the communicative context play a significant role in sign acquisition. Chief amongst these factors is the influence of communication partners on acquisition. The partners of sign users can facilitate and inhibit sign acquisition in significant ways. Many learning-disabled subjects do not make the transition to multi-sign utterances, but continue to use one-sign utterances (von Tetzchner and Martinsen 2000). Although in some cases cognitive and linguistic impairments may hinder the development of multi-sign utterances, it is increasingly clear that communication partners may constrain sign use, albeit unwittingly, through certain patterns of interaction with sign users. Learning-disabled subjects are often passive in interaction. This passivity is reinforced by communication partners through their assumption of the role of questioner in interaction. In this role, partners can decide both the duration and the topic of conversation. Importantly, they can also restrict the user's responses to one-sign utterances through their choice of questions – yes-no questions tend to dominate these exchanges, with open questions rarely being used. The reader is referred to section 2.3.3.2 in chapter 2 for a fuller discussion of how the interaction styles of communication partners may restrict the output of sign users.

Interaction styles aside, communication partners have also been shown to influence the signing behaviour of others through their own use of signs. In a study of 49 children with severe learning difficulties, Grove and McDougall (1991) found a significant but weak positive association between the frequency of Makaton signing in these children and their classroom teachers. Also, the frequency of signing by children in a teacher-directed setting was positively associated with the quality of the signing environment, with children using Makaton signs more often in high than low signing classrooms. In a study of multi-sign utterances produced by a group of 10 intellectually impaired children, the Mean Length of Sign Turn in children (1.84) was similar to the mean number of signs per clause (1.45) used by teachers (Grove et al. 1996). It is interesting to note that two-sign utterances, which are normally lacking in learning-disabled individuals, were also rarely used by teachers in this study. (Four children had a Mean Length of Sign Turn above 2.0 and only two teachers regularly produced multi-signed clauses with a manual sign density of over 2.0.) On the basis of these findings, it is reasonable to suppose that the failure of learning-disabled subjects to acquire two-sign utterances may be related to low levels of sign use by communication partners.

Ultimately, the only way to assess the effect of sign system features, cognitive and other attributes of sign users and the interactive style and signing behaviour of communication partners on sign acquisition is to submit each of these groups of factors to systematic investigation. Recent work in augmentative and alternative communication is doing just that. Experimental studies are now routinely used to compare different AAC systems. In this way, Foreman and Crews (1998) investigated the use of Makaton signing and the COMPIC system of computerised pictographs to teach the names of objects to young children with Down's syndrome. The findings of these studies provide a rational basis for clinical decisions concerning intervention. For example, the use of bimodal and multimodal methods of intervention is supported by Foreman and Crew's finding that a sign method (verbal + sign) and a multimodal method (verbal + sign + symbol) are both equally effective and more effective than verbal instruction alone and the use of COMPIC symbols in teaching DS children to name objects.

3.3 Autistic Spectrum Disorder

For a significant number of children and adults, impairments of communication occur alongside deficits in socialisation and imagination. To describe impaired functioning across these three domains, Wing and Gould in 1979 coined the expression 'triad of impairments'. Today, this expression captures the main behavioural features of a group of disorders, which clinicians have variously labelled as autistic spectrum disorders (ASDs) or pervasive developmental disorders (PDDs). While ASD and PDD are both in current use in the clinical literature, in this section we will follow the dominant tendency in British literature and use the term 'autistic spectrum disorder'. In the discussion to follow, we examine recent epidemiological findings relating to the prevalence and incidence of ASDs. As part of this examination, we discuss the finding that many more boys and men have ASDs than girls and women. We also assess whether there is any validity to the claim that there has been a large and sustained increase in ASD cases in recent years. Although the aetiological basis of ASDs is still largely unknown, and is likely to vary in individual cases, we examine the genetic and other factors that are believed to play a role in the development of these disorders. Approximately 50 per cent of autistic individuals fail to develop verbal communication. Even amongst those who do acquire speech, there are significant, lifelong impairments of communication. We examine how speech and language therapists assess and treat communication impairment in this clinical population. First, we begin by outlining in a general way each of the autistic spectrum or pervasive developmental disorders.

In the absence of biological markers for the ASDs, clinicians have developed detailed behavioural criteria for their diagnosis. These criteria are included in the *Diagnostic and Statistical Manual of Mental Disorders* (American Psychiatric Association, APA) and the *International Classification of Diseases* (World Health Organization, WHO) (ICD-10). They are continually revised as more becomes known about the phenotype of autism and other ASDs.[85] The most recent edition of the Diagnostic and Statistical Manual – DSM-IV-TR (APA 2000) – recognises five pervasive developmental disorders: autistic disorder, Rett's disorder, childhood disintegrative disorder, Asperger's disorder and pervasive developmental disorder, not otherwise specified (PDD,NOS). The ICD-10 includes eight categories of pervasive developmental disorder.[86] Although these disorders have much in common – most notably, some combination of deficits in socialisation, communication and imagination – they also differ in relation to factors such as age of onset, developmental history and prognosis. Many of these factors also assume diagnostic significance within the above classification systems and will be discussed below.

Autistic disorder, which is sometimes called 'classic' autism,[87] is the form of ASD that is most prominent amongst the general public and most researched by theorists and clinicians. According to the DSM-IV criteria for autistic disorder, an individual must exhibit six (or more) of 12 characteristic behaviours in order for this particular diagnosis to be made. These behaviours include qualitative impairments in social interaction (e.g. failure to develop peer relationships appropriate to developmental level); qualitative impairments in communication (e.g. in individuals with adequate speech, marked impairment in the ability to initiate or sustain conversation with others); and restricted, repetitive and stereotyped patterns of behaviour, interests and activities (e.g. persistent preoccupation with parts of objects). The DSM-IV criteria also state that delays or abnormal functioning in social interaction, language as used in social communication and symbolic or imaginative play must have an onset prior to the age of three years[88] and that the child's condition cannot be better accounted for by Rett's disorder or childhood disintegrative disorder. Children with autistic disorder are normally physically well developed and have good motor skills. Stereotyped and repetitive motor mannerisms (e.g. hand or finger flapping or twisting, or complex whole-body movements) are thus not related to any motor impairment. As with ASDs in general, mental retardation and other comorbid conditions (e.g. epilepsy, hearing impairment) are present in many individuals with this disorder (see section 3.3.2).

Rett's disorder[89] (also called Rett's syndrome) is a severe condition that is found almost exclusively in girls (see section 3.3.1). This disorder is characterised by a period of normal development, following which marked regression[90] occurs. Diagnostic criteria for Rett's disorder in DSM-IV reflect features of both normal development and regression in affected individuals. In this way, for a diagnosis of Rett's disorder to be made, an individual must exhibit all of the following characteristics: apparently normal prenatal and perinatal development; apparently normal psychomotor development through the first five months after birth; and normal head circumference at birth. After an initial period of normal development, onset of the following conditions must be observed: deceleration of head growth between 5 and 48 months; loss of previously acquired purposeful hand skills between 5 and 30 months with the subsequent development of stereotyped hand movements (e.g. hand-wringing or hand-washing); loss of social engagement early in the course (although often social interaction develops later); appearance of poorly coordinated gait or trunk movements; and severely impaired expressive and receptive language development with severe psychomotor retardation. Individuals with Rett's disorder are generally mentally retarded. Although the prognosis for this disorder is very poor, there may subsequently be some improvement in behaviour, alertness span and communication skills and the affected individual may go on to show more interest in her surroundings.[91]

Childhood disintegrative disorder (CDD, also known as Heller's syndrome) is a further PDD in which marked regression occurs. Diagnostic criteria for this disorder in DSM-IV require that affected children display apparently normal development for at least two years after birth, as manifested by the presence of age-appropriate verbal and nonverbal communication, social relationships, play and adaptive behaviour. Affected children must also exhibit a clinically significant loss of previously acquired skills, before 10 years of age, in at least two of the following areas: expressive or receptive language, social skills or adaptive behaviour, bowel or bladder control, play and motor skills. CDD shares social, communicative and imaginative impairment with autism. DSM-IV criteria reflect impairments in these domains by requiring that affected children display abnormalities of functioning in at least two of the following areas: qualitative impairment in social interaction (e.g. failure to develop peer relationships), qualitative impairments in communication (e.g. delay or lack of spoken language) and restricted, repetitive and stereotyped patterns of behaviour, interests and activities, including motor stereotypies and mannerisms. The final DSM-IV criterion states that the child's disturbance should not be better accounted for by another specific PDD or by schizophrenia. CDD has a variable course. It may be characterised by progressive deterioration or by a developmental plateau with little subsequent improvement. Much less frequently, marked improvement occurs. In general, the prognosis for CDD is worse than that for autism.

Asperger's disorder (also called Asperger's syndrome) is a recent addition to DSM-IV. Its inclusion as a disorder separate from autism within the wider category of PDDs has been controversial and continues to provoke much debate. One of the most disputed issues concerns the validity of Asperger's syndrome as a diagnostic category distinct from high-functioning autism (HFA): that is, autism associated with overall normal intelligence.[92] Like other PDDs examined thus far, individuals with Asperger's syndrome display social impairments and abnormal behaviour, interests and activities. Diagnostic criteria for Asperger's disorder in DSM-IV include qualitative impairment in social interaction, as manifested by at least two of the following: marked impairment in the use of multiple nonverbal behaviours (e.g. eye-to-eye gaze, facial expression); failure to develop peer relationships appropriate to developmental level; a lack of spontaneous seeking to share enjoyment, interests or achievements with other people; and a lack of social or emotional reciprocity. The DSM-IV criterion relating to restricted, repetitive and stereotyped patterns of behaviour, interests and activities requires at least one of the following to be present: encompassing preoccupation with one or more stereotyped and restricted patterns of interest that is abnormal in either intensity or focus; apparently inflexible adherence to specific, nonfunctional routines or rituals; stereotyped and repetitive motor mannerisms (e.g. hand flapping); and persistent preoccupation with parts of objects. Social and behavioural impairments in Asperger's syndrome disrupt functioning in a number of areas – another DSM-IV criterion states that 'the disturbance causes clinically significant impairment in social, occupational, or other important areas of functioning'. (The inclusion of 'occupational' reflects the fact that many more individuals with Asperger's syndrome than individuals with other forms of PDD will have the requisite skills to secure employment.)

Unlike other PDDs, language and communication skills are relatively spared in Asperger's syndrome (AS). (This is not to say, however, that these skills are entirely normal; see section 3.3.2.) To reflect the relatively intact language skills of AS individuals, a DSM-IV criterion requires that there is no clinically significant general delay in language (e.g. single words used by age two years, communicative phrases used by age three years). The intellectual functioning of AS individuals is superior to that of other PDD subjects and is usually in the normal range.[93] To this end, a further diagnostic criterion in DSM-IV states that 'there is no clinically significant delay in cognitive development'. (This criterion also states that there is no clinically significant delay in 'the development of age-appropriate self-help skills, adaptive behaviour (other than in social interaction), and curiosity about the environment in childhood'.) A final diagnostic criterion requires that criteria are not met for another specific PDD or schizophrenia.

The fifth PDD included in DSM-IV is pervasive developmental disorder, not otherwise specified (PDD,NOS,[94] also referred to as 'atypical personality development', 'atypical PDD' or 'atypical autism'[95]). An individual is assigned to this diagnostic category when there is a severe and pervasive impairment in the development of reciprocal social interaction or verbal and nonverbal communication skills, or when stereotyped behaviour, interests and activities are present. However, the full criteria are not met for schizophrenia, schizotypal personality disorder, avoidant personality disorder or for a specific PDD. In this way, cases of 'atypical autism' are included in this diagnostic category. These are individuals who present with many of the features of autism, but who fall short of a diagnosis of autistic disorder because of late age at onset, atypical symptomatology, subthreshold symptomatology, or all three of these conditions. Unlike other PDDs, the DSM-IV does not provide specific diagnostic criteria for PDD,NOS. Moreover, it is clear that PDD,NOS is to be thought of as a 'default diagnosis' that is only to be applied in those cases in which no other diagnosis is judged to be more suitable. These factors have led to a situation in which much less research is conducted into PDD,NOS than into other PDDs; also, the research that is conducted is quite difficult to assess, because often children with very different symptoms are being compared both within and between studies.

3.3.1 Epidemiology and Aetiology

Epidemiological investigations of ASDs have resulted in varying estimates of the prevalence and incidence of these disorders. Much of this variability is related to issues of case definition – different diagnostic criteria and thresholds, methods of assessing children and modes of case ascertainment (e.g. active versus passive ascertainment of cases) can all affect the number of children who are diagnosed as having an ASD and who are included within epidemiological studies. In its review of autism research, the Medical Research Council found that the average prevalence from all studies published by the year 2000 is 10 per 10,000 for autistic disorder and 2.5 per 10,000 for Asperger's syndrome (MRC 2001). These same prevalence rates for autistic disorder and Asperger's syndrome are reported by Fombonne (2003) in a recent review of the results of published epidemiological surveys. Considerably lower prevalence rates are reported for other PDDs. Fombonne (2002) reviewed 32 epidemiological surveys of autism and PDDs and found four surveys that yielded estimates for childhood disintegrative disorder ranging from 1.1 to 6.4 cases per 100,000 subjects. Fombonne concluded that the prevalence rate for CDD is 60 times less than that for autistic disorder and that only one child out of 175 children with a PDD diagnosis meets criteria for CDD.[96] Similarly low prevalence rates are reported for Rett's syndrome. Kozinetz et al. (1993) report a prevalence rate for Rett's syndrome of 0.44 cases per 10,000 females aged from 2 to 18 years of age.[97] Fombonne (2003) reports a prevalence rate of 15 cases per 10,000 persons for PDD,NOS. This prevalence rate is higher than in other types of PDD. This may be related to over-diagnosis of this condition in the absence of specific diagnostic criteria for PDD,NOS.

While most epidemiological investigations of ASDs are studies of the prevalence of these conditions, other investigations have examined the incidence of disorders on the autistic spectrum. Williams et al. (2005) examined the incidence of ASDs in children in two Australian states – New South Wales and Western Australia – between July 1999 and December 2000. Incidence was reported in five-year age bands for children aged 0–14 years. In the 0–4 years age group, the incidence of autistic disorder was 5.5 per 10,000 in Western Australia (WA) and 4.3 per 10,000 in New South Wales (NSW). The incidence was lower in older age groups – 2.4 (WA) and 1.6 (NSW) per 10,000 in the 5–9 years group and 0.8 (WA) and 0.3 (NSW) in the 10–14 years group. This was to be expected, as incidence measures the development of 'new' cases: most children received a diagnosis of autistic disorder in the 0–4 years age group (the median age at diagnosis was four years in WA and three years in NSW), with a much smaller number of cases receiving a later diagnosis. In the UK, Powell et al. (2000)[98] examined the incidence of childhood autism and other ASDs in two areas of the West Midlands between 1991 and 1996. For the combined areas, incidence per 10,000 children per year was 8.3 for all ASDs, 3.5 for classical childhood autism and 4.8 for other ASDs. Using data recorded in the UK General Practice Research Database, Kaye et al. (2001) reported an incidence rate for autism of 2.1 cases per 10,000 person years among children aged 12 and under who were newly diagnosed in 1999. No incidence figures are currently available for the US (Williams et al. 2005).

Epidemiological studies are also playing an important role in monitoring an increase in ASD cases in recent years. Some indication of the extent of this increase is provided by the following studies. Powell et al. (2000) found that incidence rates for classical childhood autism increased by 18 per cent per year between 1991 and 1996. A much larger increase (55 per cent per year) was seen for other ASDs. Kaye et al. (2001) found that the incidence of newly diagnosed autism increased sevenfold, from 0.3 per 10,000 person years in 1988 to 21 per 10,000 person years in 1999. In 1999, the Department of Developmental Services in the California Health and Human Services Agency published a report examining changes in the population of persons with autism and PDDs in the State of California from 1987 to 1998. Between 1987 and 1998, the population of persons with autism increased from 4.85 to 9.37 per cent of the total state-wide client population. The rate of increase for autism was more than four times as great as for other diagnostic categories (cerebral palsy, epilepsy and mental retardation). One example of this increase is a 16.3 per cent rise in autism cases between December 1997 and December 1998. There was a 273 per cent increase in the number of persons with autism between 1987 and 1998 and nearly a 2000 per cent increase in other PDD categories.[99] While the exact cause of this increase in ASD cases remains unknown, factors which may contribute to it include changing diagnostic thresholds and better case ascertainment. Powell et al. attribute their observed rise in incidence rates to clinicians 'becoming increasingly able and/or willing to diagnose ASDs in preschool children' (2000:624).

It has been known for some time that males account for a disproportionately large number of ASD cases.[100] Boys with the autism phenotype typically outnumber girls by at least four to one (Skuse 2000). Males constitute an even greater proportion of Asperger's syndrome cases. Gillberg (1989) reports a male to female sex ratio for Asperger's syndrome of 9–10:1. There is also evidence that the proportion of male cases of ASD has increased over time. In the 11 years from 1987 to 1998, the Department of Developmental Services of the California Health and Human Services Agency reported a 5.3 per cent increase in the proportion of males with autism. Kaye et al. (2001) found that the risk of autism in 2–5-year-old boys born between 1988 and 1993 increased nearly fourfold, from 8 per 10,000 for boys born in 1988 to 29 per 10,000 for boys born in 1993. The proportion of male cases has also been shown to vary with IQ. An influential study in this area was conducted by Wing (1981a). Using children identified in an epidemiological study that was carried out in an area of southeast London, Wing was able to show that the male:female ratio amongst children who were moderately, severely or profoundly retarded (2.1:1) was lower than the male:female ratio in those children who had language and social impairments (2.6:1). Wing concluded that the excess of males was much more marked in language and socially impaired children who were of higher ability or who had a history of typical early childhood autism. Finally, evidence of a link between ASDs and factors such as geographical region, race and socioeconomic status is at best inconclusive.

Several factors are believed to play a role in the aetiology of ASDs. Not all of these factors operate at the same level – of the genetic, neurobiological and psychological factors that have been advanced in causal explanations of autism, some have their effects on the brain, while others operate at the level of the mind.[101] In this section, we examine genetic and neurobiological factors. Although most plausible explanations of autism have tended to examine the genetic and neurobiological bases of the disorder, other possible aetiological factors have been advanced in recent years. We discuss what role, if any, these factors play in the development of autism.

That genetic factors play a key role in the aetiology of autism is suggested by several lines of evidence. First, twin studies have revealed a high concordance rate for autism in monozygotic (identical) twins. In this way, Bailey et al. (1995) report a concordance rate of 60 per cent in monozygotic twins compared with 0 per cent in dizygotic (nonidentical) twins, leading to a calculated heritability of the liability to autism of over 90 per cent. Moreover, the rate of autism in the siblings of singletons with the disorder is considerably higher than would be predicted to occur by chance. In a review of 12 family studies, Szatmari et al. (1998) calculated a pooled rate of autism among siblings of 2.2 per cent. When Asperger's syndrome and other PDDs are included, this rate can rise to 5 per cent (Szatmari et al. 1998) and ranges from 2 to 6 per cent (Bailey et al. 1998). Both of these rates are substantially higher than the population prevalence of 10 per 10,000 or 0.1 per cent. Second, there is evidence that relatives of autistic individuals may display some of the features of the behavioural phenotype of autism, such as social and language impairments. In twin studies, high concordance rates have been found for a broader phenotype of social and/or language abnormalities, with rates of 92 per cent and 10 per cent recorded for monozygotic and dizygotic twins, respectively (Bailey et al. 1995). The high rate of these milder phenotypes in the relatives and twin siblings of autistic individuals once again points strongly to a genetic basis for autism. Third, in between 10 and 30 per cent of autism cases,[102] the disorder is associated with a known medical condition. More often than not, these conditions involve single gene disorders or chromosomal abnormalities. They include untreated phenylketonuria (see note 9), tuberous sclerosis (see note 8), fragile X syndrome (see section 3.2.1), Turner's syndrome (see note 38), duplication and inverted duplication of chromosome 15q11-q15[103] and FRAXE.[104] The strongest evidence of a causal association is found for tuberous sclerosis, fragile X syndrome and inverted duplications of chromosome 15 (MRC 2001). Regardless of the exact nature of the association between these medical conditions and ASDs, the fact that ASDs frequently occur alongside conditions of a genetic or chromosomal origin is a further indication that genes play an important role in the aetiology of autistic disorders.

Advances in neuroimaging and neuropathology have transformed our understanding of the brain mechanisms in autism. Magnetic resonance imaging (MRI) has undergone considerable development in recent years as a technique for measuring brain morphology. Improvements in the post-processing of image data have allowed researchers to achieve more precise definition and measurement of neural structures. Functional MRI (fMRI) has enabled scientists to study the 'discrete brain systems that underlie the cognitive, behavioural and social-emotional deficits that define autism . . . fMRI studies are now testing the role of specific perceptual, motor, attentional, and affective systems in autism' (Volkmar et al. 2004:145).[105] At the same time, data that can shed light on the role of specific brain structures in the pathobiology of autism have continued to be generated by structural MRI, postmortem and animal lesion models. With nearly every brain structure and system implicated in the neuropathology of autism, the following discussion will examine areas in which some consensus has been achieved rather than the findings of individual studies. For a more detailed discussion, the reader is referred to Belmonte and Carper (1998).

In its recent review of autism research, the Medical Research Council (2001) describes three areas that postmortem and structural MRI studies have consistently shown to be abnormal in autism: (1) increased brain weight, (2) decreased Purkinje cell number and (3) developmental abnormalities of the inferior olive. Brain weight is one of a number of head and brain measurements that appear to be elevated in autism – others include brain volume and head circumference.[106] Schultz (2001) reports that overall brain size appears to be increased in autism by about 5–10 per cent on average. The magnitude of this size increase tends to diminish with age and amounts to a few percent at most in adolescents and adults with autism. The same cannot be said of head circumference sizes, which have consistently been found to be increased across autistic individuals of all ages (Volkmar et al. 2004). Normally, head circumference is not significantly enlarged at birth and children are usually 3–4 years of age before changes are apparent (MRC 2001). There is also evidence that increases in brain volume may not affect all neural systems and brain regions equally. In this way, studies have reported selective enlargements of individual lobes of the brain and a disproportion in the grey matter to white matter ratio, although findings are not consistent.[107] The neuropathological mechanisms that are responsible for increases in brain volume are not clear at this time but may involve an over-production of cells, which subsequently do not undergo cell death, or a failure of synaptic pruning (MRC 2001). It is also unclear what the functional significance of brain expansion may be. Certainly, variance in brain and head size does not appear to correlate with the severity of autistic symptoms or other measures of disability (Volkmar et al. 2004).

Cerebellar abnormalities have also been reported in studies of autism. There is a significant decrease in the number of Purkinje cells and granule cells in the cerebellum (Bauman and Kemper 1994). In a review of neuropathological literature on autism, Palmen et al. (2004) found a decreased number of Purkinje cells in 21 of 29 studied cases. This decrease probably occurs late in the prenatal period or early in postnatal development, although some loss may be secondary to seizures in individuals with epilepsy (MRC 2001). Other cerebellar abnormalities have also been reported. These include hypoplasia of the cerebellar vermal lobules VI–VII (Carper and Courchesne 2000). However, this particular finding has not been replicated outside Courchesne's laboratory (MRC 2001). Developmental abnormalities of the inferior olive are a common observation in autism. These abnormalities rarely occur in isolation, but are normally found in association with regions of cortical maldevelopment (MRC 2001). In a study of six autistic cases, Kemper and Bauman (1993) found large neurones in the inferior olive in the three youngest subjects who were 9, 10 and 12 years of age. In subjects older than 22 years, these same neurones were small. Kemper and Bauman 'speculate that the unusually large neurons in the inferior olive and cerebellar nuclei in the younger patients and atrophy and loss of these cells in the older individuals may be related to a persistent fetal cerebellar circuit' (1993:182).

One set of neuropathological findings, which has clear functional significance for autistic behaviour, concerns the limbic system. Bristol et al. (1996) remark that '[i]nformation from neuropathology indicates that there may be abnormalities in the amygdala, hippocampus, septum [and] mammillary bodies' (134). Schultz (2001) states that postmortem examination finds 'consistent evidence for abnormalities in size, density, and dendritic arborization of neurons in the limbic system, including the amygdala, hippocampus, septum, anterior cingulate, and mammillary bodies' (985). Bauman and Kemper (2005) report that in the limbic system, 'the hippocampus, amygdala and entorhinal cortex have shown small cell size and increased cell packing density at all ages, suggesting a pattern consistent with development curtailment' (183). Abnormalities of the limbic system, particularly the amygdala, are believed to be responsible for impaired social and emotional functioning in autistic individuals.[108] Grelotti et al. (2002) argue, for example, that amygdala dysfunction disrupts social interest and its correlate, face processing,[109] in individuals with an ASD. fMRI studies of normal subjects suggest a role for the amygdala in tasks involving social perception and cognition. In a study of healthy young adults, Schultz et al. (2003) demonstrate that in addition to the fusiform face area (FFA), the amygdala, temporal pole, medial prefrontal cortex, inferolateral frontal cortex and superior temporal sulci are significantly engaged by a social attribution task (SAT).[110] Schultz (2005) states that 'these data argue for a role of the FFA–amygdala system in social cognition more generally' and that the failure of this system to activate strongly in ASD 'points to a genuine causal mechanism involved in autism' (137).

Genetic influences and neurobiological abnormalities are not the only causal factors that have been discussed in relation to autism. A recent increase in the number of children with ASDs has led investigators to consider the role of immunisations in the aetiology of these disorders. One immunisation in particular, the mumps, measles and rubella (MMR) vaccine, has been the focus of much research, since Wakefield et al. (1998) first reported evidence of ileal-lymphoid-nodular hyperplasia followed by autistic behaviour disorders in 12 children. A number of expert review groups[111] has now considered if there is a causal link between the MMR vaccine and ASDs. One of these groups, the Medical Research Council, concluded that 'the current epidemiological evidence does not support the proposed link of MMR to ASDs' (2001:3).[112] Kaye et al. (2001) found that although the incidence of autism among 2–5-year-olds increased markedly among boys born in each year separately from 1988 to 1993, MMR vaccine coverage was over 95 per cent for successive annual birth cohorts. These data, Kaye et al. conclude, 'provide evidence that no correlation exists between the prevalence of MMR vaccination and the rapid increase in the risk of autism over time' (2001:460).

Viral infections have also been implicated in the aetiology of autism. Ghaziuddin et al. (2002) describe the case of an 11-year-old Asian boy who developed autistic symptoms following an episode of herpes encephalitis. This child continued to show the core deficits of autism at follow-up after three years. These researchers conclude that '[t]his case further supports the role of environmental factors, such as infections, in the etiology of autism' (2002:142). Yamashita et al. (2003) report the cases of two children with symptomatic congenital cytomegalovirus infection who developed typical autistic disorder. With the effective elimination of congenital rubella following the introduction of immunisation, reports of ASDs in the presence of this viral infection have decreased significantly. However, in an earlier study Chess (1977) reports a high rate of autism in a sample of 243 children with congenital rubella. Chess states that '[e]xamination of the data suggested that the rubella virus was the primary etiologic agent' (1977:69). Each of these viral infections affects the central nervous system and so their association with autism is not surprising. However, it is worth remarking that the cases examined by these studies 'were sporadic and rare and hence it is unlikely that these viruses act as triggers for the majority of individuals with ASDs' (MRC 2001:27).

Other environmental factors have been examined with a view to establishing their role in the aetiology of autism. Researchers have investigated exposure to lead and mercury, and carbon monoxide poisoning in pregnancy as possible risk factors for autism. To date, there has been no conclusive evidence to support a causal role for any of these factors in the development of autism. Indeed, in a literature review undertaken in 1999 by the Agency for Toxic Substances and Disease Registry in the US, available data suggested only a 'possible involvement' of chemical exposure in the development of autism. Physiological abnormalities affecting the gastrointestinal tract, sulphation and the serotonin and immune systems have also been investigated but, once again, there is no compelling evidence to support a causal role for these factors in autism. Further research into these abnormalities and other potential causal factors is required.

3.3.2 Clinical Presentation

For an ASD diagnosis to be made, certain behavioural criteria must be satisfied. These criteria capture the core deficits of these disorders, which usually involve some combination of impairments of socialisation, communication and imagination. The problem for clinicians who are involved in diagnosis is that these impairments can present differently in different individuals. Ascertaining the presence of autistic behaviours is complicated by the fact that many ASD individuals also have comorbid medical conditions. Conditions such as intellectual disability, sensory impairments and mental illnesses can all affect the way core autistic deficits are presented and may even serve to mask these deficits. Clinicians must be prepared, therefore, to engage in differential diagnoses and to refer to other agencies and experts when there is doubt about presenting symptoms. A multidisciplinary approach that involves a range of professionals is more likely to result in accurate diagnosis. Certainly, this approach can serve to reduce the likelihood that clinicians will identify behavioural features reflecting their own disciplinary background, while at the same time overlooking other, potentially significant features.[113] This has resulted in misdiagnoses in the past and has caused much distress to both affected individuals and their families, as valuable time is lost pursuing inappropriate intervention or not pursuing intervention at all. It is also the case that disciplines with an interest in ASDs – psychiatry, psychology, language pathology, and so on – are still trying to characterise the deficits that constitute these disorders. It will be seen below, for example, that language pathologists are actively engaged in studies designed to delineate the speech, language and communication features of ASDs. The results from these different disciplinary enquiries will help to establish more refined criteria for diagnosis.

In this section, we consider the clinical manifestations of ASDs in children and adults. Given the number of these disorders, the fact that our knowledge is greatest for two of them (classic autism and Asperger's syndrome) and the communication orientation of the current discussion, we will focus largely on the communication features of autism and Asperger's syndrome in the following paragraphs. However, we will also consider other PDDs – for example, Rett's syndrome – as individuals with these disorders must also undergo communication assessment by speech and language therapists. In the next section, we consider the different tools that are used by clinicians, both to assess ASDs and to obtain information about the nature and extent of particular deficits (e.g. checklists of language and communication skills). We begin with a discussion of the various comorbid conditions that can occur in ASD individuals. Many of these conditions can affect the presentation of autistic symptoms and the appropriateness of communication and other interventions.

3.3.2.1 Comorbid Conditions

In its 2001 review of autism research, the Medical Research Council notes the following comorbid medical conditions in ASD: epilepsy, cerebral palsy, fragile X, tuberous sclerosis, sensory impairments of hearing and vision, Down's syndrome, neurofibromatosis, congenital rubella and phenylketonuria.[114] In addition to sensory loss, Down's syndrome, epilepsy, tuberous sclerosis and fragile X, Jordan et al. (2001) list the following 'associated conditions' in ASD: language disorders, dyspraxia, learning difficulties, Tourette's syndrome, depression and bipolar disorders. Several of these conditions (e.g. fragile X) have been discussed in relation to the aetiology of autism (see section 3.3.1). Other conditions (e.g. Down's syndrome) have been examined at length in earlier contexts. Accordingly, we will describe these disorders very briefly in the present context. Of the remaining conditions, some will be examined thoroughly, as they have implications for language and communication skills in ASD individuals.

There is considerable disagreement in the literature concerning the frequency of each of the above conditions in ASD. In a recent review of epidemiological surveys of autism, Fombonne (2003) reports a median rate for fragile X of 0.3 per cent. This figure, he argues, is most certainly an underestimate, as fragile X was not recognised until relatively recently and screening for this disorder does not always take place. In this same review, median rates of 1.2 per cent and 1.3 per cent were obtained for tuberous sclerosis and visual deficits, respectively. Under an hypothesis of no association, the rate for tuberous sclerosis is about 100 times higher than expected (Fombonne 2003). An association between epilepsy and idiopathic ASDs has been recognised since the late 1960s (MRC 2001). In keeping with other studies that have recorded a high rate of epilepsy in autism, Fombonne reports a median rate for epilepsy of 16.8 per cent. The highest epilepsy rates were observed in those studies with higher rates of severe mental retardation[115] and a higher median age. There were no cases of neurofibromatosis amongst the studies reviewed by Fombonne.

In section 3.3, it was remarked that motor skills are normally intact in individuals with autistic disorder. However, it is frequently observed that subjects with Asperger's syndrome tend to exhibit motor clumsiness. Although this characterisation of these disorders is consistent with current diagnostic systems,[116] it is increasingly being recognised that problems may reside with the motor skills of both ASD groups. Ghazuiddin and Butler (1998) compared the performances of 12 AS subjects, 12 subjects with autistic disorder and 12 subjects with PDD,NOS on a standardised test of motor coordination. Coordination deficits were found in all three groups. Importantly, AS subjects were found to be less impaired than those with autistic disorder and PDD,NOS. However, after adjusting for level of intelligence, there was no longer a significant relationship between motor coordination scores and diagnosis. These researchers suggest that AS children may be less clumsy than children with autistic disorder as a result of their higher level of intelligence. In a simple motor reprogramming task, Rinehart et al. (2001) found that autistic and AS individuals display anomalies in movement preparation but have an intact ability to execute movement. However, the nature of the movement preparation problem differed in the two groups, with AS subjects displaying an atypical deficit in motor preparation, and autistic subjects showing a lack of normal anticipation.[117]

Consistent with these findings of motor deficits in AS and autistic subjects is the finding that some ASD individuals may also present with a motor speech programming disorder. At least one group of researchers proposes that a subgroup of children with ASD can also be characterised by severe developmental verbal dyspraxia (DVD). Gernsbacher and Goldsmith hypothesise that a sizeable minority of minimally verbal or nonverbal persons with ASD may also have DVD.[118] To support this claim, Gernsbacher and Goldsmith point to a number of genetic, neuroimaging and treatment considerations. Further evidence in support of a DVD subtype of ASD derives from a study by Gernsbacher et al. (2002). These researchers conducted structured telephone interviews with the primary caregivers of children with ASD. Interviews contained questions about critical oral–motor and manual–motor behaviours at 6, 12, 18, 24 and 36 months, as well as questions about traditional motor milestones. Forty typically developing (TD) children were matched for age and sex to children in the ASD group. Oral–motor and manual–motor behaviours were chosen for investigation because previous studies had suggested that these behaviours might act as markers of poor speech skills and possible dyspraxia in a subgroup of nonverbal ASD children. Gernsbacher et al. found that individual items from a group of 7 oral–motor and 21 manual–motor markers significantly differentiated the ASD and TD groups. Moreover, these markers were more successful than traditional motor milestones (e.g. walking) and, in some cases, even rivalled classic diagnostic signs (e.g. orienting to name) in distinguishing the two groups. Oral–motor and manual–motor markers predicted later speech in the ASD group, with the strongest prediction achieved when both sets of markers were combined to form composites. Manual–motor markers predicted later speech nearly as well as oral–motor markers. Importantly, Gernsbacher et al. found that these markers (so-called 'dyspraxic' markers) clustered in a subset of perhaps 15 per cent of the ASD children. It was also found that these particular ASD children were overwhelmingly nonverbal.

Several other comorbid medical conditions in ASD also have implications for the communication skills of affected individuals. Fombonne (2003) reports a median rate of hearing deficits in autism of 1.7 per cent. In a study of 199 children and adolescents with autistic disorder, Rosenhall et al. (1999) found mild to moderate hearing loss in 7.9 per cent and unilateral hearing loss in 1.6 per cent of subjects tested. In 3.5 per cent of all cases, pronounced to profound bilateral hearing loss or deafness was diagnosed. This represents a prevalence, Rosenhall et al. argue, that is considerably above that in the general population and which is comparable to the prevalence found in populations with mental retardation. A further 18.0 per cent of the autism group was diagnosed with hyperacusis. (This compares with 0 per cent in an age-matched nonautism comparison group.) The rate of serous otitis media and related conductive hearing loss was 23.5 per cent and 18.3 per cent, respectively. Rosenhall et al. found similar rates of hearing deficits at all levels of intellectual functioning in their subjects. Carvill (2001) remarks that deaf people can demonstrate some features similar to those in autism, although an association between deafness and autism has not been conclusively made.

Mental retardation is a common comorbidity in ASD/PDD. La Malfa et al. (2004) report that nearly 70 per cent of people with PDD also have intellectual disability, while 40 per cent of people with intellectual disability also present with a PDD. (This compares, La Malfa contends, with a prevalence of PDD in the general population of 0.1–0.15 per cent.) The relationship of mental retardation to autism is a complex one. First, autism is more common in subjects with severe to profound mental retardation; also, the severity of autistic symptomatology varies according to the level of mental retardation or learning disability (O'Brien and Pearson 2004). Second, individuals with a dual disability of mental retardation and autism/PDD have poorer social skills and display more maladaptive behaviour than nonautistic mentally retarded subjects. In a review of studies of adaptive behaviour in subjects with a dual disability, Kraijer (2000) found that the performance of individuals with mental retardation and autism/PDD was particularly poor in the domain of social skills and socialisation, and was somewhat less poor in communication, compared with matched nonautistic persons. Performance did not differ across subjects in the domains of self-help and daily living skills, and (gross) motor skills. Autistic mentally retarded subjects were also found to display more maladaptive behaviour. Third, not all types of ASD/PDD exhibit the same pattern or severity of intellectual disability. Differences in intellectual functioning have been used to distinguish ASD/PDD categories. The still uncertain distinction between Asperger's syndrome and high-functioning autism receives support from studies which suggest that persons with AS possess a high verbal IQ and a low performance IQ, whereas in most cases of HFA, this pattern is reversed. One such study is conducted by Ghaziuddin and Mountain-Kimchi (2004), who investigated intellectual functioning in 22 AS subjects and 12 HFA controls. These researchers found that, as a group, AS subjects showed a higher verbal IQ and higher scores on information and vocabulary subtests than those with HFA.

Other comorbid conditions, which have implications for the development of communication in autism, include Down's syndrome and cerebral palsy. In a review of epidemiological surveys, Fombonne (2003) reports a median rate for Down's syndrome in autism of 1.3 per cent. Kent et al. (1999) found a minimum comorbid rate of 7 per cent for ASDs in a study of all children with Down's syndrome in a defined population of south Birmingham, England. As with other comorbid conditions, the presence of Down's syndrome can often make it difficult for clinicians to arrive at a diagnosis of autism. This is demonstrated in a study by Rasmussen et al. (2001), who reported a considerable delay in the diagnosis of autism in 25 DS subjects compared with autistic children who did not have Down's syndrome. Fombonne's (2003) review revealed a median rate for cerebral palsy in autism of 2 per cent. In an epidemiological survey of 325,347 French children, Fombonne et al. (1997) calculated a prevalence rate for cerebral palsy of 2.9 per cent among 174 children in whom autism was identified. Nordin and Gillberg (1996) examined the prevalence of ASDs in children with mental retardation and/or motor disability in a defined geographical region over a two-year period. Among children with cerebral palsy, Nordin and Gillberg found that 10.5 per cent had an ASD. Given these high prevalence rates, clinicians must be aware of how motor impairment can influence the presentation of autistic symptoms.

3.3.2.2 Communication Features

The conditions discussed in section 3.3.2.1, we argued, present clinicians with a diagnostic challenge. This is because each of these conditions can influence how the core behavioural features of autism are presented. In some cases, this has resulted in misdiagnoses, when features of autism are incorrectly attributed to the comorbid condition (e.g. hearing impairment) or when they are masked by the severity of this condition (e.g. mental retardation).[119] In addition to displaying autistic communication features, the autistic child may be dysarthric as a result of cerebral palsy or language impaired on account of fragile X syndrome. Where autistic communication features are particularly subtle, or where an associated communication impairment is severe, a single diagnostic label (e.g. dyspraxia) can come to dominate the entire clinical picture. To the extent that a differential communication diagnosis is possible – and in complicated neurodevelopmental cases, where there are several overlapping disorders, this may not be possible – the speech and language therapist should attempt to assess the contribution of each of these disorders to the child's overall communication impairment. A communication diagnosis that is sensitive to autistic communication features, as well as to any associated communication impairments, is more likely to lead to effective intervention and to successful therapeutic outcomes. The features of associated communication impairments such as dysarthria and dyspraxia have been discussed in other contexts and will not be examined further in the present section. In the rest of this section, we examine the communication deficits that form part of the core symptoms of autism. These deficits are present to varying extents in individuals who have an ASD in the absence of comorbid conditions. However, we must also assume that these same communication deficits are present in autistic individuals who have comorbid conditions, even though the presence of these conditions serves to mask or otherwise distort how these deficits come to be manifested in these complex cases.

Abnormal vocalisation patterns are one of the earliest indications that a child's development may not be proceeding along normal lines. This is no less the case in autism than in other neurodevelopmental disorders. The developmental significance of early vocalisations is recognised by a multidisciplinary Consensus Panel[120] with responsibility for devising practice guidelines for the screening and diagnosis of ASDs. This Panel includes no babbling by 12 months of age amongst its indications for further developmental evaluation.[121] However, studies of the early vocalisation behaviour of autistic infants reveal a more complex situation than that which is captured by simple characterisations such as the presence or absence of babbling. In a study of early vocal behaviours in young children with autism, Sheinkopf et al. (2000) found that autistic children did not have difficulty with the expression of well-formed syllables (i.e. canonical babbling). These children did exhibit, however, significant impairments in vocal quality (i.e. atypical phonation). In specific terms, they produced a greater proportion of syllables with atypical phonation.[122] By observing videotapes of first and second birthday parties, Werner and Dawson (2005) examined communicative, social, affective and repetitive behaviours, as well as toy play, in three groups of children: children with early-onset autism, children who had undergone autistic regression and typically developing children. Interestingly, analyses revealed that children with autistic regression made more frequent use of words and babble than typical infants at 12 months of age. This corresponds to the period before the onset of regression. By contrast, children with early-onset autism displayed fewer of these communicative behaviours at 12 months than either the typically developing children or the children who experienced regression. Wing (1981b) suggests that questions about babbling, which, she observes, may be limited in quantity and quality in infants with Asperger's syndrome, should be asked of parents during the taking of a developmental history.

Atypical early vocalisations foreshadow later problems in speech and language development in autistic children.[123] Speech and language are late to emerge. In a study by Bartak et al. (1975), 58 per cent of autistic children had no single words by 24 months and no phrase speech by 30 months. (It is worth noting that 42 per cent of cases had a diminished or abnormal babble.) If speech and language do develop, problems in both domains are normally evident. In a case study of an 8-year-old autistic boy, Wolk and Edwards (1993) found that stops, nasals and glides were generally present and fricatives, affricates and the liquid /r/ were absent. Several phonological processes (e.g. velar fronting) were observed to persist beyond the expected age and some unusual sound changes (e.g. extensive glottal replacement and segment coalescence) also occurred. There was also evidence of 'chronological mismatch'[124] and restricted use of contrasts in this child's speech. As a result of these phonological processes, process interactions and the use of jargon, the intelligibility of this child's speech was severely reduced. In a study of 30 children with high-functioning autism, Gibbon et al. (2004) found normal articulation in 24 subjects and articulation disorders in six subjects. Amongst these six subjects, disorders ranged from mild to severe. 'Atypical' substitutions accounted for 53 per cent of the errors in this group and these subjects rarely produced errors in the 'almost mature' category. The HFA subjects with normal articulation produced a majority of errors (49 per cent) that were 'almost mature'. None of these children produced more than one 'atypical' substitution.

Articulation errors in the autistic population have also been found to extend into adolescence and beyond. Shriberg et al. (2001) examined speech and prosody characteristics of adolescent and adult subjects with high-functioning autism and Asperger's syndrome. All subjects were in the wide age range 10–50 years. When HFA and AS subjects were compared to typically developing speakers, it was found that significantly more of them had residual articulation distortion errors. It should be emphasised that other studies have failed to find evidence of articulation disorder in the autistic population. Indeed, the widely accepted clinical picture is one in which articulation skills are largely intact compared to other areas of language and communication. In a study of 89 children with autism, for example, Kjelgaard and Tager-Flusberg (2001) concluded that 'among the children with autism there was significant heterogeneity in their language skills, [but] across all the children, articulation skills were spared' (287).

Prosody plays an important role in several communicative functions, one of which is the expression of emotions or the speaker's affective state. The presence of impaired social and emotional functioning in autism has led investigators to enquire if prosodic disturbances[125] might not also feature amongst the communication deficits in this disorder. Within the small body of literature in this area,[126] most studies have examined prosodic expression. The focus of these studies is typically on stress. Shriberg et al. (2001) used the Prosody-Voice Screening Profile to examine stress[127] in male speakers with high-functioning autism and Asperger's syndrome. HFA speakers used appropriate lexical and phrasal stress in 77.3 per cent of utterances and AS speakers in 86.5 per cent of utterances. While both groups of subjects were clearly able to use stress appropriately in the majority of utterances, they still used stress appropriately less often than typically developing subjects (95.2 per cent). Much less investigation has been conducted into prosodic reception in autism.[128] A notable exception is a study by Paul et al. (2005), who examined the production and perception of three prosodic elements (stress, intonation and phrasing) in a group of ASD subjects. Each of these elements was examined in two prosodic functions: a grammatical and a pragmatic/affective function. The performance of 27 ASD subjects (average age = 16.8 years) on a series of prosodic tasks was compared with that of 13 typically developing subjects (average age = 16.7 years). Experimental group subjects consisted of 14 individuals (52 per cent) with a diagnosis of HFA, 10 individuals (37 per cent) with a diagnosis of AS and 3 individuals (11 per cent) with a diagnosis of PDD,NOS. Paul et al. found significant differences between the ASD and typically developing groups in the grammatical production of stress, as well as in the pragmatic/affective perception and production of stress. The difference between the two groups on the grammatical perception of stress also showed a trend toward significance. Ceiling effects on 5 of the 12 tasks used in this study, Paul et al. argue, prevent firm conclusions being drawn about the production and perception of intonation and phrasing in ASD subjects.

The standard view of language impairment in autism is that, although pragmatic deficits are common and constitute a significant barrier to effective communication, structural language is relatively intact. Noens and van Berckelaer-Onnes (2005) remark that '[r]eviews suggest that the development of formal and semantic aspects is relatively spared, whereas pragmatic skills are considered to be specifically impaired' (123). Recent studies, however, are beginning to challenge this standard view. Kjelgaard and Tager-Flusberg (2001) found significant impairments of vocabulary, syntax and semantics in a subgroup of autistic children whose language was defined as borderline or impaired. The pattern of these impairments, combined with other features of the performance of these children[129] (viz. good articulation skills and a difficulty with nonsense word repetition), led Kjelgaard and Tager-Flusberg to conclude that there is a distinct subgroup of autistic children with specific language impairment (SLI): 'Although, by definition, SLI may not be diagnosed in children who meet criteria for autism, in fact, our data suggest that some children with autism may have a parallel or overlapping SLI disorder, as indicated by their pattern of impaired performance on diagnostic language measures' (2001:304).

While structural language impairments have tended to be overlooked in ASD, an area that has attracted considerable clinical and research interest is pragmatics. It is frequently commented that autistic individuals fail to use language in either an appropriate or an effective way in a range of communicative situations. Pragmatic aspects of language that are disordered in ASD include the comprehension and production of speech acts, the use and understanding of nonliteral language and a range of conversational skills (e.g. turn-taking). Speech acts have received relatively little attention in research into pragmatic deficits in autism. Among the studies that have been conducted, some have construed the term 'speech acts' so widely that it is not clear what it is intended to exclude. In a study by Loveland et al. (1988), for example, behaviours as diverse as nonresponses, gesture and vocalisation were classified as types of speech acts. Recent investigations have overcome the classificatory confusion of these earlier enquiries. One study has attempted to relate the speech acts used by autistic individuals to the mental states of these speakers. Ziatas et al. (2003) examined assertive speech acts in autistic children and children with AS. Children with SLI and normally developing children acted as comparison groups. It was found that autistic children used significantly lower proportions of assertions involving explanations and descriptions than the SLI or normally developing children. Autistic children also used significantly lower proportions of assertions involving internal states and explanations than the children with AS. When mental assertions were analysed further, it was found that children with autism and AS referred predominantly to desire and made few references to thought and belief. SLI and normally developing children, however, used a higher proportion of references to thought and belief. Ziatas et al. relate these findings to theory of mind impairments in the autistic children. (For further discussion of theory of mind deficits in autism, the reader is referred to chapter 9 in Cummings (2005).)

Nonliteral language presents autistic individuals with a particular problem of interpretation. To see why this is the case, one need only consider how normal speakers and listeners interpret nonliteral language. To understand when an utterance is being used ironically or to humorous effect, a listener must be able to establish the speaker's communicative intention in producing the utterance. In order to arrive at this intention, a listener must be able to make certain inferences about the belief and other mental states of the speaker. The ability to make inferences about the mental states of others – to have a 'theory' of other 'minds' – is known to be lacking or at least impaired in individuals with autism. One consequence of this impairment in autism is difficulty in the use and understanding of irony and humour in language. Emerich et al. (2003) investigated the ability of adolescents with HFA or AS to comprehend humorous material. Typical subjects and subjects with HFA or AS were required to choose funny endings for cartoons and jokes. Results confirmed the presence of a breakdown in the comprehension of humorous material in autistic subjects. For cartoon and joke tasks combined, adolescents with autism performed significantly more poorly than typical adolescents. Only on the joke task was there a significant difference between autistic adolescents and typical adolescents. On the cartoon task, autistic subjects chose significantly more straightforward endings than other endings. There was no significant difference in the endings chosen on the joke task, but the humorous non sequitur ending was selected most often by autistic adolescents. Both these endings, Emerich et al. remark, are consistent with impairment in cognitive flexibility. It was concluded that the autistic subjects in this study had difficulty with surprise and coherence aspects of humour.

Martin and McDonald (2004) found that individuals with AS performed significantly more poorly than controls on tasks requiring the interpretation of ironic jokes. AS subjects were more likely to conclude that the protagonist in stories was lying rather than telling an ironic joke. A further aim of this study was to test which, if either, of two theories could best explain the pragmatic performance of AS subjects. The two theories in question were weak central coherence (WCC) and theory of mind (TOM). WCC did not appear to be related to pragmatic interpretation. By contrast, second-order TOM reasoning – where the subject is required to indicate what the protagonist believes about the listener's knowledge – was significantly associated with the ability to interpret nonliteral utterances. Martin and McDonald conclude that 'the ability to infer the mental states of others plays a significant role in the interpretation of non-literal language, such as irony, in individuals with AS' (2004:326).

It is widely recognised that autistic children struggle to comprehend the teasing behaviour of other children and cannot use teasing effectively in social interaction. An examination of the skills that are involved in teasing makes it clear why this is the case. The comprehension of teasing requires an ability to understand intention, nonliteral communication, pretence and social context (Heerey et al. 2005). During teasing, the teaser must convey and the recipient decipher conflicting intentions – the teaser's intention to be critical of the recipient and the intention to convey this criticism in a playful and affectionate manner. In order to establish these intentions, the recipient must be able to attribute belief and other mental states to the teaser. We described above how autistic subjects had particular difficulty with this theory of mind skill. Equally, teasing requires mastery of nonliteral communication: 'Much of the playful content of a tease is nonliteral, seen in similes, prosodic variations . . . and grammatical devices . . . that indirectly render the provocation less hostile' (Heerey et al. 2005:56). However, we have just seen how the use and understanding of nonliteral language is compromised in autism. In short, teasing and other aspects of social communication cannot be less impaired than the pragmatic language skills upon which they depend. And these skills, we have seen, represent a significant area of deficit in autistic subjects generally.

Many other aspects of pragmatics have been investigated in recent studies. Some of these studies have produced unexpected findings. Verbosity is included routinely in accounts of communication deficits in AS. Klin and Volkmar (1995) state that some authors view verbosity as one of the most prominent differential features of the disorder. However, Adams et al. (2002) found that children with AS were no more verbose during conversations that differed in emotional content than a control group of children with severe conduct disorder. Verbosity, Adams et al. remark, was 'not a reliable characteristic of the group as a whole' (2002:679). Other studies have revealed previously unacknowledged areas of pragmatic competence in autism. For example, Barry Prizant and various collaborators have demonstrated that echolalia in autism can serve a range of communicative functions. Still other studies are exploring new areas of pragmatic functioning in autism. These investigations include the work of John Richardson and colleagues, who are applying the framework of pragma-dialectics to the study of argumentation in AS (Richardson et al. 2007). For further discussion of pragmatic deficits in autism, the reader is referred to chapter 9 in Cummings (2005).

An autistic child's language abilities also reflect his or her level of intellectual functioning. Kjelgaard and Tager-Flusberg (2001) found a significant relationship between IQ and language abilities, especially as measured by vocabulary tests, across the full range of children in their study. These researchers conclude that 'IQ itself accounts for some of the heterogeneity found in language among children with autism' (2001:301). Vogindroukas et al. (2003) examined semantic errors in children with autism and mild learning disability and in children with mild learning disability only. Very few differences were found between the two groups of children in their ability to name objects, as measured by the Word Finding Vocabulary Test (Renfrew 1995). Both sets of children produced a range of paraphasias (the replacement of a word with an irrelevant one). The autistic children produced more semantic and global paraphasias and did not use underextension, although these differences were not significant. When the name of an object could not be recalled, both groups of children used similar mechanisms (e.g. description) in an effort to name pictures. Although Vogindroukas et al. urge caution in the interpretation of these results on account of the small number of participants in the study (six children were assigned to each group), it is clear that autism is a less significant determinant of semantic skills in these children than learning disability: 'As far as semantics are concerned, according to these preliminary findings, these particular language disabilities shown by children with autism did not seem to be syndrome specific, since similar disabilities were found in the children with mild learning disabilities alone' (Vogindroukas et al. 2003:201).

Language deficits are also evident in other PDDs. According to DSM-IV criteria, a diagnosis of Asperger's syndrome (or disorder) can only be made when there is 'no clinically significant general delay in language'. This delay is defined in relation to language milestones and structural aspects of language, rather than the use of language.[130] However, there is now growing evidence that language development and structural language may not fall within normal limits in AS individuals. In a recent study of adults with HFA and AS, Howlin (2003) reports that 'poor performance on language tests . . . challenges the assumption that early language development in Asperger Syndrome is essentially normal' (3).[131] Koning and Magill-Evans (2001) found significantly lower scores on the receptive subtests of the CELF-R in adolescent boys with AS than in age-matched control subjects. (Seven out of 21 boys with AS had a receptive language score more than 1SD below the mean.) In an attempt to establish if absence of speech delay could be supported as a DSM-IV criterion for AS, Mayes and Calhoun (2001) divided children with clinical diagnoses of autism or AS into two groups: those with and without a significant speech delay. No significant differences were found between children with and without speech delay on any of the 71 variables examined (expressive language being one such variable). Mayes and Calhoun conclude that 'speech delay as a DSM-IV distinction between Asperger's disorder and autism may not be justified' (2001:81).

Language impairments are common in Rett's syndrome (Lavås et al. 2006). These impairments are generally severe in nature and reflect the extent of developmental regression or of any subsequent recovery. Sandberg et al. (2000) studied language and communicative functions in eight young women with disorders in the Rett syndrome complex.[132] At the age of 29 years, one of these women was performing at the same linguistic level that she had reached at the onset of regression at 20 months (i.e. mostly single-word utterances and some two- or three-word combinations). Another subject, who had acquired two single words at the point of developmental arrest at 18 months, regained spoken language at seven years of age and was able to use fully formulated short sentences at assessment (although sometimes function words were omitted and incorrect word order was used). Her performance corresponded roughly to her mental age of 36 months and to results on the PPVT-III and TROG, leading Sandberg et al. to conclude that 'to be able to use speech after regression, subjects with forme fruste RS must function on a developmental level of 30–36 months of age' (2000:262). Comprehension of spoken language was atypical in these two forme fruste cases. (In other subjects, comprehension was limited to one's name, key words or simple sentences with visual or situational support.) Receptive abilities were judged to be commensurate with mental age in one of the subjects and restricted to simple sentences expressed orally in the other subject.[133]

3.3.3 Clinical Assessment

The assessment of communication deficits in ASD presents clinicians with something of a challenge. In high-functioning individuals, pragmatic impairment and language deficits are often subtle and are not always easily identified in a clinical setting. Conceptual confusion has meant that pragmatic phenomena have often been poorly characterised by clinicians and researchers alike (see chapter 9 in Cummings (2005) for further discussion of this point). There is also considerable disagreement amongst investigators concerning the nature and extent of communication deficits in ASD individuals. We described in the last section, for example, how some investigators have failed to find evidence of verbosity in individuals with AS, while other clinicians and researchers view verbosity as a prominent feature of the disorder. Clearly, each of these factors creates difficulties for clinicians, who must assess communication problems in ASD in order to plan effective forms of intervention.

In this section, we examine some of the methods that have been developed for the purpose of assessment. These methods include standardised tests of articulation (e.g. Goldman-Fristoe Test of Articulation) and receptive and expressive language (e.g. Clinical Evaluation of Language Fundamentals). They also include assessments of a child's pragmatic and nonverbal communication skills (e.g. eye gaze[134]). The latter assessments are often performed through the use of checklists (e.g. Children's Communication Checklist) that are completed by parents, teachers and speech and language therapists. Other important components of the assessment process include parental interviews and observation of a child's communication skills during play and other activities. These less structured components of the assessment process are a particularly effective means of obtaining information about communication skills that are beyond the scope of standardised tests. They also provide therapists with some insight into the communication skills and strategies that are used by autistic children in nonclinical contexts.

For many years, clinicians and researchers have used formal assessments to quantify the speech and language abilities of children and adults with a range of communication impairments. The standardised nature of these assessments, their ease of administration and the informativeness of the data that they provide have all helped to establish these tests as the assessment method of choice in many research studies and clinical settings. However, while structural language readily lends itself to analysis by means of formal assessments – syntactic and semantic structures, for example, can be easily tested and quantified – the same cannot be said of pragmatic aspects of language. As a consequence, few formal tools have been developed for the purpose of assessing pragmatics. Where such tools have been developed, some have been shown to be more effective than others in differentiating pragmatic impairment in the ASD population. Recently, Young et al. (2005) investigated if two formal assessment tools could be used to differentiate pragmatic language disorders in children with ASDs from controls matched on verbal IQ and language fundamentals. The tests in question – the Test of Pragmatic Language (TOPL; Phelps-Terasaki and Phelps-Gunn 1992) and the Strong Narrative Assessment Procedure (SNAP; Strong, 1998) – were administered to 34 matched ASD subjects. Results showed that ASD subjects obtained significantly poorer scores than controls on the TOPL. On the SNAP, children with ASDs performed similarly to controls in the areas of syntax, cohesion, story grammar and completeness of episodes. On the ability to answer inferential questions, controls performed significantly better than ASD subjects. Young et al. concluded that while the TOPL was effective in differentiating pragmatic language disorders in children with ASDs, the SNAP was not effective in differentiating these disorders in the two groups in this study.

Formal tools, such as those investigated by Young et al., may well be shown to have a part to play in the assessment of pragmatic language disorder in ASD subjects.[135] Certainly, Young et al. suggest that future research efforts should be directed towards developing 'formal assessment tools that target the unique language disabilities of high-functioning individuals with ASDs' (2005:62). For many clinicians and researchers, however, autistic deficits in the use of language can only be adequately assessed by means of informal methods. These methods include observation of children's communication skills in a range of contexts and discussions with parents and other professionals (e.g. teachers, social workers, etc.). Therapists and others can use these methods to complete checklists of a child's communicative skills. Informal techniques are certainly more time-consuming than formal methods of assessment. Their accuracy also relies to a considerable extent on the observation and reporting skills of other individuals, not all of whom will have the training or expertise necessary to recognise communication problems. However, these methods have a unique advantage over formal assessments in that they permit therapists to observe communication in naturalistic contexts. Pragmatic impairments will be most evident in these contexts. Furthermore, therapists are able to observe nonverbal communication (e.g. gesture), as well as record how children respond to communication breakdown. During observation sessions, therapists are also able to assess the communicative strategies that are adopted by partners involved in conversational exchanges with ASD children. Conversational partners can be important facilitators of communication in ASD individuals (see section 3.3.4). It is thus vital for the planning of intervention that therapists observe the interaction styles of conversational partners and record any strategies used by partners that facilitate or hinder communication in the ASD child or adult.

Communication checklists are increasingly being used by clinicians to assess the pragmatic impairments of ASD children. One such checklist is the Children's Communication Checklist, version 2 (CCC-2)[136] by Bishop (2003). Bishop explains the need for such a checklist as follows: 'The Children's Communication Checklist (CCC) was developed to assess aspects of communicative impairment that are not adequately evaluated by contemporary standardised language tests. These are predominantly pragmatic abnormalities seen in social communication' (1998:879). The test consists of 10 scales in speech, syntax, semantics, coherence, inappropriate initiation, stereotyped language, use of context, nonverbal communication, social relations and interests. Standard scores and percentiles are provided for each of these scales. On the bases of these scales, two composites are derived. The General Communication Composite is used to identify children who are likely to have clinically significant communication problems. The Social Interaction Deviance Composite can assist in identifying children with a communication profile that is characteristic of autism.[137] The 70 items in the checklist are designed to be completed by an adult who has regular contact with the child (e.g. parent, speech and language therapist, psychologist, paediatrician). Parent and professional ratings have been compared and show good internal consistency.[138] Checklist ratings have also been found in studies to be tightly linked to a number of PDD and other diagnoses (e.g. ADHD).[139] The CCC-2 takes 5–15 minutes to complete and is suitable for use with 4–16-year-olds.

Many pragmatic deficits in autistic children are revealed during play activities with peers and adults. By observing the autistic child in play with others, the speech and language therapist can establish if the child initiates communication. This may be attempted by a nonverbal means, which may not be particularly effective – the autistic child's play partner may not understand the behaviour in question and may not view it as an attempt to initiate communication. The autistic child's responses to communication that is initiated by others can also be observed. For example, the autistic child who does not appreciate the two-way nature of communicative exchanges may simply fail to respond, making it less likely that future opportunities for communication will even arise. Play activities are a natural context for the performance of speech acts. The autistic child may need to request a building block or present a challenge to another child during play. By placing a child's favourite toy within view but beyond reach, the therapist can create a natural situation for the elicitation of requests and other speech acts. It is equally important to assess a child's comprehension of speech acts. This can be achieved by examining a child's responses to naturally occurring speech acts during play. Where this approach is unlikely to expose the child to a sufficiently large range of speech acts, the therapist may introduce specific speech acts during play activities. The observation of play also allows therapists to assess the impact of pragmatic impairment on more sophisticated forms of language use (e.g. teasing).

Play is a particularly valuable activity in the assessment of the nonverbal autistic child. Verbal comprehension can be assessed by examining the child's responses to the questions and directives of others. The therapist can use imitative play (e.g. blowing bubbles) to assess oral motor skills. This particular activity also permits the assessment of behaviours that are vital for the development of pragmatic language skills. The therapist can observe, for example, if the child is able to take turns blowing bubbles. The child's response to the cessation of the activity should also be recorded. For example, is the autistic child able to indicate through gesture and vocalisation that he or she wishes play to continue? Or does the child passively resign himself to the termination of the activity? Cognitive abilities that are essential to the development of communication (e.g. joint attention) can also be observed during play with the nonverbal autistic child. Therapists can expect to commit considerable time to this type of communication assessment (one of the drawbacks of this approach). Adams (2002) remarks, for example, that '[a] play-based observation will be lengthy in order to allow opportunities for communicative acts to be demonstrated' (982). Other difficulties associated with this approach include the poor social interaction skills of autistic children, which may preclude all but the most familiar adults from working with the child, and the aberrant nature of play in autism.[140] We will return to play in section 3.3.4, when we come to examine its role in communication intervention.

Many clinicians and researchers, it was argued above, believe that formal tests of pragmatics have a limited contribution to make to the assessment of pragmatic language skills. Formal assessments, they claim, are necessarily restricted in what they can tell us about an individual's level of pragmatic functioning, because most pragmatic phenomena defy the type of description and quantification that is essential to formal testing. However, there is an important sense in which formal assessments of pragmatics are also misleading. Many high-functioning autistic individuals can perform well in a formal test of pragmatics and yet still manifest considerable pragmatic impairment in everyday communicative contexts. Klin et al. (2000) remark that:

> Although a formal assessment of pragmatic skills can be performed for children ages 5 to 13 using the Test of Pragmatic Language (Phelps-Terasaki & Phelps-Gunn, 1992), it is often the case that the performance of the child with [Asperger's syndrome] in such structured testing might be at a higher level than one would observe in a more spontaneous situation. Therefore, even if this battery is used, it is important that an assessment of language in social interaction is conducted in less structured situations. (326)

Once again, only informal methods can fill this assessment niche. During conversation with the high-functioning individual, the therapist can naturally introduce a range of probes to test specific pragmatic skills (e.g. comprehension of indirect requests, idioms, etc.). The successful completion of a task in a formal assessment should not blind the therapist to the possibility that certain skills may not be transferable to everyday communication. For example, the high-functioning individual who can successfully complete the verbal reasoning items in the Test of Pragmatic Language may struggle to compute the inferences that are needed to derive the implicature of an utterance in conversation. The therapist can use a recording of conversation to establish the source of his or her subjective impression that a particular exchange did not flow easily or was difficult to follow and disorganised. Any one of these subjective impressions could arise due to problems with Gricean maxims (e.g. relation, quantity), a lack of cohesive ties (e.g. pronouns) and difficulty with topic maintenance. In order to pursue effective pragmatic intervention, it is important to establish the precise causal mechanism that is responsible for each of these impressions. Many high-functioning individuals enjoy employment opportunities that are denied to more impaired subjects. Employment presents additional communicative challenges for high-functioning clients and increases the settings in which communication skills should be assessed. By speaking to work colleagues, the therapist can establish if the high-functioning client is able to use and recognise indirect and polite forms. Autistic clients must also be aware of the need for shifts in register, in order that a conversational style that is more suitable for use with friends and family does not come to dominate interactions with superiors at work. Many of the contextual variables that influence the choice of language forms and conversational styles are particularly impenetrable to individuals with HFA and AS. Colleagues are often best placed to assess the extent to which problems with these skills are undermining the effectiveness of communication in the work environment. Of course, a work informant can also address many of the same questions that are posed of individuals in other settings. For example, a request for clarification[141] that is misunderstood at work may be successfully addressed at home, where other cues render the speaker's intent transparent to the autistic client. By comparing the responses of several informants to a number of standard questions, the therapist is able to assess if there is significant cross-contextual variation in a client's use and understanding of pragmatic phenomena.

3.3.4 Clinical Intervention

There is no single prescribed technique or programme for use in communication intervention with the ASD population. Rather, the intervention methods used by therapists and teachers are as varied as the communication abilities of ASD individuals in general. For children and adults who are nonverbal or who have severe communication impairment, the establishment of an augmentative or alternative system of communication (AAC) should be the focus of intervention. The Picture Exchange Communication System (PECS) is one such AAC system that has been used successfully with ASD children since it was first developed by Bondy and Frost in the US and introduced to the UK in 1998. We will examine how PECS has been used with ASD clients below. Other communication modalities that have been used with nonverbal ASD clients (e.g. communication boards, voice output communication devices) will also be briefly considered. For the high-functioning autistic client and the individual with AS, combined social and communication skills training is often the intervention method of choice amongst practitioners. There is growing recognition that play can make a valuable contribution to the development of language and communication skills in autism. We review the findings of studies that suggest a beneficial role for play in communication intervention with ASD clients. Finally, none of these approaches to intervention can be effective if the regular conversational partners of ASD clients have not received communication training. Such training has come to assume a core role in many intervention programmes, as practitioners have seen the various communication benefits of it for ASD clients. Below, we examine the main principles that guide the communication training of conversational partners of ASD children and adults.

For many severely impaired autistic clients, verbal communication may not be attainable in either the short or long term. In order to facilitate interaction and the satisfaction of basic needs, some alternative system of communication must be established for these clients. For a significant proportion, this alternative system will be the sole means of communication for the rest of their lives. In the subjects that remain, the alternative system may eventually be displaced by verbal communication or may continue to be used to augment verbal communication skills. The selection of an appropriate alternative communication system can only be made after an extensive consultation process that involves family members, speech and language therapists and other professionals (e.g. occupational therapists). This process will seek to establish the client's communication needs, topics of interest to the client, the contexts in which communication takes place and the client's significant conversational partners. It will also include discussion of the client's skills and deficits and of how each is likely to influence the choice of AAC system. Particularly significant deficits include sensory impairments (e.g. vision and hearing), physical disabilities (e.g. limb dyspraxia), language impairments and a range of cognitive problems (e.g. memory, perception). Portability of the system is also an important consideration for the ASD individual with no physical disability who moves between settings (e.g. home, school, hospital). The system must also be readily acquired. In the ASD client with learning disability, this particular constraint on the choice of system may also be the most important one. In short, the chosen AAC system must be one that best meets the ASD client's communication needs, whilst mitigating the effects of factors such as impairments that present a barrier to effective communication.

For many teachers and therapists, PECS is the alternative communication modality that most successfully accommodates the different considerations described above. This system was developed for children with ASDs who have limited or no functional communication skills. Pictures or symbols are used to teach spontaneous communication skills in a social context. PECS employs teaching based on behavioural principles and there is particular emphasis on prompting and reinforcement techniques. Unlike other alternative communication systems, PECS requires few prerequisite skills such as joint attention, imitation or eye contact, all of which are lacking or impaired in ASD clients. PECS also differs from other systems in that children are encouraged to develop spontaneous initiation of communication. The teaching of the system is organised around six structured and hierarchical levels. At the simplest level, children are taught how to make requests by exchanging a single picture or symbol for a desired object. At the most complex level, children learn how to comment in response to a question – for example, to respond to questions like 'What do you have/see or hear?' with symbols for 'I see', 'I have' or 'I hear', and to discriminate between these questions and 'What do you want?' questions.

Recent studies have examined the effectiveness of PECS in ASD children. Improvements have been observed in several domains, including speech, language complexity and social-communicative behaviours. At the same time, studies have also reported decreases in problem behaviours and nonword vocalisations. Kravits et al. (2002) examined the effects of PECS on the spontaneous communication skills and social interaction of a six-year-old girl with autism. Both home and school environments were included in this study. These environments involved leisure and snack time in the child's home and journal time (writing/colouring in notebooks followed by play) and centre activities (free play) at school. Increases were observed in spontaneous language (i.e. requests and comments) including use of icons and verbalisations in those settings in which PECS was implemented. In two of three settings (home and journal time), intelligible verbalisations increased, while changes were observed in peer social interaction in one of the two school settings (journal time). Ganz and Simpson (2004) examined the impact of the use of PECS on the communication skills of three young children with ASD and developmental delays with related characteristics. This study aimed to establish if PECS could improve the number of words spoken, increase the complexity and length of phrases, and decrease nonword vocalisations in these children. Subjects were taught Phases 1–4 of PECS (i.e. picture exchange, increased distance, picture discrimination and sentence construction). It was found that the ASD children in this study mastered PECS rapidly and that the number of words and complexity of grammar in utterances increased. Charlop-Christy et al. (2002) examined the acquisition of PECS in three children with autism and the effects of PECS training on speech emergence in play and academic settings. These investigators also recorded ancillary measures of social-communicative and problem behaviours. Results revealed that all three children met the learning criterion for PECS and displayed concomitant increases in verbal speech. Increases in social-communicative behaviours and decreases in problem behaviours were also observed to occur.

Infrequent and unskilled use of AAC systems by communicative partners is one of the most commonly cited reasons why children fail to acquire such systems. Conversely, partners that have been trained in the use of a particular AAC system are well equipped to facilitate a child's acquisition and use of that system. This has been clearly demonstrated in the case of PECS in a study by Magiati and Howlin (2003). These researchers examined the effects of PECS training of teaching staff on the use of PECS, spontaneous communication and adaptive behaviour of 34 children with ASDs (29 boys and 5 girls). In total, 14 teachers, 22 teaching assistants, 10 care staff and one speech and language therapist undertook training, which consisted of a two-day PECS workshop and six half-day visits from PECS consultants. The level of PECS attained by the children, their PECS vocabulary and the frequency of PECS use all showed significant increases over time. The greatest improvements occurred very soon after the implementation of training, with steady but somewhat smaller increases occurring after this time. Changes in the children's general level of communication were slower and less marked. On the Wetherby and Prizant communication checklist, the average rating rose from just below 6 (i.e. giving/pointing/using pictures to indicate needs) to a mean of over 7 (i.e. using single words or echoed words to communicate). Increases in children's use of signing only just reached significance and there was a small but significant increase in children's single-word vocabulary. There was a small but statistically significant decrease in the children's scores on the communication sub-scale of the Rimland Autism Treatment Evaluation Checklist, indicating an improvement in communication. Finally, an overall improvement occurred in problem behaviours, but there were no significant changes in scores for sociability or maladaptive behaviour.

Other forms of AAC have been successfully used by ASD children and adults. This is true even in severely impaired cases. For example, von Tetzchner et al. (2004) describe the use of a graphic-mode communication intervention[142] in the treatment of a girl with intellectual impairment and autism who lacked comprehension of spoken language. Vocabulary selected for teaching reflected the girl's interests, preferences, activities and routines. In the absence of comprehension of spoken instructions, nonlanguage cues were used to teach the meaning of graphic vocabulary. Through this teaching method, the girl acquired an active use of over 80 photographs and pictograms, even though her comprehension (and hence use) of spoken language had been lacking over a three-year period. AAC intervention in autism must also address the problem of how to transfer clinically acquired skills to the many other settings in which an AAC system may need to be used. Sigafoos et al. (2004) assessed transfer of AAC skills to the home setting in a 12-year-old male with autism. This boy was taught how to use a voice-output communication device during an initial clinical trial. After learning how to use the device in this context to request access to preferred objects, intervention was transferred to home. The parent was followed up by e-mail and telephone and the child's progress was monitored by examining videotapes of initial home-based sessions. The approach employed in this study was successful in teaching the autistic child to use a portable AAC device to make requests, first in a clinical trial and then in two home-based activities.

Training of conversational partners is a core component of communication intervention in autism. There is a particular imperative for this training to take place if the autistic child is an AAC user, but the partners of verbal children must also receive instruction and guidance. One of the key objectives of training is to raise awareness in partners of the barriers to effective communication with the autistic child and of the strategies that can be implemented to facilitate communication. Where the child is an AAC user, a lack of familiarity with a particular AAC system or its unskilled use by a partner may negatively impact on the communication experiences of the autistic child. However, often it is the more mundane conversational behaviours of partners that contribute most to communication failure in autistic children. Even minor changes in these behaviours have been shown to bring about significant communication gains in autistic children. Light et al. (1998) studied partner behaviours that facilitated or hindered communication in a six-year-old autistic boy called Josh who was an AAC user. Observational data revealed that Josh responded to 0/17 spoken messages when partners did not secure his attention before speaking to him. Josh responded best when spoken input had simple content and form and was augmented by writing, typing and/or gestures. Although Josh needed 15–20 seconds to respond to a partner's instruction or question, observational data showed that partners typically only allowed him 2–3 seconds to make a response before they began to recode their question or comment. As is often the case with AAC users, Josh was a largely passive communicator. This was demonstrated by a lack of communicative initiation on Josh's part and by his tendency to take only obligatory turns (and even then, not all of them). Light et al. (1998) found that in over eight hours of interaction, Josh produced only 16 initiations. He took 68 per cent of his obligatory turns and only 10 per cent of his nonobligatory turns.

Based on the above findings, it seems clear that any intervention programme targeting Josh's communicative partners should at least aim to make them aware of the following facilitative strategies: (1) secure Josh's attention before providing instructions or asking a question, (2) when presenting instructions or asking questions, use simple sentence structures, (3) to augment spoken language input, use writing or typing on Josh's Powerbook and (4) allow Josh at least 15–20 seconds to produce a response after asking him a question or providing him with instructions. Instruction of Josh's parents and teachers was organised according to the following procedures, reproduced here from Light et al. (1998:173): (1) describe the support (the target interaction strategies) required by the individual who uses AAC; (2) discuss the impact of these strategies; (3) demonstrate the target strategies; (4) encourage facilitators to practise the strategies in role plays; (5) encourage the facilitators to use the strategies in interactions with the individual; (6) provide feedback on the facilitators' performance; (7) practise until facilitators consistently use the strategy at criterion level (e.g. 90 per cent) in their daily interactions; (8) check for generalisation to a wide range of interactions; (9) evaluate the individual's and facilitators' satisfaction with the instruction and its outcomes; and (10) conduct maintenance checks to ensure continued use of the strategies post instruction. As a result of these procedures, Josh's partners at follow-up nearly two years after initial AAC assessment were routinely obtaining his attention before speaking to him. They augmented complex spoken input by using sentence strips (for classroom instructions) or by typing on Josh's Powerbook (for individual instructions). Josh's partners also consistently provided him with more time to communicate.

Although the above procedures relate to partner training in the case of an autistic child who is an AAC user, they embody a number of general principles that are equally applicable to the training of partners of verbal autistic children. Like the partners of the AAC user, the partners of the verbal child may exhibit a tendency to dominate communication through selection of topics, relentless questioning and other behaviours. Partners may also determine the duration of communication by deciding when to terminate a particular exchange with the child. Unwittingly, partners may also limit the autistic child's opportunities for communication by speaking on the child's behalf or avoiding social situations. Each of these behaviours must be addressed directly during partner training. As a first step, partners need to be made aware of how their behaviour is impacting negatively on the autistic child's communication. Video recordings of partner-child interactions are particularly effective in raising partners' awareness of the habitual behaviours that are detrimental to communication in the autistic child. Having identified these behaviours, partners can then set about modifying them under the guidance of a speech and language therapist. For example, rather than dominating exchanges in the ways outlined above, partners can be taught techniques to encourage greater conversational participation on the part of the child. These techniques may involve the use of open as opposed to closed questions, the creation of situations in which the child is compelled to make requests and express choices, and the use of cueing strategies when a child fails to respond or produces an inadequate response. At first, the therapist can demonstrate these techniques in isolation. Video recordings showing the therapist using these techniques with the child in question or with other autistic children can also be particularly helpful at this stage. The focus of training, however, should very quickly turn to the partner's proficient use of these techniques in communication with the autistic child. At this stage, feedback from a therapist who has directly observed partner-child interactions or who has analysed a video recording of these interactions is integral to the success of partner training. Feedback can assist partners in monitoring and improving their use of target techniques and strategies. It also has an important role to play in motivating partners, who are more likely to continue using specific techniques if they can be shown to produce communication gains in autistic children. Ongoing feedback is also essential if partners are to be successful in transferring modified communication behaviours to other nonclinical contexts. Of course, time and resources permitting, significant conversational partners of the child in these other contexts should also receive communication training.

The communication needs of children and adults with HFA or AS have often been overlooked by professionals. A traditional emphasis on structural language skills explains at least part of this neglect – because these children and adults exhibit few problems with phonology, syntax and semantics, their language and communication problems are somehow judged to be less severe than those of individuals with deficits in these areas. However, an even more significant cause of this neglect is the fact that few therapists and other professionals feel equipped to treat communication problems in individuals with significant social disabilities.[143] This lack of practical expertise is reflected in the relatively small number of training packages that have been developed for use with high-functioning individuals. Moreover, many of the social and communication skills packages that have been developed have yet to be properly evaluated or have failed to lead to generalised improvements in target skills. (For example, training based on theory of mind principles has led to improvement in children's performance on experimental tasks, but not in general social and communication competence.) Given their knowledge of conversation and pragmatics, it seems clear that speech and language therapists will be integral to future efforts to develop and implement intervention programmes for use with high-functioning autistic clients:

> the professionals who would appear to be at the greatest advantage to play the central role in this area are speech and language therapists with a special interest in pragmatics or conversational skills, although other mental health or educational professionals could certainly be equally proficient. (Klin and Volkmar 2000:351)

Below, we examine the main components of such a programme.

Any social and communication skills training programme should aim to raise the autistic individual's metalinguistic awareness of the skills that underpin effective communication. Individuals with HFA or AS have the requisite cognitive and language abilities to reflect on the features of good and bad conversation and to discuss the cause(s) of communication failure. This is most effectively achieved in small group work with other high-level subjects, although individual sessions may also be required initially to establish target behaviours and to review progress at regular intervals during intervention. Group sessions permit an exchange of ideas about the interpretation of a video-recorded behaviour or situation. They also enable the autistic client to rehearse problematic social situations before tackling them in real, and potentially more threatening, contexts. The activities pursued during intervention will vary with the age and abilities of the clients in this group. For the older client, it may well be appropriate to rehearse the social and communicative strategies that will be needed in an interview; for the adolescent client, it may be more important to concentrate on developing topics of conversation that are of interest to a peer. (This is often a particular problem for the high-functioning individual, whose restricted interests lead to conversations on topics that fail to engage same-age conversational partners.) Even activities contained in published training packages must be assessed for suitability against the skills and deficits of individual clients. For example, Hodgdon (1995, 1996) proposes the use of visual tools and resources to help the autistic child communicate more effectively and to understand the communication demands of the surrounding social environment better. However, many of these activities will not be appropriate for the autistic child with poor visual-spatial processing skills.[144] In what follows, we discuss the skills and behaviours that should be targeted during social and communication skills training with the high-functioning client. For discussion of techniques and activities that may be used for this purpose, the reader should consult more practically oriented texts.

The implicit knowledge that normal speakers use in conversation and social interaction with others must be explicitly taught to high-functioning subjects. This knowledge can be broadly classified as (1) knowledge of the structure of conversation, (2) knowledge of the mental states of other participants in conversation and interaction, and (3) knowledge of whether the subject's own conversational and social performance conforms to typical conversational structure on the one hand and the expectations (mental states) of other participants on the other hand. We examine each type of knowledge in turn and consider the various skills and behaviours that draw upon this knowledge. Discussion of the structure of conversation should emphasise the reciprocal nature of communicative exchanges. This reciprocity is embodied first and foremost in the turn-taking structure of conversation. However, it is also reflected in our commonsense assumptions about conversation: for example, that conversation should involve a mutual exchange of interests and opinions, that all participants should have equal opportunity to contribute topics for discussion and so on. For many autistic individuals, these assumptions are not commonsense and they must, therefore, be made explicit and examined. Notions like reciprocity (or user-friendly, 'two-way communication') can form themes for group discussions with high-functioning clients. Clients can be encouraged to view video recordings of conversation and to compile lists of behaviours that are facilitative or obstructive of reciprocity in conversation. Where a particular behaviour is judged to be unacceptable, the group should discuss how the behaviour in question limits the reciprocity of the exchange. For example, the verbose speaker who violates the maxim of quantity is effectively denying other participants their turn in conversation. Of course, once clients are made aware of problematic behaviours in conversation, they must eventually come to apply this newly acquired knowledge to their own use of conversation. This requires clients to assume a critical stance on their own conversational performance. This can be achieved initially by the client and therapist jointly viewing video recordings of the client in conversation with others – by pausing the recording, specific behaviours that are detrimental to the reciprocity of the exchange can be identified. Eventually, however, the aim should be for the client to establish effective self-monitoring of conversational behaviour in real time. Other conversational themes (e.g. appropriateness) can undergo the same reflective and critical processes outlined here for reciprocity.

Even if the autistic client is successful in acquiring certain 'rules' of conversation, these rules can only be successfully applied in conversation if they are grounded in knowledge of the mental states of other participants. A fundamental problem for autistic subjects is that they fail to regard behaviours that are readily understood by normal speakers as revealing anything about the mental states of the subjects that produce them. These behaviours include facial expressions, gestures and prosodic features of speech (e.g. stress), to name but a few. Such linguistic and paralinguistic behaviours serve as cues to the mental states of speakers for normal subjects but are often overlooked or misunderstood by autistic subjects. In this way, nonautistic individuals can readily detect from the facial expression of an addressee that a change of topic or the termination of a conversation is desired. The autistic client may overlook this same nonverbal cue and may continue to talk about a topic that is no longer of interest to other participants in the conversation. While normal speakers can make intuitive judgements about the meaning of such cues, autistic clients must be explicitly taught the significance of these cues for the development of a conversational exchange or social interaction.[145] A range of techniques can be used for this purpose. By viewing and pausing video recordings of conversational exchanges, specific visual cues can be emphasised and their significance for the interpretation of those exchanges discussed. Autistic clients should also receive instruction in the use of these cues to signal their own emotional and mental states. The client who is unable to use eye contact appropriately, for example, may be negatively evaluated by conversational partners, who may regard this behaviour as indicating a lack of interest in, or even hostility towards others. By rehearsing social situations such as greeting familiar and unfamiliar people, autistic clients can learn to make more accurate and consistent use of social cues such as eye contact. They can also acquire an understanding of how factors such as setting, social distance of speakers and so on can influence the use of language forms and paralinguistic behaviours in those situations. The client's monitoring of his or her verbal and nonverbal behaviour during these exercises may be aided initially by examination of video recordings of practice sessions. Problematic behaviours such as excessive speaking volume and inappropriate body proximity may be drawn to the attention of the client and can form the focus of future exercises. Eventually, the client should be able to independently monitor his or her use of social cues across a range of contexts.

Play-based interventions are increasingly being used to stimulate language development and communication in autistic children. The effectiveness of play as an intervention technique has recently been demonstrated in a number of studies. Schuler (2003) reported language and communication gains in a nine-year-old autistic girl called Teresa who participated in adult-facilitated peer play. Teresa took part in play groups, which occurred twice weekly for 30 minutes. Prior to her participation in these groups, Teresa's speech consisted of immediate but mostly delayed echolalic utterances that were frequently repeated in a ritualised fashion. Within the first six months of her play group experiences, Teresa was using a greater variety of linguistic forms and functions, including socially referenced communication and self-regulatory language use. Kok et al. (2002) examined the effect of structured and facilitated play conditions in promoting spontaneity and responsiveness in communication in eight children with autism (mean chronological age = 64.1 months). In general, there was an increase in appropriate communication after the implementation of these play conditions. Six of the children showed more appropriate communicative responses in the structured play conditions. Three subjects displayed more appropriate initiations in the facilitated play conditions compared with the structured play conditions. Also in the structured play conditions, three participants showed more inappropriate responses. Bernard-Opitz et al. (2004) compared traditional behavioural approaches and natural play interventions for young children with autism. Eight children, who were aged between 28 and 44 months, received five weeks of training in each of the two conditions (10 weeks' training in total). Improvements in play, attention, compliance and communication were observed in both intervention procedures. Communication gains were also confirmed by video data of the child's interaction with the clinician and the parent. Of four verbal children, three increased the percentage of responsive and spontaneous communication. When pre-post changes across interaction partners and conditions were examined, it was found that improvements in verbal communication of 55 per cent, 45 per cent and 20 per cent occurred in three children. During intervention, a previously nonverbal child began to talk.

Play is also being used to address the sensory processing problems that are experienced by autistic children. Mistry et al. (2004) describe the use of play activities in a summer school for children with ASD. The school was a bidisciplinary project involving occupational therapists and speech and language therapists. All the children who attended were known to occupational therapy services, mainly for sensory processing difficulties. Amongst other activities (e.g. the use of PECS), intervention included structured messy play sessions that were designed to provide the children with an intense tactile experience.

Although it was not possible to measure improvements in sensory integration during a week-long summer school, therapists were able to establish if improvements had occurred in the organisation of behaviour, attention control and participation in sensory activities. Improvement could also be indicated by whether a reduction had occurred in the level of sensory input that was provided by occupational therapists to the children (e.g. proprioception, vibration and tactile desensitisation through deep pressure). Amongst a number of sensory improvements recorded, it was observed that two children who were initially identified as tactile-defensive had been able to progress to free exploration of dry textures.

Notes

1. Mental health clinicians have defined four degrees of severity of mental retardation or learning disability based on IQ score. These are mild learning disability (IQ range 50–55 to about 70), moderate (IQ range 35–40 to 50–55), severe (IQ range 20–25 to 35–40), and profound (IQ level below 20–25). Mild learning disability accounts for some 85 per cent of cases. Approximately 10 per cent of learning disabled cases have a moderate impairment. Severe and profound learning disability account for 3–4 per cent and 1–2 per cent of learning-disabled cases, respectively.
2. Founded in 1946, Mencap is the leading UK charity working with children and adults with a learning disability and their families and carers.
3. One of the main characteristics of Prader-Willi syndrome is a voracious appetite, which can lead to morbid obesity if it is not adequately controlled. Early severe hypotonia can cause articulation problems, feeding difficulties and hypernasality due to velopharyngeal insufficiency. Language, particularly expressive language, is generally delayed. Severe hypotonia can make the initial signs of language delay and cognitive impairment appear worse than they really are. After early delay, considerable gains can be made in both language and intellectual development (Shprintzen 2000).
4. Williams syndrome (WS) is caused by an interstitial deletion from the long arm of chromosome 7 that encompasses the elastin gene, ELN. Articulation skills are good in many cases. However, articulation may be slurred and speech rate is often rapid (Shprintzen 2000). Problems in the social use of language contrast with strengths in lexical and morphosyntactic domains. Expressive language skills generally exceed verbal comprehension abilities. WS individuals often echo phrases and sentences spoken by their interlocutor in the absence of their comprehension (echolalia) (Rondal and Edwards 1997). Also see note 51 in this chapter.
5. Down's syndrome is the result of an extra chromosome 21, which is found in all cells (trisomy 21) or in only some cells (mosaic), or which is attached to another chromosome (translocation). Trisomy 21 is the most common form of Down's

syndrome, affecting 94 per cent of cases. Translocation and mosaic forms of Down's syndrome account for 4 per cent and 2 per cent of cases, respectively.

6. Cri du chat syndrome is so called because crying in the affected infant resembles the cry of a cat. This is not related to structural anomalies in the larynx. This syndrome has an estimated population prevalence of 1 in 50,000. The severe mental retardation that occurs in this syndrome precludes the development of communication in most cases. The majority of individuals with cri du chat do not develop speech. Where cleft lip and palate also occurs, communication is further impaired. Cleft lip and palate and hypotonia complicate early feeding. Typically, language fails to develop or is very severely impaired (Shprintzen 2000).

7. Angelman's syndrome and Prader-Willi syndrome both involve the deletion of the long arm of chromosome 15. However, in Angelman's syndrome the deletion occurs in the maternal chromosome, while in Prader-Willi syndrome the deletion involves the paternal chromosome. Angelman's syndrome also occurs if there is a deleted segment on the maternal chromosome 15 and two such segments on the paternal chromosome 15 (paternal uniparental disomy). Similarly, Prader-Willi syndrome can be caused by maternal uniparental disomy. Despite involving the same chromosome deletion, Prader-Willi syndrome and Angelman's syndrome have very different phenotypes. Individuals with Prader-Willi syndrome develop speech and language, while those with Angelman's syndrome do not (Shprintzen 2000).

8. In addition to mental retardation, tuberous sclerosis is associated with seizures, distinctive skin lesions, benign, tumour-like nodules (hamartomas) of the brain and other organs, and cyst-like areas within certain skeletal regions. Tuberous sclerosis may arise spontaneously for unknown reasons or it may be inherited as an autosomal dominant trait. The gene mutations that cause tuberous sclerosis are gene TSC1 on the long arm of chromosome 9 and TSC2 on the short arm of chromosome 16.

9. Phenylketonuria (PKU) has a prevalence of approximately 1 in 10,000 live births (Sebastian 2002). PKU is caused by mutations of the PAH gene (phenylalanine hydroxylase) on chromosome 12. Phenylalanine hydroxylase is an enzyme that converts the amino acid phenylalanine in the diet to the amino acid tyrosine during phenylalanine metabolism. In the absence of this enzyme's activity, phenylalanine builds up in the bloodstream, causing hyperphenylalaninaemia and brain damage.

10. The last US rubella epidemic occurred in 1964–5. Since the introduction of a rubella vaccination programme in 1969, rubella incidence has rapidly declined in the US. In 2002, an annual total of 18 rubella cases was reported. There has been a similar decline in the number of congenital rubella syndrome (CRS) cases. From a figure of 67 cases in 1970, the number of CRS cases has fallen to an average of 5–6 annually since 1980 (CDC, National Immunization Program).

11. The meningococcus causes two types of illness: meningitis (inflammation of the meninges) and septicaemia (blood poisoning by meningococci). The fatality rate of meningococcal septicaemia is 10 times that of meningococcal meningitis (National Meningitis Trust 1996). The combined case fatality rate for both meningococcal meningitis and septicaemia has varied little in the UK between 1991 and 1995, ranging from 12.2 per cent in 1991 to 10.1 per cent in 1995 (Stuart 1996).

12. The term foetal alcohol effects (FAE) has been used to describe children who have all the clinical signs of FAS, but at mild or less severe levels. In 1996, the Institute of Medicine in the US replaced FAE with the terms alcohol-related neuro-developmental disorder (ARND) and alcohol-related birth defects (ARBD). Individuals with ARND have functional or mental impairments that are related to alcohol exposure. These impairments include behavioural problems (e.g. poor impulse control) and/or cognitive abnormalities (e.g. learning difficulties, memory and attention deficits). Children with ARBD have problems affecting the heart, kidneys, bones and/or hearing.

13. This meeting was held in March 2004 and was convened by the Department of Health and Human Services and the CDC.

14. Hawley et al. (2004) found that 10–18 per cent of children with mild head injury presented with frequent behavioural, emotional, memory and attention problems when they were followed up on average at 2.2 years post-injury. This figure increased considerably among children who were severely and moderately injured. Hawley et al. found that one third of their severe group and one quarter of their moderate group exhibited frequent behavioural, emotional, memory and attention problems. Importantly, Hawley et al. found no evidence that there was a level of injury severity below which the risk of late sequelae could be safely discounted. In another study, McKinlay et al. (2002) observed long-term psychosocial deficits in children who had sustained a mild head injury before the age of 10. These authors remark that 'the view that all mild head injuries in children are benign events requires revision and more objective measures are required to identify cases at risk' (281).

15. According to the United States Cancer Statistics for 2001, the incidence rate of ALL for the age group 0–19 years was 3.1 per 100,000 persons. The second most common form of cancer was tumours of the brain and nervous system, which had an incidence rate of 2.8 per 100,000 persons. Excluding combined leukaemia deaths, brain and nervous system cancers were the most common cause of death related to cancer (0.6 per 100,000 persons), with deaths from ALL the second most common cause (0.4 per 100,000 persons).

16. The United States Cancer Statistics indicate that, in 2001, the incidence rates for astrocytomas, primitive neuroectodermal tumours (which include medulloblastomas) and ependymomas in the 0–19 age group were 13.4, 5.4 and 2.2 per one million persons, repsectively.

17. Boring et al. (1991) report that survival rates for children with brain and nervous system tumours in the US have shown considerable improvement, from 35 per cent during 1960–3 to 59 per cent during 1981–6. Other studies suggest that there has been little improvement in survival rates in recent decades. Jenkin (1996) examined outcomes for 1,034 children who received radiation treatment in the management of a brain tumour at the University of Toronto Institutions from 1958 to 1995. It was concluded that 'despite improvements in imaging, neuro-surgical technique, and radiation treatment, children treated during the last 20 years did not have a significantly improved outcome when compared to children treated earlier' (Jenkin 1996:715).

18. Murdoch et al. (1999) remark that 'it is also important that health professionals and parents are aware that, although a child treated for cancer with radiotherapy might have an intelligence quotient (IQ) that falls within the average range, their IQ post-treatment may actually be significantly below the pre-treatment level' (28).

19. Chemotherapy may be used as CNS prophylaxis (in the case of ALL, for example) or as an initial treatment to reduce the size of a large tumour. It may also be administered after an intracranial tumour has been removed from an infant, in order to reduce the risk of metastatic spread and to control the growth of residual or recurrent tumours until such time as a child is considered old enough to undergo radiotherapy. High-grade tumours may warrant the use of combined radiochemotherapy, as has been advocated in the treatment of medulloblastomas. Chemotherapy may be reserved for the treatment of recurrent disease or as a form of palliative therapy when it is clear that further intervention is unlikely to be successful (Murdoch et al. 1999).

20. The three main structural changes that occur in the brain of ALL patients who undergo CNS prophylaxis are leukoencephalopathy (destruction of white matter), cortical atrophy (wasting of the cortex's grey matter) and microangiopathy (calcification of cerebral blood vessels).

21. Dubowitz's syndrome is a rare genetic syndrome that has an autosomal recessive pattern of inheritance. The gene responsible for this syndrome has not yet been mapped or identified (Shprintzen 2000). Cognitive impairment may be variable, ranging from normal intellect to severe mental retardation. Other features associated with this syndrome include low birth weight and postnatal growth retardation, microcephaly, hoarse cry, small facies, shallow nasal bridge, telecanthus, ptosis and micrognathia. Speech, voice and resonance can be compromised in this syndrome.

22. In a study of 28 subjects with Opitz–Frias syndrome, Wilson and Oliver (1988) identified oesophageal dysmotility in 69 per cent of cases. Laryngotracheal clefts were identified in 44 per cent of cases, cleft palate or bifid uvula occurred in 34 per cent, and mental retardation was present in 38 per cent of subjects. Twenty-three of these subjects were published cases who had dysphagia.

23. The pharyngeal phase of swallowing is disrupted most by the presence of a tracheotomy tube. Specific problems include a delayed swallow response, a lack of superior excursion of the entire larynx in the neck, especially the arytenoids and epiglottis (the tracheotomy tube mechanically fixates the larynx in the neck), delayed closure of the laryngeal vestibule leading to laryngeal penetration and closure of the larynx that is delayed until after the upper oesophageal sphincter has relaxed. Pressure transmitted from a cuffed tracheotomy tube to the oesophagus can also interfere with swallowing. An inability to generate intrathoracic pressure can result in a blunted or absent cough reflex when a tracheotomy tube is in position (Arvedson and Brodsky 2002).

24. 'Gastroesophageal reflux also is relatively common and may become evident following placement of a gastrostomy tube in a child with a head injury or any other kind of neurologic impairment' (Arvedson and Brodsky 2002:446).

25. Both static and progressive forms of encephalopathy have responded well to the use of highly active antiretroviral therapy (HAART) since it was first introduced in 1996. The AIDS Institute of the New York State Department of Health estimates that HAART has reduced the rates of progressive encephalopathy found in clinical practice to approximately 5–10 per cent.

26. Epstein et al. (1986) described progressive encephalopathy in 36 children with HIV infection. Progressive encephalopathy developed in 16 of 21 children with AIDS, 3 of 12 children with AIDS-related complex and 1 of 3 asymptomatic seropositive children. The presence of progressive encephalopathy correlated with a poor, usually fatal, outcome. The incubation period from initial HIV infection in the perinatal period to the onset of progressive encephalopathy varied from two months to five years. Progressive encephalopathy was found to be the result of primary and persistent infection of the brain with this retrovirus.

27. Andy presented at three months with oral and oesophageal candidiasis and failure to thrive. Davis–McFarland also attributes feeding problems in children with HIV infection to xerostomia (dry mouth), which is a side effect of some medications.

28. In HIV encephalopathy, three patterns of cerebral atrophy have been identified through CT or MRI: (1) ventriculomegaly, which is out of proportion to the degree of cortical atrophy, (2) generalised atrophy and (3) necrotising encephalopathy with an associated cardiomyopathy (Jeanes and Owens 2002).

29. In a study of 12 women who consumed ethanol (alcohol) in orange juice prior to breast feeding their infants, Mennella and Beauchamp (1991) found that infants consumed between 0.5 and 3.3 per cent (mean, 1.7 ± 0.3 per cent) of the maternal alcohol dose.

30. All 21 children studied by Cornwell et al. (2003a) had their tumour pathology confirmed following surgery. Eleven children had medulloblastoma, 8 had astrocytoma and 2 had ependymoma. Treatment involved surgery alone in 8 subjects, surgery and radiotherapy in 5 subjects, surgery and chemotherapy in 2 subjects

and combined surgery, radiotherapy and chemotherapy in 6 subjects. Only 11 of the 21 subjects who received treatment for cerebellar tumour displayed dysarthric speech and were included in the study.

31. These differences include the severity of the dysarthria, localisation of the cerebellar lesion and the age of participants. For example, excess and equal stress is more commonly found in severe dysarthria, while the subjects in Cornwell et al.'s study had mild dysarthria. Also, children are more likely to have a localised cerebellar lesion than adults, who more often experience cerebellar degeneration (Cornwell et al. 2003a).

32. Cornwell et al. (2003a) report ataxic and lower motor neurone components in the mild dysarthria of their child subject AC. AC was 7.5 years old at the time of the study. She had received treatment for a recurrent posterior fossa tumour. Her speech and swallowing were assessed two years and four months following the completion of treatment. For a discussion of AC's dysphagia, the reader is referred to section 3.2.2.1 of this chapter.

33. Tongue-reduction surgery has been conducted in an effort to improve the articulatory proficiency of Down's syndrome (DS) speakers. However, the effectiveness of this surgery has yet to be clearly demonstrated. For example, Parsons et al. (1987) studied articulation in 18 DS children who underwent tongue-reduction surgery. Articulation was examined pre- and postoperatively and at a six-month follow-up. No significant differences were found in the number of articulation errors produced by these DS individuals before and after surgery. Moreover, the articulation scores of the DS children who underwent surgery were not significantly different from the scores of DS children who did not receive surgery.

34. Pryce (1994) found that DS subjects used more energy to initiate voice (131.57 microvolts) than subjects with functional dysphonia (116.89 microvolts), subjects with learning disability (125.53 microvolts) and normal control subjects (72.52 microvolts). Pryce also found that only 13 per cent of DS subjects consumed four or more drinks daily (compared to 86 per cent and 83 per cent of normal controls and subjects with functional dysphonia, respectively). Reduced fluid intake compounds the dehydrating effect of an open mouth posture in Down's syndrome individuals.

35. Hoarseness is a common sequela of velopharyngeal incompetence in children with a 22q11.2 microdeletion. This is because the laryngeal mechanism and vocal cords particularly are used excessively in an effort to compensate for faulty velopharyngeal valving. However, many other phonatory problems have been reported in this clinical population, including high pitch, strained or strangled voice and vocal fatigue.

36. Velopharyngeal impairment was present in the majority of these subjects and was so severe in over half the subjects that surgery either had been conducted or was considered necessary. A high level of correct place and manner of consonant

articulation was only observed in children from six years of age. Stops and fricatives were the consonants most often misarticulated. Glottal articulation occurred
less commonly than had been expected, given earlier studies. Intelligibility was
extensively reduced in this group of subjects, with only 17 per cent of the children
aged 5–10 years judged to be intelligible all or most of the time.

37. Wolf-Hirschhorn syndrome (WHS) is caused by a deletion of a portion of the
     short arm of chromosome 4. Well over 10 per cent of cases are related to translo-
     cations in the paternal chromosome 4 (Shprintzen 2000). This syndrome has an
     estimated incidence of 1 in 50,000 births (Gorlin et al. 2001). WHS is a multiple
     malformation disorder in which hypertelorism (increased distance between the
     eyes), highly arched eyebrows, oral/facial cleft and 'Greek helmet' facies consti-
     tute the syndrome's abnormal craniofacial features. The cardinal features of this
     syndrome are prenatal-onset growth retardation, failure to thrive, microcephaly,
     severe mental retardation, seizures and congenital heart malformations (Van
     Borsel et al. 2004).

38. Turner's syndrome has a population prevalence of approximately 1 in 2,500
     (Shprintzen 2000). This syndrome is caused by the absence of one of the X
     chromsomes (hence, the use of the terms XO syndrome, 45X syndrome and
     monosomy X for this disorder). In mosaic cases, not all cells lack an X chromo-
     some. The expression of this disorder is most severe in cases where there is a large
     percentage of cells with a missing X chromosome. If 100 per cent of the cells have
     an X chromosome monosomy, affected individuals exhibit an absence of sec-
     ondary sexual characteristics, an absence of gonads and short stature. The pres-
     ence of neck webbing is variable (Shprintzen 2000). Individuals with Turner's
     syndrome are also at risk for learning disabilities and communication disorders
     (Van Borsel et al. 1999).

39. Although he is careful to avoid the suggestion of a causal relationship between
     cognitive development and phonemic acquisition, Ingram (1976) relates phono-
     logical development to Piaget's cognitive stages. However, Rondal and Edwards
     (1997) remark that 'to the best of our knowledge, he is the only one to have pro-
     posed such a direct relationship between cognitive and phonological develop-
     ments' (157).

40. This study also examined phonatory parameters of this child's noncry vocalisa-
     tions. The fundamental frequency (F_0) of these vocalisations did not decrease
     during the 8–26-month age period, unlike in normal infants. Interutterance F_0
     variability was quite small compared to that which occurs in normal subjects and
     failed to show the systematic decreases reported to occur in normal infants.

41. In addition to conductive, sensorineural and central hearing losses, Church and
     Kaltenbach (1997) describe a fourth type of hearing disorder in FAS – develop-
     mental delays in the maturation of the auditory system. Delayed maturation of the
     auditory system can be demonstrated by the auditory brainstem response. Church
     et al. (1997) found that 2 of 13 FAS subjects who underwent ABR testing had

abnormal prolongations of interpeak latencies, suggesting impaired transmission of neural information along the brainstem portion of the central auditory pathway.

42. In a study of 1,218 normal school-age children, Bess et al. (1998) report a prevalence of minimal sensorineural hearing loss (SNHL) of 5.4 per cent. Church and Kaltenbach (1997) state that the rate of sensorineural hearing loss in FAS subjects is similar to the SNHL rates observed in other children with craniofacial anomalies assessed in their clinic – Down's syndrome (24 per cent), overt cleft palate (47 per cent) and submucous cleft palate (26 per cent).

43. Church et al. (1997) found that otitis proneness extends into adulthood in FAS subjects, unlike in other children with craniofacial anomalies, in whom the incidence and severity of recurrent serous otitis media decreases with increasing age.

44. The increased otitis proneness of FAS subjects is unrelated, according to some researchers, to the presence of cleft palate in these subjects. Church et al. (1997) found that the incidences of otitis proneness among their FAS subjects with (83 per cent) and without (70 per cent) histories of cleft palate were both very high and not significantly different from each other. However, Church and Kaltenbach (1997) remark that

> [t]his is not unique. There are several craniofacial syndromes that are not strongly associated with cleft palate, but that are frequently accompanied by RSOM [recurrent serous otitis media]. These include Down's, Crouzon's, Apert's and Turner's syndromes, and patients with dentofacial abnormalities. (504)

45. For a review of the findings of human and animal FAS studies, the reader is referred to Church and Kaltenbach (1997).

46. It is impossible to eliminate the role of cognitive deficits and cleft palate in the development of speech and language problems in Church et al.'s FAS subjects. Cognitive skills were not assessed by Church et al., and while the presence of cleft palate was not associated in Church et al.'s subjects with any significant increase in the rate of either sensorineural hearing loss or otitis media (itself linked to conductive hearing loss), it is still possible that cleft palate could operate independently of a hearing disorder to cause speech and language problems in these FAS subjects. The reader is referred to sections 2.2.2.2 and 2.2.2.4 in chapter 2 for a discussion of the effect of cleft palate on speech and language development.

47. In their study of eight children with foetal alcohol syndrome, Becker et al. (1990) found that FAS children demonstrated a significantly poorer ability to store linguistic elements in short-term memory when compared to younger chronological age controls. However, when a comparison of memory abilities was based on mental age, statistical significance was not achieved.

48. However, this is unlikely to be a case of exceptional language, where language performance surpasses that which can be expected given an individual's cognitive

level. Van Borsel et al.'s WHS subject had a smaller deletion and a milder phenotype of this syndrome. It is thus likely that the unexpectedly good language
performance of this subject was related to a less severe cognitive impairment than
is normally encountered in individuals with this syndrome. It should be noted
that, although Van Borsel et al. reported the cognitive level of their subject –
testing at 9;3 years using the Dutch version of the McCarthy Developmental
Scales revealed a mean cognitive score below the 50th percentile and scores on the
verbal and performance scale below the 22nd percentile – these researchers did
not attempt to relate the subject's language performance to this cognitive level.

49. The phenotype in Williams syndrome (also known as Williams-Beuren syndrome or elfin facies with hypercalcaemia) includes a facial dysmorphology that
is commonly described as elf-like in appearance, malformations of the connective
tissue, cardiac anomalies (e.g. supravalvular aortic stenosis), and abnormalities of
calcium metabolism (infantile hypercalciuria and hypercalcaemia). Also see note
4 in this chapter.

50. The situation is quite different in WS adults, who are widely recognised as having
impressive vocabularies compared to other populations with equivalent general
cognitive impairments. In fact, vocabulary scores in WS adults are often closer to
the chronological age of these adults than to their general mental age (Stevens and
Karmiloff-Smith 1997).

51. Paterson (2001) cautions against basing estimates of early language performance
in disorders such as Williams syndrome on the adult language phenotype of
affected individuals. Her caution is justified by the quite different receptive
vocabulary performances of the infants and adults with Down's syndrome and
Williams syndrome in her study. The results of a visual preference experiment
revealed that DS and WS infants aged 24–36 months were equally able to match
a word to its referent. However, DS adults had a greater vocabulary impairment
than WS adults, as measured by the British Picture Vocabulary Scale (Dunn et al.
1982). Paterson remarks that '[t]he pattern of language abilities seen in the Down
syndrome and Williams syndrome groups in this infant study is not the same as
that seen in adulthood. This important fact would have been missed if infant performance had been simply inferred from the adult data' (2001:82).

52. As in normal controls, WS subjects showed greater latencies when monitoring
words (shown in capitals) that follow an auxiliary violation (e.g. It could have been
very embarrassing. We didn't realise he *might expecting* SPEECHES at the . . .) or
a phrase structure violation (e.g. Susan seems much happier. I expect *special the*
PILLS she got from the doctor . . .) than when no such grammatical violation
occurs. However, unlike normal controls, WS subjects did not display increased
latencies when monitoring words that followed a subcategory violation (e.g. The
burglar was terrified. He continued *to struggle the* DOG but he couldn't break free).

53. Tyler et al. (1997) also acknowledge that off-line experiments involve metalinguistic processes that affect the performance of individuals with cognitive deficits.

To minimise these metalinguistic demands, Tyler et al. use an on-line task –
semantic priming – in their study of the semantic structure of the lexicon in
Williams syndrome.

54. On the block of test items that examined comprehension of comparatives (e.g. the
knife is longer than the pencil), the WS subjects exhibited an error rate of 27.5
per cent. A similar error rate (27.9 per cent) was obtained by the WS subjects on
test items that examined comprehension of prepositional phrases. However, by
far the highest error rates occurred on those items that examined comprehension
of embedded structures. For example, WS subjects displayed an error rate of 67.9
per cent and 38.3 per cent on test items that assessed the comprehension of relative clauses (e.g. the book the pencil is on is red) and subordinate clauses (e.g. the
pencil is on the book that is yellow), respectively.

55. While many recent studies have demonstrated that syntax is an area of considerable deficit in Williams' syndrome, other studies have revealed phonology to be
an area of strength in the language of WS subjects. Volterra et al. (1996) found
that WS subjects between 4;10 and 15;3 years of age performed significantly
better than controls on the Phonological Fluency Test (Semel et al. 1980). The
apparent skills of WS subjects in recalling and reproducing foreign words have
led to the claim that phonological short-term memory is an area of particular
strength in these subjects. To investigate this claim, Grant et al. (1996) carried
out a test of phonological short-term memory that used nonce words which
obeyed the phonotactics of a language unknown to the WS and control subjects.
WS subjects performed significantly worse than English-speaking (group 1) and
French-speaking (group 2), normally developing 6-year-olds. Grant et al. argue
that the aforementioned proficiencies of WS subjects do not stem from mere
mimicry of auditory input by these subjects, but reflect these subjects' developing knowledge of the phonological systems of their native tongue.

56. The Children's Communication Checklist (Bishop 1998) consists of a series of
statements to which raters respond with one of the following: (a) does not apply,
(b) applies somewhat, (c) definitely applies or (d) unable to judge. Statements are
organised within nine sections that examine particular linguistic, pragmatic and
social skills: (A) Speech output (e.g. 'people can understand virtually everything
he says'), (B) Syntax (e.g. 'tends to leave out words and grammatical endings'), (C)
Inappropriate initiation (e.g. 'talks to anyone and everyone'), (D) Coherence (e.g.
'it is sometimes hard to make sense of what he is saying because it seems illogical
or disconnected'), (E) Stereotyped conversation (e.g. 'will suddenly change the
topic of conversation'), (F) Use of conversational context (e.g. 'tends to repeat
back what others have just said'), (G) Conversational rapport (e.g. 'tends to look
away from the person he is talking to: seems inattentive or preoccupied'), (H)
Social relationships (e.g. 'is popular with other children') and (I) Interests (e.g. 'has
one or more overriding specific interests'). These sections sample three correlated
but dissociable domains – language structure, social use of language and interests.

Developmental disabilities are associated with deficits in one or more of these domains. (For example, in autism there are impairments in all three domains.)

57. The investigation of DS infants by Ramruttun and Jenkins (1998) belongs to a group of studies that

> applied a pragmatic model to the analysis of communicative patterns and placed emphasis on interactive, as opposed to linguistic, qualities of communication behavior. As such, communicative competence is viewed in terms of how effectively one conveys a message, and the degrees to which social processes and functions are evident, such as intentionality (i.e., purposeful signaling to others), joint focus, and reciprocation. (Sarimski 2002:485).

Sarimski (2002) adopts a similar pragmatic model in his analysis of the communicative behaviours of 13 children with Cornelia de Lange syndrome.

58. Cornelia de Lange syndrome is a rare disorder with an incidence of 1 case in every 10,000–50,000 live births (Tekin and Bodurtha 2002). Individuals with this syndrome have severe cognitive limitations. Kline et al. (1993) found an average IQ of 53 (range from below 30 to 85) in their study of 122 patients with clinically confirmed Brachmann-de Lange syndrome (another name for the disorder). Other anomalies include microcephaly, growth failure, distinctive facies, anomalies of development of the hands and feet and excessive growth of hair. As there are currently no biochemical or chromosomal markers for this syndrome, diagnosis is based solely on clinical grounds.

59. Only two of the CdLS subjects attained level V (symbolic interactions) on a developmental model of cognitive competencies. In typical development, level V is reached by 18 months, while the mean age of the CdLS subjects was 5.0 years.

60. Child behaviours were used to examine intentionality in play and included coordinated acts (e.g. filling containers), exploration (e.g. taking objects out of a container), observation/visual regard (e.g. inspection of objects), off-task behaviour (e.g. leaving the chair to walk away) and guided acts (acts performed with guided assistance from the adult). Intentional communication acts were categorised into proto-imperatives or requests (e.g. stretches hand toward entity), proto-declaratives or comments (e.g. picks up object and immediately shows it to an adult), responses (an act that served to fulfill an obligation, e.g. an answer to a question) and protests (e.g. resisting the adult offering a toy).

61. Sarimski (2002) captures these first two points as follows:

> While direct behaviours, which are deliberate enactments of a person's needs and interests, are not symbolic and do not constitute a formal language system, they must be recognized as perhaps the most effective communication means for many individuals with severe cognitive disabilities. One implication of this finding is that it is as critical for those designing or providing

interventions to recognize direct behaviours as having communicative value as it is to teach those skills and behaviours which are more closely associated with conventional forms of language. (485)

62. Calandrella and Wilcox (2000) examined natural interactions between 25 developmentally delayed toddlers and their mothers at three observation points over a 12-month period. Thirteen of the toddlers had Down's syndrome, while the remaining 12 toddlers had developmental delay of undetermined aetiology. Results indicated that the rate of intentional nonverbal communication at the beginning of the 12-month period was a predictor of spontaneous word productions at the end of this period. It was also found that the rates of intentional communication and of gestural indicating behaviour at six months predicted subsequent language outcomes, as measured by the Sequenced Inventory of Communication Development – Revised (Hedrick et al. 1984). In a study of 58 toddlers with mild to moderate developmental delays, McCathren et al. (1999) found that rate of joint attention and rate of communication at the start of the study were statistically significant predictors of expressive vocabulary one year later. Prior to testing, all children had fewer than three words in their expressive vocabularies and exhibited at least one instance of intentional prelinguistic communication.

63. Various criteria have been adopted by investigators to distinguish preintentional and intentional communicative behaviours in the prelinguistic period. Two such criteria are (1) the ability to coordinate visual attention between an interactive partner and a communicative referent and (2) the use of gestures, vocalisations and/or eye contact to direct the attention or actions of an interactive partner. Calandrella and Wilcox (2000) use criterion (1) to define their set of intentional nonverbal communication acts.

64. Yoder and Warren (2002) describe canonical vocal communication as 'nonword vocalization with a consonant-vowel syllable that is combined with a gesture or attention to the message recipient' (1160). Yoder and Warren used canonical vocal communication acts as a measure of vocal development.

65. Peterson et al. (2005) examined the effectiveness of teaching parents to use milieu language teaching procedures with children who belonged to families with multiple risk factors. Two sets of milieu language teaching skills were taught: responsive interaction and incidental teaching. Peterson et al. found that parents were able to acquire these skills and maintain their use after the completion of intervention. Child comments and correct response to parental questions both increased as a result of the use of these procedures. Children's mean length of utterance and scores on the Sequenced Inventory of Communication Development also increased. Responsive interaction skills were more likely to encourage child comments, while incidental teaching was more likely to promote correct responses from children.

66. Rondal and Edwards (1997) defend this particular emphasis of intervention in terms of language modularity:

> Language organization is basically modular. Remediation probably cannot be made in any truly effective way outside the modularity approach. This means defining particular intervention strategies corresponding to various language components. The specificity of the major language components is such that attempts to implement multipurpose remediation procedures are bound to generate mediocre effects. (214)

67. Rondal and Edwards (1997) state that '[i]ntervention programmes might work better when the child's aetiology is among several important characteristics considered in designing remediation. This objective can be fully met when more data have been gathered on the various syndromes leading to mental retardation' (214).

68. Thomas and Karmiloff-Smith (2005) capture this point as follows:

> Cross-syndrome comparisons have indeed identified apparent dissociations in the development of language components. For example, in comparing Down's syndrome, Williams syndrome, autism and fragile X, Fowler (1998) described dissociations between phonology, lexical semantics, morphosyntax, and pragmatics. These disorders illustrate that different etiologies can have dramatically different linguistic profiles. (66)

69. 'Later intervention in late adolescence and early adult years should be recommended, particularly for the lexical and the pragmatic language aspects' (Rondal and Edwards 1997:215).

70. An emphasis on pragmatic and social skills will be particularly important in intervention with learning-disabled subjects who display autistic behaviours. Learning disability and autistic spectrum disorders are common co-occurring conditions (see section 3.3.2.1 for further discussion).

71. Dementia caused by Alzheimer's disease is more common in individuals with Down's syndrome than in the general population. In 2001, the Mental Health Foundation and the Foundation for People with Learning Disabilities published a briefing for commissioners. This briefing states that at least 36 per cent of people with Down's syndrome aged between 50–59 years and 54.5 per cent aged 0–69 years are affected by dementia. This compares to a prevalence rate of 5 per cent in the general population aged over 5 years.

72. The learning-disabled child who is attending a mainstream school will have very different language needs (e.g. literacy training) from those of the severely learning-disabled individual who is being cared for in a residential setting. The professionals encountered by each will also differ (e.g. teachers versus nursing staff).

73. In relation to children with Down's syndrome, Buckley and Le Prevost (2002) remark that 'visual short-term memory is not impaired relative to non-verbal mental abilities and is described as a relative strength' (71).

74. In key-word signing, speech and manual signs from the Makaton Vocabulary and the British Sign Language for the Deaf are used simultaneously to support key words in an utterance.

75. The Total Communication approach advocates that all modes of communication be made available to the person with communication difficulties as appropriate. This can involve the complementary use of speech, manual signs, photographs and pictorial symbols alongside all the usual elements of non-verbal and paralinguistic communication. (Powell and Clibbens 1994:127)

76. DS children exhibit a specific impairment of auditory short-term memory (Chapman 1999). However, visual short-term memory is an area of relative strength (Buckley and Le Prevost 2002). The most effective speech remediation tasks are thus likely to be those that make use of visual prompts and other visual information. Indeed, there is evidence that DS children can use their skills in visual memory to compensate for weaknesses in auditory memory (Broadley et al. 1995).

77. Leddy and Gill (1999) describe the very different therapy and educational experiences of children and adults with Down's syndrome – the former receiving 'thousands of hours of intervention' that were largely denied to DS adults when they were children. This lack of early intervention has led professionals to assume incorrectly that little progress could be made in improving the language skills of DS adults: 'Professionals have been pessimistic about what could be accomplished with adults who have cognitive disabilities because these individuals have aged beyond the developmental years, beyond the time when traditional treatment was thought to be effective' (206).

78. 'Because the visual channel is often a strong channel through which to learn, the use of reading to aid in language development should be considered' (Kumin 1996).

79. Kim and Lombardino (1991) compared the use of script-based and nonscript-based treatments on the comprehension of semantic constructions in four learning-disabled children. In the script-based treatment, semantic constructions were rehearsed within three thematic or goal-oriented sequences – popcorn-making, pudding-making and milkshake-making. For example, an action-object-locative construction was rehearsed within a milkshake-making routine through the use of utterances like 'Put the cup on top of the ice box.' No such sequences or themes were used in nonscript-based treatments. Comprehension of semantic constructions was monitored using daily probes. The script-based treatment was found to be more effective than the nonscript-based treatment in establishing these constructions in three of the four subjects.

80. In a study of argument structure in DS children, Grela (2003) found that DS children were more likely to omit subject arguments in comparison to direct object arguments during transitive verb productions. As normal children develop an understanding of the properties of tense, they also become aware of the need to use subject arguments in tensed clauses. Prior to this point, normal children are in an optional subject (OS) period. Because of their difficulties with syntax and morphology, the DS children in Grela's study are late in acquiring a knowledge of tense. These children are still likely to be in the OS period, which explains their greater omission of subject arguments. Grela remarks that

> the results of this study can provide useful information about intervention for children with DS. If children's omission of subject arguments is closely related to the knowledge that tense is required in main clauses in English, then intervention may focus on facilitating the children's acquisition of tense markers along with subject omission. If children become aware of the link between tense and subject use, then as they use tense more consistently we should expect to see children move beyond the OS period. (2003:276)

81. DS children are delayed in acquiring a productive vocabulary. On average, first words are spoken at 18 months. (Normally developing children produce their first word between 11 and 12 months; Buckley 1999.) DS children are on average 27 months of age by the time they have produced 10 words. (Normally developing children have produced 10 words by 18 months.) A productive vocabulary of 50 words – the point at which two-word phrases are produced – is acquired by DS children at 37 months and by normally developing children at 19 months (Buckley 1999). Productive vocabulary deficits extend into the teenage years and have serious implications for the education of DS children. Buckley and Le Prevost (2002) state that 'many secondary school pupils with Down syndrome will have small productive vocabularies (800 words or even less)' (74).

82. The parents of DS children have often been first to recognise the wider language gains that can be achieved through reading. In 1979, Leslie Duffen wrote to Sue Buckley to inform her of the progress of his daughter, Sarah, who was attending mainstream school. Leslie attributed Sarah's good progress to her early experience of reading – Sarah had been introduced to reading from the age of three years. Leslie's observations were subsequently investigated and confirmed by Buckley and her colleagues (Buckley 2002:1).

83. The argument based on mutual output constraints states that nonword repetition appears to be correlated with expressive language because both activities involve the assembly of articulatory instructions, among other output processes.

84. As well as iconicity affecting the ease with which a sign system may be acquired, sign iconicity has also been shown to influence judgements about the intelligibility of speech. Powell and Clibbens (1994) found that in two poor speakers with

Down's syndrome, only words that were paired with iconic signs received an intelligibility rating by a naive rater and a skilled rater with no knowledge of sign (a speech and language therapist who worked in a different speciality). All other words were judged to be 'not understood'.

85. The evolving nature of these classification systems can be seen in the inclusion of Asperger's syndrome for the first time in DSM-IV (APA 1994). Following a large, international field trial involving over a thousand children and adults with autism and related disorders (Volkmar et al. 1994), it was decided that Asperger's disorder could be included in DSM-IV as a diagnostic category distinct from autism within the wider class of pervasive developmental disorders.

86. The ICD-10 (WHO 1993) includes the following PDD categories: childhood autism, atypical autism, Rett's syndrome, other childhood disintegrative disorder, overactive disorder associated with mental retardation and stereotyped movements, Asperger's syndrome, other pervasive developmental disorders and pervasive developmental disorder, unspecified.

87. Dr Leo Kanner, a psychiatrist at Johns Hopkins University, was the first person to describe autism in children. In 1943, he applied the term 'early childhood autism' to a group of 11 children who were self-absorbed and who had severe social, communication and behavioural problems. The expression 'classic' autism is a reference to this early work. In the years since Kanner's original description of the disorder, the term autism has been defined and classified in various ways. In 1968, the American Psychiatric Association defined autism as a single disorder, rather than a syndrome consisting of behavioural and medical features. In recent years, there has been an attempt to reclassify autism as one type of PDD.

88. Parents are usually first to notice abnormalities in their child's behaviour. In a recent review of autism research by the Medical Research Council (2001), it was found that the majority of parents are aware that something is not quite right in the months leading up to the second birthday. However, there is often a considerable lapse of time between parents first noticing something wrong with their child's behaviour and a diagnosis of autism being made. In a study of individuals aged from 2 to 49 years, Howlin and Moore (1997) found that the average age at which parents first became aware of problems in their child's development was 1.69 years, while the average age at final diagnosis was 6.11 years.

89. It should be noted that although Rett's disorder is classified as a pervasive developmental disorder, it is not part of the autistic spectrum: 'This last disorder [Rett's disorder], although showing similarities with ASDs in its early stages, shows characteristic progressive physical regression, and is not currently conceptualised as part of the autism spectrum' (Medical Research Council 2001:11).

90. The regression phase in Rett's disorder is generally taken to consist of four stages. Stage I (early-onset stage) begins between 6 and 18 months of age. This stage may be overlooked, as symptoms are quite vague and a subtle slowing of development may not be noticed by parents and doctors. Infants may exhibit less eye contact

and show less interest in toys. Gross motor skills, such as sitting and crawling, may be delayed. Deceleration of head growth and hand-wringing are present. This stage usually lasts a few months, but can also persist for more than a year. Stage II (rapid destructive stage) usually begins between 1 and 4 years and may last for weeks or months. Onset may be rapid or gradual. As its name suggests, this stage involves the greatest loss of skills (e.g. purposeful hand movements, spoken language, social interaction). This stage is characterised by abnormal hand movements (e.g. hand-wringing and clapping), breathing irregularities (e.g. apnoea, hyperventilation), general irritability and sleep irregularities. Gait is unsteady and it may be difficult for the child to initiate motor movements. Deceleration of head growth is normally noticed in this stage. Stage III (plateau or pseudo-stationary stage) usually begins between the ages of 2 and 10 and can last for years. During this stage, apraxia, motor problems and seizures are evident. Many girls remain in stage III for most of their lives. Stage IV (late motor deterioration stage) can last for years or even decades. Previously mobile girls can experience reduced mobility. Prominent features of this stage include muscle weakness, rigidity, spasticity, dystonia and scoliosis. While there is a reduction in mobility, there is no decline in cognition, communication and hand skills during this stage. Eye gaze usually improves and repetitive hand movements may decrease.

91. These improvements occur in stage III of Rett's disorder (see note 90).

92. In a study comparing the neuropsychological profiles of subjects with Asperger's syndrome and high-functioning autism, Klin et al. (1995) found that 11 neuropsychological deficits discriminated between these two conditions. Of these 11 deficits, six were shown to be predictive of Asperger's syndrome: fine motor skills, visual motor integration, visual spatial perception, nonverbal concept formation, gross motor skills and visual memory. The remaining five deficits were predictive of non-Asperger's syndrome: articulation, verbal output, auditory perception, vocabulary and verbal memory. These researchers also found a high level of concordance between Asperger's syndrome (but not HFA) and a neuropsychological characterisation of the Nonverbal Learning Disabilities (NLD) syndrome. On the basis of this finding, Klin et al. suggest that NLD can be seen as an adequate neuropsychological marker of Asperger's syndrome.

93. Although most individuals with Asperger's syndrome function in the normal range of intelligence, some have been reported to be mildly retarded (Wing 1991). A universal finding reported by Klin et al. (1995) was that verbal IQ was higher than performance IQ in their group of AS subjects.

94. PDD,NOS should not be confused with PDD – the former term is a diagnosis, whereas the latter term is a class of conditions, to which PDD,NOS belongs.

95. Within a wider assessment of the state of the science in autism, scientists at the National Institutes of Health reviewed current diagnostic categories of autism. In relation to PDD,NOS, they concluded that '[a] category such as Pervasive

Developmental Disorder – Not Otherwise Specified (PDD–NOS) is still needed, but would be more appropriately entitled 'Atypical Autism' for cases that meet some, but not all of the criteria for autism' (Bristol et al. 1996:123). See the main text for a brief discussion of atypical autism.

96. These figures are calculated on the basis that autism affects 10 cases per 10,000 persons and that PDD has a prevalence rate of 30 cases per 10,000 persons. The Medical Research Council (2001) reviewed five studies reporting prevalence for CDD. Its prevalence rate of between 0.1 and 0.6 cases per 10,000 is similar to the rate obtained by Fombonne (2002).

97. Kozinetz et al. (1993) obtained this figure from the Texas Rett Syndrome Registry, the largest population-based registry of cases and potential cases of Rett's syndrome in the world. It is worth remarking that this prevalence rate was obtained prior to the discovery in 1999 of the gene responsible for Rett's syndrome: the MECP2 gene on the X chromosome (see section 3.3.1 in the main text). It is expected that the discovery of this gene will lead to greater diagnostic precision in the identification of Rett's cases. What effect this will have on earlier prevalence rates of Rett's syndrome still remains to be seen.

98. Powell et al. remark that the ascertainment of ASD cases in the UK is complicated by the fact that the care of these children is shared by both the health and the education systems. For this reason, Powell et al. restricted their study to preschool children (children under five years) who were detected through medical services: namely, child development centres.

99. The report by the Department of Developmental Services includes several other noteworthy findings: (1) there has been a 5.3 per cent increase in the proportion of males with autism in the 11 years from 1987 to 1998, (2) the median age of the population of persons with autism dropped from 15 years to 9 years during this period, (3) there was a significant change in the percentage of persons with autism who have no mental retardation – the 1998 population contained significantly more persons with no or mild mental retardation and far fewer persons with severe to profound mental retardation.

100. Kopp and Gillberg (1992) argue that the autism phenotype might be different in males compared with females. In support of this claim, they discuss the cases of six girls who presented with a picture that was clinically difficult to categorise and who met criteria for autistic disorder at one time during development. It is argued that if these cases are considered for a diagnosis of autism – as well as females who are given diagnoses of anorexia nervosa, paranoid disorder or obsessive compulsive disorder but who can be shown to have the same kind of social impairment as that seen in autism – then the typically high male to female ratio encountered in autism might drop considerably.

101. The type of causal mechanism that is envisaged in the main text is adequately captured in the following statement: 'The aim for research must be to uncover causal pathways from one or more possibly interacting causes, through their

effects on the brain, and sequelae in the mind, to the effects in observed behavioural deficits and abilities' (MRC 2001:21).

102. The lower figure of 10 per cent is proposed by Rutter and colleagues; Gillberg and colleagues advance the higher figure of 30 per cent. Barton and Volkmar (1998) reviewed records on 211 subjects with autism and other developmental disorders. They found that the prevalence of medical conditions with a suspected aetiological relationship with autism varied between 10 and 15 per cent, depending on the system used to diagnose autism.

103. Schroer et al. (1998) found that in the first 100 cases of autism enrolled in the South Carolina Autism Project, abnormalities of chromosome 15 emerged as the single most common cause of the disorder. Deletions and duplications of proximal 15q were identified. In all cases, these deletions or duplications occurred on the chromosome inherited from the mother.

104. The FRAXE disorder has no distinct dysmorphology, which makes clinical diagnosis difficult. A phenotype of mild mental retardation and severe language delay is associated with expansions of the FMR2 gene. Females with FMR2 expansions are typically normal, suggesting that this disorder may follow an X-linked pattern of expression.

105. fMR1 studies of autism have largely examined aspects of the 'social brain', with similar studies of other areas of functioning such as language, working memory, attention and motor functioning tending to lag behind (Volkmar et al. 2004).

106. It is important to consider brain size apart from head circumference, as the latter correlates only about .50 with brain size (Volkmar et al. 2004).

107. In some cases, findings may even be contradictory. For example, Piven et al. (1996) report a selective enlargement in autism of occipital, parietal and temporal lobes, but not of the frontal lobes. However, Carper et al. (2002) found the frontal lobe to be the most enlarged in their study.

108. 'The universal impairment in social cognition found in neuropsychologic studies of autism suggests involvement of certain brain regions known to mediate social and emotional behaviour, namely, regions of the limbic system, such as the amygdala and orbital frontal cortex' (Bristol et al. 1996:135).

109. One of the most consistent findings to emerge from face processing studies in autistic subjects is that while normal individuals focus on eyes during face recognition, autistic individuals are much more likely to attend to the mouth. Klin et al. (2002) observed a similar pattern during a task that required normal controls and autistic subjects to view naturalistic social situations. These researchers found that control subjects visually fixated on the eye region two times more than did the subjects with autism. Interestingly, visual fixation on the mouth in autistic subjects predicted improved social adjustment and less autistic social impairment, while more fixation time on objects predicted the opposite relationship. Another finding to emerge from studies of face perception in autism is that autistic individuals tend to use compensatory perceptual-encoding mechanisms, some

of which are more typical of object perception. This is confirmed in a study by Schultz et al. (2000), who found that individuals with ASDs demonstrated a pattern of brain activity during face discrimination that is consistent with feature-based strategies typical of nonface object perception.

110. The SAT involves perception of human-like interactions among three simple geometric shapes. While normal subjects are able to describe the movements of these shapes through a social lens and in human terms (e.g. shapes chase one another, etc.), individuals with autism fail to impose social meaning on these movements. Schultz et al. (2003) remark that

> [u]se of simple shapes to display human social interactions without percep-
> tual representations of real people strips the social event down to the essen-
> tial elements needed to convey social meanings. In this regard, the SAT is an
> ideal neuroimaging probe for assessing social cognitive and social perceptual
> processes in a way that is not confounded by perceptual processes that would
> be provoked if actual images of faces or people were used. (416)

111. In addition to the Medical Research Council, the question of whether or not there is a causal link between the MMR vaccine and ASDs has been considered by the American Medical Association, the Institute of Medicine, USA, the World Health Organization, the American Academy of Pediatrics, the Population and Public Health Branch of Health Canada and the Irish Department of Health and Children.

112. The Institute of Medicine states that '[this] conclusion does not exclude the pos-sibility that MMR vaccine could contribute to ASD in a small number of children, because the epidemiological evidence lacks the precision to assess rare occurrences of a response to MMR vaccine leading to ASD' (Stratton et al. 2001:6).

113. This is more likely to happen when deficits are subtle, such as occurs in high-functioning individuals. Bishop (2000b) remarks that

> when relatively high-functioning children present with subtle deficits affecting
> a range of different behaviors, one has the impression that the particular diag-
> nosis, and consequently the type of intervention received, may be more a func-
> tion of the discipline of the specialist who is the point of first referral than of
> the particular symptom profile. The same child might receive a diagnosis of
> PDD-NOS or atypical autism from a psychiatrist, of developmental language
> disorder (semantic-pragmatic type) from a speech-language therapist, or right-
> hemisphere learning disability from a neuropsychologist. (274–5)

114. Congenital rubella and untreated phenylketonuria are nowadays so rare that we will not give further consideration to them. Indeed, in a recent review of epi-demiological surveys of autism, Fombonne (2003) reports that congenital rubella and phenylketonuria account for almost no cases of autism.

115. This reflects a more general pattern, in which medical conditions occur more frequently in autism when the latter is accompanied by severe or profound mental retardation. In their review of the literature in this case, Rutter et al. (1994) state that '[k]nown medical conditions are much more common when autism is accompanied by severe retardation and especially if there is profound retardation' (315).

116. Rinehart et al. (2001) state that

> [m]otor clumsiness is referred to in the ICD-10 ... as a symptom often found in Asperger disorder; however no mention of motor clumsiness is made in the clinical description of autism. No mention of clumsiness is made in the DSM-IV for autism or Asperger's disorder. (80)

117. It was implicit in the motor reprogramming task in this study that subjects would receive a single oddball response, after which movement perception could be expected to be faster. While subjects in the control groups prepared the first movement after the oddball movement faster than they prepared movements occurring before the oddball, AS subjects were slower to prepare for the movement which occurred after executing the oddball response (the 'atypical deficit' in motor preparation referred to in the main text). A movement preparation advantage was not shown by the autistic subjects, who displayed similar preparation time for all movements (i.e. they lacked a normal anticipatory pattern).

118. Gernsbacher and Goldsmith do not claim, however, that DVD constitutes in and of itself a subtype of ASD.

119. O'Brien and Pearson (2004) state that

> a diagnosis of autism becomes difficult in individuals with profound learning disability, because it is almost impossible to determine whether the impairments observed are due to gross cognitive delay or to autism . . . [i]n that case one could argue that the diagnosis of autism may be of less relevance, because of the extent to which the severity of their learning disability dominates the presentation. (126)

120. The Consensus Panel included representatives of nine professional and four parent organisations, with liaisons from the National Institutes of Health. The Panel came about as the result of a proposal by the Child Neurology Society and the American Academy of Neurology to formulate practice parameters for the diagnosis and evaluation of autism for their memberships. In developing these parameters, the Panel analysed over 2,500 scientific articles. The Panel's recommendations are reported by Filipek et al. (1999).

121. Other indications for further developmental evaluation advanced by the Panel include no pointing or other gestures by 12 months of age, no single words by 16 months of age, no two-word spontaneous phrases by 24 months of age and loss of previously learned language or social skills at any age.

122. A further finding was that autistic children in this study displayed a deficit in joint attention behaviours. However, atypical vocal behaviours were found to be independent of individual differences in joint attention skill.

123. It should be emphasised that this only applies to autistic children who acquire verbal communication. The Yale Child Study Center states that speech (spoken language) is absent in about 50 per cent of autism cases.

124. 'Chronological mismatch' is used by Grunwell (1981) to describe a child who uses very early normal processes alongside later normal processes. For example, if syllable-initial cluster reduction were to persist while the use of complex syllable-final clusters had become well established, such a pattern would be a chronological mismatch.

125. Schultz et al. (2000) relate prosodic disturbances in autism to amygdala dysfunction: 'failure of the amygdala to transmit social-emotional information to cognitive and motor output centers of the frontal lobe would result in abnormal responses to social stimuli, such as faces, and difficulties conveying social emotional information (e.g. prosody)' (190).

126. In a review of studies of prosody in ASDs, McCann and Peppé (2003) found that only 16 papers had been published in this area between 1980 and 2002.

127. The Prosody-Voice Screening Profile (Shriberg et al. 1990) contains codes for two types of inappropriate stress: inappropriate stress at the word or lexical level and inappropriate stress at the phrase and utterance level. The latter category includes reduced stress on typically stressed syllables. It also includes a type of monostress in which unstressed syllables are articulated with greater force (i.e. excessive/equal) or stress is shifted from expected syllables and words to elsewhere in the utterance (i.e. misplaced stress).

128. In their review of prosody research in autism, McCann and Peppé (2003) remark that 'the understanding of prosody is seriously under researched: very few studies address this, and none in the context of expressive abilities' (348). Since McCann and Peppé's review, a study by Paul et al. (2005) has examined the perception and production of prosody in speakers with ASDs (see main text).

129. In keeping with a method used in the SLI literature, Kjelgaard and Tager-Flusberg (2001) divided the autistic children in their study into normal, borderline and impaired subgroups according to their performance on one of the language measures used – either the Peabody Picture Vocabulary Test-III (PPVT-III) (Dunn and Dunn 1997) or the Clinical Evaluation of Language Fundamentals (CELF) (Wiig, Secord and Semel 1992). Among the children whose language was defined as borderline (more than 1SD below the mean) or impaired (more than 2SD below the mean), it was found that vocabulary skills were superior to knowledge of syntax and semantics, as measured by the CELF. Articulation skills, as measured by the Goldman-Fristoe Test of Articulation (Goldman and Fristoe 1986), were in the normal range for all three language groups. However, in children with low vocabulary and CELF scores, nonsense

word repetition was impaired. (Nonsense word repetition was assessed using a subtest from the NEPSY, a developmental neuropsychological assessment (Korkman et al. 1998).) From these findings, Kjelgaard and Tager-Flusberg conclude that '[t]he profile of language performance among the children with autism who have borderline or impaired language abilities mirrors what has been reported in the literature on SLI' (2001:304).

130. One of the DSM-IV criteria for Asperger's disorder states that single words should be used by two years of age and communicative phrases by three years of age. Bartlett et al. (2005) remark that '[a] definition of characteristics such as the acquisition of first words and phrases reflects a syntactic perspective of language' (206). Bishop (2000b) states that this DSM-IV criterion 'is defined in relation to mastery of language milestones and in terms of sentence length and complexity rather than to how language is used' (258).

131. Eisenmajer et al. (1996) found that among the subjects in their study with a diagnosis of AS, 43.1 per cent were reported to have experienced a delay in language onset. Only 10.8 per cent of AS subjects were reported by parents as communicating normally.

132. Of the 8 subjects with Rett's syndrome (RS) studied by Sandberg et al., 3 subjects had classical RS and 5 subjects had forme fruste RS. Forme fruste is a variant of RS and comprises about 80 per cent of all atypical cases (Sandberg et al. 2000). Other variants in the RS complex include congenital-onset RS, infantile seizure-onset RS, late-regression RS and preserved/regained speech RS. All atypical cases or variant forms of RS contrast with classical RS in terms of either age of onset, severity of symptoms or both (Sandberg et al. 2000).

133. More general language findings were that receptive ability exceeded expressive ability in 7 of the 8 subjects in this study. Also, all eight subjects displayed normal onset of babbling and appearance of first words.

134. Impairments of nonverbal communication are common in ASD. Stone et al. (1997) found that two- and three-year-old children with autism were less likely to point, show objects or use eye gaze to communicate than children with developmental delays and/or language impairments. Control and autistic subjects in this study were matched on chronological age, mental age and expressive vocabulary level.

135. Adams (2002) states that '[f]ormal testing of pragmatics has limited potential to reveal the typical pragmatic abnormalities in interaction but has a significant role to play in the assessment of comprehension of pragmatic intent' (973). Adam's comments are not limited to ASD children, but apply to children in general with communication impairments.

136. The CCC-2 is the most recent version of an assessment that has been in development for 10 years. Earlier research versions of this checklist included the CCC, the Checklist for Language-Impaired Children (CLIC) and CLIC-2. None of these earlier versions was standardised. The CCC-2 has been standardised on a UK population aged from 4 to 16 years.

137. The CCC-2 may be used to identify pragmatic impairments in children who have already received an ASD diagnosis. Equally, the checklist may be used to identify children who may merit further assessment for an ASD.

138. Bishop and Baird (2001) found that reliability, as measured by internal consistency, was 0.7 or higher for most scales, when checklists were completed by parents and professionals. For individual pragmatic scales, however, correlations between ratings for parents and professionals were in the range of 0.30–0.58, with a correlation of 0.46 for the pragmatic composite. This correlation increases considerably when professionals complete the checklist. In a study in which the checklist is completed by teachers and speech and language therapists, Bishop (1998) reports inter-rater reliability and internal consistency of around 0.80 on the five pragmatic subscales of the CCC.

139. Geurts et al. (2004) examined whether children with attention deficit hyperactivity disorder (ADHD) and children with high-functioning autism (HFA) could be differentiated using the Children's Communication Checklist. It was found that parent and teacher ratings on the CCC correctly predicted group membership in 73–78 per cent of cases, respectively. The pragmatic composite score of the parent CCC was a good measure for case identification. Bishop and Baird (2001) found a relation between diagnostic category and scores on the pragmatic composite of both parent and professional checklists. For both types of rater, the pragmatic composite was lowest for children with a diagnosis of autism (a low rating on the CCC suggests impairment), intermediate for those with a diagnosis of AS, PDD,NOS or ADHD, and highest for those with a diagnosis of specific learning disability. The relation between pragmatic composite scores and diagnosis was at its strongest when ratings from parents and professionals were combined.

140. Numerous studies have found evidence of play impairments in autism. Blanc et al. (2005) found that the regulation of pretend play was very disordered in children with autism. Autistic children exhibited breaking off, dissociation and instability of actions. However, during directed play the actions of autistic children were more structured and corresponded to a better developmental level. Williams et al. (2001) compared the functional play of children with autism to that of developmentally matched children with Down's syndrome and typical infants. These groups of children did not differ in the proportion of total play time spent in functional play or in the number of functional acts performed. However, the functional play of the autistic children was shown to be less elaborated, less varied and less integrated than that of controls. Baranek et al. (2005) examined the duration and highest level of object play present in autistic, developmentally delayed and typically developing infants. Object play was classified according to four hierarchical categories – exploratory, relational, functional and symbolic play. Baranek et al. found similar levels of engagement with objects in these three groups of children. Also, there were no statistically significant differences in the duration of

exploratory play in these groups. However, when the highest levels of play in these three groups were compared, it was found that only typically developing infants engaged in functional play.

141. Volden (2004) examined how nine school-age, high-functioning children with ASD responded to a stacked series of requests for clarification (RQCLs). Like language age-matched control children, ASD children were able to respond to RQCLs and employed a variety of repair strategies. ASD children were also similar to controls in that they added increasingly more information in response to successive RQCLs. However, compared to control subjects, ASD children were significantly more likely to respond to a request for clarification with an inappropriate response (i.e. a response that was bizarre, shifted the topic or was an attempt to discontinue the interaction).

142. The two graphic methods used in intervention were photographs and pictograms. Photographs were 10×15cm in size and featured objects and activities relating to three situations: meals, special training and the play area. The subject in this study was attending a special preschool in Norway. Reflecting the widespread use of the system of Pictogram Ideogram Communication (Maharaj 1980) in Norway, pictograms were also used in intervention.

143. Klin and Volkmar (2000) remark that

> the number of professionals trained to implement such a curriculum, or even to train educational professionals on the fundamentals of this approach, is still quite minimal, leaving both educational managers and parents in a dire quandary, namely, how to include what is being promoted as the most important component of any program for individuals with social disabilities without access to the knowledge base in this area, and even less access to professionals who feel comfortable carrying out the social-skills-building program. (351)

144. Shields et al. (1996) examined the performance of the following four groups of children on tests of right hemisphere function: children with high-level autism; semantic-pragmatic disorder (SPD); phonologic-syntactic disorder and normal children. Visual-spatial processing was an area of weakness for the autistic and SPD children, with both groups of children attaining significantly lower scores than normal controls and children with phonologic-syntactic disorder on the Visual Object and Space Perception Test (Warrington and James 1991).

145. Klin and Volkmar (2000) remark that

> [t]he meaning of eye contact, gaze and various inflections, as well as tone of voice and facial and hand gestures, at times, needs to be taught in a fashion not unlike the teaching of a foreign language; that is, all elements should be made verbally explicit and appropriately and repeatedly drilled. (354)

4

Disorders of Speech and Language Development

4.1 Introduction

The acquisition of speech and language is an unproblematic developmental process for the large majority of children. However, there is a sizeable minority of children for whom speech and language acquisition is considerably delayed and/or markedly deviant. In these children, delayed and deviant speech and language acquisition occurs in the presence of normal intellectual, social and imaginative functioning and normal nonverbal communication skills. These children thus present a very different clinical picture from the children examined in chapter 3. In some cases, children may struggle to use sounds contrastively in language, even when they can articulate these sounds in isolation or in imitation of the therapist. Such children have a phonological disorder. In other cases, children may have difficulty programming their articulators to perform the movements that are required to produce speech sounds. The speech disorder in these children is that of dyspraxia. In still other cases, breakdown occurs in a number of structural language levels in addition to phonology (e.g. syntax, semantics). For example, the child may struggle to produce certain syntactic constructions (e.g. passive voice) or comprehend the constructions used by others. In these children, the communication disorder is one of specific language impairment (SLI). Still other children exhibit communication disorders that are not so clearly developmental, in that considerable speech and language development has taken place. However, this development is interrupted long before the child can be said to have anything like a complete mastery of language. (In this sense, the disorder is not acquired either.) The severe communication problems that attend the rare condition Landau–Kleffner syndrome is one such disorder. In this chapter, we examine

the following developmental speech and language disorders: dyspraxia, phonological disorder and specific language impairment. (The developmental speech
disorder dysarthria was examined at length in chapter 2.) The unique profile
of communication impairments that occurs in Landau–Kleffner syndrome will
also be discussed.

4.2 Developmental Verbal Dyspraxia

Developmental verbal dyspraxia (DVD)[1] is a motor speech disorder that can
seriously compromise intelligibility in the children whom it affects. Although
definitions of this disorder vary, there is general agreement amongst clinicians
that volitional speech movements are particularly affected (nonspeech movements are intact, unless there is an accompanying oral dyspraxia[2]) and that the
disorder must not be caused by an underlying neuromuscular deficit. In this
way, Strand (1995) remarks that '[i]n DAS, a child has difficulty carrying out
purposeful voluntary movement sequences for speech in the absence of a paralysis of the speech musculature' (127). These characteristics set DVD apart
from another motor speech disorder, developmental dysarthria, in which
speech and nonspeech movements are equally affected and a neuromuscular
impairment is responsible for the speech disorder. Other definitions of DVD
contain an implicit reference to speech production models, in which DVD is
characterised as a breakdown between language (phonological) and speech
(phonetic) levels in these models. Hayden (1994), for example, states that '[i]n
its purest form DAS is a disorder of the ability to translate phonemic and linguistic codes to differing planes of movement over time' (120). These models
posit discrete, but interrelated, planning and programming stages during
speech production. These stages are emphasised in some definitions of DVD.
Caruso and Strand (1999) claim that '[i]t is our view that the term developmental apraxia of speech is a motor level of impairment. Specifically, we posit
that the speech characteristics of these children are due to disruption of sensorimotor planning or sensorimotor programming' (16–17).

4.2.1 Epidemiology and Aetiology

Although many figures are available for the prevalence of developmental dyspraxia in general,[3] few studies have investigated the prevalence of developmental verbal dyspraxia in particular. Shriberg et al. (1997a) state that DAS
affects 1–2 children per thousand. It is thus a less common childhood communication disorder than either phonological disorder (see section 4.3) or specific
language impairment (see section 4.4). However, DVD has been reported to
occur more frequently in a number of specific populations. Spinelli et al. (1995)
examined word-finding difficulties, verbal paraphasias and verbal dyspraxia in

10 individuals with fragile X syndrome. These investigators state that 'verbal dyspraxia can be a common feature within the spectrum of this syndrome' (39). Scheffer et al. (1995) describe the presence of oral and speech dyspraxia in nine members of the one family. All individuals presented with a new epilepsy syndrome, autosomal dominant rolandic epilepsy. The electroclinical features of this new syndrome resemble those of benign rolandic epilepsy, a common inherited epilepsy of childhood. McLaughlin and Kriegsmann (1980) describe a case of severe developmental speech dyspraxia in a member of a family that is typical of other reports of X-linked mental retardation without physical abnormality (Renpenning's syndrome). Motor or speech dyspraxia was also evident in other family members. These investigators state that '[o]ther reports of X-linked mental retardation have mentioned "verbal disability", which suggests that developmental dyspraxia may be quite common in these families' (84). Hall, Jordan and Robin (1993) followed a child with developmental apraxia of speech who had Robinow's syndrome.

Little is known about the aetiology of DVD. However, the similarity of symptoms in DVD to those found in children who develop verbal dyspraxia as a result of a stroke, tumour or head injury suggests the presence of a neurological aetiology.[4] Belton et al. (2003) found several bilateral grey matter abnormalities in a family with a large three-generational pedigree, in which half of the members presented with a verbal and oro-facial dyspraxia. Reduced grey matter density was observed bilaterally in the caudate nucleus, the cerebellum and the left and right inferior frontal gyrus. Additionally, increased grey matter density was found in the planum temporale bilaterally. These grey matter abnormalities could only have arisen by means of genetically mediated neurodevelopmental processes. Indeed, Belton et al. relate the verbal and oral dyspraxia of members of the KE family to a point mutation in the $FOXP_2$ gene.[5] (Fisher et al. (1998) also discuss the KE family; see section 4.4.1.)

Clearly, the aggregation of verbal and oro-facial dyspraxia cases[6] in the family studied by Belton et al. and the presence of DVD in various genetic syndromes point strongly to the operation of genetic factors in the aetiology of this disorder. Other features of DVD have also led researchers to look to genetic factors to explain this speech disorder. The first of these features is that DVD is more common in boys than in girls. Although the boy:girl ratio varies from study to study, Hall et al. (1993) found an average ratio of approximately 3:1 in a review of 24 group studies and 11 single-subject studies. Some of these studies found that the number of boys affected was as high as 100 per cent. The second feature relates to the interaction between the sex of individuals with DVD and the severity of the disorder. Hall et al. report roughly equal numbers of girls and boys with DVD in their diagnostic clinic. They also observe that their clinic receives a larger proportion of severely disordered children than is found in the typical caseload. To explain the fact that girls make up a greater proportion of severe cases of DVD than less severe cases, Hall et al. employ the concept of a threshold model from genetics. Using this model, Hall et al. suggest that the threshold for expression of DVD is higher in females than in males. This higher threshold prevents less severe forms of the disorder from being expressed in females. However, the greater loading of factors that is needed for this threshold to be reached in females also means that when expression of the disorder does occur in females, it is likely to be severe.

There is increasing evidence that DVD may be caused by certain metabolic disorders. One such disorder, galactosaemia, has been studied extensively in this regard. Galactosaemia is an autosomal, recessively inherited inborn error of metabolism in which patients lack a milk enzyme that is needed to convert galactose to glucose. This disorder affects 1:60,000 children born in the US (Hall et al. 1993). Nelson et al. (1991) studied the speech characteristics of 24 patients who were treated for galactosaemia. It was found that 54 per cent of these patients had verbal dyspraxia. These investigators conclude that '[t]he findings indicate the association of a specific and unusual speech defect with a specific and rare metabolic disorder' (346). Hansen et al. (1996) examined eight galactosaemic patients who were between 9 months and 19 years old at the time of the study. None of these patients had undergone neonatal screening for galactosaemia. Delayed language development was present in the majority of these subjects and three subjects were classified as having verbal dyspraxia. Hansen et al. conclude that '[g]alactosaemia appears to be associated with significant risks of developmental and language delays in this unscreened population' (1197). More recently, Robertson et al. (2000) investigated a genotype/phenotype relationship between DVD and a common missense mutation, Q188R, of the galactose-1-phosphate uridyltransferase (GALT) gene. Forty-three patients with galactosaemia – 38.1 per cent of the patients investigated – were classified as having DVD. Robertson et al. conclude that 'homozygosity for Q188R mutations in the GALT gene is a significant risk factor for DVD' (142).

4.2.2 Clinical Presentation

Even a brief survey of the literature on DVD can leave one with the impression that the clinical features of DVD are as numerous as the studies that have investigated them. Moreover, amongst these studies, there is little agreement on the features of this speech disorder. The result is a bewildering array of clinical characteristics, the diagnostic significance of which is often contested. With a definitive list of diagnostic criteria not possible at the present time, my aim in this section is the altogether more modest one of describing those features of DVD that have been consistently reported in the literature. Some of these features relate to the consistency with which these errors are produced and the groping or silent posturing that is frequently observed to accompany articulation. The question of how clinicians assess these features will be considered in section 4.2.3. We will also discuss the extent to which these characteristics can be used to distinguish DVD from other developmental speech disorders in that section.

A range of consonant and vowel errors can result in reduced speech intelligibility in children with verbal dyspraxia. Consonant errors include the deletion of initial and final consonants, cluster reductions, voicing errors and substitutions. Thoonen et al. (1997) found an overall higher rate of singleton consonant errors (substitutions, omissions, distortions) and cluster errors (cluster reductions) in 11 children with developmental apraxia of speech than in 11 normal-speaking children. Moreover, the substitution rate, particularly during real word imitations – the children in this study were also required to imitate nonsense words – was shown to correlate significantly with the severity of the DAS children's speech disorder, as rated by two speech and language therapists. Shriberg et al. (1997b) found that omissions accounted for 42 per cent of the consonant errors that were produced by children with developmental apraxia of speech, compared to 25 per cent in children with speech delay. More recently, Lewis et al. (2004) examined the speech and language skills of children with suspected childhood apraxia of speech (CAS group), children with isolated speech-sound disorders (S group) and children with combined speech-sound and language disorders (SL group). The errors of initial and final consonant deletion, syllable deletion and cluster reduction occurred in higher proportions in the CAS group than in the other two groups. Specifically, 100 per cent of CAS subjects produced final consonant deletion errors, compared to 25 per cent and 38 per cent of the S and SL groups, respectively. In relation to syllable deletion and cluster reduction, it was found that 90 per cent of CAS subjects deleted syllables and 60 per cent simplified clusters. This compared to 8 per cent and 15 per cent for the S and SL groups, respectively, for syllable deletion and 0 per cent and 8 per cent of the S and SL groups for cluster reduction. In a study of three children with childhood apraxia of speech, Jacks et al. (2006) found that omissions and substitutions were the most frequent error types, occurring with a mean frequency across sessions of 42 per cent and 34 per cent, respectively. Final consonants were omitted more often than either initial or medial consonants. Retroflex and cluster errors were less frequent, occurring with mean frequencies of 14 per cent and 9 per cent, respectively. Finally, in an analysis of consonant production in 11 children with DVD, Thoonen et al. (1994) found that DVD children show low percentages of retention for place and manner of articulation and voicing due to high substitution and omission rates. These children also showed a particularly low percentage of retention of place of articulation in words which, along with error rate, was found to be strongly related to the children's severity of involvement.

Other significant aspects of consonant production in DVD concern the relationship of consonant errors to syllable structure and the changes that occur in these errors over time as children develop. That DVD children have difficulty perceiving and processing syllable structure has been amply demonstrated in recent studies. Marquardt et al. (2002) examined the performance of three children with developmental apraxia of speech on a range of syllable tasks. DAS subjects and three age- and gender-matched children with normal speech and language development were required to identify the number of syllables in words, judge intrasyllabic sound positions and construct syllable shapes (single versus consonant cluster arrangements) within monosyllabic frames. It was found that the DAS participants in this study displayed impaired performance on all these tasks. Marquardt et al. conclude that the '[r]esults of this study showed that children with moderate to severe DAS demonstrate an apparent breakdown in the ability to perceive "syllableness" and to access and compare syllable representations with regard to position and structure' (42). Jacks et al. (2006) investigated the relationship between syllable structure and consonant accuracy in three subjects with CAS. It was found that syllable shape accuracy accounted for 87 per cent of the variance in consonant accuracy and that syllable shape accuracy and consonant accuracy were positively related – low syllable shape accuracy predicted low consonant accuracy and high syllable shape accuracy predicted high consonant accuracy. Jacks et al. also demonstrated that frequency of polysyllables accounted for 47 per cent of the variance in consonant accuracy and that high occurrence of polysyllables predicted lower consonant accuracy. These investigators conclude that '[a]lthough consonant errors do not necessarily result in syllable shape errors, in this study of children with CAS, consonant accuracy is strongly linked with syllable construction errors and patterns of syllable production' (437). Other studies have failed to find a relationship between syllable structure and aspects of consonant production. Nijland et al. (2003b) examined the production of high and low frequency of occurrence syllable utterances in six children with DAS and six normally speaking children. Anticipatory coarticulation was analysed using second formant trajectories. Although stronger coarticulation was found in the DAS children than in the normally speaking children, neither group of children displayed a systematic effect of syllable structure on the second formant trajectory.

Few longitudinal studies of children with DVD have been undertaken. Yet, these studies are essential if we are to gauge progress in DVD children and if we are to understand the developmental stages through which these children pass. One study that has attempted to characterise the speech features of DVD children over time is the investigation by Jacks et al. (2006), described above. Consonant and syllable production data were obtained from three English-speaking male children with CAS at one-year intervals (time 1–time 3) between the ages of 4.6 and 7.7 years. The three children – P_1, P_2 and P_3 – displayed different patterns of improvement during the course of the study. The child with the most severe speech disorder at the start of the study, P_3, was the only subject to show a clear pattern of improvement over time. Improvement was inconsistent for P_1 and P_2. For example, P_1's performance was poorest at time 2, while P_2's best performance was recorded at time 2. Also, while segmental variability decreased over time for P_3, variability was highest for P_1 at time 2 and lowest for P_2 at time 2.[7] Early developing consonants /m,b,j,n,w,d,p,h/ were more accurate than middle developing consonants /t,ŋ,k,g,f,v,tʃ,dʒ/, which were more accurate than late developing consonants /ʃ,θ,s,z,ð,l,r,ʒ/. However, there was an exception to this pattern – P_2 at times 2 and 3 produced middle developing sounds slightly more accurately than early sounds. There were also changes in consonant errors (omissions, substitutions, cluster errors and retroflex errors) across time. The relative frequency of omissions decreased over time for all participants. A more complicated pattern was observed for substitutions, with the relative frequency of these errors decreasing over time for only one subject (P_2). In P_1 and P_3, substitution errors were greatest at time 2. Cluster errors increased across time for P_2 and were greatest at time 2 for P_1 and P_3. Retroflex errors increased over time for P_1 and P_2 and were at their lowest level at time 2 in P_3. In keeping with wider variability in performance in these children, it is clear that there is no general trend towards reduction in the frequency of consonant error types in children with DVD.

Vowel errors are a common cause of speech unintelligibility in DVD children. Lewis et al. (2004) found that 100 per cent of a group of children with CAS produced vowel errors. This compared to only 1 per cent of child participants with isolated speech-sound disorders (S group) and 1 per cent of participants with combined speech-sound and language disorders (SL group). These findings were based on the Goldman–Fristoe Test of Articulation (Goldman and Fristoe 1986), which was conducted when the children were of preschool age (4–6 years). When these children were subsequently assessed at school age (8–10 years), a similar pattern of results emerged. An analysis of conversational speech samples revealed that 90 per cent of CAS participants produced vowel errors compared to only 8 per cent and 0 per cent of S and SL participants, respectively. As well as demonstrating the frequency of vowel errors in DVD children, studies have also examined the type of vowel errors that is produced and the effect of phrase length and word complexity on vowel accuracy. Davis et al. (2005) charted the vowel inventory and accuracy patterns of three children with suspected DAS over a three-year period. The children, who were between 4;6 and 7;7 years, received treatment during the study. These children's vowel inventories were generally complete, with the exception of rhotic vowels. Vowel accuracy was impaired in all children during the study, although accuracy did show a moderate increase from a range of 61–75 per cent at the first data recording to 71–85 per cent at the final data recording. Errors consisted mainly of vowel substitutions and de-rhoticisation. No consistent pattern of errors was found in the substitutions. Also, errors that involve small changes in vowel quality in the same area of vowel space (e.g. tensing/laxing) were also observed to occur more commonly than other errors. Although other studies have reported extensive diphthong reduction in DVD children (Pollock and Hall 1991; Davis et al. 1998), substantial diphthong reduction was not found in this investigation. Vowel accuracy did not decrease with increasing utterance length and there was only a slight trend towards decreasing accuracy with increasing syllable and word complexity. Other recent findings include the demonstration of poorer perception of vowels in apraxic children than in control children (Maassen et al. 2003) and the (unexpected) finding of an improvement in vowel quality in DAS children during the use of a bite block (Nijland et al. 2003a).

Prosodic disturbances, particularly anomalies of stress, have been frequently reported in studies of children with DVD. Munson et al. (2003) examined the acoustic correlates of stress and perceptual judgements of accuracy of stress production in five children with suspected developmental apraxia of speech (sDAS) and five children with phonological disorder (PD). Although no group differences in the production of stress were found, listeners judged that the nonword repetitions of children with sDAS matched the target stress contour less often than the repetitions produced by the PD children. Shriberg et al. (2003a) investigated whether a lexical stress ratio (LSR) that quantified the acoustic correlates of stress (frequency, intensity, duration) in bisyllabic word forms could distinguish 11 children with suspected apraxia of speech (sAOS) from 24 children with speech delay. LSR scores of children with sAOS were found to differ from those of children with speech delay. Of the six scores at the upper and lower extremes of the distributions of LSR scores, five of these scores (83 per cent) were from speakers with sAOS. Odell and Shriberg (2001) compared prosody-voice patterns in adults with apraxia of speech (AOS) and children with suspected apraxia of speech and inappropriate stress (AOSci). Compared to AOS speakers, speakers with AOSci had significantly more utterances meeting criteria for inappropriate stress and significantly fewer utterances that met criteria for inappropriate phrasing and inappropriate rate of speech. Shriberg et al. (1997b) compared the speech and prosody-voice profiles of 14 children with suspected DAS and 73 children with speech delay. These investigators found that inappropriate stress was the only linguistic domain that differentiated these two groups of children. This finding was cross-validated by a second study that used retrospective data obtained from a sample of 20 children with suspected DAS who had been evaluated in a university phonology clinic during a 10-year period. A third study by Shriberg et al.

(1997c) used conversational speech samples that were obtained from 19 children with suspected DAS to examine the use of stress. These samples were provided by five DAS researchers at geographically diverse diagnostic facilities in North America. Across these three studies, Shriberg et al. (1997c) found that 52 per cent of 48 samples from 53 children with suspected DAS had inappropriate stress. Of 71 samples from 73 age-matched children with speech delay of unknown origin, only 10 per cent had inappropriate stress. Other prosodic disturbances are reported by Nijland et al. (2003b), who found that normally speaking children produced metrical contrasts that were not realised by DAS children. Finally, Shriberg et al. (2003c) found higher coefficient of variation ratios in children with sAOS than in children with normal speech acquisition and in children with moderate to severe speech delay of unknown origin. This finding indicated that there was proportionally more variation in the duration of pause events and/or less variation in the duration of speech events in the sAOS children than in the normal speech or speech-delayed children.

A commonly described phenomenon in DVD is the inconsistency of speech errors. Marquardt et al. (2004) found high levels of error token variability in the speech of three children with DAS who were examined in a three-year longitudinal study. Jacks et al. (2006) report similar levels of variability in a later study of these same children. These investigators conclude that their results are 'suggestive of high session-to-session variability in children with CAS in addition to within-session variability' (2006:433). In a feature analysis study of singleton consonant errors in 11 children with DVD, Thoonen et al. (1994) found that these children were inconsistent in their feature realisation and feature preference. In a study of the diagnostic criteria used by 75 speech-language pathologists to establish a diagnosis of DAS, Forrest (2003) found that inconsistent productions constituted one of six characteristics that accounted for 51.5 per cent of responses. We return to the role of error inconsistency in the differential diagnosis of DVD in section 4.2.3.

Other commonly reported characteristics of DVD include articulatory groping and poor sequencing of sounds and syllables. Nijland et al. (2003b) state that groping (what they term 'articulatory searching behaviour') is 'typical' of DAS. Groping/effortful productions and poor sequencing of sounds were two of the most commonly reported characteristics used by speech-language pathologists to diagnose DAS in Forrest's (2003) study. These behaviours were reported with a frequency of 9.3 per cent and 6.2 per cent, respectively. Lewis et al. (2004) examined sequencing of syllables in 10 children with CAS. The sequencing of syllables in real and nonsense multisyllabic words was assessed in the preschool years and school years using the Multisyllabic Word Repetition task (Catts 1986), the Nonsense Word Repetition task (Kamhi and Catts 1986) and the Fletcher Time-by-Count Test of Diadochokinetic Syllable Rate (Fletcher 1978). Problems with syllable sequencing in the preschool years (only two CAS children were able to repeat diadochokinetic sequences) continued into the school years, with CAS children showing little improvement in the sequencing of syllables in real and nonsense multisyllabic words.

Individuals with DVD often experience language and other speech problems. Oral apraxia, feeding and general motor difficulties are also encountered in this clinical group. The CAS children studied by Lewis et al. (2004) displayed persistent receptive and expressive language deficits, with receptive skills consistently superior to expressive language skills. Even though some gains in language were made by the CAS children between preschool and school years, progress was less than that made by children with isolated speech-sound disorders and by children with combined speech-sound and language disorders. Relative to normative standards, most children with CAS lost ground in language skills and had deficient reading comprehension. CAS children performed even more poorly on the measure of spelling than on the reading measures.[8] Reduced mean length of utterance and poorer expressive than receptive language were among the characteristics used by speech-language pathologists to diagnose DAS in Forrest's study. (These two characteristics, however, only accounted for 0.8 per cent of the responses obtained.) Robin (1992) states that '[a]lthough [DAS] children often have language impairments, particularly in the expressive realm, these language-learning problems should be considered concomitant symptoms and *not* part of the apraxia' (21; italics in original). Clinicians must also be aware that speech problems such as dysarthria can occur in children with DVD. This can create something of a diagnostic problem for clinicians, who must decide if such a disorder is present in order to initiate an appropriate programme of intervention. That such a differential diagnosis is not easy to achieve is evident in the finding that dysarthric elements in the speech of DVD children are quite often overlooked. For example, Forrest (2003) reports how four in a group of 10 children referred to her university clinic following a diagnosis of DAS by area speech-language pathologists had signs of dysarthria. Two of these children had abnormally high velar air flow, while the other two children exhibited excessive laryngeal resistance. These clinical anomalies, Forrest argues, may explain the treatment failure that was noted by referring clinicians.

Robin (1992) states that 'one of the most frequent symptoms mentioned in the literature on DAS is the presence of oral apraxia' (20). Affected individuals have difficulty performing a range of nonspeech oral movements, such as tongue protrusion and elevation. Forrest (2003) found that general oral-motor difficulties were the second most common characteristic used by speech-language pathologists to diagnose DAS, accounting for 9.3 per cent of clinicians' responses. The role of feeding problems in DVD is disputed, with some clinicians treating deficits in this area as central to the diagnosis of DVD and other clinicians rejecting any place for feeding difficulties in the disorder. This is evident in the characteristics investigated by Forrest. A range of feeding and feeding-related difficulties were reported by the speech–language pathologists in this study – swallowing problems, feeding coordination problems and drooling/excessive saliva collectively accounted for 1.8 per cent of clinicians' responses. However, another characteristic – motor problem for speech with normal movement for feeding – accounted for a further 0.9 per cent of responses. Finally, verbal dyspraxia often occurs as part of a wider dyspraxia in which problems of motor coordination and clumsiness are evident (Bowens and Smith 1999). Lewis et al. (2004) believe that these motor problems may account for their finding that school-age children with CAS had a lower mean performance IQ than either children with isolated speech-sound disorders or children with combined speech-sound and language disorders: 'the lower Performance IQ of the CAS group may reflect a more general motor dyspraxia' (132). In particular, differences were observed between the CAS group and the group with speech-sound and language disorders on subtests of the Wechsler Intelligence Scale for Children (WISC) (Wechsler 1991) that required manual dexterity.[9] Also, Forrest (2003) found gross and fine motor difficulties and motor weakness among the characteristics used by speech-language pathologists to diagnose DAS – these characteristics accounted for 1.8 and 0.4 per cent of clinicians' responses, respectively.

4.2.3 Assessment and Diagnosis

Assessment of the DVD child covers the same areas that would be investigated during an initial evaluation of any child with a communication disorder. These areas are early history, hearing status, play skills and language, speech and motor abilities. However, some special considerations also apply to the assessment of these areas in DVD. A detailed early history can be particularly revealing of DVD. Velleman and Strand (1994) describe several features of this history that are characteristic of DVD. They include the late onset of babbling or minimal babbling, which may reflect an early difficulty in organising consonantal and vocalic elements within a simple canonical syllable. Velleman and Strand note that '[p]aucity in syllable variation is another hallmark of the early history of children with DVD' (1994:122). For example, the child may use only CV syllables such as [ba], [da], [bʌ] and [dʌ]. Parents often observe frustration on the part of the young child during communication on account of the gap between relatively intact comprehension skills and poor speech and expressive language skills. Some parents may report the use of elaborate natural gesture systems by the child as he or she tries to compensate for speech production problems. The child who can sequence these gestures is displaying knowledge of word order. In general, DVD children are reported to be communicative, despite their severe speech problems, and are often observed to use their parents as interpreters in situations that are unfamiliar to them or that are otherwise pressurised (Velleman and Strand 1994).

The assessment of a DVD child must include the results of a complete audiological evaluation to establish if there is any concomitant hearing impairment. Although figures do not exist, it seems likely that conductive and sensorineural hearing impairments are as prevalent in DVD children as in the child population as a whole or in children with other motor speech disorders. Certainly, their presence is a significant complicating factor in any remediation that aims to achieve motor learning. The child who has subnormal hearing or difficulty discriminating speech sounds is unlikely to acquire the motor patterns required to articulate speech sounds. An examination of representational play skills in the young DVD child is often revealing of the extent of the child's wider deficit in selecting, planning and organising motor patterns. Velleman and Strand (1994) state that

> [i]t has been our observation that many young children with DVD may be able to complete single functional play elements (e.g., comb a doll's hair, feed a doll) but have difficulty organizing a series of play elements into an integrated pretend play sequence (e.g., cook food, feed the doll, then put the doll to bed). This inability to organize and sequence play elements, in our view, is one more outward manifestation of their underlying praxis 'frame' deficit. (123)

These investigators also observe that, although the performance of DVD children on standardised tests of symbolic play has not been systematically compared to that of normally developing children, '[i]t seems possible that a distinctive profile would emerge if this were done' (1994:123).

Language skills must be assessed and deficits in phonology, syntax, semantics and pragmatics identified. A range of standardised tests can help the clinician to establish if discrepancies exist between known nonverbal cognitive abilities and the child's receptive performance on each of the language levels. Expressive language skills in DVD children are typically inferior to these children's receptive language abilities. Hodge and Hancock (1994) state that 'children who are first diagnosed with DAS are typically between 2.5 and 3.5 years of age and are still in the first 50-word stage in spoken language development' (104). This limited output, particularly in young children, has implications for how expressive language can best be assessed. In the young DVD child, assessment is usually restricted to estimating the size of the child's spoken vocabulary through parental report or spontaneous speech samples. These samples, along with samples elicited through object or picture naming, can be used to obtain the child's phonetic repertoire and to perform a phonological analysis.

At higher levels of expressive language development, clinicians can transcribe and analyse spontaneous language samples and use standardised tests to assess phonology, syntax and semantics. The child's metaphonological awareness (e.g. ability to rhyme words, break words into syllables) and skills in reading, writing and spelling (or exposure to preliteracy experiences, such as listening to nursery rhymes, if the child is not yet of school age) are also important components of a language assessment in DVD.

A wide-ranging assessment of speech skills must not only describe the nature and severity of any impairment, but also include an examination of the child's physiological support for speech. Procedures for assessing a child's phonetic inventory and phonological system are discussed elsewhere (see section 4.3.3) and will not be considered in the present context. Speech actions can be assessed by means of spontaneous and elicited speech samples. Observation of the child during spontaneous speech can reveal motor programming and coordination difficulties. These problems usually manifest themselves as groping behaviour and dysfluencies, such as prolongations and hesitations. Attempts at self-correction during spontaneous speech should also be noted. The phonological analysis can be examined for errors that are characteristic of DVD (see section 4.2.2) and for the effect of factors such as word length on error frequency. If sounds are absent from the child's phonetic inventory, the clinician should test their stimulability. The clinician provides a model of the target sound, which the child is then encouraged to imitate. If a sound is not immediately stimulable, additional cues may be used to encourage production. Hodge and Hancock (1994) suggest a hierarchy of cues which move from acoustic information only (the lower half of the examiner's face is covered), to visual and acoustic information and then, finally, to auditory, visual and tactile information, the latter in the form of placement or position cues (and on the condition, of course, that the child is not hypersensitive to touch).

Sounds that involve the sequencing of articulatory movements are often disrupted in DVD (e.g. diphthongs and affricates). Voicing and oral-nasal contrasts are also problematic for DVD children. In each case, one articulatory movement (either vocal fold adduction or opening of the velopharyngeal port) must be timed to coincide with another articulatory movement. Hodge and Hancock state that '[t]he precise timing demands for intercomponent coordination in these sound classes may present increased production difficulty' (1994:107). The child's performance on these potentially difficult sound classes should be recorded. The ability to sequence speech actions is itself influenced by a number of factors, each of which must be controlled for during assessment. If novel speech actions are used (i.e. sounds not in the child's phonetic inventory), then it may be difficult for the clinician to distinguish between an inability to generate a new motor programme and an inability to sequence a series of actions. Sequencing of actions is also influenced by the cognitive and linguistic demands of the task. If the child is having to direct processing resources to remembering lengthy instructions or unfamiliar target words, then motor performance can be expected to deteriorate. Sequencing sounds within syllables should be considered apart from sequencing of syllables within multisyllabic structures. Sounds within the child's phonetic inventory should be used in monosyllabic sequences. The child's ability to produce syllable shapes of increasing complexity should also be assessed. The same hierarchy of cues that was used to elicit individual sounds should also be used to elicit syllables. The clinician should record the most complex syllable shapes that can be produced by the child and the type of cue that is needed to elicit them.

When assessing the child's production of multisyllabic structures, the clinician should begin with sounds and syllable shapes that are within his or her phonetic repertoire. The child's ability to repeat the same syllable should be assessed first and then repetition of different syllables. The production of sequences such as /pəpəpə/ and /pətəkə/ can be timed to obtain diadochokinetic rates for the child. Real words can also be used to assess the child's ability to sequence syllables (e.g. baby, puppy). If the child tries to maintain articulatory accuracy by reducing speaking rate, diadochokinetic rates can be expected to increase with increasing motor demands of sequences. If, on the other hand, speaking rate is maintained as the motor demands of sequences increase, the child may begin to misarticulate individual sounds and produce syllables in the wrong sequence. The child's ability to sequence syllables in contexts where target sounds and words are controlled to avoid undue stress on motor programming, should be compared to sequencing ability in spontaneous speech. The greater linguistic and memory demands of spontaneous speech may reveal problems of syllable sequencing that are not evident in single-word contexts. As with the assessment of individual sounds, the clinician should note the type and frequency of cues needed to elicit syllable sequences, the level at which sequencing abilities break down (e.g. single word, spontaneous speech), the factors that trigger this breakdown (e.g. linguistic load) and any conditions that facilitate sequencing of syllables (e.g. rate reduction). Where possible, the clinician should also compare the child's motor performance to normative data (e.g. diadochokinetic rates).

Assessment should also examine the child's oral-motor abilities. The clinician can engage the child in activities designed to encourage the movement of vocal tract components (e.g. lips, tongue, mandible, velopharynx, larynx). If the child fails to produce a particular movement or sequence of movements on command, a visual model can be provided. A scoring system should be adopted. This may involve little more than rating a particular movement as 'normal' or 'abnormal'. However, a more detailed system might require the clinician to note if a demonstration of the movement was required and the accuracy, latency and completeness of the child's response. During an assessment of speech and oral-motor abilities, signs of neuromuscular involvement should be recorded. Such signs are important in helping the clinician make a differential diagnosis – neuromuscular damage compromises speech and nonspeech (oral) movements, a clinical picture that is more consistent with dysarthria than developmental verbal dyspraxia. Signs of neuromuscular involvement that should be noted include poor control of oral secretions, muscle weakness, abnormal muscle tone (either low or abnormally increased), involuntary movements, slow or inaccurate movements and, depending on the level of impairment, muscle atrophy (Hodge and Hancock 1994). Attention should also be paid to any structural abnormalities of the oral cavity that may compromise speech production.

The process of assessment results in a diagnosis of the child's speech disorder. However, it is still not particularly clear which assessment findings should lead clinicians to make a diagnosis of DVD. Almost every characteristic of DVD examined in section 4.2.2 has been credited with some diagnostic significance by investigators. Forrest (2003) captured the extent of this diagnostic problem in her recent survey of the criteria used by speech-language pathologists to reach a diagnosis of DAS. A total of 50 different characteristics were identified. Forrest concluded that her results were 'consistent with the general ambiguity of the diagnostic criteria of DAS' (2003:376). The number and type of vowel and consonant errors, the inconsistency or variability of sound errors, speech timing and aberrant patterns of stress are some of the most commonly reported features of DVD believed to have diagnostic significance. Although Davis et al. (2005) found that vowel accuracy and the frequency of vowel types used in substitution errors were not highly correlated in their study of three children with suspected DAS, these investigators suggest that such an accuracy-frequency relationship 'may provide another fruitful area for further inquiry regarding potential differential diagnostic indicators for DAS' (270). Maassen et al. (2003) found that a combination of vowel perception measures had a high differential and clinical value for the assessment of children with apraxic speech problems. Thoonen et al. (1994) quantified diagnostic characteristics relating to consonant production in DVD. This quantification consisted of (1) low percentages of retention for place and manner of articulation and voicing, (2) a low percentage of retention of place of articulation in words which, along with error rate, is related to the severity of the disorder, (3) inconsistency in feature realisation and feature preference and (4) a high syntagmatic (feature assimilation) error rate.

Error inconsistency is widely believed to have diagnostic significance for DVD. However, although reports of inconsistency abound, clinicians have generally not attempted to measure aspects of articulatory error inconsistency. Recently, Betz and Stoel-Gammon (2005) developed three formulae for this purpose. The formulae in question were proportion of errors, overall consistency of error types and consistency of the most frequently used error type.

These investigators report significant differences between children with DAS and children with phonological delay on the first of these formulae – proportion of errors – but not on the remaining two formulae. They conclude that '[f]uture research is needed with children with DAS and PD to determine whether error consistency is a defining characteristic of DAS' (2005:65). Shriberg and co-workers have based diagnostic markers for DAS on features such as temporal regularity and stress. Shriberg et al. (2003c) developed a metric known as the coefficient of variation ratio to capture DAS children's relative temporal variation in speech events and pause events within utterances (see section 4.2.2). Shriberg et al. (2003a) proposed a lexical stress ratio for suspected apraxia of speech (see section 4.2.2). This ratio was found to distinguish reliably children with suspected apraxia of speech from children with speech delay. Other findings of inappropriate stress in DAS children by Shriberg et al. (1997b,c) have led these investigators to conclude that 'inappropriate stress is a diagnostic marker for a subtype of DAS' (1997b:306). Not all studies have found evidence of stress anomalies in DVD. For example, Munson et al. (2003) found no group differences in the production of stress in children with suspected DAS and children with phonological disorder.

4.2.4 Clinical Intervention

Treatment of DVD involves a range of techniques that are more often used in combination than in isolation. Some of these techniques target speech sounds directly, usually in the form of intensive drills of increasing motor complexity. Other techniques aim to improve speech motor learning in children through delivering enhanced feedback to the speech mechanism. The PROMPT technique – Prompts for Restructuring Oral Muscular Phonetic Targets (Chumpelik 1984) – and the adapted cueing technique (Klick 1985) are two such forms of intervention. Still other techniques set out to improve speech intelligibility by modifying features of spoken prosody. In a small number of reported cases, prosthetic intervention has brought about gains in speech intelligibility in dyspraxic children. Augmentative and alternative communication may be used to support speech production in the dyspraxic child or as a substitute for speech in the severely unintelligible child. Children with DVD require frequent, intensive intervention to make significant gains in speech intelligibility. We conclude this section by addressing issues relating to the frequency and intensity of treatment in DVD.

The production of speech sounds is directly targeted in most forms of dyspraxia intervention. The nature of speech sound intervention varies between individual approaches, but there are a number of common features between these approaches. Most clinicians[10] are in agreement that therapy sessions must provide the dyspraxic child with the maximum number of opportunities to practise target sounds. This is normally achieved through the use of intensive, systematic and frequent drills, which may provide the child with well over a hundred repetitions of a target sound in a single session. Such intensive rehearsal is required to achieve learning of new articulatory motor patterns. The sound hierarchies that are used in practice must be selected with care. Decisions about which sounds and sound combinations to treat first are influenced by a number of considerations, including the developmental sequence of sounds (teach early sounds first), the stimulability and frequency of sounds (frequently occurring sounds are more likely to affect intelligibility) and the visibility of sound production (sounds that are clearly visible during production are easier to teach than sounds which lack a visual aspect). Sound practice should move quickly from the production of phonemes in isolation to production of the target sound within syllables of increasing complexity. All practice words and phrases should be familiar to the child or at least within his or her language abilities to avoid any increase in the child's linguistic load – unfamiliar words and syntactically complex sentences will diminish the processing resources at the child's disposal for motor learning. Many of these features, and others besides, are incorporated in the Nuffield Dyspraxia Programme. This programme is used to treat children with DVD who are aged three years and older. Vowel and consonant sounds are targeted through drill/play exercises that build from sounds in isolation to their use in simple alternating sequences and eventually in phrases. To aid learning, each sound has an associated visual referent – a picture of a toy drum for /d/, a parrot for the diphthong /ɒɪ/ and a mouse for /i/.

For clinicians who subscribe to the view that DVD is related to a failure of feedback in the speech production mechanism,[11] techniques that augment feedback and/or provide alternative modes of feedback are the remediation method of choice. The two techniques that will be examined here are PROMPT and Klick's adapted cueing technique. However, in practice many other techniques, including the use of a mirror to provide visual feedback to a child on the position of his or her articulators, operate by enhancing feedback in the speech production mechanism. As Square (1994) describes the PROMPT technique, it involves 'the dynamic delivery of tactile and kinesthetic cues to the speech mechanism to signal place of articulation, timing of respiratory, laryngeal, and velopharyngeal activity, and the durations of valving constrictions or vocal tract postures' (157). PROMPT avoids many of the methods employed in more traditional forms of therapy for DVD, including oral-motor exercises, speech drill and developmental speech hierarchies. Square et al. (2000) have demonstrated the efficacy of PROMPT intervention in children with speech-motor deficits. Six male children with unintelligible speech and a history of minimal progress in traditional therapy received PROMPT treatment in a 90-minute group session twice weekly for 12 weeks.

It was found that PROMPT treatment produced perceptually improved speech in these children even on untrained words. Additionally, functioning in several other domains (overall behaviour, social interactions and language skills) was also shown to improve significantly.

Klick's adapted cueing technique (ACT) uses visual cues to facilitate speech production. The emphasis of this approach is on the sequential production of phonemes: 'cues are presented in such a way as to suggest sequential, coarticulatory movement in an overall pattern of motion' (Klick 1994:183). The clinician's hand moves forward and back along the side of his or her face, while specific speech sounds are indicated through finger movements that are loosely based on the manual alphabet for the hearing-impaired. Cueing of phoneme sequences occurs along three dimensions: place, manner and vowel–related mandibular motion. Vowel production is cued along two parameters, the focal point of resonance and mandibular closure. In her original paper on this technique, Klick (1985) described how one child, a girl of 5;6 years called J, responded to treatment based on ACT. Prior to treatment, J had jargon–like speech and only 2–4 true words, and used nonoral communication in a variety of situations. After three months of treatment, J's oral communication skills had improved. She was using several carrier phrases and 12 single words. J's oral-motor control for verbal imitation had also improved. By six months, J was beginning to use novel utterances and her parents reported an increase in the amount and intelligibility of her speech at home. The use and presentation of ACT changed over time to reflect J's changing need for facilitative cues. As treatment continued and J became less reliant on cueing, the role of ACT was reduced.

Melodic intonation therapy[12] (MIT) aims to improve the speech of dyspraxic children by targeting spoken prosody. The three elements of spoken prosody upon which this technique is based are the melodic line, tempo and rhythm, and points of stress. Helfrich–Miller (1994) explains that

> [i]n an intoned utterance, the tempo is lengthened, the rhythm and stress are exaggerated, and the constantly varying pitch of speech is reduced and stylized into a pattern involving the constant pitch of several whole notes. A typical intoned utterance only varies by one whole note, much like chanting. (176)

Melodic intonation therapy does not target the production of individual speech sounds. Helfrich–Miller states that '[i]t is not designed to replace other therapy approaches but to supplement and augment them' (1994:175). Like other treatments for dyspraxia discussed in this section, few studies have examined the efficacy of MIT in dyspraxic children.[13] Those studies that have been performed are so fraught with procedural and methodological problems that one cannot reliably base claims about the effectiveness of this technique upon them. Recently, Roper (2003) examined only three published studies[14] that included information on the characteristics and consequences of melodic intonation therapy. The duration of MIT intervention in the six child participants in these studies ranged from 2 to 33 months, while the frequency of sessions ranged from once a week to three times a week. The studies differed considerably in terms of the treatment protocols that were used (only three children completed all levels of MIT and modifications were made to the paediatric version of MIT) and the outcome measures that were adopted. Other perceived weaknesses in these studies include small dose–response effects (there was little change in relation to the amount of intervention provided), threats to statistical validity and multiple treatment interference. Roper concludes that

> [t]he small number of studies, small number of participants, lack of treatment fidelity measures, possible threats to external and internal validity, and individual modifications that were made in the MIT procedures, all converge on the fact that the empirical evidence to support Melodic Intonation Therapy with children with apraxia is meager at best. (2003:4)

On some occasions, prosthetic intervention may be used to improve specific speech defects in DVD, such as hypernasality. Hall et al. (1990) remark that DAS children '[o]ften . . . continue to be perceived as excessively hypernasal sounding, even as their speech skills improve. In such cases physical management techniques may need to be considered' (455). These investigators conducted a case study of a child whom they had followed for a period of 11 years since the age of seven. This child, known as TB, had many of the speech characteristics that are associated with DAS (e.g. vowel omissions or misarticulations, inconsistent errors). Additionally, she had features that are known to accompany DAS (e.g. oral apraxia for nonspeech movements). During initial evaluation, TB exhibited significant nasal emission of air on nearly all plosives, fricatives and affricates. Significant hypernasality contributed to her lack of intelligibility. TB's soft palate was asymmetrical at rest and moved to the right upon phonation. There was also some lateral pharyngeal wall movement. Despite intensive remediation using a motor-programming therapy approach, TB continued to exhibit nasal airflow and a failure of velar movement during isolated vowel productions. The construction of a palatal lift prosthesis was recommended to help TB impound intra-oral air pressures and, in doing so, improve her articulatory skills. With the assistance of the lift, TB was able to improve her articulation skills markedly. Hall et al. (1990) conclude that '[p]alatal lift management seems effective with DAS children exhibiting velopharyngeal closure problems' (458).

In cases of severe dyspraxia, augmentative and alternative communication is often an essential component of intervention. DVD presents some unique challenges for AAC intervention, not least of which is that additional motor problems may restrict the type of system that can be used by the dyspraxic child. If manual signs are to be used, they must be easy for the dyspraxic child to perform (von Tetzchner and Martinsen 2000). Several case studies have demonstrated the efficacy of AAC intervention in dyspraxic children. Bornman et al. (2001) examined the language and communication skills of a dyspraxic child who used a Macaw Digital voice output device. The subject's mother was trained in how to use the device to give her child access to higher levels of language functioning. The specific benefits that derived from the use of this digital device included an increase in the number and cognitive complexity of questions that were directed to the child. It was also found that the number of appropriate answers, communication modalities and communication attempts by the child increased. Bornman et al. (2001) conclude that '[d]igital voice output devices can be used as a method to facilitate higher cognitive functioning and have various positive impacts on the functioning of a child with DAS' (623). Cumley and Swanson (1999) conducted case studies of three children diagnosed with DAS. These children received a multimodal AAC intervention that consisted of speech, gestures, manual signs and various AAC aids. Some of these aids used low technology (i.e. communication boards, remnant books and symbol dictionaries), while others used high technology (i.e. voice output communication aids and print output communication aids). The child's natural speech in each case was supplemented through the use of these AAC aids and strategies. AAC intervention also increased opportunities for facilitating language development, communicative competence and academic achievement. Through the use of AAC aids and strategies, the children with DAS had greater opportunities to initiate and maintain interactions and repair breakdowns in communication in different situations with familiar and unfamiliar partners.

The generalisation of clinically acquired skills to novel situations and behaviours is widely taken to indicate the success of a particular intervention. Many clinicians have remarked upon the lack of generalisation to follow from interventions for DVD. Ballard (2001) states that '[s]everal treatment approaches have been developed to remediate this motor programming impairment . . . but their success in terms of response generalization has been limited' (4). Clearly, an urgent question for clinicians and researchers is which factor or group of factors leads to the generalisation of motor speech skills in the child with DVD. Inevitably, this question has led investigators to examine factors such as the frequency and intensity of intervention and the mode of delivery of intervention. It is frequently remarked in the literature that the number of sessions that is required to achieve significant speech gains in children with phonological disorder is not sufficient to produce marked gains in the speech of DVD children. Using a General Communication Outcome Questionnaire (Campbell 1998), Campbell (1999) reported that while phonologically disordered children required, on average, 29 individual treatment sessions (range: 21–42 sessions) to be rated by their parents as having about three-fourths of their speech understood by an unfamiliar listener, children with apraxia of speech required 151 individual sessions (range: 144–168 sessions) to attain a similar level of parental estimated intelligibility. On the basis of these figures, Campbell (1999) concludes that apraxic children need 81 per cent more individual treatment sessions than children with phonological disorder to achieve a similar functional outcome.

Clearly, DVD children require more intervention in total than children with phonological disorder. Studies have also demonstrated that intervention needs to be delivered in shorter, more frequent sessions than longer, less frequent sessions. Most clinicians and researchers now advocate the use of distributed over mass practice in DVD. Strand and Skinder (1999) state that

> for children with significant motor planning or programming problems, distributed practice will likely result in better motor learning. For example, if 2 hours of therapy per week are recommended, sessions should be scheduled four times per week for half an hour, versus two times a week for an hour. (121)

Skinder-Meredith (2001) proposes the use of 'frequent short sessions' – four times per week for 30 minutes a session is recommended – and remarks that 'children with phonologic delay progress more quickly than children with DAS. This means that the child with DAS will need these intensive services longer' (8). Hall et al. (1993) concur with the need for 'intensive services' in the treatment of DVD children. However, in their clinic these services take the form of a summer programme in which children are in residence for six weeks and receive four hours of remediation for five days each week: 'It is our experience that these intensive summer sessions result in greater gains in remedial goals than children with DAS experience when they receive services once or twice weekly for half-hour or hourly sessions'(125). Simms and Schum (2000) state that '[c]hildren who have oral-motor deficits, especially speech apraxia, require intensive speech and language therapy' (156).

Finally, although group therapy has many positive benefits for children with communication disorders, it is generally agreed that DVD children require individual therapy if significant speech gains are to be made. Hall et al. (1993) state that these children 'seem to require a great deal of professional service, typically done on an individual basis' (125). Strand and Skinder (1999) argue that 'it seems logical to assume that individual treatment sessions go much further in offering the child the opportunity to practice the movement gestures with enough frequency for the motor learning to be retained' (121). Each of the 45-minute treatment sessions described by Campbell (1999) was conducted on an individual basis.

4.3 Developmental Phonological Disorder

There is an important group of childhood speech disorders that has been discussed extensively in the clinical literature. Although a large number of terms has come to be used of this disorder,[15] we will adopt the term developmental phonological disorder (DPD) throughout this discussion. This disorder is set apart from other childhood speech disorders (e.g. developmental dysarthria) by its lack of a known origin. Specifically, there is no identifiable neurological impairment or anatomical malformation that can account for the child's speech disorder, and hearing, intelligence, and social, emotional and behavioural skills are all within normal limits. In this section, we consider what is known about the prevalence of DPD and other epidemiological features of this disorder. We examine the speech characteristics of DPD as well as discuss additional impairments in language that have been found to occur in this disorder. Issues in the assessment and treatment of DPD will also be addressed. We consider, for example, the use of sampling techniques in phonological assessment and examine the efficacy of treatment methods. We begin by examining the epidemiology and aetiology of DPD.

4.3.1 Epidemiology and Aetiology

A considerable number of studies has examined the prevalence of DPD – in their own prevalence study, Shriberg et al. (1999) state that over 100 such investigations have been conducted. These studies have produced widely differing prevalence estimates and reviews of these investigations have uniformly concluded that there is no consensus on the prevalence of this disorder (Shriberg et al. 1999). Shriberg (1994) reports how he and his colleagues have found that approximately 60 per cent of the preschool children in their local populations have speech delay without associated involvements. Using the US national prevalence figure of 2.5 per cent, they calculate that this translates to a population estimate of 1–2 children per hundred with a form of DPD called speech delay. Shriberg et al. (1999) report that the prevalence of speech delay in a group of 1,328 monolingual English-speaking six-year-old children in the US is 3.8 per cent. Law et al. (2000) examined prevalence figures for speech delay in a recent review of literature. Among 21 studies meeting full criteria for inclusion in the review, prevalence figures ranged from 2.3 to 24.6 per cent.

Gender findings display the same variability as the more general prevalence figures just examined. Shriberg et al. (1999) found that speech delay was approximately 1.5 times more prevalent in boys (4.5 per cent) than girls (3.1 per cent). This sex ratio, these investigators argue, is lower by as much as 100 per cent than earlier estimates that range from 2:1 to 3:1 in samples of preschool children with speech delay. Shriberg (1994) reports the higher figure of 75 per cent boys in their samples. In their literature review, Law et al. (2000) state that '[a] propensity for marked speech . . . delays to be more common in males than females is generally confirmed by the studies reviewed here' (173).

Familial aggregation data are playing an increasingly important role in genetic explanations of DPD. Studies are now revealing the presence of speech and language impairments amongst the biological relatives of individuals with DPD. Felsenfeld et al. (1995) used a battery of tests to assess the articulation, language and nonverbal reasoning abilities of the offspring (children over three years) of 24 adults with a documented history of a moderate phonological-language disorder. These investigators found that the children of these adult subjects performed significantly more poorly than control children on all measures of language expression, although scores generally fell within normal limits when compared to test norms. A similar pattern was found on articulation scores – proband children attained lower scores which were still within the average range when compared to normative data. Additionally, 40 per cent of proband children were judged to have had a speech production problem at some time, compared to only 7 per cent of control children. In total, it was found that 53 per cent of proband families had one or more offspring with a developmental articulation or language disability. This compares to a population rate for these disorders of only 4 per cent and a control group rate of 0 per cent.

Although DPD is, by definition, a speech disorder of unknown origin, it is looking increasingly likely that some type of genetic mechanism may ultimately be responsible for at least one subtype of the disorder. Shriberg et al. (2005) state that '[c]onverging evidence supports the hypothesis that the most common subtype of childhood speech sound disorder (SSD) of currently unknown origin is genetically transmitted' (834). These investigators examined two groups of children with speech delay of unknown origin. One group had a high genetic load for the disorder (these children had two or more family members with current and/or prior speech-language disorder). The other group had reduced genetic load for speech delay (no affected family members). The speech error patterns of these children differed significantly in three ways. The children with a high genetic load for speech delay displayed (a) a significantly higher proportion of relative omission errors on the late-8 consonants /ʃ,θ,s,z,ð,l,r,ʒ/ (b) a significantly lower proportion of relative distortion errors on these same consonants, and particularly the sibilant fricatives /s,z,ʃ/ and

(c) a significantly lower proportion of backed /s/ distortions. It is argued that these speech error patterns have validity as a three-part diagnostic marker for a genetic subtype of speech delay. It seems likely that, as more studies of this type are performed, and further aetiological mechanisms underlying speech delay are revealed, the classification of DPD as a disorder of unknown origin will have to be substantially revised.

4.3.2 Clinical Presentation

Speech sound (segment) errors in children with DPD can be described in terms of distinctive features[16] or phonological processes. Reflecting the dominant use of process analysis in clinical phonology,[17] this section will examine the types of process that occur in disordered phonology and review the findings of studies in the area. Stoel-Gammon et al. (2002) describe three basic types of phonological process. The first type affects the syllable structure of words and includes final consonant deletion ('bat' pronounced [bæ]), cluster reduction ('swim' pronounced [wɪm]) and weak syllable deletion ('banana' pronounced [nænə]). The second type of process involves changes in the place, manner or voicing of consonants and includes velar fronting ('gun' pronounced [dʌn]), palatal fronting ('sheep' pronounced [sip]), stopping ('sun' pronounced [tʌn]), gliding ('red' pronounced [wɛd]), prevocalic voicing ('pen' pronounced [bɛn]) and final devoicing ('bag' pronounced [bæk]). In the third type of process, one consonant assimilates to (that is, becomes like) another consonant in the word. Assimilatory processes include velar assimilation ('dog' pronounced [gɔg]) and labial assimilation ('top' pronounced [bɑp]).

Each of the simplification processes described above can be found in the speech of children who are developing phonology along normal lines. The question for clinicians and researchers, then, is how to distinguish children with phonological disorders from children in whom these processes resolve as part of normal maturation. Yavaş (1998) describes several characteristics that researchers have proposed in order to set apart children with a disordered phonological system from children in whom phonology is developing normally. The first of these characteristics is the persistence of normal processes. Processes such as prevocalic voicing and consonant harmony (assimilation) are normally expected to resolve by three years of age (Stoel-Gammon and Dunn 1985). However, in children with disordered phonology, these processes may persist to four years and beyond (Yavaş 1998). A child's pattern of speech errors may reveal chronological mismatch (see note 124 in chapter 3). The child with disordered phonology may also exhibit variable use of processes in relation to one and the same target structure. For example, the child may delete final consonants on some occasions, but replace them with a glottal stop [ʔ] on other occasions. Systematic sound preference is another feature of disordered phonology. This is where a child may use only one or two sounds to replace a group of sounds that share the same manner of articulation. An example is the use of [tɪn] for each of the target words 'thin', 'sin', 'fin' and 'skin'. Clearly, substitutions of this type have significant implications for the intelligibility of a child's speech as they eliminate a number of contrasts. Finally, children with disordered phonologies are more likely to make use of unusual/idiosyncratic/ atypical processes. Yavaş (1998) lists the following simplification processes that are rarely found in children with normal phonological development: backing of alveolars ('pat' → [pæk]), gliding of fricatives ('fig' → [wɪg]), glottal insertion ('ladder' → [læʔər]), frication of stops ('ban' → [væn]), unusual cluster reduction ('train' → [ren]) and initial consonant deletion ('tape' → [ep]).

Many of the processes that have been described in this section have also been analysed in recent studies of phonological disorder in children. Stoel-Gammon et al. (2002) examined a four-year-old boy, referred to as Eric, whose score on the Assessment of Phonological Processes – Revised (APP-R; Hodson 1986) gave him a rating of 'severe' phonological disorder. An analysis of Eric's speech revealed the following processes: final consonant deletion, velar fronting, stopping, cluster reduction and gliding of liquids. Each of these processes occurred more than 40 per cent of the time, as measured on the APP-R. Powell et al. (1999) present longitudinal data on the phonological systems of five children with phonological disorders. At 5;2 years, one of these children, Keith, displayed evidence of velar fronting in word-initial position but not in word-final position ('comb' [toʊm]; 'duck' [dʌk]). A second child, Sally (3;10 years), displayed the same pattern of velar fronting as Keith. Analysis revealed extensive stopping of fricatives in word-initial position and intervocalically ('soup' [tup]; 'nosy' [noʊdi]). Sally also omitted fricatives in word-final position ('teeth' [ti]). Sally's nonidentical twin sister, Suzy, similarly stopped fricatives, with the exception of /v/, which was realised as [t] ('vase' [tɛt]). In Suzy's phonological system, the omission of fricatives in word-final position was optional ('ice' [aɪ]; but 'glove' [tʌt]). Both affricates were realised as [t] ('cheese' [ti]; 'jeep' [tip]). The voicing distinction was a source of difficulty for Suzy, with devoicing occurring in both word-initial and word-final positions (see production of 'vase'). Both twins omitted /ŋ/ and used [h] for liquids and glides in prevocalic and intervocalic positions ('yawn' [hɔn]; 'leafy' [hiti]). Postvocalically, liquids and glides were realised as vowels. Both girls used nasal assimilation when a syllable ended in a nasal ('drum' [nʌm]). A fourth child, John (5;0 years), used a number of unusual substitutions, including the use of [v] for liquids in the context of a [f] and [ð] for liquids in other contexts ['laugh' [væf]; 'leg' [ðeɪg]). The fifth child studied by Powell et al., Chad (5;9 years), was the only child to use [s] in pretreatment. However, [s] production was restricted to postvocalic position, was replaced by [l] in prevocalic position and was omitted within words. The use of [l] was a more general feature of Chad's phonological system, where it was used in word-initial position for targets other than stops or nasals.

Disordered phonological systems often display a high degree of variation, with the same sound in the same position being realised in several different ways. Miccio and Ingrisano (2000) described the phonological system of a girl of 5;3 years who was diagnosed with a severe phonological disorder. This girl, referred to as K, displayed a number of variable productions. For example, although the glide /j/ was correctly realised on some occasions ('yes' [jɛt]), different substitutions were observed in 'yellow' [ʔɛlo] and 'yard' [hɑrd]. Similarly, /h/ was correctly realised on some occasions ('hide' [haɪd]; 'hat' [hæt]) but was substituted with a glottal stop on other occasions ('house' [ʔaʊt]). K's other phonological processes included fronting ('cut' [tʌt]), stopping ('sock' [tɑt]), consonant harmony ('dog' [dɑd]) and /s/ cluster reduction ('swim' [wɪm]). Other consonant clusters were present, even if they were not always correctly realised ('frog' [prɑg]; 'blow' [bloʊ]). As is often the case in phonological disorder, K's speech did not contain vowel errors.[18] As well as variation within individual phonological systems, there are considerable differences between systems. Miccio et al. (1999) examined the phonological systems of four children who were aged between 3;10 and 5;7 years. Although processes such as stopping were found in all four subjects, the types of sound affected by this process and the position of these sounds within words varied considerably between subjects. In this way, participant 1 used /v/ → [b] in word-initial position and /ð/ → [d] in intervocalic position. Where only two fricatives succumbed to stopping in participant 1's phonological system, all fricatives were replaced by [d] in word-initial position in participants 2's system. In intervocalic position, fricatives were replaced by the glottal stop [ʔ]. In participant 3's system, all fricatives but one – /ð/ – were replaced by stops. Additionally, however, affricates were also replaced by stops. Finally, participant 4 also stopped fricatives and affricates. Unlike participant 2, who used different substitute stops in word-initial position and intervocalic position – [d] and [ʔ], respectively – participant 4 used only one stop in these positions (the stop [d]) and used [t] in word-final position. The individual differences in these four cases reflect the type of variation that occurs between phonologically disordered systems and should not be viewed as exceptional.[19]

The presence of language deficits in children with phonological disorders is now clearly attested to in the literature.[20] Investigators have found evidence of impaired lexical acquisition in children with phonological disorders. Storkel (2004) reported that children with functional phonological delays displayed a common sound sequence disadvantage in lexical acquisition, while younger, phonologically matched children showed a common sound sequence advantage. Specifically, where common sound sequences facilitated phonological processing and speeded lexical acquisition in the younger children in this study, these same sound sequences led to lexical competition in children with phonological disorder and a concomitant reduction in these children's ability to create unique lexical representations. Additional language deficits have also been found to persist into adulthood. Felsenfeld et al. (1992) examined 24 adults with a documented history of moderately severe phonological disorder. These adults performed significantly more poorly than a group of 28 control adults on all measures of articulation and expressive and receptive language. These investigators conclude that 'many adults with a childhood history of delayed phonological development will continue to experience linguistic outcomes that are less favourable than those of controls' (1992:1114).

Language-based academic problems are also commonly encountered in children with phonological disorders. These problems centre on literacy skills, such as reading and spelling. Larrivee and Catts (1999) examined 30 children with expressive phonological disorders and found that they performed significantly less well on tests of reading achievement than 27 children with normally developing phonology and language (although considerable within–group variability was noted). When subjects with phonological disorders were split into two groups – children with good and poor reading outcomes – it was found that the poor reading outcomes group had more severe expressive phonological disorders, poorer phonological awareness[21] and poorer language skills than the children with good reading outcomes. Using hierarchical multiple regression, Larrivee and Catts found that expressive phonology and phonological awareness accounted for significant amounts of variance in reading achievement. Bird et al. (1995) studied 31 children with expressive phonological impairments at 70, 79 and 91 months. These children scored well below control children on assessment of phonological awareness and literacy. Bird et al. also found that the severity of phonological impairments in relation to age was an important determinant of literacy outcome: 'children who have severe expressive phonological impairments at the time they start school are at particular risk for reading and spelling problems' (1995:446). Lewis et al. (2000) followed 52 children, who had been identified as having moderate to severe expressive phonology disorder at 4–6 years, into the third and fourth grades. The children were divided into two groups depending on whether a phonological disorder occurred in isolation (P group) or in combination with language problems (PL group). At follow–up, the PL group exhibited poorer performance than the P group on measures of phoneme awareness, language, reading decoding, reading comprehension and spelling. The spelling skills of the P group were poor relative to their reading and language abilities. Finally, Bernhardt and Major (2005) used a battery of speech, language, cognitive and academic tasks on 12 children who had participated in a phonological and metaphonological intervention programme three years earlier. Five of these children had residual phonological impairment. Although only two children had below average reading performance (decoding and comprehension), five children displayed below average spelling performance.

4.3.3 Phonological Assessment

An assessment of phonological disorders in children must include consideration of a vast range of factors which are known to influence speech sound production. A detailed case history, with the child's parent as an informant, enables the clinician to establish which aspects of a child's development and wider environment may have contributed to the disorder. Much of the information that is gleaned through history taking will also have a bearing on how the child is likely to respond to treatment, if intervention is required (e.g. the extent of parental support). Bleile (2002) recommends that a case history should examine the child's communication development, birth and medical history, social development and educational history. A lack of babbling and delays in achieving communication milestones (e.g. first words, two-word utterances) are often the first signs that a child is at risk for speech production problems. Recurrent episodes of otitis media may necessitate referral of the child to other professionals (e.g. audiologist, otolaryngologist) and have implications for speech development. The clinician must establish if the child is receiving communication opportunities within the home environment. For example, an older sibling may be dominating communication at home or speaking on behalf of the speech-impaired child. If the child is receiving additional or special services in schools, the clinician must enquire about them. At the very least, the therapist should talk to the child's teacher (nursery worker, if the child is of preschool age), who will be able to provide information on how the child is communicating with his or her peers.

Following the completion of a case history, attention turns in assessment to the evaluation of skills necessary to communication. Good speech production skills require a sound oral mechanism and normal hearing levels. The structure and function of the oral mechanism should be assessed using both speech and nonspeech tasks. Owing to the invasive nature of at least part of this examination, this particular evaluation is more appropriately undertaken some time into the assessment session, when the child is more relaxed in the presence of the clinician. A range of abnormalities may be observed and their significance for speech production assessed. For example, drooping or parted lips and involuntary chewing movement or fasciculations may indicate possible neuromuscular dysfunction (Miccio 2002). Structural abnormalities may also be discovered, including palatal fistulae or a submucous cleft palate. In such cases, a neurological or craniofacial referral may be required. Due to the flexibility and adaptability of the speech mechanism, only gross abnormalities are likely to interfere with speech production (Bleile 2002). Hearing assessments, including pure tone audiological screening and tympanometry, are conducted.[22] If a child fails to achieve a threshold of 20dB across the frequencies 500, 1000, 2000 and 4000 Hz, then a referral for a complete audiological evaluation can be made (Miccio 2002). An oral examination and hearing screening are vital in arriving at a differential diagnosis of speech sound disorders in children – significant positive findings on these sections of the assessment have traditionally been taken to preclude a diagnosis of functional phonological disorder (i.e. phonological disorder of unknown origin).

Given the presence of wider language deficits in children with phonological disorders, assessment must go beyond an evaluation of speech sounds to include an examination of structural language skills. Standardised and non-standardised procedures are commonly used to examine speech and language skills. The advantage of standardised tests is that they allow the clinician to compare the child's performance to normative data. This can provide a useful baseline for intervention – by repeating the test on later occasions, the child's progress can be charted. Also, the results of these tests often satisfy the enquiries of parents, who want to know how their child is performing. Additionally, standardised procedures are often more easily administered and quickly scored than nonstandardised procedures. A drawback of standardised procedures is that they provide a mere snapshot of a child's speech and language abilities. Tests that examine a child's pronunciation of single words or that evaluate a child's comprehension of phrases and sentences are often not able to reveal fully how a child uses speech and language in more spontaneous settings. For this reason, the results of standardised tests should always be interpreted alongside findings obtained from an analysis of a spontaneous conversational speech sample.

Published phonological assessments are now in abundance. Yavaş (1998) lists nine such assessments that use a phonological process analysis alone. Phonological tests vary considerably along a number of parameters. Even amongst the nine assessments listed by Yavaş, the Assessment of Phonological Processes – Revised (Hodson 1986) examines 40 processes, while Weiner's (1979) Phonological Process Analysis and Shriberg and Kwiatkowski's (1980) Natural Process Analysis assesses 16 and 8 processes, respectively. Tyler and Tolbert (2002) recommend the Bankson–Bernthal Test of Phonology (Bankson and Bernthal 1990) as the instrument of choice for standardised articulation/phonology testing. This assessment provides standard scores and percentile ranks and allows the clinician to establish quickly the child's phonetic inventory as well as sounds in error and phonological error patterns (Tyler and Tolbert 2002). Hodson et al. (2002) advocate the use of the Assessment of Phonological Patterns-3 (HAPP-3; Hodson 2004) when evaluating highly unintelligible children. Omissions, Hodson et al. argue, have the greatest negative impact on unintelligibility. The HAPP-3 reflects this fact by weighting omissions more heavily than substitutions in the analysis. A number of investigators recommend assessing phonological awareness skills in children, because of the widely reported link between poor phonological awareness, expressive phonological disorders and later reading problems. Hodson et al. (2002) suggest the use of the Assessment of Metaphonological Skills – Preschool (Hodson 1995) for this purpose. This assessment examines word/syllable blending (e.g. 'pop' plus 'corn'), rhyme matching (e.g. 'Which word rhymes with cat? "Ball" or "bat"?') and syllable segmentation (e.g. 'How many parts are in 'birthday'?). Hodson et al. (2002) also recommend performing an assessment of the child's speech rate, because of a purported link between rate, phonological awareness deficits and later literacy difficulties. To this end, they suggest measuring diadochokinetic rates – the child is asked to say 'buttercup' or /pə, tə, kə/ as rapidly as possible.

Tests of the type just described vary considerably in terms of sample size. The number of words tested can range from 50 or fewer (e.g. Goldman–Fristoe Test of Articulation (Goldman and Fristoe 1986); Assessment of Phonological Processes (Hodson 1986)) to more than 300 (e.g. procedures described by Elbert and Gierut 1986). Concerns about the sample size of these tests has led Miccio (2002) to use them as screening tools, from which she goes on to elicit a supplementary probe (multiple tokens of questionable sounds are obtained) or use a play routine to elicit a spontaneous speech sample: 'I view all articulation tests as screening devices because of the limitations in the size of the sample and because of the way the sample is obtained' (224). In addressing the question of what constitutes an acceptable sample size, Grunwell (1985:7) acknowledges that no 'hard and fast guidelines can be laid down' but that a comprehensive analysis requires a '*minimum*' (Grunwell's italics) of 100 different words. Theoretical considerations can also influence sample size. For example, two key concepts in nonlinear phonological theory are hierarchy and autonomy. Hierarchy describes the representation of phonological form from phrase at the top of the hierarchy to feature at the bottom. This concept is motivated by the observation that constraints at one level in the hierarchy (e.g. syllable structure) can affect other levels (e.g. the presence of segments). The child who deletes weak initial syllables (e.g. 'balloon' ['lũːn]) but is able to produce [b] and [ə] on other occasions is displaying a top-down effect from syllable level to segment level. There is also a degree of autonomy between levels, as when a child says [būːn] for 'balloon'. Although the child cannot produce the initial weak syllable, the [b] of that syllable is retained while the medial consonant [l] is lost, so syllable and segment levels are somewhat independent of each other. In relation to hierarchy and autonomy, Bernhardt and Holdgrafer (2001) remark that '[t]he two major concepts of nonlinear phonology . . . underline the importance of eliciting a sample that addresses all levels of the hierarchy in order to see autonomous patterns at each level as well as the interactions between levels' (22).

Having completed testing of speech sounds, the clinician should now have at hand a range of information. He or she should have a complete phonetic inventory for the child, including each sound that the child produces in different word positions. It should be possible to tell if syllable or word structure is a problem for the child. The clinician will also be aware if there are patterns underlying the child's sound substitutions or if substitutions are entirely random in nature. Although this information is vitally important in making diagnostic and intervention decisions, it still cannot tell us about the child's intelligibility in spontaneous speech. Given that the severity of the child's speech disorder will be judged by others on how well he or she communicates through speech in everyday settings, and not on how single words are pronounced out of context, the clinician must also examine the child's spontaneous speech skills. A sample of the child's spontaneous speech can be obtained during play. Miccio (2002) uses a hide-and-seek routine as a means of giving the child multiple opportunities to produce later-developing consonant sounds, syllable structures and lexical stress patterns. Prompts can be naturally included in the play routine to encourage spontaneous use of speech by the child. If these are not successful, Miccio uses a prompting hierarchy in which the child is first asked a question ('What's that?'), then a question containing a forced choice ('Is this a ___ or a van?') and finally, if an answer is still not forthcoming, the child is presented with a target word which he or she is then required to imitate ('It's a ___. Say ___.'). Spontaneous speech samples may also be collected through the use of wordless picture books, in which the clinician first tells the story and the child is then asked to retell it. One advantage of the latter method, particularly in the case of a highly unintelligible child, is that the clinician is likely to be aware of the target words that the child is attempting to produce. The spontaneous speech sample should contain at least 50 utterances, but if the child is talkative, 100–200 utterances can be collected (Tyler and Tolbert 2002).

With a spontaneous speech sample in place, the clinician must proceed to use an analysis of it to address several questions about the child's speech and language skills. Intelligibility ratings are a useful way of assessing the severity of the child's speech disorder and can be meaningfully communicated to parents and professionals alike. Intelligibility ratings may be obtained in several ways. Hodson et al. (2002) play the sample to a listener who knows the context but is not familiar with the child. The listener orthographically transcribes each word that can be understood and uses a dash when a word is totally unintelligible. The number of words identified by the transcriber is divided by the total number of words in the sample to obtain a percentage of intelligible words. If the child is so severely unintelligible that word boundaries cannot be identified, Hodson et al. divide by the number of syllables instead. Tyler and Tolbert (2002) also use intelligibility ratings, but avoid a percentage figure 'because this implies a numerical calculation' (219). For these investigators, intelligibility ratings of good, fair or poor are based on parent reports of how well they understand the child with and without context, other professional judgements reported prior to assessment and the clinician's assessment of intelligibility with and without context.

A spontaneous speech sample also allows clinicians to examine important interactions between phonology and semantics and phonology and morphosyntax. In terms of treatment planning, it is relevant to ask if a child's phonological errors are related to increases in linguistic load. These linguistic interactions cannot be observed on standardised tests, where lexical and syntactic interactions with phonology are excluded by virtue of the single-word format of these tests.[23] Lexical, semantic and syntactic structures can be directly examined in a spontaneous sample and findings compared with the results of formal language tests. The child's use of grammatical morphemes (e.g. past tense -ed), prepositions, articles, auxiliary and main verbs and pronouns should be noted. Tyler and Tolbert (2002) calculate a mean length of utterance (MLU) for comparison to Miller and Chapman's (1981) reference data. If the child is highly unintelligible, it may be impossible to determine the number of morphemes in an utterance. In this case, Hodson et al. (2002) suggest the use of the mean length of response (Bloodstein 1979) until such time as a valid MLU can be obtained. In terms of receptive language, the clinician can establish if the child is able to follow simple instructions (e.g. put the brick in the box) or if contextual cues are needed for the instruction to be executed (e.g. the clinician holding the brick up for the child). Pragmatic abilities, such as turn-taking in conversation and understanding the intended meaning of utterances (e.g. that the clinician who says 'Can you put the toys away?' is making a request and not asking a question) can be readily assessed using a spontaneous speech sample. This sample also allows the clinician to assess prosodic factors such as rate, rhythm, intonation, pitch and loudness, as well as make an evaluation of the child's use of resonance and overall quality of voice. Finally, fluency can also be assessed on the basis of a spontaneous speech sample, with the clinician taking care to note if the child's dysfluency frequency exceeds 2 per cent or if episodes of dysfluency are not typical of normal nonfluencies (Tyler and Tolbert 2002).

Stimulability testing is also an integral part of assessment. Stimulability describes 'a child's ability to imitate a sound absent from his/her phonetic inventory immediately following an examiner's model' (Miccio 2002:225). The procedures and format used to elicit such imitation vary considerably. Tyler and Tolbert (2002) suggest using (1) models of sounds that are missing from the child's inventory, first in isolation and then, if correct, in CV and VC syllables, (2) models of sounds in positions in syllables and words in which they are incorrect and (3) models of sounds that are produced inconsistently at word level in words and sentences. If a child is unable to imitate an auditory model, Hodson et al. (2002) introduce tactile cues. Should a correct production of the word still not be forthcoming, these investigators use slight amplification. The clinician first speaks the word into a microphone while the child is wearing earphones. The child is then given the microphone so that his or her own production of the word can be heard. Hodson et al. have found that 'amplification is a great tool for facilitating stimulability. The amplification seems to help the child focus on how the target sounds rather than continuing to rely solely on how the production feels' (2002:238). The results of stimulability testing play an important role in intervention planning. Many clinicians believe that stimulable sounds should be directly targeted in therapy. Bleile (2002) argues that '[a]ll other things being equal, since most preschoolers are remarkable for a low frustration point in the face of clinic failure, I often select therapy targets for which a client shows some production capacity' (247). Miccio (2002) believes that stimulable sounds may not require direct treatment. She supports this claim with two findings: (1) nonstimulable sounds are less likely to change in the absence of direct treatment and (2) stimulable sounds undergo most change in the absence of direct intervention. Miccio concludes that '[t]hese results suggest that stimulable sounds are being acquired naturally and may not require direct treatment' (2002:225).

With the results of standardised testing and findings from a speech and language sample analysis in place, the clinician must decide if the child's problem is sufficiently severe to warrant intervention and, if so, the form that this intervention should take. The decision to initiate intervention is based upon a number of factors, including poor performance on the part of the child in relation to same-age peers, reports of academic disadvantage as a result of the disorder, and significant psychological distress and social isolation caused by the disorder. An equally diverse set of considerations is involved in deciding which treatment method to use with phonologically disordered children. In the next section, we examine some of the intervention methods currently in use as well as consider the efficacy of different techniques.

4.3.4 Phonological Intervention

In this section, we consider some of the techniques that clinicians use to treat phonological disorders in children. We begin by examining a treatment method that is based on phonological processes, Hodson and Paden's cycles approach. Recently, Williams (2000a,b) has used the approach of multiple oppositions to treat children with moderate, severe or profound phonological disorder.[24] We discuss this approach and examine its use in the treatment of a phonologically disordered child. Many treatment approaches have a perceptual focus. We examine several studies in which perceptual-based treatments have been used.

Ingram and Ingram (2001) advocate the use of a whole-word approach to phonological assessment and remediation. We examine the claims of this approach and discuss its implications for treatment. Some clinicians have used feedback techniques to treat specific speech errors in children with phonological disorder. We review one study that used electropalatography to remediate a persistent phonological process in a eight-year-old boy. We begin by considering an issue that must be addressed by all clinicians embarking on intervention, the issue of which sounds to target in treatment.

Decisions about the sounds to target during phonological intervention are based on several considerations. Traditionally, clinicians have tended to follow a developmental model in selecting sound targets. In this case, features that affect earlier-developing phonemes are targeted before features that affect later-developing phonemes. If the analysis of a child's sound errors has used phonological processes, processes that are suppressed early in a child's sound system are targeted before those that are suppressed later. (Final consonant deletion is treated before gliding, for example.) A developmental model is still influential in treatment planning. For example, Ingram and Ingram (2001) state that '[w]ithin a whole-word approach . . . the actual targets selected can follow a developmental model' (281). However, as more is known about the effects of treatment on the disordered phonological system, it no longer seems inevitable that clinicians should select sound targets on the basis of their order of acquisition during development. Sounds are now equally likely to be targeted during intervention if they fulfil other, nondevelopmental criteria. A focus on intelligibility may lead clinicians to treat sounds (or processes) that are contributing most to the child's unintelligibility: 'Processes that occur with high frequency are likely to affect intelligibility and are targeted initially by most clinicians' (Stoel-Gammon et al. 2002:8). The significance of stimulability for the selection of sound targets is also not as straightforward as was once thought. (That is, stimulable sounds are targeted during treatment and show greater improvement than nonstimulable sounds). Many clinicians subscribe to the view that treatment should target stimulable sounds, while some clinicians believe that stimulable sounds will be acquired regardless of intervention and that their direct treatment is therefore unnecessary (see section 4.3.3). Moreover, a lack of pretreatment stimulability does not mean that a nonstimulable sound cannot show improvement during treatment – Rvachew et al. (1999) found that the probability of a reasonable treatment outcome was 0.50, even for those sounds that had poor pretreatment perception and/or stimulability. Finally, and somewhat contrary to expectation, it has been found that by targeting more complex sounds, clinicians can actually effect more significant gains in a child's phonological system than would be possible if less complex sounds were targeted: '[T]reatment of more complex properties of the phonological system appears to result in the greatest generalization and change. This effect of complexity on learning has been shown to hold across converging studies, populations and perspectives' (Gierut 2001:229).

Hodson and Paden's approach to therapy is one of the most fully articulated intervention techniques that is based on phonological processes (Stoel-Gammon et al. 2002). The emphasis of this approach is not on the correct production of phonemes but on targeting phonological patterns (e.g. the structure VC, if final consonants are lacking). These patterns are treated in successive cycles. During a cycle, a phonological pattern is targeted for 2–6 hours. It is then 'rested' while another pattern is targeted. After all the primary patterns are targeted, the Hodson Assessment of Phonological Patterns (Hodson 2004) is administered to determine which of these patterns needs to be recycled. Secondary patterns are not targeted until the child is able to use alveolars and velars contrastively, /s/ clusters are emerging in conversation, liquids in words are not being substituted by glides and there are no omissions involving early-developing patterns: for example, singleton consonants in word-initial and/or final position (Hodson et al. 2002). Stoel-Gammon et al. (2002) used a pattern-based intervention to treat phonological disorder in a four-year-old boy called Eric. Five phonological processes occurred more than 40 per cent of the time in Eric's productions: final consonant deletion, velar fronting, stopping, cluster reduction and gliding of liquids. As such, these processes were targeted in Eric's first cycle of treatment. This cycle consisted of five phases, each targeting a different process over four sessions of 50 minutes (sessions taking place twice weekly). Although Eric made progress during this first cycle, his results on the APP-R (Hodson 1986) showed little change from his pretreatment scores. A second cycle of treatment was initiated. This cycle contained some new exemplars (target words) and patterns. By the end of this cycle, administration of the APP-R revealed that final consonant deletion was occurring less than 40 per cent of the time. As a result this process was dropped as a target in the third cycle. Although several processes continued to occur 40 per cent or more of the time at the end of the third cycle, the APP-R showed that most processes had reduced frequencies of occurrence. After two years of cycles treatment, Eric had only a mild level of severity on the APP-R.

Williams (2000a,b) uses a multiple oppositions approach to treat phonological disorder in children. In a traditional contrastive approach to phonological intervention, a pair of words is selected that differs in a single consonant or vowel. This pair of words will be produced by the child as homonyms (e.g. 'sip' and 'tip' as [tɪp]). In a multiple oppositions approach, a larger number of sounds within a phoneme collapse is targeted simultaneously in an effort to reduce homonymy: 'Multiple oppositions addresses homonymy directly with the use of contrastive pairs while using larger treatment contrast sets than are used with the singular contrastive approach of minimal pairs' (Williams 2000a:282). Williams (2000a) reports the use of multiple oppositions in the treatment of a child called Michelle (3;5 years) who had a functional speech disorder of a nonorganic nature. Pretreatment phonological analysis revealed that Michelle collapsed glides and /s/ and /ʃ/ in word-initial position to the liquid [l]. Accordingly, minimal contrast therapy was initiated to remediate word-initial [s,ʃ,w]. During this treatment, Michelle's performance on [w] continued to improve – she had inconsistently produced [w] correctly before therapy. However, performance on [s] and [ʃ] remained low for nine treatment sessions (five weeks). The focus of intervention was changed from minimal pairs to multiple oppositions, in which [s,ʃ,w] were all contrasted with [l]. A single oppositional set found 'lock' contrasted with 'sock', 'shock' and 'wok'. Five such sets were used in total. Following the initiation of treatment using multiple oppositions, Michelle demonstrated significant and immediate improvement. Treatment criteria for all target sounds were met and treatment moved from word to sentence level. Michelle's accuracy on [ʃ] began to decline at this point, with [s], a sound close to the target, used instead of the original [l] substitution. After 15 treatment sessions, phonological analysis revealed improvement not only in trained sounds in trained positions but also in targeted and untargeted sounds in untrained positions. The three phoneme collapses targeted during intervention were either eliminated or significantly reduced.

Interventions with a perceptual focus are commonly used to treat phonological disorders in children. Rvachew et al. (2004) used a perceptual approach to treat preschool children with moderate or severe expressive phonological delays. Thirty-four preschoolers received 16 treatment sessions in addition to their regular speech and language therapy. An experimental group received a perceptual intervention consisting of training in phonemic perception, letter recognition, letter-sound association and onset-rhyme matching. Rvachew et al. found that this group showed greater improvements in phonemic perception and articulatory accuracy, but not in phonological awareness, than a control group who listened to computerised books. Wolfe et al. (2003) used sound identification training in preschool children with severe phonological disorders. Nine children were randomly assigned to two groups for the treatment of stimulable sound errors. In one group, children received concurrent production and sound identification training, while in the other group children received production-only training. For sounds with low pretraining sound identification scores, greater progress was made with articulatory errors after the combined production and sound identification training. For sounds receiving production training only, it was found that perception of error sounds prior to treatment may affect the degree of improvement and that production training may improve perception of error sounds. Similar findings were reported by Rvachew et al. (1999), who examined the relationship between stimulability, speech perception ability and phonological learning in phonologically disordered children. In the first of two studies, three phono-logical processes were targeted during nine group treatment sessions that used the cycles approach. For sounds that were stimulable prior to treatment, those sounds that were well perceived pretreatment made the greatest progress. In the second study, each child received three individual treatment sessions followed by six group sessions. During the individual sessions, children were trained in phonetic placement and perception of target sounds. It was found that most phonemes improved as a result of treatment, including those that were poorly perceived or nonstimulable before treatment. Clearly, pretreatment speech perception is a good predictor of treatment outcome, at least for stimulable sounds, and treatments that include speech perception can achieve reasonable gains in production accuracy.

Ingram and Ingram (2001) recommend the use of whole-word phonology to assess and treat phonological disorders in children: 'We advocate a whole-word approach to assessment and remediation, building on the assumption that children are word-oriented, not segment-oriented' (271). Ingram and Ingram claim that the goal of phonological acquisition is the attainment of word productions that are in close proximity to and will eventually match adult target vocabulary. To assess the extent to which this goal is being achieved in an individual child, these investigators propose examining four aspects of word production: whole-word correctness, complexity, intelligibility and variation. Ingram and Ingram propose specific measures for these aspects. For example, the proportion of whole-word proximity is advanced as a measure of intelligibility. The emphasis in remediation is on whole-word goals. Ingram and Ingram suggest three whole-word treatment goals for a 42-month-old boy called John. The first goal was to increase John's whole-word correctness, as analysis showed that he had few whole words correct. John's second goal was to increase his phonological mean length of utterance (a measure of whole-word complexity) to stage III from its current level of 3.85 (stage II). The third whole-word goal for John's treatment was to use words with a phonological mean length of utterance from 5.5 to 8.0. This was undertaken in order to increase John's proportion of whole-word proximity. A necessary note of caution, which is also echoed by Ingram and Ingram, concerns the current lack of research to support the efficacy of this approach: 'A whole-word approach takes the emphasis of the minimal unit of change (phoneme) and puts more emphasis on whole-word production and inner motivation to match the adult target. Whether this results in efficacious therapy remains to be seen' (2001:281).

All therapy approaches to phonological disorder use feedback to some degree. Typically, this involves auditory feedback in the form of spoken models of target sounds and visual feedback through the use of a mirror. For some phonologically disordered children, a therapy approach that gives emphasis to feedback during training can achieve significant speech gains, particularly in substitution patterns that have failed to resolve following more conventional treatments. Gibbon et al. (1999) describe the case of a child called Robbie (8;2 years), who at 5 years 9 months was assessed as having a moderately severe speech disorder on the Goldman–Fristoe Test of Articulation (Goldman and Fristoe 1986). Assessment showed that Robbie consistently backed /t/, /d/ and /n/ to a velar place of articulation in all phonetic contexts and that /tʃ/ and /dʒ/ were realised as velars in the majority of examples. It was also found that /r/ was realised as a uvular fricative [ʁ]. Between 6;7 years and 7;5 years, Robbie received 33 conventional speech therapy sessions (23 individual and 10 group sessions). As a result of this intervention, Robbie was able to produce /n/ and /r/ targets correctly in spontaneous speech. However, he continued to retract alveolar stops and affricates. To eliminate this persistent backing pattern in Robbie's speech, his speech-language pathologist recommended the use of electropalatography. Between 8;2 years and 8;8 years, Robbie received a total of 32 treatment sessions using electropalatography. From sessions 1–7, Robbie received visual feedback via a portable training unit. This was withdrawn in subsequent sessions when Robbie was able to produce /t/ and /d/. The remaining sessions concentrated on incorporating /t/ and /d/ into increasingly natural speech contexts. The speech-language pathologist discharged Robbie after 32 sessions on the grounds that his productions of alveolar plosives and affricates were perceptually normal and he was using these sounds in naturalistic speech contexts.

4.4 Specific Language Impairment

There is a significant number of children who have a severe and persistent disorder of language in the absence of an identifiable aetiology (e.g. hearing loss, neurological impairment, socio-emotional deficits). Although a large number of terms have been used to describe this population of children,[25] clinicians and researchers have in recent years tended to adopt the label 'specific language impairment'. This term reflects the fact that, while language development fails to proceed along normal lines in these children, other domains of functioning are within normal limits (i.e. the developmental disorder is *specific* to language). Typically, these children exhibit poor language performance alongside normal nonverbal intelligence. Motor and sensory skills are unimpaired and children do not present with the severe socialisation impairments that are evident in autistic spectrum disorders. Language impairment is not secondary to craniofacial anomalies (e.g. cleft lip and palate) and is not the result of a genetic or chromosomal syndrome. Against intact structure and function in each of these areas, there exists a language disorder that is so severe that children must often be educated in special language units.

In this section, we discuss a number of epidemiological findings in relation to specific language impairment (SLI). As well as examining the general prevalence of this language impairment in children, we discuss studies that reveal a greater prevalence of the disorder in boys than in girls. Although the label 'specific language impairment' is applied to children who have a language disorder in the absence of a clear aetiology, there is now growing evidence of a genetic basis for the disorder. One particularly important source of evidence in this regard is provided by family studies. We review several family studies that indicate higher than expected levels of language impairment in the biological relatives of SLI children. The language deficits in SLI children have been extensively discussed in the literature and include breakdown in phonology, morphology, syntax, semantics and pragmatics. We examine deficits in each of these language levels, as well as discuss the literacy problems that occur in SLI. Intervention and treatment issues in this clinical population will be considered. Finally, we conclude this section with a discussion of the cognitive problems that some researchers believe are responsible for the language deficits in SLI.

4.4.1 Epidemiology and Aetiology

Few studies have examined the prevalence of SLI – in a review of studies that examine the prevalence of primary speech and/or language delays, Law et al. (2000) report just two studies of this type. In one of these studies, Tomblin et al. (1997) obtained an estimated overall prevalence rate of SLI in monolingual English-speaking kindergarten children of 7.4 per cent. On the basis of this prevalence rate, and using information from the 1990 US Census, Tomblin et al. estimate that 273,025 of the 3,689,533 five-year-old children in the US present with SLI. This disorder, these investigators conclude, is a 'common condition among kindergarten-age children when compared with the prevalence of many developmental disorders' (1997:1258). In their review of prevalence studies, Law et al. (2000) report separate estimates for expressive and/or receptive language delay. For combined expressive and receptive delay, a prevalence estimate between 2 and 3 per cent, which remains constant across the age range, was found. For expressive delay only, prevalence figures range from 2.34 to 4.27 per cent over the age range 3–7 years. The prevalence figures for receptive delay only range from 2.63 to 3.95 per cent. These prevalence figures are similar to those reported by the American Psychiatric Association in DSM-IV – prevalence estimates of 3–5 per cent and 3 per cent are recorded for production deficits and combined production and comprehension deficits, respectively.

Epidemiological studies of SLI suggest greater male susceptibility for this disorder. Although figures vary from study to study, the prevalence of SLI in males is consistently reported to be greater than that in females. Tomblin et al.

(1997) obtained prevalence estimates for boys and girls of 8 per cent and 6 per cent, respectively. Robinson (1991) reports a boy:girl sex ratio of 3.8:1 amongst children attending a residential school in Surrey, England.[26] Cheuk et al. (2005) found that males accounted for 75.2 per cent of SLI cases below five years of age referred over a four-year period to the Duchess of Kent Children's Hospital in Hong Kong. SLI cases were defined as those children 'with a language quotient more than one standard deviation below the mean and below the general developmental quotient in children with normal general developmental quotient, but without neurological or other organic diseases' (2005:303). Cheuk et al.'s figure produces a male:female sex ratio of approximately 3:1.

A growing number of studies is revealing an increased prevalence of language impairments in the biological relatives of SLI children. Tallal et al. (2001) examined the language-related abilities of all biological, primary relatives (mother, father, siblings) of 22 SLI probands and 26 control subjects. The overall rate of language impairment in family members was significantly higher for the SLI probands (31 per cent) than the control subjects (7.1 per cent). Rates of maternal impairment, paternal impairment and sibling impairment were all higher in SLI families than in control families. Amongst all mothers identified as language-impaired, 12.5 per cent were mothers of SLI probands and 6.3 per cent were mothers of control subjects. Also, 14.9 per cent of language-impaired fathers were the fathers of SLI probands. (Only 2.1 per cent were the fathers of controls.) The majority of language-impaired siblings were the siblings of SLI probands (18.2 per cent) – only 2.6 per cent were siblings of control children. Rice et al. (1998) examined the histories of 31 families identified through SLI probands who were known to have particular limitations in a stage of grammatical acquisition known as extended optional infinitive. The rates of speech and language difficulties and language-related difficulties (e.g. reading) in these families were compared to rates in 67 control families. The rate of speech and language difficulties was significantly higher amongst nuclear proband family members (mothers, fathers, brothers and sisters) than in nuclear control family members – 22 per cent and 7 per cent, respectively. A similar pattern was observed for extended family members (aunts, uncles, cousins and grandparents), with 14 per cent of extended proband family members reported to have speech and language difficulties compared to 6 per cent of extended control members (a significant difference). Rates of reading/spelling/learning difficulties were not significantly higher in nuclear proband family members than in nuclear control members. A similar finding was obtained for reading/spelling/learning difficulties in extended proband and control family members. Conti-Ramsden et al. (2006) used two methods – investigator-based interview and direct language assessment – to examine the prevalence of language and literacy disorders in the families of 93 children with a history of SLI. High prevalence rates of language and literacy difficulties were reported for all family members, using both interview data (35.5 per cent) and direct assessment (35 per cent). Maternal, paternal and sibling prevalence rates, as ascertained by direct assessment, revealed no significant differences. Few significant differences in prevalence rates amongst family members were obtained using the interview method. (Older brothers and younger siblings had significantly higher prevalence rates than sisters and parents, respectively.)

The findings of familial aggregation studies lend support to the view that the aetiology of SLI is genetic in nature. Additional confirmation of a genetic aetiology is provided by findings of higher concordance rates of SLI in monozygotic (identical) versus dizygotic (nonidentical) twins. Bishop et al. (1995) examined concordance rates for 63 monozygotic and 27 dizygotic same-sex twin pairs, who were aged seven years and over. Twin pairs were selected because at least one member of the pair satisfied diagnostic criteria for specific speech or language disorder. Bishop et al. found that when the phenotype was broadened to include a less marked discrepancy between verbal and nonverbal ability and a past history of disorder, the concordnace rate for monozygotic twins was close to 100 per cent, while the rate for dizygotic twins was approximately 50 per cent. Furthermore, amongst concordant twins, there was close similarity for type of disorder. Bishop et al. conclude that '[t]here is good evidence that genetic factors play a role in the aetiology of speech and language impairment' and that 'twin data may help us arrive at a clearer conception of the phenotype as well as quantifying the extent of the genetic contribution' (1995:56).

Investigation of the genetic basis of SLI is now proceeding apace. Bartlett et al. (2002) have found a major susceptibility locus for SLI located on 13q21. The SLI Consortium (2002) conducted a full genome scan in 98 nuclear families, all of which contained probands with standard language scores greater than or equal to 1.5SD below the mean for their age. Two regions on chromosomes 16 and 19 were linked to language-related measures – 16q was linked to nonword repetition and 19q was linked to expressive language score on the Clinical Evaluation of Language Fundamentals – Revised. O'Brien et al. (2003) used samples from SLI children and their family members to examine linkage and association of SLI to markers within and around the forkhead box P_2 (FOXP$_2$) gene on chromosome 7q31. These investigators also examined samples from 96 SLI probands to determine if there were mutations in exon 14 of FOXP$_2$. Although no such mutations were found, a strong association was found to two markers that are adjacent to FOXP$_2$. Warburton et al. (2000) used two chromosome rearrangements involving band 7q31 to support linkage of autism and SLI to 7q3. Fisher et al. (1998) identified a region on chromosome 7 which co-segregates with speech and language disorder found in a family (called 'KE') with a large, three-generation pedigree. (Belton et al. (2003) also discuss the KE family; see section 4.2.1.)

While most investigative effort has been directed towards establishing a genetic aetiology of SLI, a smaller number of studies has examined aspects of brain structure in SLI children. Gauger et al. (1997) used MRI to make quantitative comparisons of the planum temporale (Wernicke's area) and pars triangularis (Broca's area) in 11 children with SLI and 19 age- and sex-matched controls with normal language skills. Subjects also received a neurolinguistic battery of tests. Gauger et al. found that pars triangularis was significantly smaller in the left hemisphere of SLI children than in normal language controls (an average length of 2.4cm and 3.2cm, respectively). Also, SLI children were more likely to have rightward asymmetry of language structures. Moreover, anomalous morphology in these language areas was found to correlate with depressed language performance. Gauger et al. conclude that '[t]hese findings support the hypothesis that language impairment is a consequence of an underlying neurobiological defect in areas of the brain known to subserve language' (1997:1272).

4.4.2 Clinical Presentation

In this section, the linguistic manifestations of SLI will be examined. We consider the findings of studies that report deficits in phonology, morphology, syntax, semantics and pragmatics. We will also discuss the significant impairments in literacy skills that are now widely reported in SLI children. It is often assumed that speech impairment in SLI children is related to these children's phonological difficulties; that is, the origin of speech impairment is linguistic in nature. However, we begin by reviewing a study which suggests that phonetic deficits may play a much greater role in the early expressive problems of SLI children than was previously thought.

Speech delay often occurs alongside SLI in children. Shriberg et al. (1999) report a comorbidity rate of speech delay with SLI of 0.51 per cent in monolingual English-speaking six-year-old children. They also found that approximately 5–8 per cent of children with persisting SLI had speech delay. A question of some contention is the extent to which linguistic (phonological) and phonetic factors have a role to play in this delay. Rescorla and Ratner (1996) address this question by comparing the vocal behaviours of typically developing children to those of children with specific expressive language impairment (SLI-E). Spontaneous language samples were obtained from 30 24-month-old toddlers with SLI-E and 30 age-matched typically developing toddlers. Rescorla and Ratner used these samples to examine the vocalisation patterns, phonetic inventories and syllable formation patterns of both groups of toddlers. Toddlers with SLI-E vocalised significantly less often than typically developing toddlers (51.4 versus 118.2 vocalisations, respectively). SLI-E toddlers also had proportionately smaller consonant and vowel inventories than typically developing toddlers (8.6 consonants and 7.3 vowels (SLI-E) compared to 17.4 consonants and 12.4 vowels (controls), a significant group difference). Toddlers with SLI-E also used a more restricted and less mature array of syllable shapes than typically developing toddlers (V and CV shapes as opposed to CV and CVC syllables and nonreduplicated two-syllable productions). Rescorla and Ratner performed a vowel-by-vowel comparison of averaged rates but found no significant differences in vowel usage between the two groups. When the use of consonants in different word positions was examined, significant differences were found between the groups. In control children, one consonant was never observed in word-medial position and two consonants were never observed in word-final position. However, in SLI-E children, one consonant [ɵ] was missing in word-initial position, five were missing in word-medial position and eight were never observed in word-final position. Rescorla and Ratner conclude that '[s]uch patterns of vocal and phonetic behaviour confirm earlier reports of phonetic delay in SLI-E, and suggest that non-grammatical factors contribute to the development of expressive language deficits in toddlers' (1996:153).

Phonological deficits are also common in SLI children.[27] The phonology of three-year-old SLI children and same-aged children with language delay was examined by Aguilar-Mediavilla et al. (2002). Two control groups of children – an age control and a language level control – were also included in the study. SLI children were significantly less accurate than age and language controls in their production of vowel sounds and significantly less accurate than age controls in their use of laterals. SLI children were markedly less accurate than age controls in their use of stops and nasals and only slightly less accurate than language controls in their use of nasals. Although differences were not significant, SLI children used stops less accurately than language controls. There were significant differences between SLI children and age controls on the following syllabic structures: CV, VC, CVV, CCV, CVC, other syllables and total number of correct syllables. The structure CV produced significant differences between SLI children and language controls. SLI children produced significantly more inaccuracies on three-syllable words than age controls. In terms of simplification processes, SLI children used more syllabic and nonsyllabic cluster reduction and initial and final consonant deletions than age controls. SLI children also deleted medial consonants significantly more often than age controls. As for word simplification processes, SLI children deleted unstressed syllables in initial position significantly more than both control groups. Aguilar-Mediavilla et al. (2002) state that these results suggest that 'the development of SLI phonology is deviant' (573).

Roberts et al. (1998) examined vocalisation rate, verbalisations, fully intelligible utterances, phonetic inventories, percentages of consonants correct, phonological processes and mean length of utterance in the group of SLI-E children that were examined at age two years by Rescorla and Ratner (1996). By age 3 years, these SLI-E children were producing the same number of vocalisations as age-matched, normally developing peers. However, other areas of phonological development were still not age-appropriate in the SLI-E children by three years of age. Measures of intelligibility – namely, rate of verbalisations and fully intelligible utterances – were still significantly delayed in certain SLI-E children (those with 'continuing delay') compared to control children and SLI-E children described as 'late bloomers'. On the phonetic inventory measure, the late bloomers performed significantly better than the continuing delay group but were still behind the normally developing children. Both groups of SLI-E children were still behind normally developing children in their percentages of consonants correct at three years of age. Finally, although late bloomers produced significantly longer MLUs than children with continuing delay, they still did not attain the MLUs of normally developing children. It is clear that while significant phonological gains are made by some children with SLI-E between that ages of 2 and 3 years (the late bloomers in this study), there is still a significant number of SLI-E children for whom phonology remains an area of considerable deficit.

Deficits in morphosyntax have been extensively reported in SLI. Tense-marking morphemes are particularly vulnerable to impairment in this clinical population. Rice et al. (1998) found that morphemes that share the property of tense marking (third person singular -s; past tense -ed; 'be' and 'do') are mastered by age four years in typically developing children and after seven years in SLI children. Rice and Wexler (1996) examined this same set of morphemes in three groups of preschool children: 37 children with SLI, 40 MLU-equivalent children and 45 age-equivalent children. These investigators found three kinds of evidence to support the use of tense as a clinical marker for SLI. First, mean levels of accuracy for each of these morphemes reliably differentiated SLI children from children in the control groups. Second, affectedness was only evident for those morphemes defined by the linguistic function of tense. (Morphemes that do not mark tense were not affected.) Third, most subjects in the normative comparison group master these tense-marking morphemes by age five, while the majority of SLI children performed below 50 per cent. Leonard et al. (2003) found that SLI children used past tense -ed and passive participle -ed in fewer obligatory contexts than age-matched and MLU-matched normally developing children. Only SLI children had greater difficulty with past tense -ed than passive participle -ed. Eadie et al. (2002) report that SLI children performed significantly more poorly than children with typical language development on composite measures of tense, tense inflections and nontense morphemes. Rice et al. (2000) examined regular and irregular past tense verb acquisition in SLI children between 5 and 8 years. During this period, the acquisition of regular past tense -ed by SLI children fell behind that of younger control children. Growth of percentage correct of irregular past tense forms in SLI children was found to parallel that of younger children.[28] Bedore and Leonard (1998) found that a finite verb morpheme composite, consisting of regular past tense inflections, regular third person singular present inflections, and copula and auxiliary 'be' forms, discriminated SLI children and age-matched controls with high levels of accuracy. (This composite showed sensitivity exceeding 85 per cent and specificity of 100 per cent.)[29] Not all studies have found deficits in the use of tense-marking morphemes in SLI children. Beverly and Williams (2004) found that eight boys with SLI (42–58 months old) had a significantly higher percentage of 'be' use in obligatory contexts (46 per cent) than younger, MLU-matched controls (27 per cent).[30]

Other grammatical findings are also noteworthy. Redmond and Rice (2001) found that SLI children and language-matched controls had similar production and acceptance rates of past tense over-regularisations (e.g. he falled) and higher rates than age-matched controls. SLI children were also more likely to produce and accept infinitive forms in finite positions (e.g. he fall off) and accepted more finite form errors in VP complement positions (e.g. he made him fell) than control subjects. Rice et al. (1995) found that SLI children used nonfinite forms of lexical verbs or omitted 'be' and 'do' more frequently than MLU-matched children and age-matched children. Grela and Leonard (2000) report that children with SLI in their study omitted more auxiliary 'be' verbs than either MLU or age controls. Like MLU controls, SLI children were more likely to omit auxiliary forms when sentences contained greater argument-structure complexity. Leonard (1995) examined the following functional categories in the spontaneous speech of 10 children with SLI: determiner, inflection, complementiser. SLI children were able to use each of these functional categories. Examination of samples revealed the presence of three different types of determiner articles (a, the), prenominal determiners (this, that) and pronominal possessive forms (e.g. my, his). Several examples of the inflection category were also in evidence: third-person singular or regular past verb inflection, some form of copula 'be', some form of auxiliary 'be', the modal forms 'can' and 'can't', the auxiliary form 'don't' and three different pronouns reflecting nominative case. The complementiser category was also represented in the SLI samples in the form of auxiliary inversion and an utterance-initial wh-phrase that could not be construed as the subject of the sentence (e.g. What is he making?). Although SLI children showed evidence of these functional categories, Leonard found that these children used the grammatical elements associated with these categories to a more limited degree than MLU controls.

Studies have repeatedly shown that SLI children have significant deficits in lexical semantics. Lahey and Edwards (1999) found that SLI children made more errors in naming pictures than children with no language impairment. (The difference between the groups was significant.) Moreover, proportionally more of the SLI errors than the errors of the normal language children were names of objects that were associated with the pictured object (e.g. shoe/foot) and that were phonologically related to the target. McGregor et al. (2002) report that SLI children made significantly more errors when naming age-appropriate objects than normally developing age-matched controls. Semantic misnaming and indeterminate responses (e.g. 'don't know' or nonspecific responses) formed the predominant error types for both groups of subjects. McGregor et al. relate the poor naming performance of SLI children to impoverished semantic representations in these children: 'This study demonstrates that the degree of knowledge represented in the child's semantic lexicon makes words more or less vulnerable to retrieval failure and that limited semantic knowledge contributes to the frequent naming errors of children with SLI' (2002:998). As well as having expressive impairments in lexical semantics, SLI children have also been shown to have receptive impairments. To investigate receptive difficulties in SLI children, Alt et al. (2004) used a computer task during which SLI children and age-matched subjects with normally developing language were exposed to novel objects and actions with novel names. These investigators found that, when asked questions about the semantic features of these objects and actions, SLI children recognised fewer semantic features than the children with normal language. Moreover, SLI children also performed poorly relative to normal language children on a lexical label recognition task.

Extensive investigations have been conducted into word learning in SLI children. These studies demonstrate that SLI children have reduced word-learning ability compared to normal language subjects. Oetting et al. (1995) examined quick incidental learning of novel vocabulary in SLI children. Twenty novel words, that referred to one of four semantic classes (object, attribute, action and affective state), were introduced to SLI and normal language children in videotaped stories. A picture-pointing task was used to measure word learning. Although SLI children demonstrated some word-learning ability, their gain was significantly less than that of normal language children. A particularly low gain was observed among SLI children on words belonging to the action class. Researchers have also investigated the factors that may contribute to poor word learning in SLI children. Gray (2004) found that phonological memory and semantic knowledge contributed to word-learning difficulty in SLI children. These investigators examined a group of eight poor word learners, seven of which were SLI children. Poor word learners appeared overall to have enough semantic information to draw objects that they were learning to name and to comprehend their names, but had difficulty producing them. This was taken to indicate that poor word learners had sufficient semantic knowledge of target objects but insufficient phonological representation to produce the word consistently. Existing lexical knowledge, as measured by the Peabody Picture Vocabulary Test (Dunn et al. 1997), predicted comprehension and production performance on a fast-mapping task and predicted the number of words children learned to comprehend during word learning.

Studies have considered if SLI children are able to use syntactic cues to facilitate word learning. Rice et al. (2000) examined the syntactic bootstrapping abilities of two groups of SLI children, one group aged five years, the other group aged seven years. The ability of these children to learn novel count and mass nouns presented in a videotaped story was compared to the performance of two control groups, one group matched to SLI subjects on MLU and the other group matched on chronological age. Syntactic cues were provided in one condition of the experiment, while in a second condition syntax was neutral. Only five-year-old control children showed evidence of using the syntactic cues. Comparable scores were achieved by five-year-old SLI children and three-year-old control children. Oetting (1999) examined if SLI children were able to use argument structure cues to facilitate verb learning. Six-year-old SLI children and control children matched for either language or age participated in two tasks. One task examined the children's use of cues to interpret novel verbs during viewing of single action scenes. In a second condition, the role of cues for novel verb interpretation and retention was examined through a story viewing task. Oetting found that SLI children were able to use argument structure cues to interpret verb meaning – in the first task, scores of SLI children were not significantly different from the scores of either control group; in the second task, SLI scores exceeded chance and were not different from those obtained by language-matched controls. However, on verb retention SLI children achieved lower scores than both control groups. Moreover, SLI scores did not exceed chance even after repeated exposure to stimuli and additional testing. Oetting states that '[s]pecific deficits with the storage and retrieval of grammatical information within the lexicon, general working memory/ capacity limitations, or both are posited as plausible, but unconfirmed explanations for the verb retention difficulties of the children with SLI' (1999:1261).

The use of syntactic cues to facilitate word learning by SLI children is a language-based word-learning strategy. Nonlinguistic factors have also been shown to aid word learning in SLI children. Riches et al. (2005) examined the effect of frequency of presentations (12 or 18 presentations) and spacing of presentation (all presentations in one session or spread over four days) on word learning in SLI children. Twenty-four SLI children and 24 language-matched control children were taught novel verbs during play sessions. Comprehension and production probes were conducted after the final session and one week later. Although no frequency and spacing effects were observed in the control children, SLI children were found to benefit significantly from frequent and widely spaced presentations. Gray (2003) examined the relationship between fast mapping and word learning and between comprehension and production of new words in 30 preschool SLI children and 30 age-matched controls with normal language. She found that, while both groups performed similarly on the fast-mapping task, normal language children comprehended and produced significantly more words than SLI children. Moreover, they achieved this in fewer trials. Gray concludes that '[s]ome children with SLI may need to hear a new word twice as many times as their [normal language] peers before comprehending it' (2003:56).

Traditionally, it has been assumed that pragmatic language skills are an area of strength in SLI children. Alternatively, investigators have argued that if pragmatic language deficits do exist in SLI children, these are merely secondary to the structural language problems of these children.[31] However, an increasing number of studies is beginning to demonstrate that both these positions are mistaken. In several studies, Bishop and co-workers have presented the case for a subgroup of SLI children in whom pragmatic deficits are not simply the consequence of problems with language form and content (Bishop 1998, 2000a; Bishop et al. 2000). Previously known by the term 'semantic pragmatic disorder', children with pragmatic language impairment (PLI) are described as being poor at inferencing, over-literal, neglectful of their listener's perspective and displaying a tendency to use socially inappropriate and/or stereotyped conversational responses (Bishop 2000a). Even children with more typical SLI are not necessarily free of pragmatic language deficits (Bishop et al. 2000). Below, we examine the findings of studies that have examined pragmatic impairments in PLI and SLI subjects. For a more detailed discussion of pragmatic impairments in the SLI population, the reader is referred to chapter 9 in Cummings (2005).

All pragmatic interpretation involves the use of inferencing. Botting and Adams (2005) examined this key skill in 25 children with SLI and 22 children with primary pragmatic difficulties (PD), all of whom were aged 11 years at the time of study. Subjects participated in an inferential comprehension task, during which they were asked a series of literal and inferential questions. Inferential questions required subjects to compute logical (text connecting) inferences, bridging (gap-filling) inferences and elaborative inferences. Children in both clinical groups scored more poorly than age-matched peers on this task, but showed no significant differences from younger children aged seven and nine years. Perhaps of most significance in the present context is the finding that SLI children performed similarly to the children with primary pragmatic difficulties on this inferential comprehension task – the mean scores of the SLI and PD children were almost identical (15.2 and 15.1, respectively). This similarity in performance of these two groups extends more widely than this study. Botting and Adams remark that 'other studies examining inferential ability have also struggled to measure any difference between those known to have pragmatic language difficulties and those with more typical SLI' (2005:60).[32] This raises the possibility that in relation to this key skill for pragmatic functioning, SLI children may share certain primary pragmatic deficits with PD children.

Laws and Bishop (2004) examined pragmatic aspects of language in four groups of subjects: children and adults with Williams syndrome, children and adults with Down's syndrome, children with SLI and typically developing children. Pragmatic language skills were assessed in these groups by means of the Children's Communication Checklist (Bishop 1998), which was completed by teachers and speech and language therapists in the case of SLI children. All three clinical groups scored significantly less than controls on the pragmatic composite (PC) of the CCC. However, there were no statistical differences in PC scores among the three clinical groups. Although the mean PC score of the SLI group (133.4) was slightly above the cut-off point of 132 for pragmatic impairment, seven children with SLI (41 per cent of the SLI group) scored 132 or less on the pragmatic composite. SLI children showed significantly more evidence of stereotyped conversation than controls. It is clear from the results of this study that SLI children have impaired pragmatic language skills compared to normal language subjects and that PLIs are at least as severe in SLI children as those found in other clinical populations.

Many SLI children experience additional problems with reading and writing. Flax et al. (2003) found that 68 per cent of SLI probands in their study also met diagnostic criteria for reading impairment.[33] Catts et al. (2005) examined the overlap between SLI identified in kindergarten and dyslexia identified in second, fourth or eighth grades in a sample of 527 children. These investigators found a limited but statistically significant overlap between SLI and dyslexia. Catts et al. conclude that this finding 'supports the view that SLI and dyslexia are distinct but potentially comorbid developmental language disorders' (2005:1378). Nation et al. (2004) examined the oral language skills of eight-year-old children with impaired reading comprehension. A range of tasks was used to examine phonology, semantics, morphosyntax and broader language skills. With the exception of tasks tapping phonological skills, children with poor reading comprehension were impaired across all language measures relative to control children who were matched for age and decoding ability. Nation et al. argue that 'a substantial minority can be classified as having specific language impairment' (2004:199). A smaller number of studies has examined written language impairments in children with SLI. Mackie and Dockrell (2004) conducted standardised measures of language production, writing and reading decoding in 11 children with SLI. On a writing assessment, these investigators found that the SLI group wrote fewer words and produced proportionately more syntax errors than age-matched controls. However, SLI children did not differ from these controls on a measure of the content of written language or on the proportion of spelling errors. SLI children also produced proportionately more syntax errors than language-matched controls. Boudreau and Hedberg (1999) found that preschool SLI children performed more poorly than peers matched for age, gender and socioeconomic status on tasks measuring knowledge of rhyme, letter names and concepts related to print.

Clinicians and researchers are increasingly reporting the presence of dysfluencies in the speech of SLI children. To address the question of the rate and type of dysfluencies in SLI children, Boscolo et al. (2002) examined narratives elicited from 22 pairs of nine-year-old children. Half of these children had histories of specific expressive language impairment (HSLI-E), while the other half had typical developmental histories. Children with HSLI-E and typically developing children produced average rates of 4.56 per cent and 3.3 per cent dysfluent words, repectively. There was a significant difference in the total dysfluency rates of HSLI-E and typically developing children – rates ranged from 2.1 per cent to 7.7 per cent and from 1.0 per cent to 5.2 per cent, respectively. Children with histories of language impairment did produce significantly more stutter-like dysfluencies than typically developing children (an average of 0.76 per cent words with stutter-like dysfluencies compared to 0.33 per cent). Also the number of children exhibiting some stutter-like dysfluencies was higher for the HSLI-E group (78 per cent) than for the typically developing group (52 per cent). This difference in proportional usage of stutter-like dysfluencies was significant. HSLI-E children produced seven times as many blocks and three times as many part-word repetitions as typically developing children.

4.4.3 Clinical Intervention

The techniques that clinicians use to treat language deficits in SLI children are increasingly being shaped by the results of intervention studies. In this section, we examine the findings of some of these studies. Much is now known, for example, about the factors and methods that can facilitate word learning in SLI children. Also, aspects of grammar can be successfully targeted during intervention in these children. Word learning and grammatical interventions will be considered below. Parents play an essential role in any programme of intervention in SLI children. We discuss a technique that parents can use to bring about morphosyntactic gains in their SLI children. Finally, a successful language intervention is one that results in the generalisation of newly acquired knowledge and skills to untrained domains and contexts. How such generalisation can be achieved in the case of SLI children will be considered.

Techniques to facilitate word learning in SLI children have been the focus of a number of intervention studies. Kouri (2005) examined the use of two interactive treatment approaches to train late-talking preschoolers with SLI in the production of target vocabulary. In one procedure (mand-elicited imitation), elicitations and imitative prompts were used. In the second procedure, auditory bombardment and play modelling were adopted and there were no response demands placed on children. Kouri found that mand-elicited imitation was relatively more effective than auditory bombardment and play modelling in facilitating frequency and rate of target word learning in the treatment setting. However, there were no significant differences between these techniques in the number or percentage of target words generalised to the home setting. Lexical productivity was balanced across settings in the children who received mand-elicited imitation, while children who received auditory bombardment and play modelling produced more target words that were restricted to the home setting. Gray (2005) examined the use of phonological and semantic encoding cues in promoting word learning in SLI children. Twenty-four preschool SLI children and 24 age- and gender-matched children with normal language participated in phonological and semantic treatment conditions. While normal language subjects displayed similar performance across both conditions, SLI children comprehended more words in the semantic condition and produced more words in the phonological condition. Gray also found that normal language subjects required significantly fewer trials than SLI subjects to produce words in the semantic condition and to comprehend words in the semantic and phonological conditions. This confirms the findings of other studies that have demonstrated a significant effect of frequency of presentation on word learning (see Riches et al. (2005) and Gray (2003) in section 4.4.2).

Given the widespread occurrence of syntactic deficits in SLI children, any language intervention programme must have the treatment of syntax as one of its priorities. Fey et al. (2003) present 10 principles which they regard 'as essential in developing state-of-the-art grammatical interventions for children with SLI' (4). The basic goal of any grammatical intervention, Fey et al. argue, is to confer on the child 'greater facility in the comprehension and use of syntax and morphology in the service of conversation, narration, exposition, and other textual genres in both written and oral modalities' (principle 1). Clinicians should target other aspects of language and communication in addition to grammatical form (principle 2) and select intermediate goals that reflect grammatical categories, principles and operations rather than teach specific language forms (principle 3). The specific goals that are selected must be ones for which the child is cognitively, socially and linguistically prepared and for which there is some need (principle 4). Intervention should manipulate aspects of context to create greater opportunities for grammatical targets (principle 5) and exploit different textual genres and the written modality (principle 6). Clinicians should manipulate the linguistic context in order to achieve salience of target forms in pragmatically felicitous contexts (principle 7). For example, by stressing capitalised 'is' in the sentence 'That boy is working hard. He really IS,' the clinician can increase the salience of this auxiliary verb in a way that is not pragmatically anomalous. (Compare 'That boy IS working hard'.) Through the use of sentence recasts (see below), clinicians should systematically contrast the child's grammatical forms with mature grammatical forms from adult grammar (principle 8). Grammatical models should always be presented in well-formed phrases and sentences – telegraphic speech, in which grammatical functors are omitted in order to highlight relationships between content words, should be avoided (principle 9). Finally, Fey et al. (2003) recommend the use of elicited imitation both to make target forms more salient and to give the child practice with phonological patterns that are difficult to access or produce (principle 10).

Sentence recasts have attracted considerable interest from clinicians and researchers who are involved in language intervention in SLI children. There are two reasons for this interest. First, intervention studies have shown that recasts are an effective means of achieving grammatical gains in SLI children in a clinical context. Nelson et al. (1996) compared the relative effectiveness of conversational recast treatment and imitative treatment in SLI children aged 4;7 to 6;7 years and younger, language-normal children who were matched on language levels. Recasts were defined as 'replies to child utterances that specifically incorporate a challenge to the child's current language level but maintain the child's central meaning in the adult recast' (1996:850). An appropriate adult recast for the child who lacks auxiliaries and says 'The pony running' would be 'Yes, the pony is running.' Three grammatical targets were selected for each child. Three of these targets were absent from the child's expressive language, while the other three were only partially mastered. Nelson et al. found that target acquisition was more rapid under conversational recast treatment than under imitative treatment for both groups of subjects. Moreover, this outcome was observed both for targets that were initially absent from the child's expressive language and for targets that were partially mastered. Nelson et al. state that '[t]he results of the current study . . . suggest excellent learning capacity in the SLI children, particularly when conversational recast input was provided' (1996:857).

Second, given that recast use is an effective means of facilitating morphosyntactic development in SLI children, it is likely that the use of recasts by parents will prove to be at least as effective in generalising language gains to the home environment of these children. Certainly, studies are beginning to provide clinicians and researchers with information about the nature and extent of recast use by the parents of SLI children. Contrary to previous reports of reduced recast usage by the parents of SLI children (e.g. Conti-Ramsden et al. 1995), Fey et al. (1999) found no difference in sentence recast usage of the parents of SLI children and the parents of 10 younger children with typical language at two points in time. Proctor-Williams et al. (2001) examined the use of copula and article recasts by 10 parents of children with SLI and 10 parents of younger language-matched children with typical language. These children's productions of copulas and articles were assessed at three points across an eight-month period. Both groups of parents produced copula and article recasts at similar rates and in a similar manner across time. However, only in the typical language group were parental copula recasts significantly correlated with child copula rate and accuracy. Notwithstanding similar parental rates of recasts in both groups, it seems that SLI children are less able than typical language children to use these recasts to learn certain grammatical targets. Proctor-Williams et al. (2001) conclude that 'children with SLI can benefit substantially from the grammar-facilitating properties of recasts, but only when the recasts are presented at rates that are much greater than those available in typical conversations with young children' (155).

The success of any language intervention is ultimately judged by how well it achieves the generalisation of newly acquired language skills. Generalisation involves the transfer of skills and knowledge from items that have been directly trained in one context, usually a clinic, to untrained items in many different contexts. Swisher et al. (1995) addressed the question of generalisation by comparing two methods used to train a novel bound morpheme, /u/, in SLI children and children with normal language. The 'rule' that governed the expression of the bound morpheme was that the morpheme was used in relation to large animate and inanimate figures (e.g. gacku, pimu). When the smaller versions of these figures were used, the bound morpheme was dropped from the vocabulary stem (e.g. gack, pim). In the 'implicit-rule' condition, this rule was conveyed to the children by means of contrasts between affixed and unaffixed words. In the 'explicit-rule' condition, the rule was verbalised by the trainer ('The pimu was a big creature. When it is small you say pim, but when it's big you have to say [u], pimu'). Swisher et al. found that the SLI children generalised the bound morpheme less often than the normal language children under the explicit-rule condition. Generalisation did not differ significantly between SLI and normal language children in the implicit-rule condition. These investigators conclude that 'the explicit presentation of metalinguistic information during training may be detrimental to bound-morpheme generalization by preschool-age children with SLI' (1995:168–173).

Leonard et al. (2004) examined morpheme generalisation in 31 children with SLI who were aged 3;0 to 4;4 at the beginning of the study. These children participated in 48 intervention sessions during which they received treatment either for the third-person singular -s or the auxiliary is/are/was. Two control morphemes (nonthematic 'of' and the infinitival complementiser 'to') and past tense -ed were also examined. The target morphemes marked tense and agreement. Past -ed marked tense and was designed to assess across-morpheme generalisation. The control morphemes were developmentally comparable to the target morphemes and did not mark tense or agreement. Leonard et al. found that gains in the use of target morphemes were significantly greater than gains on control morphemes. Importantly, these investigators found that untreated verb forms that mark tense and agreement showed more change during intervention than did past -*ed*. Leonard et al. conclude that 'by gaining skill in the use of morphemes that mark both tense and agreement, the children were able to identify and acquire other morphemes in the language that mark both of these features. This increase in sensitivity did not appear to apply to forms in the language that express tense only' (2004:1363). Kiernan and Snow (1999) found that SLI children required more training sessions than normal language children to achieve criterion-level bound-morpheme generalisation. SLI children also learned to produce significantly fewer words and affixed forms than normal language children during training. However, poorer bound-morpheme generalisation was neither associated with, nor dependent upon, the learning of words and affixed forms in SLI children.

4.4.4 SLI and Cognitive Deficits

Researchers have tended to look to underlying linguistic deficits on the one hand and cognitive deficits on the other hand in accounts of the aetiology of SLI: 'Current theories of specific language impairment in children fall into 2 general classes: those that attribute SLI to processing limitations and those that attribute the disorder to deficits in grammatical knowledge' (Deevy and Leonard 2004:802).[34] In this section, we discuss what is known about the cognitive deficits or 'processing limitations' that are believed to underlie SLI. We consider the findings of several recent studies that have addressed the question of the role of cognitive deficits in SLI. Some of these studies relate language impairment in SLI to limited processing capacity, while other studies make more specific claims about the contribution of verbal (phonological) working memory deficits in the language impairment of SLI children. We begin with two studies that report a significant effect of the rate of linguistic input on the performance of SLI children.

Many investigators have explained performance deficits in SLI children in terms of reduced processing speed. Fazio (1998) found poorer recognition of serial patterns in SLI children than age-matched peers under short presentation conditions. However, under long presentation conditions the performance of SLI children was similar to that of age-matched peers. The serial memory deficits of these SLI children were not specific to phonological processing – recognition of common objects, which could be easily recoded into a phonological form, was not impaired relative to visual tasks that were less likely to be recoded. Fazio concludes that serial memory in these SLI children was affected by the duration of presentation and that '[t]he findings from this study are further support for general speed of processing problems in children with SLI' (1998:1380). Weismer and Hesketh (1996) investigated the effect of rate of linguistic input on performance in a novel word-learning task in 16 children with SLI and 16 normal-language controls matched on mental age. Rate effects were most evident on production of novel words – SLI children produced significantly fewer words that had been produced at fast rate during training than normal-language children. Weismer and Hesketh conclude that '[f]indings from the present study are consistent with the claim that processing capacity limitations, especially temporal processing constraints, appear to be at least one component of the difficulty that these children are experiencing' (1996:188).

Other studies have also found evidence of reduced speed of processing in SLI children. Miller et al. (2001) examined the mean response times of SLI children and children with normal language on tasks involving linguistic and nonlinguistic activities. They found that SLI children responded more slowly across all task conditions and also when linguistic and nonlinguistic tasks were analysed separately. Miller et al. state that '[t]he results of the group analyses support the hypothesis that speed of processing in children with SLI is generally slower than that of children with normal language' (2001:416). Lahey and Edwards (1996) found that SLI children aged 4–9.5 years were significantly slower than age-matched children with no language impairment on naming and responding to nonlinguistic stimuli. These investigators relate SLI children's speed of naming to slower nonlinguistic response processing and not to speed of linguistic or perceptual processing. Edwards and Lahey (1996) found that SLI children were significantly slower than age-matched, typically developing peers in recognising sequences of sounds that represent words in their lexicon (auditory lexical decision). Slower nonlinguistic processing speed was one of two explanations that Edwards and Lahey used to account for the longer lexical decision times of SLI children.

Amongst the cognitive deficits investigated by SLI researchers are impairments of verbal (phonological) working memory. Montgomery (2000) examined the effect of a verbal working memory task on sentence comprehension in SLI children.[35] In this task, children tried to recall words under three processing load conditions – a no-load condition, a single-load condition (words were recalled according to the physical size of word referents) and a dual-load condition (words were recalled by the semantic category and physical size of word referents). Redundant (longer) and nonredundant (shorter) sentences were used in the comprehension task. Montgomery found that SLI children recalled fewer words than normally developing, age-matched controls in the dual-load condition and comprehended fewer redundant and nonredundant sentences than these controls. These results were taken to indicate that SLI children have less functional verbal working memory capacity (i.e. ability to coordinate storage and processing functions) than age-matched peers. Briscoe et al. (2001) found that the mean scores of SLI children on tests of phonological short-term memory were significantly poorer than those of age-matched controls. Weismer et al. (1999) used the Competing Language Processing Task, developed by Gaulin and Campbell (1994), to examine verbal working memory capacity in SLI children. These children performed similarly to normal language controls on true/false comprehension items, but displayed significantly poorer word recall than these controls. These researchers conclude that 'findings from this investigation indicate that children with SLI evidence greater deficits in verbal working memory capacity than normal language peers' (1999:1258). Other studies that have found evidence of deficits in working memory in SLI children include Marton and Schwartz (2003), Gillam et al. (1998) and Hoffman and Gillam (2004).

4.5 Landau–Kleffner Syndrome

The disorders that have been discussed so far in this chapter have certain features in common. They arise when speech and/or language skills fail to develop along normal lines, often in the absence of an identifiable aetiology or clear onset. Other communication disorders have an onset during childhood and can be linked to an organic aetiology. The communication problems that result from traumatic brain injury and neoplastic conditions (e.g. cerebellar tumour) or that attend Landau–Kleffner syndrome are cases in point. The implications of neoplastic conditions and traumatic brain injury for communication and feeding have been discussed in earlier sections (3.2.1, 3.2.2.1 and 3.2.2.2 in chapter 3) and will not be considered further in the present context. In the rest of this section, we consider the communication characteristics and other features of Landau–Kleffner syndrome.

Landau–Kleffner syndrome (LKS) is a rare disorder that was first described in 1957 by Dr William M. Landau and Dr Frank R. Kleffner. Other terms that are used for this disorder include infantile acquired aphasia, acquired epileptic aphasia and aphasia with convulsive disorder. These terms variously reflect the late onset of the disorder (it is 'acquired' during childhood) and the fact that the aphasia is associated with epileptiform activity (the aphasia is 'epileptic' or occurs in the presence of a 'convulsive' disorder). The disorder is rare.[36] Simms and Schum (2000) report a prevalence estimate for LKS of 0.2 per cent of all childhood epilepsy. Higher prevalence rates are reported in special settings. In a residential school in Surrey, England, that is attended by children aged 8–16 years with severe, specific disorders of speech and language, Robinson (1991) reported that 6 per cent of children presented with LKS. Boys are affected more often than girls (Gordon 1997). Apart from a small number of reports of

LKS occurring in siblings and twins (Temple 1997), little is known about the familial characteristics of LKS.

Although an exact cause of LKS has not been established, the association of this disorder with epileptiform activity suggests that seizures are the proximal aetiology of the language impairment in LKS. Simms and Schum (2000) state that

> LKS is associated with an EEG pattern that shows electrical status epilepticus during slow-wave sleep. Such abnormalities may be unilateral or bilateral and may fluctuate from the right to the left hemisphere, although characteristically they are located over the temporal and parietal areas. (150)

Although the presence of epileptic activity in the EEG of LKS children is a constant finding (Gordon 1997), as many as 25 per cent of these children do not have overt seizures (Tuchman 1997). Gordon (1990) reports that a family history of epilepsy is found in 12 per cent of LKS cases. Brain regions that are important to language processing have recently been reported to have reduced volume in LKS. Takeoka et al. (2004) performed MRI volumetric analysis of various neocortical regions and subcortical structures in four children with typical LKS. In areas where receptive language is localised, volume reduction of 25–63 per cent (planum temporale) and 25–57 per cent (superior temporal gyrus) was recorded. The brain infection, encephalitis, has been considered a possible cause of LKS by some investigators – one of the LKS children in Robinson's (1991) study developed the disorder after presumed viral encephalitis at three years. Findings such as the increased occurrence of epilepsy in family members of LKS children and the presence of LKS in the siblings of affected children and in twins[37] make it likely that the distal aetiology of this disorder will be genetic in nature. Landau (1992) claims that 'the possibility of genetic liability cannot be rejected' (353).

Onset of LKS can vary widely from 18 months to 13 years, with a peak incidence between four years and seven years (Temple 1997). Loss of language can occur abruptly or insidiously, with receptive language first to be affected. Expressive language is also impaired. Expressive deficits usually occur later than receptive deficits and are thus considered to be secondary to the receptive impairment (Honbolygó et al. 2006). Affected children no longer recognise spoken words. The auditory agnosia is often confused with sudden deafness, although hearing is normal when assessed. A diagnosis of LKS may not be considered if the child has not had any recognised clinical seizure, the onset is very gradual, the symptoms are transient or mild and if there is spontaneous recovery (Deonna 2000). Additional impairments can also occur alongside deterioration in language. These include behavioural problems like hyperactivity and aggressiveness as well as cognitive deficits. Some cases of LKS may not conform to the clinical picture described here. Tutuncuoglu et al. (2002) describe the case of a 3.5-year-old girl who was referred to their clinic with stuttering. She had no verbal agnosia but had a history of epilepsy. An EEG revealed multiple spike and wave discharges. Stuttering commenced three months after anti-epilepsy drugs were discontinued.

A growing number of studies is investigating the nature and extent of language impairment in LKS children. Metz-Lutz et al. (1996) examined language skills in four children with onset of LKS between 3 years and 6 years 3 months. Epileptic aphasia varied in duration from 22 months to 51 months. A wide range of tests was used to assess language skills every six months during follow-up. Performance on these tests revealed that impairments in auditory short-term memory and phonological processing were the main aphasic consequences of LKS. Moreover, deficits in phonological processing 'may account for impairments in lexical growth, acquisition of reading and writing and comprehension of abstract words and syntax, usually observed following Landau and Kleffner syndrome' (Metz–Lutz 1996:150). Doherty et al. (1999) examined prosodic aspects of expression and perception in a 7.5-year-old girl with LKS. This girl was unable to use or perceive phonemes meaningfully.[38] However, she was able to convey emotional and propositional intent by varying the fundamental frequency, duration and intensity of utterances (prosodic expression). She was also able to discriminate the prosodic contours of a male adult voice to an age equivalent to 5.5–6.5 years (prosodic perception). Doherty et al. conclude that 'this case report raises the possibility that such an important aspect of non-verbal communication in speech is preserved in Landau–Kleffner syndrome' (1999:233). Baynes et al. (1998) describe the language skills of a 27-year-old woman who had chronic auditory agnosia as a result of LKS diagnosed at 4.5 years. This woman (called T.M.) was only able to name 28 of 60 items, although she recognised most items and had alternate names for some of them. She was able to use signs for 30 items. On the Peabody Picture Vocabulary Test – Revised, T.M. scored at the level of a 6.4-year-old (auditory administration) and 7.7-year-old (written administration). On an assessment of written language, T.M. demonstrated impairment in vocabulary and spelling. Her performance improved considerably when written language tasks became more conceptual in nature. T.M.'s comprehension of conceptual-semantic relations was normal. Language production revealed a profound impairment of stress and intonation.

Baynes et al.'s subject, T.M., had a significant language impairment many years after clinical seizures had resolved. (She discontinued anticonvulsants at age 12 without experiencing a return to seizures.) Moreover, at the time of study a neurological examination, EEG and MRI scan were all normal. The persistence of language deficits, many years after the epileptiform activity that precipitated the disorder has resolved, has prompted investigators to ask which factors are predictors of language outcome. Factors that have been examined include age at onset of the disorder, intensity of epileptic activity (persistent or intermittent) and duration of disorder (weeks, months or years). Electrical status epilepticus in sleep (ESES) was examined by Robinson et al. (2001) in a study of course and outcome of LKS in 18 children at a mean length of 67 months' follow-up. These investigators found that the length of ESES correlated strongly with the length of time between illness onset and onset of recovery and with eventual receptive and expressive language. Only 3 of the 18 children had a language outcome in the normal range. No child with ESES for longer than 36 months had normal language outcome. Rossi et al. (1999) examined 11 LKS children with a mean follow-up of nine years and eight months. Only 18.2 per cent of subjects displayed complete language recovery – 9.1 per cent of cases had a severe language outcome and 72.7 per cent had moderate or severe language impairment. In 36.4 per cent of cases, the early onset of aphasia compromised language acquisition. In two subjects, the duration of bitemporal electrical status epilepticus during sleep (BTESES) and intercalated electrical status epilepticus during sleep (IESES) and their continuity without fluctuations had negative effects on language and cognitive functions. Rossi et al. state that

> [t]he prognosis of LKS in our cases may depend on the interaction of different negative factors such as onset of aphasia before 4 years, its duration for longer than 1 year, long-lasting duration and continuity without fluctuations of BTESES/IESES, and probably preexisting mild speech delay. (1999:90)

Of course, poor long-term prognosis in LKS can be minimised through prompt intervention. Treatment includes the use of anti-epileptic drugs, such as valproic acid, and corticosteroid therapy. In cases where patients have not responded to multiple medical therapies, neurosurgical techniques such as multiple subpial transection have been employed (Mikati and Shamseddine 2005). This technique has led to a marked improvement in language skills and behaviour in LKS children.[39] Early speech and language therapy, which includes signing amongst other techniques, is essential for LKS children. Unfortunately, few treatment studies have been conducted in this clinical population (see chapter 9 in Lees (2005)).

Notes

1. In keeping with the dominant usage in British literature, the label developmental verbal dyspraxia, or simply DVD, will be used throughout this chapter. The reader should be aware, however, that a number of other labels are used of this disorder.

Popular terminology in American literature includes developmental apraxia of speech (DAS) and childhood apraxia of speech (CAS). The labels developmental articulatory dyspraxia and oral motor planning disorder are also used, albeit less commonly, of this disorder.

2. Dyspraxia is a general term that refers to an impairment in the organisation and planning of complex movement. When this disorder affects particular parts of the body, the term 'dyspraxia' assumes a range of other labels – limb dyspraxia (movements of the arms and legs), oral dyspraxia (nonspeech, oral movements) and verbal dyspraxia (speech movements).

3. In a recent review of research into childhood dyspraxia, Bowens and Smith (1999) state that most studies place the prevalence of dyspraxia between 5 and 10 per cent, with boys and girls affected by a ratio of around 4:1.

4. Caruso and Strand (1999) state that '[c]hildren may exhibit acquired apraxia as a result of a stroke, tumour, or more diffuse neurologic damage that occurs after head injury' and that '[s]ymptoms of acquired and developmental apraxia of speech overlap quite a bit' (14, 16).

5. FOXP$_2$ ('forkhead box P$_2$') is the first gene to have been implicated in a developmental communication disorder (MacDermot et al. 2005). A mutation in this gene in multiple members of the KE family has been found to cause problems in the sequencing of muscle movements for speech (DVD), as well as impairments in linguistic and grammatical processing.

6. Hall, Jordan and Robin (1993) discuss the aggregation of DVD cases within families. They state that '[c]hildren with DAS are often not alone in coping with their communication problems – many children find themselves in families where multiple other family members also experience, or have experienced, such problems' (87). In demonstration of this claim, Hall et al. report the case of a severely apraxic client who was treated in their clinic. This client had six family members across three generations who presented with communication difficulties. These difficulties included a speech sound disorder that included velopharyngeal difficulties (older sister), delays in communication skills (preschool sister), severe articulation and language problems (mother and aunt), speech problems (a second aunt) and a severe articulation disorder (maternal grandmother).

7. This variability in performance was also evident in an earlier three-year longitudinal study of these same children. Marquardt et al. (2004) found that, although longitudinal patterns were indicative of decreasing token variability and increasing token accuracy, change was not consistently unidirectional for two of the three children in the study.

8. Lewis et al. (2004) used the Test of Written Spelling – Third Edition (Larsen and Hammill 1994) to assess written spelling. Reading was assessed by two subtests of the Woodcock Reading Mastery Tests – Revised (Woodcock 1987) and the Reading Comprehension subtest of the Wechsler Individual Achievement Test (Wechsler 1992).

9. The WISC subtests in question were the Coding, Block Design and Object Assembly tests.

10. That is, most clinicians who subscribe to the view that DVD is a motor rather than a linguistic problem. Robin (1992) takes this view when he claims that 'phonological approaches to speech sound remediation are inappropriate and are doomed to failure. Rather, development of techniques that focus on training the acquisition of specific speech sounds and speech sound sequences should be more efficacious' (21).

11. Square (1994) subscribes to such a view of DVD. She remarks that

> DAS . . . is conceived here as a sensorimotor impairment. The sensorimotor impairment is based on reduced or aberrant reafference. Thus, tactile or kinesthetic methods of treatment, as well as treatment techniques that may facilitate the processing of peripheral sensation (such as slowed speech), have been proposed as being the most facilitative. (151)

12. Melodic intonation therapy was originally developed as a form of intervention in adults with aphasia (Albert et al. 1973). However, the technique is now being extensively used with children who have DVD. Roper (2003) states that 'websites . . . training . . . and college curricula . . . all recommend the use of MIT with children with apraxia' (1).

13. Ballard (2001) states that '[a]lthough there is a range of treatment approaches for AOS, there are surprisingly few well-controlled treatment efficacy studies available in the literature' (4).

14. The three studies in question are Miller and Toca (1979), Krauss and Galloway (1982) and Helfrich-Miller (1994).

15. Shriberg et al. (1999) state that '[s]ome of the most common terms are *functional articulation disorder* and *developmental phonological disorder*; hybrids such as *articulation/phonology disorder*; and less theoretically committed terms such as *multiple phoneme disorder, speech delay,* or *intelligibility impairment*' (1462; italics in original).

16. In a distinctive feature analysis, segments are described in terms of a number of binary features which are either present or absent. These features can be used to describe error patterns in children with disordered phonology. For example, the child who produces [du] for 'zoo' has performed the substitution z→d. In terms of distinctive features, this substitution represents two feature changes, + strident → − strident and + continuant → − continuant. For discussion of distinctive feature analysis and its application to disordered phonology, the reader is referred to chapter 4 in Yavaş (1998).

17. Yavaş (1998) states that

> [t]he literature is quite rich on processes, and their impact is very significant in the investigation of disordered child phonology. In addition to numerous

applications in several case studies of children with disordered phonology that have appeared in professional journals and textbooks, several assessment procedures are based on phonological process analysis. (146)

18. Yavaş (1998) states that

[i]t is quite obvious from our exposition that an overwhelming majority of studies in disordered phonology have focused on consonants, and vowel disorders largely have been ignored. The main reason behind this is the fact that there are far fewer vowel errors. (157)

19. In relation to earlier case studies of phonologically disordered children, which claimed to reveal idiosyncratic systems, Powell et al. (1999) remark that 'the diversity of these case studies attests to the individual differences that exist among children with speech sound production disorders and such cases should not be viewed as exceptions to the rule, but as commonly occurring variations that must be accommodated by theory' (165).

20. Studies have failed to agree on the comorbidity rate of language impairment and phonological disorder. In their prevalence study of six-year-old children, Shriberg et al. (1999) report comorbidity of speech delay and language impairment of 1.3 per cent. This figure, these investigators argue, is lower than that reported in other studies and is consistent with or marginally higher than the comorbidity percentage that could be expected by chance. Across 10 studies providing comorbidity data for children from 5 to 7 years of age, Shriberg et al. report figures ranging from 9 per cent to 77 per cent.

21. Phonological awareness skills are now widely believed to be impaired in children with phonological disorders and concomitant literacy problems. Rvachew et al. (2003) compared the phonological awareness abilities of four-year-old children with moderately or severely delayed expressive phonological skills to those of children with normally developing speech and language. The phonologically delayed children had significantly poorer phonemic perception and phonological awareness skills than their normally developing counterparts. Gillon (2000) found that children with expressive phonological difficulties and early reading delay made significantly more gains in their phonological awareness skills and reading development when treated with an integrated phonological awareness intervention approach than two other groups of phonologically disordered children who received other treatments (traditional speech–language intervention and a minimal intervention). Rvachew and Grawburg (2006) examined variables that may contribute to poor phonological awareness skills in preschool children with speech sound disorders. These investigators found that speech perception is a key variable that has a direct effect on phonological awareness. They also found that phonological awareness skills predict emergent literacy skills.

22. In the US, speech-language pathologists can perform various hearing screening tests. The nature and extent of the speech-language pathologist's role in audiological screening is set out in the document *Scope of Practice in Speech-Language Pathology* (American Speech-Language-Hearing Association 2001). This document states that the practice of speech-language pathology involves '[s]creening hearing of individuals who can participate in conventional pure-tone air conduction methods, as well as screening for middle ear pathology through screening tympanometry for the purpose of referral of individuals for further evaluation and management' (I-29).

23. Hoffman and Norris (2002) state that 'a child's phonological performance is typically better when labeling pictures and speaking individual words than when organizing syntactically more complex utterances as parts of narratives or when speaking in conversations' (230). Hoffman and Norris propose assessing phonology as part of the overall structure and use of language: 'This methodology allows us to assess . . . speech production as part of . . . overall production of language within contexts that typically result in children producing more speech errors than in single word naming responses' (2002:231).

24. In the study by Williams (2000b), which will not be reviewed in the main text, 10 children with moderate to profound phonological impairments received different models of intervention (multiple oppositions, minimal pairs and naturalistic speech intelligibility training) in different structures of treatment (vertical, horizontal and cyclical).

25. Schuele and Hadley (1999) list some of these terms as follows: speech/language delay, speech/language disorder, speech/language impairment, childhood aphasia, developmental dysphasia, developmental language disorder and language learning disability.

26. This study demonstrates a problem in all prevalence studies of SLI, that of including only those children who meet strict clinical criteria for the disorder. As Robinson (1991) describes the entry criteria for attendance at this residential school, it is clear that they correspond to the criteria used to identify SLI:

> The entry criteria specify that the children should be aged from eight to 16 years and have severe, specific disorders of speech and language. They must have non-verbal intelligence within the average range, no hearing loss greater than 40dB and no major physical disability. Their primary problem must not be behaviour disturbance, autism or stammer. (944)

However, also included in this study are some children with an acquired speech/language disorder and three children with a history of cleft palate. As Robinson remarks, 'both these small groups would be excluded by the definition of specific developmental language disorder' (1991:944).

27. If children with phonological problems can be classed as having an SLI, the question naturally arises of how these children can be set apart from those with phonological disorder (see section 4.3). Leonard (1998) responds as follows:

> children with phonological disorders are included in the category of SLI only if they perform poorly on other measures of language . . . the exclusion of certain children with phonological problems does not mean that phonology is ignored. Because phonological abilities are so often limited in children otherwise meeting the criteria for SLI, this area of language receives a good deal of attention. (13–14)

28. In another longitudinal study, Goffman and Leonard (2000) examined changes in finite verb morphology in nine preschool SLI children between the ages of 3 and 5 years. Compared to normally developing children, the production of finite verb morphology continued to be significantly delayed during the preschool years in SLI children. Finite verb morphology was assessed by means of a composite consisting of percentage correct production of regular past -ed, present third person singular -s and both the copula and auxiliary forms of 'is', 'are' and 'am'.

29. Marchman et al. (1999) examined productivity in the past tense in SLI children. They found that SLI children produced significantly more errors than normal language children of equivalent chronological and mental age. Moreover, a greater proportion of these errors resulted from zero-making (e.g. go) than suffixation (e.g. goed).

30. A number of morphological strengths are also discussed by Oetting and Horohov (1997). Although SLI children were found by these investigators to be less accurate than MLU-matched controls and age-matched controls in their productive marking of past tense, SLI children produced the same patterns of past-tense marking as a function of a word's phonological composition and inflectional frequency as MLU-matched controls.

31. Leonard (1998) argues that

> [g]iven the criteria for SLI, it would be natural to assume that any pragmatic difficulties observed in these children were secondary to problems of linguistic form or content . . . Indeed, some of the evidence of pragmatic difficulties in children with SLI is of this type. In other instances, however, the basis of the problem is not so clear. (78)

32. One such study is conducted by Norbury and Bishop (2002). These investigators examined the story comprehension abilities of children with typical specific language impairment (SLI-T), children with pragmatic language impairments who were not autistic (PLI), high-functioning autism children and typically developing controls. During a story comprehension task, children were required to answer

literal and inferential questions. Inferential questions required subjects to make text-connecting inferences and gap-filling inferences. Norbury and Bishop found that SLI and PLI children and children with HFA had more difficulty answering literal and inferential questions than age-matched controls. However, there was no significant difference between the clinical groups, SLI and PLI specifically included, on this inferencing task (although there was a trend for the HFA group to do more poorly than other clinical groups on questions requiring inferences, particularly gap-filling inferences).

33. Flax et al. (2003) conducted two family studies, the findings of which confirm many of the epidemiological features of SLI that were discussed in section 4.4.1. In their first study, these investigators found that the rates of language and reading impairments amongst the family members of SLI probands were significantly higher than those of control family members. Affected members of SLI families were more likely to have combined language and reading impairment than either impairment in isolation. In Flax et al.'s second study, there was a high degree of co-occurrence of language and reading impairments amongst the family members of SLI probands (46 per cent), while 25 per cent and 23 per cent had isolated language and reading impairments, respectively. Also, more males were found to have both language and reading impairments than females.

34. Deevy and Leonard (2004) examine the relative contribution of processing limitations and deficits in grammatical knowledge to the performance of SLI children in a study of wh-question comprehension. To comprehend subject and object wh-questions, SLI children must have knowledge of grammatical movement. By varying the length of questions, these investigators were able to vary the processing demands placed on these children. Deevy and Leonard found that SLI and typically developing children performed similarly on short questions, with high accuracy achieved by both groups in subject and object conditions. However, on long object questions the SLI children showed poorer performance than on long subject questions. The performance of SLI children on long object questions was also less accurate than that of typically developing children. It is clear from these results that the SLI children performed more poorly than typically developing children when questions combined a more difficult structure and additional length (long object questions) than when either of these factors occurred alone. (Long subject questions and short object questions were comprehended at similar rates in SLI and typically developing children.) Deevy and Leonard conclude that '[a]n explanation in terms of syntactic knowledge alone will not explain these results; however, an explanation that incorporates linguistic processing resources – especially one pertaining to working memory – seems more successful' (2004: 813–14).

35. In an earlier study, Montgomery (1995) examined the influence of phonological working memory on sentence comprehension in SLI children. SLI children and children with normal language participated in a nonsense word repetition task (an index of phonological working memory) and a comprehension task that used

redundant and nonredundant sentences. SLI children repeated significantly fewer three- and four-syllable nonsense words than normal-language children and comprehended significantly fewer redundant (longer) sentences than nonredundant (shorter) sentences. Also, performance on nonsense word repetition and sentence comprehension tasks was positively correlated. Montgomery concludes that 'children with SLI have diminished phonological working memory capacity and that this capacity deficit compromises their sentence comprehension efforts' (1995:187).

36. In 1997, Tuchman reported that over 160 cases of LKS had been reported in the medical literature. More recently, Smith and Hoeppner (2003) recorded a total of 198 published cases of LKS.

37. Temple (1997) reported the first case of LKS in monozygotic twins. In her account of these children, she provides a full medical and developmental history as well as information on the onset and course of language impairment.

38. Honbolygó et al. (2006) found that automatic phoneme discrimination was preserved in a boy with LKS. Discrimination of altered stress patterns was deficient in this subject.

39. Irwin et al. (2001) assessed the effect of multiple subpial transection (MST) on language and cognitive ability, behaviour, seizures and EEG abnormalities in five children with LKS. After surgery, behaviour and seizure frequency improved dramatically in all children. Although none of the children improved language to an age-appropriate level, improvement nevertheless occurred in all children. Electrical status epilepticus in sleep was eliminated in all five children by means of surgery. Grote et al. (1999) investigated speech and language outcomes in 14 LKS children who underwent MST. Significant postoperative improvement on measures of receptive or expressive vocabulary was reported in 11 of the children.

5

Acquired Communication and Swallowing Disorders

5.1 Introduction

In adults, previously normal speech and language skills can be impaired through injury and disease. A cerebrovascular accident (CVA) or stroke may disrupt language. The resulting aphasia can affect the comprehension and expression of spoken language to a greater or lesser extent. Written language may also be affected with impairments of reading (dyslexia) and writing (dysgraphia) in evidence. As well as CVAs, degenerative conditions such as multiple sclerosis (MS), motor neurone disease (MND) and Parkinson's disease (PD) adversely affect neuromuscular function. The resulting impairments of speech, feeding and swallowing require prompt assessment and treatment. We examine the dysarthrias that occur in these conditions and describe the management of dysphagia in neurological disorders. Many of the same neurological events and traumas that cause aphasia and dysarthria in adults also give rise to apraxia. We discuss what is known about this motor speech programming disorder in adults. While dysarthria, aphasia and apraxia in adults are communication disorders of neurological origin, other communication disorders with an onset in adulthood lack a clear neurological aetiology. The significant communication impairments that attend schizophrenia are a case in point. We conclude this chapter with discussion of these impairments.

5.2 Acquired Dysarthria

By definition, the term 'dysarthria' applies only to speech disorders that have a neurogenic origin. In 'acquired' dysarthria, the onset of the neurological condition or injury that causes speech impairment is significant in at least two respects. First, in individuals with acquired dysarthria speech development is complete. It is therefore mature speech abilities that are disrupted. (Compare with the disruption of developing speech skills in developmental dysarthria.) Second, the mature brain lacks the neural plasticity of a developing brain and is likely to mount a different response to disease and injury. This response will affect the nature and extent of any speech recovery. For both these reasons, acquired dysarthria and developmental dysarthria should be treated as distinct disorders, notwithstanding certain similarities in their presentation. In this section, we examine the epidemiology of a range of conditions that are known to cause dysarthria in adults – reliable incidence and prevalence figures for dysarthria itself are not available. We discuss the neurodegenerative changes that are responsible for dysarthria in disorders like MS and MND. The speech features of dysarthria will be examined. We will also consider assessment and treatment issues in relation to this speech disorder.

5.2.1 Epidemiology and Aetiology

CVAs, commonly known as strokes, are a leading cause of dysarthria in adults. A stroke occurs when a blood clot (embolus) forms somewhere in the body (usually the heart) and travels in the bloodstream to the brain where it blocks a blood vessel (embolic stroke). Also, a blood clot (thrombus) may form in one or more of the arteries supplying blood to the brain and disrupt the flow of blood to the brain (thrombotic stroke). Often, clots form in response to fatty deposits and cholesterol that line the inside of blood vessels over a period of years (athero-sclerosis). Alternatively, a blood vessel in the brain may rupture and bleed (haem-orrhage). A haemorrhagic stroke may be caused by long-standing high blood pressure and cerebral aneurysms (weak spots, which are usually congenital, in the wall of a blood vessel).[1] There are two types of haemorrhagic stroke. In an intracerebral haemorrhage, a blood vessel within the brain bleeds. Hypertension (high blood pressure) is the primary cause of this haemorrhage. In a subarach-noid haemorrhage, an aneurysm bursts in a large artery on or near the arachnoid membrane (the middle membrane of three membranes (meninges) that cover the brain and spinal cord). Blood leaks into the subarachnoid cavity, the space between the arachnoid and pia mater (innermost meninx).

Stroke is one of the major causes of death and disability in developed coun-tries. Considerable efforts have thus been undertaken to obtain a thorough understanding of the epidemiology of stroke. Carroll et al. (2001) used data from the Fourth National Morbidity Survey to estimate the incidence of first ever and recurrent strokes in England and Wales. These investigators estimated that in 1999, 87,700 people had a first ever stroke and 53,700 had a recurrent stroke. Age-adjusted rates for first ever or recurrent strokes were 0.20 per cent in males and 0.16 per cent in females. The American Heart Association reports that each year in the US about 500,000 people have a first stroke and 200,000 experience a recurrent attack. The Association claims that men's stroke incidence rates are 1.25 times greater than women's rates. Of all strokes, 88 per cent are ischaemic (blood-clot strokes), 9 per cent are intracerebral haemorrhage and 3 per cent are subarachnoid haemorrhage. The majority of strokes occur in people aged 65 years and older. Carroll et al. (2001) found that 81 per cent of the individuals in their study who suffered a first ever or recurrent stroke were over 64 years of age. It should not be overlooked, however, that babies and children can also suffer a stroke.[2]

Less commonly, dysarthria in adults is caused by disorders such as MS, MND and PD. MS is a chronic, frequently progressive disease in which the body's immune system attacks and breaks down the fatty insulating sheath (myelin) that envelopes the axons of nerve cells. Myelin facilitates the propagation of electrical impulses along the axons of neurones and its destruction disrupts the transmission of impulses to muscles. As well as being damaged, myelin may become inflamed in MS. Inflammation of myelin can lead to lesions in many different sites throughout the central nervous system. There is also evidence that axons themselves may be damaged in MS, even in the earliest stages of the condition. The effect of these neuropathological changes in MS varies with the site of lesions. If the spinal cord is involved, as occurs in primary progressive MS (see below), walking and bowel, bladder and sexual function may be impaired. If the brain is involved or the optic nerve is damaged, cognitive problems and visual disturbances may occur, respectively.

Four types of MS are recognised by neurologists: benign, relapsing/ remitting, primary progressive and secondary progressive. The benign form of the condition affects about 10 per cent of MS individuals. These are people who experience few relapses with little or no residual disability over a period of 15 years or more. In the relapsing/remitting form of MS, a series of relapses or attacks is interspersed with periods of remission. Relapses and remissions are of variable duration. Relapses can last from 24 hours to a period of weeks or months. They occur, on average, approximately once or twice every two years. Remissions may extend from months to decades. During a remission, symptoms that caused disability in a relapse may resolve. If there is some residual damage after a relapse, incremental disability may occur. The relapsing/ remitting form occurs in about two-thirds of MS individuals. While people with relapsing/remitting MS may experience their first symptoms in their early twenties, individuals with primary progressive MS develop their first symptoms in their forties or later. This form of MS affects about 10 per cent of MS patients. There are no relapses or remissions. Rather, symptoms gradually worsen over a period of years. A substantial number of people with relapsing/remitting MS go on to develop secondary progressive MS – it is estimated that by 15 years, 65 per cent of people with relapsing/remitting MS will have become secondary progressive. For a diagnosis of secondary progressive MS to be made, there needs to be clear evidence of a sustained deterioration that lasts for six months or more and which is completely independent of relapses. This diagnosis is made more difficult by the fact that some people with secondary progressive MS continue to have relapses.

Although epidemiological studies of MS in England and Wales have produced different prevalence estimates, the average prevalence is estimated to be 110 MS individuals per 100,000 population (Richards et al. 2002). Prevalence rates increase with distance from the equator. Grytten et al. (2006) report, for example, a prevalence rate of 150.8 per 100,000 population in Hordaland County, Norway. Overall, more women than men develop MS. The female:male sex ratio that is most frequently cited in relation to MS is 2:1. This figure is reasonably well supported by Grytten et al.'s finding that MS affects 191.3 per 100,000 among women and 109.8 per 100,000 among men. However, while relapsing/remitting MS is twice as common in women as it is in men, primary progressive MS appears to affect women and men in similar numbers.

Investigators have reported high prevalence rates of dysarthria in MS subjects. Hartelius et al. (2000) examined 77 individuals drawn from an MS population. In this cohort, the prevalence of mild to severe dysarthria was 51 per cent. All components of speech production – respiration, phonation, prosody, articulation and nasality – were affected in these subjects. Klugman and Ross (2002) examined 30 individuals with MS, 56.7 per cent of whom reported that they experienced speech problems. Hartelius and Svensson (1994) conducted a survey of approximately 460 patients with PD or MS. Among the MS subjects, 44 per cent had experienced speech and voice problems following the onset of disease. For 16 per cent of MS subjects, the speech disorder was considered to be one of the greatest problems that they experienced. It should also be noted that only 2 per cent of MS subjects had received speech therapy. Clearly, dysarthric speech deficits are a prominent, yet inadequately addressed, clinical feature of MS.

MND in adults[3] is not a single disorder, but a group of progressive neurological disorders. This group includes amyotrophic lateral sclerosis (ALS),[4] progressive bulbar palsy, pseudobulbar palsy, primary lateral sclerosis and progressive muscular atrophy. These disorders differ in terms of underlying neuropathology, age of onset and survival time. In ALS, the most common of these disorders,[5] there is degeneration of the anterior horn cells of the spinal cord and the motor cranial nuclei. Upper motor neurone findings include hyperreflexia and spasticity and lower motor neurone findings include weakness, atrophy and fasciculations. Average age of onset of ALS is 56 years, although patients may develop the disorder between 40 and 60 years (Clem and Morgenlander 2006). Median survival is between 3 and 5 years, but it is not uncommon for individuals to survive longer than five years. (Thirty per cent of patients are still alive five years after diagnosis and 10–20 per cent survive for more than 10 years.) Respiratory muscle weakness leads to death with aspiration pneumonia and problems associated with immobility contributing to morbidity.

The epidemiology of MND varies with the population investigated and form of the disorder. In a study of Hong Kong Chinese MND subjects, Fong et al. (2005) report an adjusted incidence rate of 0.60/100,000/year and an adjusted point prevalence of 3.04/100,000. The average age of MND onset in these subjects was 58.76 years with a peak age of onset between 60 and 64 years. The male:female ratio was 1.72:1. Higher incidence and prevalence figures are reported by the ALS Association (2004) in the United States. The Association states that the incidence of ALS is two cases per 100,000 population per year and the prevalence is between 6 and 8 cases per 100,000 population. Using the higher prevalence estimate and data from the 2000 US census, the Association reports that nearly 22,600 Americans are living with ALS at any one time. The mean age of onset is between 55 and 65 years of age with an incidence in the sixth decade of 3–4 cases per 100,000 population per year (ALS Association 2004).

Dysarthria is a common feature of MND and a major disability for affected individuals. The Motor Neurone Disease Association (2005) in the UK reports that 80 per cent of MND individuals will eventually be affected by dysarthria. In ALS, there is a mixed spastic–flaccid dysarthria reflecting upper motor neurone (UMN) and lower motor neurone (LMN) disease (Duffy 1995). The contributions of each type of dysarthria change as the disease progresses. Flaccid dysarthria generally becomes more prominent as the individual becomes increasingly weak (Yorkston et al. 1999). All components of the speech system may be affected. Fukae et al. (2005) report the case of a 43-year-old woman in whom hoarseness due to bilateral vocal cord paralysis was the first manifestation of ALS. The changing nature and severity of dysarthria in MND demands a staged approach to intervention (see section 5.2.4).

PD is the second most common neurodegenerative disorder after Alzheimer's disease.[6] The main symptoms of this disorder – tremor, stiffness and slowness of movement (bradykinesia) – are also the main symptoms of a number of other disorders that are grouped under the label 'parkinsonism'. These other disorders are called multiple system atrophy, progressive supranuclear palsy and drug-induced parkinsonism. They are considerably less common than idiopathic PD which occurs in 85 per cent of cases. (The term 'idiopathic' indicates that the cause is unknown.) In idiopathic PD, there is a progressive loss of dopaminergic neurones in the substantia nigra and nigrostriatal pathway of the midbrain. Many PD patients eventually lose 80 per cent or more of their dopamine-producing cells. About 7 per cent of people with parkinsonism develop their disorder following treatment with drugs that block the action of dopamine (so-called dopamine antagonists). These neuroleptic drugs are used to treat schizophrenia and other psychotic disorders, such as behaviour disturbances in people with dementia. Parkinsonism may also be caused by a stroke (vascular or arteriosclerotic parkinsonism). Prior head injury with amnesia or loss of consciousness has also been associated with an increased risk of PD (Goldman et al. 2006).

As with the other neurodegenerative disorders that we have examined, figures for the incidence and prevalence of PD vary from study to study. Reported standardised incidence rates of PD are 8–18 per 100,000 person years (De Lau and Breteler 2006). Clough et al. (2003) state that a widely accepted figure for the prevalence of PD is 200 per 100,000. Peters et al. (2006) report a lower prevalence based on an Australian population. They obtained an estimated prevalence of diagnosed idiopathic PD in Queensland of 146 per 100,000. This lower prevalence may be explained by the fact that a further 51 per 100,000 people were thought by doctors to have idiopathic PD but had not received a formal diagnosis. Also, another 51 per 100,000 may have non-idiopathic parkinsonism. The Parkinson's Disease Society estimates that there are more than 120,000 people in the UK who have the disorder and that around 10,000 people are diagnosed each year. PD is largely a disorder of older age. The disorder affects one person in 100 over the age of 65 and one in 50 over the age of 80. It should not be overlooked, however, that many younger people also develop PD – one in 20 people with PD is under 40 years old when diagnosed and one in seven is under 50 (Parkinson's Disease Society 2002). PD is more common in males than females – Fall et al. (1996) obtained a male:female ratio of 1.5:1 in a Swedish community.

Researchers estimate that 89 per cent of people with PD have a speech or voice disorder, including disorders of articulatory, laryngeal and respiratory function (Trail et al. 2005). The principal speech disorder in PD is hypokinetic dysarthria. This type of dysarthria is associated with basal ganglia pathology. (The substantia nigra, the dopamine-producing cells of which degenerate in PD, is an important basal ganglia structure.) Vocal and laryngeal abnormalities are also common in PD. In a survey of 258 PD patients, Hartelius and Svensson (1994) found that the most frequently indicated voice problems are a weak, hoarse and/or monotonous voice. Dysphonia can also be the first presenting sign of PD (Merati et al. 2005). Ho et al. (1998) classified speech impairment in 200 patients with PD according to severity, type (voice, articulation, fluency) and extent. Voice was the leading deficit in these patients. It was the most frequently affected speech feature and was impaired to a greater extent in the initial stages of the disease than other features. Articulation and fluency deficits were manifested later, with articulation impairment matching voice impairment in both frequency and extent at the severe stage. Articulation was the most frequently impaired feature at the lowest level of performance in the final stage of profound impairment.

Many other neurological events and disease can result in dysarthria in adults. Myasthenia gravis is an acquired autoimmune disorder of neuromuscular transmission in which antibodies attack acetylcholine receptors in the postsynaptic membrane of the neuromuscular junction (Pourmand 1997). Kluin et al. (1996) examined eight elderly men with myasthenia gravis and found fatigable flaccid dysarthria in all of them. Huntington's disease is a hereditary disorder (autosomal dominant transmission) in which symptoms usually appear between 30 and 50 years of age. Affected individuals experience choreiform movements, psychological changes and dementia as a result of selective neuronal loss in the cortex and striatum (Cajavec et al. 2006). Savvopoulos et al. (1990) reviewed 17 cases of Huntington's disease and found that dysarthria occurred in 95 per cent of subjects. Guillain-Barré syndrome (GBS) is an autoimmune acute peripheral neuropathy. Onset often occurs days or weeks after a patient has had symptoms of a respiratory or gastrointestinal viral infection. In severe cases, breathing and swallowing are compromised and the patient will require ventilation and tube feeding. Wada et al. (2006) describe the case of a 19-year-old woman who developed acute oropharyngeal palsy following enteritis. The first sign of GBS in this woman was an increasing nasal voice. Neurological examination on day seven of her course confirmed paretic dysarthria.

Traumatic brain injury is a common cause of acquired dysarthria. In a study of 33 patients who sustained head injury, Zebenholzer and Oder (1998) reported dysarthria in 39 and 33 per cent of patients at four and eight years postinjury, respectively. Brain tumours can also cause dysarthria in adults. Mukand et al. (2001) examined common neurological problems in adults with brain tumours admitted for inpatient rehabilitation at an acute rehabilitation centre. A range of tumour types was included amongst the 51 consecutive adult patients that were studied (glioblastoma (31.3 per cent), meningioma (25.5 per cent) and metastatic (25.5 per cent)). The incidence of dysarthria in these adult patients was 27 per cent. Dysarthria in adults can also be caused by infections. Lopez et al. (1994) describe ataxic dysarthria in six patients who developed speech motor control problems after HIV infection. Dysarthria in these patients appeared to be related to cerebellar dysfunction. Gustaw and Mirecka (2001) report a case of dysarthria due to mononeuropathy of the left hypoglossal nerve in a 65-year-old man. This mononeuropathy was a chronic consequence of *Borrelia burgdorferi* infection[7] which had caused meningitis in this subject in 1999.

Dysarthria may also be caused by medical intervention (so-called iatrogenic dysarthria). Sengupta et al. (1999) describe the case of a 35-year-old woman who developed hypoglossal nerve palsy with dysarthria following surgery of the upper cervical spine. Hypoglossal nerve palsy with dysarthria may also be caused by laryngectomy. In a study of 21 patients who underwent total laryngectomy, Clevens et al. (1993) report that speech failure was attributable to hypoglossal nerve palsy in 5 per cent of cases. Recurrent laryngeal nerve (RLN) palsy with hoarseness may occur as a result of thyroidectomy. Tomoda et al. (2006) examined 1,376 patients who were identified to be at risk from RLN palsy during thyroidectomy. These investigators identified 80 cases of temporary vocal cord palsy and 21 cases of permanent vocal cord palsy on postoperative evaluation. Although uncommon, unilateral vocal cord paralysis due to damage of the recurrent laryngeal nerve may result from oesophagectomy (Wright and Zeitels 2006). Finally, radiation therapy for head and neck carcinomas may also cause dysarthria. King et al. (1999) studied 21 patients with hypoglossal nerve palsy who received radiation therapy for nasopharyngeal carcinoma. In 14 patients (67 per cent), radiation-induced neuropathy was the probable cause of hypoglossal nerve palsy.

5.2.2 Clinical Presentation

In section 5.2.1, we discussed a range of neurological diseases and events that cause dysarthria in adults. Dysarthria was attributed to lesions and other anomalies in the central and/or peripheral nervous systems. This neurological approach to the dysarthrias was dominant until the late 1960s, when Darley et al. (1969a, 1969b, 1975) first introduced a perceptually based system to classify dysarthric speech disorders. The emphasis in a perceptual approach is on the speech characteristics that are associated with the dysarthrias. More recently, technological developments have allowed clinicians to measure dysarthric speech in a range of more objective ways. These measures, which include acoustic and physiological techniques, have been used to complement clinicians' judgements about dysarthric speech and, on occasion, to revise those judgements. The combination of neurological and perceptual approaches and acoustic and physiological measurements has enabled clinicians and researchers to provide increasingly detailed accounts of the dysarthrias in a range of neurological disorders. In this section, we examine the dysarthrias that occur in MS, MND and PD. Dysarthrias with other aetiologies, such as stroke and Huntington's disease, will also be discussed. We then turn to consider how acquired dysarthrias are assessed and treated by clinicians.

Speech and voice disturbances are common in MS (see section 5.2.1). When they do occur, they present as a spastic-ataxic dysarthria with disorders of voice quality and intensity, articulation and intonation (Merson and Rolnick 1998). Murdoch et al. (1998) examined articulatory function in 16 adults with MS. A physiological analysis was performed using lip and tongue transduction systems. These investigators found that MS speakers had significantly reduced tongue strength, endurance and rate of repetitive movements. Also, when compared to control subjects, nondysarthric MS speakers showed preclinical signs of lingual dysfunction on endurance and rate tasks. No lip dysfunction was found on either perceptual or physiological assessments. Hartelius and Lillvik (2003) compared clinical dysarthria test scores on lip and tongue function in dysarthric and nondysarthric MS speakers and normal controls. Tongue function was significantly more severely affected than lip function in the MS subjects. Moreover, tongue function (but not lip function) was also more severely affected in the nondysarthric MS subjects than in the control subjects. In the dysarthric MS subjects, test items that required increased rate of movement (oral and verbal diadochokinesis) were significantly more severely affected than items requiring force and range of movement. Tongue and lip function was also found to correlate moderately with neurological deficit scores, number of years in disease progression and perceptually perceived consonant and vowel precision.

Feijo et al. (2004) examined dysphonic symptoms in 30 MS patients. Quantitative acoustic parameters in MS and normal individuals were compared. These investigators observed dysphonia in 70 per cent of the MS patients and 33 per cent of controls. An association was found between MS and dysphonia. Fundamental frequency was higher in the MS patients. MS women (but not men) displayed significantly higher fundamental frequency deviation than controls. Jitter was also higher in MS men than in other groups. Feijo et al. conclude that 'MS seems to intensify gender effect on fundamental frequency deviation, noise, and jitter, with MS women presenting fewer voice variations than men' (2004:341). Hartelius et al. (1997) examined phonatory instability in 20 individuals with MS. Sustained vowel phonations underwent fundamental frequency and intensity analysis and were subjected to spectral analysis. All measures reliably distinguished MS from control subjects. MS subjects were distinguished from control subjects on critical frequency bands of instability corresponding to wow (1–2Hz), tremor (around 8Hz) and flutter (17–18Hz).

All speech production subsystems are eventually disrupted in MND. Langmore and Lehman (1994) used strain gauge force transducers placed on the lower lip, jaw and tongue tip to ascertain physiological deficits in the orofacial musculature of 14 ALS patients and to relate these deficits to the perceived severity of dysarthria. Maximum strength and maximum rate of repeated contractions were measured and diadochokinetic rates for repeated /pe/ and /te/ were also determined. Compared to normal controls, ALS patients were impaired on all tasks. Some measures even revealed impairment in ALS patients who were not yet dysarthric. Performance varied with the type of ALS, with bulbar patients more severely affected than either corticobulbar or spinal patients. The tongue was the most severely affected structure in all ALS patients. Perceived severity of dysarthria was found to be more highly correlated with measures of repeated contraction rate than with measures of strength. Langmore and Lehman conclude that 'more severe dysarthria may be largely due to slower movement of the orofacial structures until substantial muscle strength has been lost' (1994:28).

Tomik et al. (1999) used a computer-based acoustic method to evaluate dysarthria in 53 patients with definite or probable ALS. Three computer-analysed speech sound tests were completed for all patients. These investigators were able to construct specific dysarthria profiles for two groups of ALS patients – bulbar (dysarthric) and limb (nondysarthric) – based on the most significantly affected vowels. Tomik et al. conclude that it is possible to monitor the progression of ALS using an acoustic analysis of only several sounds and that abnormalities detected in the dysarthria profile may appear before the onset of clinical symptoms. Tjaden et al. (2005) investigated the vowel space area formed by the lax vowels /ɪ/, /ɛ/ and /ʊ/ in ALS speakers, speakers with PD and healthy controls. Only vowel space areas for ALS speakers differed from those of controls.

Speech and voice disturbances in PD have been extensively investigated. Whitehill et al. (2003) obtained a perceptual speech profile for 19 Cantonese speakers with PD and hypokinetic dysarthria. Amongst 21 speech dimensions that were rated by listeners, the 10 that were most severely affected were, in descending order of severity, rough voice, strained-strangled voice, monoloudness, bizarreness, monopitch, breathy voice, understandability, imprecise consonants, hypernasality and irregular articulatory breakdown. Three PD speakers had an unusually rapid speaking rate and six had an unusually slow rate. Perez et al. (1996) investigated laryngeal abnormalities in 22 patients with idiopathic PD and seven patients with Parkinson's-plus syndromes. Trained viewers conducted visual-perceptual ratings of endoscopic and stroboscopic examinations. Most of the 29 PD patients had tremor in one or more of these conditions – rest, normal pitch and loudness, or loud phonation. Amongst the patients with idiopathic PD, 55 per cent had tremor, with the primary location being vertical laryngeal tremor. In the Parkinson's-plus patients, 64 per cent had tremor. The primary location of tremor in these patients was the arytenoid cartilages. Perez et al. remark that laryngeal tremor was an early feature of disease in the PD patients. Abnormal phase closure and phase asymmetry were the most striking stroboscopic findings for the idiopathic PD patients. Yunusova et al. (2005) examined within-speaker fluctuations in speech intelligibility in 10 dysarthric subjects with PD or ALS. Dysarthric and control subjects read a passage aloud that was then separated into consecutive breath groups for estimates of individual breath group intelligibility. Intelligibility was assessed by 60 listeners. Results showed that the intelligibility of individual dysarthric subjects fluctuated across breath groups. Also, the breath groups of dysarthric subjects had fewer average words and reduced interquartile ranges for the second formant (a global measure of articulatory mobility).

Ackermann et al. (1995) conducted an acoustic analysis of rapid syllable repetitions in 17 patients with idiopathic PD. All PD subjects exceeded the normal range on at least one of four measures of diadochokinesis: mean number of syllables per train, median syllable duration with its variation coefficient and articulatory imprecision in terms of the percentage of incomplete closures. Furthermore, PD patients exhibited a highly specific profile of diadochokinesis performance. They produced long repetition trains, which comprised mostly incomplete closures, at a normal syllabic rate. Speech timing and articulatory rate have also been studied in PD. McAuliffe et al. (2006) used electropalatography (EPG) to examine temporal aspects of articulation in nine subjects with PD. As well as objective measurement of segment, word and sentence duration, perceptual investigation of speech rate was also performed. These investigators found that speech rate in PD speakers was impaired on perceptual assessment. However, this was not confirmed objectively – EPG investigation revealed segment durations in PD speakers to be consistent with those of control speakers.[8] A single exception was the release phase for /la/, the duration of which was significantly increased in PD subjects compared to aged and young controls. McRae et al. (2002) examined the effect of voluntary articulatory rate modification in idiopathic PD speakers on (1) perceptual impressions of severity and (2) acoustic measures of segmental and global timing and acoustic working space for select vowels and consonants. The vowels and consonants of interest were /i/, /æ/, /u/, /ɑ/, /s/ and /ʃ/. Subjects read a passage at habitual, fast and slow speaking rates. PD subjects showed a tendency toward slightly faster rates than healthy control speakers, but in all other respects temporal acoustic measures changed in the expected direction across rate conditions. Although measures of acoustic working space were not strongly affected by rate in PD speakers, there was a tendency for slower speaking rate to be associated with larger measures of acoustic working space. In terms of the impact of rate on perceptual impressions of speech severity, there was a significant main effect for group. More severe ratings were obtained for the PD group, particularly on the slow and fast conditions.

Clinicians and researchers have also investigated dysarthrias associated with other aetiologies. Hertrich and Ackermann (1994) examined syllable lengths, vowel durations and voice–onset–time (VOT) in 13 subjects with Huntington's disease (HD). Findings included increased variability of utterance duration and/or VOT in all 13 subjects. A subgroup of these subjects also displayed reduced speech tempo that was concomitant with over–proportional lengthening of short vowels. Hertrich and Ackermann relate these deviations to slowed movement execution (bradykinesia) and delayed between–movement transitions. A further HD subject, whose speech did not undergo acoustic analysis, produced barely intelligible, truncated, diphthongised sentence utterances. A similar pattern was observed in two other HD subjects whose speech was analysed. All three subjects had a long disease duration, leading these investigators to conclude that these features may be typical of advanced-stage dysarthria in HD. Ackermann et al. (1995) examined rapid syllable repetitions in 14 patients with HD. Compared to controls, HD subjects showed lowered syllabic rate, i.e. increased syllable duration. Ackermann et al. relate the slowed syllabic rate of HD subjects to the same pathomechanism that is responsible for bradykinesia and delayed transitions in upper limb motor control in HD.

Stroke is a major cause of dysarthria in adults (see section 5.2.1). Urban et al. (2006) studied the auditory perceptual features of dysarthria in 62 consecutive patients who had sustained a single, non-space-occupying cerebral infarction. Speech recordings of all patients were made within 72 hours of stroke onset and were analysed by two experienced speech and language therapists. Articulatory, phonatory and prosodic features of speech were assessed. Factor analysis revealed that the impairment of articulation mainly influenced the severity of dysarthria. The production of consonants was particularly impaired. At follow-up, 15 of 38 patients (39.5 per cent) showed normal speech while the severity of dysarthria was mild in the remaining 23 patients. Dagenais et al. (2006) examined the effect of altering speech rate on the intelligibility and acceptability of dysarthric speech. The speech of four dysarthric subjects, three of whom had sustained a stroke, was played at three different rates to normal adult listeners. Increasing and decreasing speech rate by 30 per cent had no impact on intelligibility. Dagenais et al. suggest that this undermines the assumption that by slowing speaking rate, dysarthric speakers can achieve better coordination for speech production and, hence, more intelligible speech. The most significant gains in acceptability of increased rate were found in the two speakers with higher intelligibility. Dagenais et al. state that this finding indicates that 'the articulatory patterns of these higher intelligibility speakers tend toward the normal range' (2006:147). Nishio and Niimi (2006) examined speaking rate, articulation rate and alternating motion rate (AMR) in 62 dysarthric speakers, 29 of whom had cerebrovascular disease. All three rate measures were markedly lower in dysarthric subjects than in controls. There were also marked correlations between these measures in the dysarthric subjects. AMR distinguished dysarthric and control subjects. AMR was considerably lower than articulation rate in dysarthric subjects, but not in controls. Nishio and Niimi conclude that 'AMR is a more easily detected sign of abnormal articulation than speaking rate and articulation rate' (2006:114).

5.2.3 Dysarthria Assessment

Assessment is an important component in the management of a client with acquired dysarthria. Clinicians can draw upon a range of techniques to assess dysarthria in adults. These techniques include perceptual, acoustic and physiological methods of assessment. In this section, we examine how dysarthria is assessed using these various techniques. We discuss recent studies that have used these techniques to assess dysarthric speech. We also consider the merits and drawbacks of each of these assessment approaches. The changing neurological status of many traumatic brain injury (TBI) and neurodegenerative patients means that dysarthria is not a static disorder in these clients. We examine the implications of change in a client's neurological status for the assessment of dysarthria.

Perceptual assessments are based on a clinician's impression of the auditory-perceptual attributes of a client's speech. One of the most widely used perceptual assessments of dysarthria is the Frenchay Dysarthria Assessment (FDA; Enderby 1983). The FDA is, according to Duffy (1995), the only standardised published test which 'quantifies dysarthria in a manner that distinguishes among dysarthria types' (87). Normative data are reported for normal adults and for dysarthric patients. Clinicians are able to compare the results of individual patients with those of known dysarthric groups. The test is divided into 11 sections: reflexes, respiration, lips, jaw, palate, laryngeal, tongue, intelligibility, rate, sensation and associated factors. Other perceptual assessments include the Dysarthria Profile (Robertson 1987) and the Assessment of Intelligibility of Dysarthric Speech (Yorkston et al. 1984). The latter is a tool for quantifying single-word intelligibility, sentence intelligibility and speaking rate in adolescent and adult dysarthric speakers. As well as using these formal assessments of dysarthric speech, many clinicians also implement their own assessment procedures. These informal techniques also depend on a perceptual analysis of the client's speech and voice by the assessing clinician.

The FDA is used extensively in clinical practice and research studies. McKinstry and Perry (2003) used the FDA to assess speech functions in 20 subjects (aged 47–76 years) who were all newly diagnosed with a cancer of the head and neck. All subjects completed a self-report questionnaire relating to speech intelligibility and were assessed on subscales of the FDA prior to the commencement of treatment. The specific speech dimensions examined were respiratory ability and functions of the lip, soft palate, larynx and tongue. McKinstry and Perry found that the head and neck cancer patients had a greater reduction in speech intelligibility and nearly all aspects of speech compared to the normal population. Furthermore, these investigators concluded that this study 'has also shown the usefulness of the Frenchay Dysarthria Assessment as a practicable, valid and reliable protocol of motor speech assessment for the head and neck cancer population' (2003:31). Auzou et al. (1998) adapted the FDA for use in French dysarthric patients. These researchers used the adapted FDA to examine speech production in 100 patients with four types of dysarthria (spastic, ataxic, hypokinetic and mixed). Gustaw and Mirecka (2001) used a dysarthria scale based on Robertson's Dysarthria Profile to describe speech abnormalities in a 65-year-old man with a seven-month history of articulation disturbances. This subject's dysarthria was related to hypoglossal nerve mononeuropathy that was a consequence of neuroborreliosis (see note 7). Cahill et al. (2004) used perceptual and instrumental techniques to determine the effectiveness of a treatment for impaired velopharyngeal function in 3 TBI adults. Perceptual evaluation consisted of the FDA, the Assessment of Intelligibility of Dysarthric Speech and a speech sample analysis.

Traditionally, perceptual techniques have been the assessment method of choice for clinicians and researchers.[9] Several features of these assessments have contributed to their widespread clinical use. First, they involve minimal expenditure – simply the cost of the assessment – and can be competently executed by all trained speech and language therapists. Second, perceptual techniques permit an assessment of a speaker's intelligibility, which is the yardstick by which acceptable speech is measured. Third, there is evidence that these assessments can successfully distinguish different types of dysarthria. Enderby (1983), for example, reported that more than 90 per cent of cases tested on the FDA were predicted to belong to their correct diagnostic category. Notwithstanding the merits of these techniques, perceptual assessments are also associated with a number of significant drawbacks. Perceptual judgements are subjective in nature. Their accuracy is based entirely on the assessing clinician's experience of listening to and transcribing disordered speech. This experience is often highly variable amongst clinicians, as most of it is acquired after qualification when similar clinical backgrounds are less easily guaranteed. Perceptual assessments are also difficult to standardise in relation to both the patient and the setting in which assessment is conducted. One speech symptom may also influence the perception of other symptoms. This confound, Murdoch et al. (2000) report, has been described in relation to the perception of resonatory disorders, articulatory deficits and prosodic disturbances. Finally, perceptual assessments are limited in what they can tell clinicians about the pathophysiological basis of the speech symptoms in dysarthria. For example, distorted consonants can be the result of quite distinct physiological anomalies – inadequate respiratory support for speech, velopharyngeal incompetence and weak tongue musculature – and knowledge of these specific anomalies is essential for treatment planning. In the worst scenario, a programme of intervention that is based exclusively on perceptual assessment may lead to the setting of inappropriate treatment goals.

Recent technological developments have led to a rapid expansion in acoustic assessments of dysarthric speech. Acoustic analyses can now be used to confirm a range of perceived deviant speech dimensions, including aberrant speech rate, consonant imprecision, breathy voice, voice tremor and reduced variability of pitch and loudness. Clinicians and researchers are able to characterise dysarthric speech according to several acoustic parameters. These parameters include fundamental frequency measures, amplitude measures, noise-related measures, temporal measures, perturbation measures, formant measures, measures of articulatory capability and evaluations of manner of voicing (Murdoch et al. 2000). Researchers are using these measures not only to distinguish dysarthric speech from normal speech but also to develop 'acoustic signatures' for different types of dysarthria (see Rosen et al. 2006 below). These signatures may be found to have potential diagnostic significance for dysarthria. Below, we examine several studies in which acoustic analyses of dysarthric speech have been performed. We then consider a number of benefits and limitations of the acoustic assessment of dysarthria.

Voice disorder is a common and prominent symptom of dysarthria in adults. Yet, assessments of voice are both difficult on their own terms and complicated by the presence of co-occurring impairments of articulation, resonance and respiration in dysarthria. Recent developments in voice analysis technology have provided clinicians and researchers with a better understanding of voice anomalies in dysarthria than has been possible using conventional (perceptual) techniques. One such development has been the Multi-Dimensional Voice Program (MDVP; Kay Elemetrics 1993). MDVP is a software tool for quantitative acoustic assessment of voice quality. It can calculate more than 22 acoustic parameters on a single vocalisation, including fundamental frequency, jitter, shimmer and turbulence. The number and range of these parameters reflect the fact that one or two voicing parameters are often not adequate to describe an aberration in a patient's voice. For example, a patient may have a breathy voice and yet jitter values may be within normal limits. Kent et al. (2003) review acoustic data obtained from MDVP for dysarthria associated with PD, cerebellar disease, ALS, TBI, unilateral hemispheric stroke and essential tremor. These investigators also discuss procedures and standards for the acoustic analysis of voice.

Since Kent et al.'s (2003) review, several other studies have performed acoustic analyses of dysarthrias of different aetiologies. Rosen et al. (2006) used acoustic analysis to identify acoustic signatures of hypokinetic dysarthria associated with idiopathic PD. Twenty healthy controls and 20 PD subjects repeated three isolated sentences and two minutes of conversational speech. Measures of contrastivity were calculated using a MATLAB-based program. These measures included speech–pause ratio, intensity variation, median and maximum formant slope, formant range, change in the upper and lower spectral envelope and range of the spectral envelope. Rosen et al. found that in sentence repetition and conversational speech, hypokinetic dysarthria can be consistently distinguished from the speech of healthy controls on the basis of intensity variation and spectral range. Goberman and Elmer (2005) used acoustic analysis to examine differences in conversational and clear speech in PD subjects. These investigators found that PD subjects were able to use some of the same clear speech strategies that are used by nonimpaired speakers. Specifically, decreased articulation rate, increased mean fundamental frequency (F_0) and increased speaking F_0S.D. (standard deviation of F_0) characterised clear speech in PD subjects. In a study of subjects with TBI, Wang et al. (2005) performed acoustic analyses of syllable repetitions and sentence speech samples. Acoustic measures confirmed the perception of abnormal speaking rate and emphatic stress in these subjects. Wang et al. remark that this study 'illustrates the ability of acoustic measures to give a picture of the dysprosody related to TBI-induced dysarthria' (2005:231).

Acoustic analyses have proven value in the assessment of dysarthric speech. As well as confirming clinicians' perceptual judgements of deviant speech, acoustic analyses can highlight those aspects of the speech signal that are contributing to the perception of deviance (Murdoch et al. 2000). For example, the slow speaking rate of TBI subjects in Wang et al.'s study was related to a smaller phonation proportion and larger pause proportion in these subjects. Acoustic assessments also allow clinicians to provide objective measurement of the effects of intervention and disease progression on speech production. Notwithstanding these benefits of acoustic assessment, there are a number of drawbacks associated with the use of these techniques. The technology used in acoustic analysis can be expensive. The least expensive way to get MDVP is as part of Multi-Speech or Sona-Speech and even this costs 2,500 to 3,000 USD, including local hardware (personal communication, KayPENTAX, 17 July 2006). For smaller centres and clinics, this expense may be prohibitive. Also, acoustic techniques demand considerable expertise on the part of the assessing clinician. Clinicians must not only be trained in the use of acoustic technology, but they must also know how to interpret the various acoustic measurements that are obtained through this technology. They must understand, for example, how particular acoustic findings relate to perceptual speech features and how they translate into appropriate goals of intervention. This extensive knowledge base is normally to be found in specialist therapists. Financial and training considerations aside, it appears likely that acoustic techniques will play an increasingly important role in dysarthria assessment in the years to come.

Perceived speech defects in dysarthria may be the result of impairment in one or more of the speech production subsystems. However, perceptual techniques of assessment are generally powerless to locate deficits in any one particular speech subsystem. In an effort to understand the pathophysiological basis of disordered speech, clinicians and researchers have developed a range of instrumental techniques of assessments. These techniques include the use of nasometry to assess velopharyngeal function, EPG to assess tongue–palate contacts, electroglottography (EGG) to assess laryngeal function, and lip and tongue pressure transducers to assess articulatory function. In the rest of this section, we examine how instrumental techniques have been used to assess dysarthria in adults. We conclude with a few remarks about the merits and drawbacks of these techniques.

Bartle et al. (2006) used electromagnetic articulography (EMA) to examine spatio-timing aspects of tongue–jaw coordination during speech in TBI subjects. Spatio-timing aspects did not differ significantly between TBI and non-neurologically impaired subjects. EMA results confirmed perceptual data, in that TBI adults with severe articulatory disturbances also exhibited the most deviant spatio-timing tongue–jaw coordination patterns. McAuliffe et al. (2006) used EPG to examine the articulatory timing disturbance in PD. Although perceptual assessment confirmed impaired speech rate in the PD subjects in this study, EPG analysis revealed that the segment durations of PD subjects were consistent with those of aged and young controls. The one exception was the duration of the release phase for /la/, which was significantly increased in PD subjects. Goozee et al. (2001) used a tongue pressure transducer system to examine tongue strength, endurance, fine pressure control and rate of repetitive movement in 20 subjects with dysarthria related to TBI. TBI subjects displayed reductions in tongue endurance and rate of repetitive movement, but not in tongue strength and fine pressure control, compared to age- and sex-matched control subjects. These investigators found only weak correlations in TBI subjects between the physiological nonspeech tongue parameters and deviant perceptual articulatory features. Lip and tongue force transduction systems were used by Theodoros et al. (1995) to examine lip and tongue function in 18 dysarthric subjects who sustained a closed-head injury (CHI). Compared to controls, CHI subjects had a significant impairment of lip and tongue function on measures of strength, endurance and rate of repetitive movements. The rate of repetitive lip and tongue movements was found to be significantly reduced in CHI subjects. Although lip function was significantly impaired on several measures of strength and endurance, tongue function was still more severely compromised.

The main advantage of physiological (instrumental) assessments is that they allow clinicians to target during intervention the specific physiological anomalies that are responsible for dysarthric speech. Weak pressure consonants in dysarthria may be related to inadequate respiratory support for speech or to velopharyngeal incompetence, resulting in loss of oral air pressure. Instrumental analysis can tell the clinician if intervention should focus on techniques which increase respiratory support for speech or on techniques which improve velopharyngeal function. However, many instrumental assessments do not have widespread clinical application. Techniques such as the pressure transducer systems discussed above are still largely used in the context of research studies. Other instrumental techniques involve invasive appliances that may not be tolerated by dysarthric clients (e.g. the artificial palate in EPG). Radiographic techniques such as videofluoroscopy involve exposing the dysarthric client to radiation, albeit a small dose. They also require the involvement of additional staff, principally radiographers. Such techniques are thus likely to be beyond the expertise and facilities of most smaller clinics and centres. Notwithstanding the cost and training implications of many instrumental techniques, it remains the case that physiological methods have a significant role to play alongside perceptual and acoustic techniques in the assessment of dysarthric speech.

5.2.4 Dysarthria Intervention

In a recent review of interventions for dysarthria due to nonprogressive brain damage,[10] Sellars et al. (2005) produce a comprehensive list of techniques that are in current use by speech and language therapists. These interventions include: (1) articulation, voice and prosody training, (2) behavioural interventions, (3) the use of sign language as a supplement or alternative to speech, (4) prosthetic devices, (5) assistive communication devices, (6) listener training programmes and (7) listener advice. Limitations of space preclude a detailed discussion of each of these interventions. Moreover, many of these techniques were discussed at length in section 2.3.3.2 in chapter 2 in the context of developmental dysarthria. In the rest of this section, we examine the use of voice techniques in the treatment of dysarthria. Specifically, the Lee Silverman Voice Treatment has been used extensively in recent years in patients with PD and we discuss what is involved in this method. In order to achieve a good therapeutic outcome, behavioural and prosthetic interventions are usually employed in combination. We review two studies in which prosthetic devices have been used successfully in the treatment of dysarthric patients. The permanent and progressive nature of neurological impairment in many dysarthric adults precludes the restoration of functional speech. These individuals will be dependent in part or in whole on an augmentative and alternative communication (ACC) system. We examine briefly the use of AAC techniques in an acquired dysarthric population. Finally, there is now widespread acknowledgement amongst clinicians that dysarthric clients can make communication gains when the partners of these clients receive training in and advice on effective communication. We consider the types of issue that should be addressed during the training of communicative partners.

The Lee Silverman Voice Treatment (LSVT) was developed by Ramig and her colleagues as a technique designed for use with PD clients. LSVT emphasises high-effort loud phonation to improve respiratory, laryngeal and articulatory functions during speech in PD patients (Ramig et al. 2001). Intensive phonatory training takes place in 16 sessions over a month (four one-hour sessions per week for four weeks). The PD client is encouraged to appreciate the level of effort that is required for speaking. The efficacy of this technique has been demonstrated in numerous studies. Ramig et al. (2001) found that LSVT produced a statistically significant increase in the sound pressure level (SPL) of the voice of PD subjects. These investigators observed an increase of an average of 8dB between baseline and post-treatment and of 6dB between baseline and six months follow-up in PD patients but not in two groups of controls (untreated PD subjects and age-matched, nondisordered subjects). LSVT has also been shown to produce swallowing as well as voice gains in PD patients. Sharkawi et al. (2002) used LSVT to treat swallowing and voice problems in eight patients with idiopathic PD. A modified barium swallow and voice recording were conducted before LSVT and after one month of LSVT. LSVT had a statistically significant effect on vocal intensity during sustained vowel phonation and passage reading. LSVT achieved a 51 per cent reduction in the number of swallowing motility disorders. Other gains included significant reductions in some temporal measures of swallowing and in the amount of oral residue after 3ml and 5ml liquid swallows (see section 5.5 for further discussion of dysphagia). LSVT has also been successfully used to treat patients with other types of dysarthria and with disorders other than PD. Sapir et al. (2003) used LSVT to treat a woman with ataxic dysarthria who had cerebellar dysfunction secondary to thiamine deficiency. An analysis of perceptual and acoustic measures recorded at three points (before and after treatment and at nine months follow-up) revealed short- and long-term improvement in phonatory and articulatory functions, speech intelligibility and overall communication.[11]

Prosthetic devices, often combined with behavioural techniques, have also been successfully used to treat dysarthria in adults. Ono et al. (2005) used a palatal lift prosthesis and palatal augmentation prosthesis to treat velopharyngeal incompetence and articulation in a 71-year-old man who had sustained a stroke 2 years and 5 months earlier. Speech behavioural management of this patient involved self-monitoring and biofeedback training using the See-Scape.[12] These behavioural techniques helped promote an improvement in speech intelligibility to a functionally sufficient level following prosthetic intervention for velopharyngeal incompetence. Esposito et al. (2000) conducted a retrospective study of 25 patients with ALS to determine the effectiveness of palatal lift and/or augmentation prosthesis in the treatment of speech function and intelligibility. Of these 25 patients, 21 (84 per cent) were treated with a palatal lift. These patients demonstrated an improvement in dysarthria and specifically a reduction in hypernasality. For 19 patients (76 per cent), there was a moderate benefit for six months. A further 10 patients were treated with a combination palatal lift and augmentation prosthesis. Of these patients, six exhibited improvement in articulation. Most patients reported that they could speak with less effort when the prosthesis was worn. Esposito et al. acknowledge that prosthetic speech interventions are not frequently requested by neurologists. However, on the basis of these findings, these investigators suggest that palatal lift/augmentation prosthesis should be considered in dysarthric ALS patients.

When dysarthria is severe or is likely to become worse over time, an AAC system may represent a client's best chance of attaining functional communication. The neurological impairments that attend TBI have implications not only for motor speech production, but also for the many skills and abilities that are required for the successful use of AAC. Impairments of hearing, vision[13] and upper limb control restrict the type of AAC system that can be used with TBI clients. Many TBI patients have additional cognitive and language problems that must be considered when planning AAC intervention. Fager et al. (2006) remark that

> [i]ndividuals with TBI pose a unique challenge because, although they may have retained spelling ability and may appear to have relatively sophisticated communication skills, their substantial deficits in memory, attention, and cognitive flexibility greatly impact their use of encoding techniques. (44–5)[14]

Language impairments in TBI clients can also influence the choice of message formulation strategy.[15] In a study of AAC acceptance and use patterns of 25 TBI adults, Fager et al. found that a majority of subjects (86 per cent) used letter-by-letter spelling as their primary method of message formulation. TBI subjects who formulated messages picture by picture did so on account of severe language impairment.

In TBI, the severity of neurological impairment often precludes speech recovery and necessitates the use of AAC. In neurodegenerative diseases such as MND, the progressive nature of dysarthria means that some type of AAC system will eventually have to be used to augment or replace speech. The changing neurological condition of patients with progressive disorders requires that clinicians stage dysarthria treatment in these clients.[16] AAC techniques are used in the latter stages of treatment when natural speech is no longer a functional means of communication. Hirano et al. (2006) recorded the various means of communication used by 27 patients in the advanced stages of ALS.[17] In 6.4 per cent of patients, ocular muscles only were used to communicate. The remaining patients used ocular muscles in combination with lip-reading or vocal communication, written communication, a character sheet or computer-assisted communication. In the advanced stages of many neurodegenerative diseases, patients are often dependent on invasive mechanical ventilation.[18] The clinician must also consider the communication needs of ventilator-dependent patients, many of whom are experiencing a range of distressing emotions at a time when they are least able to communicate with others. Hirano et al. found that the use of computer assistance in communication by advanced ALS patients correlated inversely with patient frustration as a result of an inability to express thoughts and feelings. Furthermore, computer-assisted communication[19] was also associated with more sources of psychosocial support and happiness. These findings provide support for a central role for AAC management in the palliative care of neurodegenerative patients (Klasner and Yorkston 2000).

The successful implementation of AAC demands as much participation from communication partners as from the clients themselves. Where an AAC system is high-tech or involves considerable learning, clinicians can expect to direct as much time and effort to the training of partners as to the training of the client. However, there is now widespread recognition amongst therapists that even when an AAC system is not in use, partners play a vital role in facilitating communication in speech- and/or language-impaired adults. Their centrality to the communication process demands special consideration by therapists who now routinely conduct training programmes for and offer advice to partners. The first component of this training must be on raising the partner's awareness of the conditions that will cause the client adversity during speaking. These conditions may not always be immediately apparent to speech-intact partners, who subconsciously make adjustments to environmental adversity (e.g. increase speaking volume in response to background noise). There are now a number of studies, some of which have been conducted on neurodegenerative populations, that provide an objective basis for the advice that clinicians offer to partners. For example, Ball et al. (2004) studied 25 patients with ALS who were required to rank social situations according to their level of communicative difficulty. ALS patients rated 'speaking in a quiet environment to a familiar person' and 'speaking in a quiet environment with an unfamiliar listener' as the most effective and second most effective communication situation, respectively. The three least effective communication environments were 'speaking in a noisy environment', 'speaking before a group of people' and 'speaking for prolonged periods of time'.

Partner training programmes are an essential component of intervention in dysarthric adults. These programmes have been informed in large part by studies that have examined the communication needs and strategies of speech-impaired adults. One such study has been conducted by Murphy (2004), who examined 15 Scottish ALS patients and their families in a three-year investigation. Through video recordings, narratives and field notes, Murphy discovered that the principal purpose of communication in these patients was not to indicate needs and wants or to transfer information, but to establish and maintain social closeness. This was achieved in these subjects by a number of means, including speaking/conversation/nonverbal strategies and low-tech AAC. Speaking strategies involved simply repeating what had been said, using spelling and emphasising key words (client strategies). Conversation strategies ranged from the use of the partner as an interpreter – a strategy that may have the adverse consequence of encouraging clients to 'opt out' of communication – to the partner's greater reliance on context and topic cues to aid their understanding of the client. To overcome the unintelligibility of ALS patients, partners also made greater use of gesture, facial expression and eye contact. The positioning of clients and partners was also important. The partner who could make good eye contact with the client was more likely to use a range of nonverbal cues to understand speech. Low-tech AAC was also employed by clients. This involved the use of alphabet charts, communication charts and pen and paper. The effectiveness of these strategies is demonstrated by the fact that client-partner dyads that did not use them experienced anger and frustration during communication. It is perhaps a sign of how much work we still have to do as a profession in this area of dysarthria intervention that only one of the ALS clients in this study received help with communication strategies. (This was despite the fact that 14 clients had contact with a speech and language therapist.)

5.3 Apraxia of Speech

Often, the same neurological diseases and injuries that cause dysarthria in adults can also cause apraxia of speech. Yet, this speech disorder still receives relatively little discussion compared to other neurogenic communication disorders. In this section, we describe the features of this motor speech disorder. We also consider how clinicians assess and treat apraxia of speech. We begin with a brief discussion of the epidemiology and aetiology of this disorder.

5.3.1 Epidemiology and Aetiology

Epidemiological studies of the incidence and prevalence of apraxia of speech are lacking. In their absence, clinicians and researchers have had to rely on less direct sources of figures. These sources include incidence and prevalence figures for neurological disorders that are associated with apraxia of speech. Incidence and prevalence data for many of these disorders were presented in section 5.2.1. Another indirect source of evidence is provided by studies of the prevalence of apraxia in general (i.e. not apraxia of speech in particular). Zwinkels et al. (2004) examined the prevalence of apraxia in 100 patients with a first stroke admitted to a rehabilitation centre. In the total group, the prevalence of apraxia was 25.3 per cent. Amongst patients with left- and right-hemisphere strokes, the prevalence was 51.3 per cent and 6 per cent, respectively. Donkervoort et al. (2000) investigated the prevalence of apraxia in 492 patients who had sustained a first left-hemisphere stroke. They found that the prevalence in rehabilitation centres and nursing homes was 28 per cent and 37 per cent, respectively. Pedersen et al. (2001) examined the prevalence of manual and oral apraxia in 618 acute stroke patients. Manual apraxia and oral apraxia occurred in 7 per cent and 6 per cent of patients, respectively. Oral apraxia occurred in 9 per cent of left-hemisphere strokes and 4 per cent of right-hemisphere strokes.

The focal nature of many adult brain lesions, particularly those associated with CVAs, has allowed researchers to study the neurogenic origins of apraxia of speech. Josephs et al. (2006) performed single photon emission tomography and MRI in 17 subjects with an initial diagnosis of degenerative aphasia or apraxia of speech. These subjects had various pathological diagnoses, including progressive supranuclear palsy (six subjects), corticobasal degeneration (five), frontotemporal lobar degeneration (five) and Pick's disease (one). Josephs et al. found that the premotor and supplemental motor cortices were the main cortical regions associated with apraxia of speech. Ogar et al. (2006) studied 26 patients who sustained a single, left-hemisphere CVA. Eighteen of these patients had apraxia of speech. These investigators found that all the patients with apraxia of speech had lesions in the superior precentral gyrus of the insula. None of the patients without apraxia had lesions in this region. Josephs et al. (2005) examined four cases of atypical progressive supranuclear palsy (PSP) which presented as apraxia of speech with progressive nonfluent aphasia. These investigators found a shift in pathology away from subcortical grey and brainstem regions, which are commonly affected in typical PSP, towards neocortical regions. Josephs et al. conclude that this shift 'accounts for the presentation of progressive nonfluent aphasia and apraxia of speech observed in [these] patients, as well as the lack of classic features of PSP' (2005:283).

5.3.2 Clinical Presentation

Researchers and clinicians have devoted considerable energy towards characterising the speech features of apraxia of speech (AOS). The impetus for such characterisation is both theoretical and practical in nature. First, theoretical controversy still exists concerning the status of AOS vis-à-vis aphasia and dysarthria. It is expected that ever more sophisticated analyses of apraxic speech will enable investigators to compile a list of speech features that is diagnostic of AOS. At the same time, these features will help resolve the issue of the exact nature of AOS. (For example, is AOS a linguistic phenomenon similar to aphasia or a motor speech disorder with similarities to dysarthria?) Second, and related to the theoretical status of AOS, different conceptions of AOS require different forms of intervention. Decisions about whether to implement linguistic, phonetic or motor programming approaches to intervention can only be taken once it is known what types of speech error are occurring in AOS. A characterisation of the speech error in apraxia is thus essential for treatment planning. With these considerations in mind, we examine what is known about the speech characteristics of AOS.

Given the theoretical significance of a characterisation of the speech errors in AOS, it is unsurprising that many studies should seek to compare the speech features of AOS, aphasia and dysarthria. Seddoh et al. (1996) examined temporal parameters of speech in normal speakers and speakers with AOS and conduction aphasia. Using acoustic analysis, these investigators measured stop gap duration, voice onset time,[20] vowel nucleus duration and consonant-vowel duration. Apraxic speakers exhibited longer and more variable stop gap, vowel and consonant-vowel durations than either aphasic or normal speakers. Apraxic speakers also displayed greater token-to-token variability than other subjects. Moreover, this variability was significantly correlated with perceptual judgements of apraxic speech. Odell et al. (1991) examined single-word imitations by apraxic, conduction aphasic and ataxic dysarthric speakers. Based on these imitations, judgements of prosody were made and narrow phonetic transcriptions were performed. Vowel error patterns were similar in the apraxic and dysarthric subjects and included errors in low, tense and back vowels, more distortions than other types of vowel error and errors predominantly in initial position of words and in monosyllabic words. Apraxic and dysarthric subjects also produced syllabic stress errors and had more difficulty initiating than completing word production. Odell and Shriberg (2001) examined prosody-voice characteristics in 14 adults with AOS. AOS speakers had significantly more utterances meeting criteria for inappropriate phrasing and inappropriate speech rate, and significantly fewer utterances meeting criteria for inappropriate stress, than children with suspected AOS.

Instrumental techniques have also been used to examine the speech disturbance in AOS. Hough and Klich (1998) used electromyography (EMG) to investigate the timing of lip muscle activity during vowel production in two subjects with marked to severe AOS. Production of /u/ was examined in the context of monosyllabic words embedded in phrases and in word stems of varying lengths. Hough and Klich (1998) found that the relative amounts of time used for the onset and offset of EMG activity for lip rounding are disorganised in AOS. The timing of the onset of muscle activity was affected by word length in both the apraxic speakers and two normal speakers. The offset of muscle activity was also affected by word length, although the effect was less systematic in the apraxic speakers. Strand and McNeil (1996) found length and linguistic complexity effects on temporal acoustic characteristics of the imitative speech of AOS speakers. Vowel duration and two between-word segment durations were examined in a total of eight experimental conditions. These conditions manipulated the length of the apraxic speaker's response, and also the linguistic complexity of that response. Across all conditions, Strand and McNeil found significantly longer vowel and between-word segment durations in apraxic speakers than in controls. In apraxic speakers, vowel and between-word segment durations were consistently longer in sentence contexts than in word contexts. Apraxic speakers also displayed greater intrasubject and intersubject variability for between-word segment durations in sentence than in word conditions. Control subjects displayed greater homogeneity in sentence production. Finally, nonspeech motor control of oral structures has also been examined in AOS. McNeil et al. (1990) examined the isometric force and static position control of four articulators in apraxic speakers – upper lip, lower lip, tongue and jaw. Results of force and position tasks indicated that apraxic speakers tended to produce significantly greater instability than normal speakers.

The studies discussed above capture a number of the key speech characteristics of AOS. The findings of these investigations revealed the presence of vowel distortions in apraxic speech. Prosodic disturbances, such as stress errors and inappropriate phrasing and speech rate, were also in evidence. Speech production in AOS speakers showed word length and linguistic complexity effects. A number of studies revealed speech abnormalities of a temporal nature, including longer vowel and consonant-vowel durations. Variability in speech production, not only between apraxic speakers but also within apraxic speakers, was also demonstrated. However, these findings are by no means exhaustive of the speech characteristics of AOS. Yorkston et al. (1999) report several others, including difficulty in volitional movement for speech, while volitional nonspeech movements, such as chewing and swallowing, are intact. Additional articulatory features include sound substitutions and additions, transposition of sounds and syllables, perceived voicing errors (which may be related to mistiming), affricates and fricatives more problematic than stops or nasals and more difficulty with consonant clusters than singleton consonants. Yorkston et al. also report greater difficulty on novel or less practised utterances than well-practised utterances, and more errors on nonsense words than real words. Groping, silent posturing and trial-and-error movement behaviour are also common in AOS. Apraxic speakers also have difficulty imitating and maintaining articulatory configurations, particularly for initial sounds, and difficulty making movement transitions in and out of spatial targets (Yorkston et al. 1999).

A range of other deficits can occur alongside AOS. These associated deficits include aphasia, dysarthria, oral apraxia, limb apraxia, apraxia for phonation and right-hemiparesis. Aphasia and dysarthria share certain perceptual features with AOS. These disorders must therefore be considered in a differential diagnosis of AOS (see section 5.3.3). Oral apraxia is the inability to perform nonspeech movements of the oral articulators on command or in imitation. An affected individual may be unable to perform actions such as lip rounding on command or may be unable to use the tongue tip to touch the upper lip in an imitative task. Yet, these same movements may be performed effortlessly during a reflexive activity such as eating. Limb apraxia is the inability to perform volitional movements of the arms in the absence of any reduction in the strength and range of motion. In an imitative context, an individual with limb apraxia may struggle to touch his or her mouth or nose. However, these same movements can be effortlessly executed in nonimitative situations: for example, during coughing and sneezing, when the hand can cover the mouth and nose, respectively. Limb apraxia has clinical significance for the speech and language therapist, who must be fully aware of its implications for the use of gesture as an augmentative form of communication. Apraxia for phonation is an inability to produce voice, even for short sustained phonations or the production of syllables. It sometimes occurs immediately after a stroke and can last for two or three weeks (Yorkston et al. 1999). There is no abnormality of the laryngeal mechanism, as evidenced by normal vocal fold adduction during a reflexive cough and laughter. Finally, the same left-hemisphere damage that causes AOS may also lead to weakness of the right side of the body (right hemiparesis). This is because many of the motor fibres that originate in the left hemisphere cross over to the right side of the body. A right hemiparesis also has implications for the use of signing and gesture by affected individuals.

5.3.3 Assessment and Intervention

Notwithstanding the greater availability and more widespread use of speech technology, assessment of AOS still proceeds for the most part by means of perceptual techniques. These techniques require that clinicians listen to the patient's speech and observe a range of oral motor movements. However, as the discussion of section 5.3.2. demonstrated, acoustic and instrumental techniques also have an important role to play in the assessment of AOS. These techniques operate best alongside perceptual methods of assessment. Their purpose is often to provide acoustic confirmation of the perceptual features of disordered speech and, in the case of instrumental techniques, to explain perceived speech anomalies. In this section, we discuss how clinicians and researchers apply these techniques to the assessment of AOS. We also address the different factors that must be considered in a differential diagnosis of AOS. We then turn to examine techniques of intervention in this clinical population.

Perceptual techniques form the cornerstone of AOS assessment. One such technique is the Motor Speech Evaluation suggested by Wertz et al. (1984). This is a screening tool which takes less than 20 minutes to administer. A wide range of tasks is used to reveal apraxic errors. They include conversation, vowel prolongation, repetition of monosyllables with /p/, /t/, /k/, repetition of these monosyllables in sequence, repetition of multisyllabic words, multiple trials with the same word, repetition of words that increase in length, repetition of monosyllabic words that contain the same initial and final sound, repetition of sentences, counting forward and backward, picture description, repetition of sentences used volitionally to determine consistency of production and oral reading. Performance on the Motor Speech Evaluation can be scored descriptively (e.g. 'A' for apraxic production, 'P' for paraphasia) or using the PICA[21] 16-point scale. Narrow or broad phonetic transcription may be used. The only normed and standardised test for AOS is the Apraxia Battery for Adults (Dabul 2000). This battery includes an inventory of 15 articulation characteristics of AOS.[22] Many of these characteristics are similar to those noted by Wertz et al. and assessed on the Motor Speech Evaluation. However, the Apraxia Battery for Adults also includes more specific articulatory errors that may be perceived by a listener (e.g. phonemic anticipatory errors, perseverative errors, transposition errors).

To the extent that the client with AOS may also have an accompanying dysarthria and/or an apraxia for nonspeech, oral movements, the latter movements must also be examined during AOS assessment. The client is prompted to perform a number of oral movements, first by using verbal instruction alone and then, if he or she fails to perform the target movement, by performing a demonstration of the movement which the client then imitates. Target movements include tongue protrusion, elevation, lowering and lateral movement. Lip, jaw and velar movements should also be assessed. Velar elevation can be examined by encouraging the client to puff out his or her cheeks. The ability to sequence oral movements must also be assessed. For example, to test the client's ability to round and spread his or her lips successively, the client should be encouraged to pucker and smile alternately. The strength, range and speed of all oral movements should be noted. Features such as muscle tone, tongue fasciculations and muscle weakness and atrophy are particularly important in a differential diagnosis of motor speech disorders and should also be recorded. Although many clinicians implement their own procedures for the assessment of oral motor functions, commercially available protocols may also be used. One such protocol is the Dworkin–Culatta Oral Mechanism Examination (Dworkin and Culatta 1980).

If at all possible, perceptual assessments should be accompanied by acoustic and instrumental analyses of speech. These additional analyses may be used to explain the pathophysiological basis of perceived speech anomalies. They may also provide insight into the particular acoustic parameters that give rise to a perceived speech defect; for example, slow speech rate may be related to increased vowel duration. We saw in section 5.3.2 that Seddoh et al. (1996) used acoustic analysis to investigate temporal parameters of speech, while Hough and Klich (1998) used EMG to assess the timing of lip muscle activity during vowel production. Other recent studies that have used acoustic techniques to analyse apraxic speech include an investigation by Shuster and Wambaugh (2000) of the speech errors in two individuals with AOS and aphasia. These researchers found that both subjects produced perceived substitutions and perceived distortions. Errors on initial stops tended to be categorised as substitutions, while those on initial fricatives were more often classified as distortions or distorted substitutions. These perceptual judgements were confirmed and augmented by acoustic analyses. Haley et al. (2000) used acoustic techniques to examine the precision of fricative place of articulation production in speakers with AOS and aphasia. Articulatory precision was determined on the basis of acoustic consistency across repeated productions of the same target words and on the acoustic distinction between similar fricative targets. Subjects produced words beginning with voiceless alveolar and palatal fricatives. The Bark-transformed first spectral moment was computed in the middle of the fricative. While this measure varied little across repetitions and target fricatives were clearly distinguished in normal speakers, there was substantial spectral variability and overlap between targets for aphasic speakers with AOS. Haley et al. state that '[t]he observed spectral imprecision is consistent with impaired phonetic motor control, not only in the temporal, but also in the spatial domain of speech production' (2000:619). Marquardt et al. (1995) compared the stress-marking strategies of AOS and normal speakers across acoustic variables of fundamental frequency, syllable duration and vocal intensity. Results showed that, regardless of whether the first or second syllable is stressed, AOS speakers were capable of producing the acoustic distinctions between stressed and unstressed syllables in disyllabic words. This was the case for words produced both in sentences and in isolation.

The specialist equipment and knowledge that are needed to undertake investigations of the type described above have tended to find acoustic techniques restricted to research studies and to a few major clinics and centres. The same is largely true of instrumental methods of assessment such as EMG. Strauss and Klich (2001) examined the effects of word length on the timing of lip EMG activity for production of the vowel /u/ and the relationship of this activity to vowel duration in two AOS speakers. In AOS and normal speakers, the length of time in which lip muscle activity was present prior to the onset of voicing for /u/ systematically decreased as word length increased. However, only in normal speakers did the length of time from the onset of voicing for /u/ to the onset of the reduction of EMG activity during the vowel decrease as word length increased. Strauss and Klich suggest that the former finding reflects a linguistic influence on the timing of motor activity underlying lip rounding. Moreover, this linguistic influence is resistant to lesions that cause AOS. The latter finding indicates that, while normal speakers systematically reduce the percentage of time used to end muscle activity as word length increases, this effect is less noticeable for apraxic speakers. Sugishita et al. (1987) used EPG to examine omission errors in the speech of two AOS speakers. Three kinds of omission error were observed: true omissions, in which there was no palatolingual contact; omissions with incorrect contact, in which there was palatolingual contact for a different sound or undifferentiated sound; and omissions with correct contact, in which there was correct palatolingual contact for a target sound. Sugishita et al. found that the latter two types of omission error occurred for initial consonants and were probably caused by a delay in air flow. One of the two consonants /t, tʃ/ also tended to be a substitute for other sounds, which suggested that the AOS speakers had difficulty inhibiting tongue activity.

In section 5.3.2, we described how aphasia and dysarthria can often occur alongside AOS in adults. Many of the perceptual characteristics of these disorders are similar to the perceptual features of AOS. For example, sound substitutions and distortions can occur in all three communication disorders. This creates a diagnostic problem for clinicians, who must establish the contribution, if any, of these other disorders to the client's speech problems in order to institute effective intervention. Factors that distinguish apraxic speech errors from the literal paraphasic errors of aphasia include dysprosody (more marked in AOS than aphasia), groping behaviour (evident in AOS), difficulty initiating utterances in AOS, more predictable speech errors in AOS than in aphasia, and less 'off-target' errors in terms of place and manner of articulation in apraxia than in aphasia. AOS speakers will also attempt to correct articulatory errors and may produce sounds that are perceived to be non-English – the sound errors in literal paraphasias are always English phonemes. Several factors distinguish AOS from dysarthria. First, the AOS speaker does not experience muscle paralysis or weakness due to problems with the innervation of muscles. In this way, the range, strength and speed of oral movements for nonspeech tasks is unimpaired, as are chewing, swallowing and coughing. The underlying neuromuscular impairment in dysarthria means that all oral movements are weak and have limited range, strength and speed. Second, the primary impairment in AOS is articulatory in nature. Prosodic impairments may result from the attempt to compensate for articulatory deficits. The AOS speaker may also be apraxic for phonation (see section 5.3.2), but in this case phonation is normal for reflexive acts such as coughing and laughter. All speech subsystems – articulation, phonation, respiration, prosody and resonance – are affected in dysarthria. Moreover, vocal fold movement is as impaired during reflexive actions as it is during phonation. Third, apraxic speech is influenced by features of the utterance. The AOS speaker has greater difficulty producing novel or unpractised utterances than those which have been said often. Also, articulatory errors in AOS increase as the phonetic complexity of utterances increases. Dysarthric speech features such as hypernasality and sound distortions occur consistently, regardless of these features of utterances.

Several treatment techniques have been developed for use with AOS clients. These techniques include traditional articulation therapy, the use of instrumental methods and, in severe cases, AAC devices. Despite the widespread use of these techniques and other treatment programmes (e.g. PROMPT), little data still exist to support the efficacy of these different approaches to AOS intervention.[23] In the rest of this section, we examine a number of AOS treatment techniques. We address the question of the efficacy of these techniques. However, the reader is referred to other sources for more detailed reviews of treatment efficacy (West et al. 2005; Wambaugh and Doyle 1994; Wambaugh 2002).

The articulatory and prosodic deficits that are so prominent in AOS are the target of some treatment approaches to this motor speech disorder. Wambaugh et al. (1998) treated sound errors in three speakers with chronic AOS and aphasia. The treatment approach adopted by these investigators combined the use of minimal contrast pairs with traditional sound production training techniques such as integral stimulation[24] and articulatory placement cueing. These techniques were applied sequentially to sounds that were consistently in error prior to training. Wambaugh et al. reported increased correct sound productions in trained and untrained words for all speakers. However, response generalisation effects across sounds and stimulus generalisation effects were limited for most speakers. Positive maintenance effects were observed, although there was some loss of treatment gains following the termination of treatment. Treatment techniques that teach AOS clients how to regulate the prosodic features of speech have also produced speech gains. Wambaugh and Martinez (2000) examined the effects of a rate and rhythm control treatment on the accuracy of consonant production in a speaker with AOS and aphasia. This subject was trained to produce multisyllabic words using metronomic rate control and hand-tapping. Treated words contained three syllables with primary stress on the first syllable. Wambaugh and Martinez examined generalisation to (1) untreated exemplars, (2) three–syllable words with different stress patterns, (3) four–syllable words and (4) s-blend words. Both trained and untrained words displayed positive sound changes. When treatment was extended to a set of words with incomplete generalisation, additional improvement was noted.

The focus on rhythm control in Wambaugh and Martinez's study is also integral to another prosodic intervention, melodic intonation therapy (MIT). The intoning of phrases in this approach is achieved through rhythmic tapping patterns which the client first imitates. Eventually the tapping and intoning of cues can be faded, as the client continues to produce the utterance. Interventions that target contrastive stress have also been used to improve speech production and prosody in AOS adults. Yorkston et al. (1999) report that they have found this method to be most effective for speakers with mild to moderate AOS who need to improve the naturalness of speech through the use of intonational contour and stress patterning in sentence production or conversational speech. The client is encouraged to produce sentences with primary or emphatic stress on a particular word. The word usually contains a phonetic string that is targeted for the client. For example, if a vowel + /r/ or /r/ + vowel combination is targeted, the clinician can ask the question 'Are you going out today?', to which the client responds 'I am going out *tomorrow*.' This technique can be used to stabilise articulatory skills in the context of appropriate stress and prosody (Yorkston et al. 1999). It can also be used to improve prosodic aspects of connected speech. The client can be encouraged to vary the emphatic stress in a sentence by producing responses to a series of questions. For example, after showing the client a picture in which a boy is hitting a ball, the clinician asks 'Is the girl hitting the ball?' The client should respond with emphatic stress on the word 'boy' – 'No, the *boy* is hitting the ball.' By posing a different question, the clinician can vary the place of emphatic stress in the response. For example, by asking 'Is the boy throwing a ball?', the client is encouraged to respond 'No, the boy is *hitting* the ball' (Yorkston et al. 1999).

A treatment technique that was first developed in the late 1970s for use with children but which has also been used to treat AOS adults is Deborah Hayden's PROMPT technique (see also section 4.2.4 in chapter 4). PROMPT (Prompts for Restructuring Oral Muscular Phonetic Targets) uses tactile cues that are 'designed to provide apractic patients with sensory input regarding place of articulatory contact, extent of mandibular opening, voice, tension, relative timing of segments, manner of articulation, and coarticulation' (Freed et al. 1997:365). Bose et al. (2001) examined the effects of PROMPT therapy on the precision and automaticity of speech movements in an individual with AOS and Broca's aphasia. Treatment effects were examined in three sentence types: imperatives, active declaratives and interrogatives. On trained and untrained imperatives and active declaratives, there was an improvement in speech precision and sequencing of movements. However, PROMPT therapy failed to have any effect on interrogatives. This result is explained in terms of the higher linguistic demand of interrogatives, which reduced the resources that the subject had available for motor speech production. Freed et al. (1997) examined the effect of PROMPT therapy on the acquisition and maintenance of a functional core vocabulary in a severe apractic-aphasic speaker. Thirty functional, personally relevant words and short phrases, chosen by the patient and his family, were targeted during therapy. Results showed that target words and phrases were produced accurately during the treatment phases of the study. (An 80 per cent treatment criterion was attained for all words and phrases.) Also, this subject produced these words and phrases accurately after the discontinuation of treatment. (The overall mean score on the maintenance probes was 78.2 per cent.)

Instrumental techniques have been successfully used to provide AOS speakers with biofeedback during treatment. Katz et al. (1999) used electromagnetic articulography (EMA) to remediate [s]/[ʃ] articulation deficits in the speech of an adult with AOS and Broca's aphasia. The subject received two treatments in a counterbalanced procedure over one month. In one treatment, EMA was used to provide the subject with visually guided biofeedback on the position of the tongue tip. In the other treatment – a foil treatment – a computer program delivered voicing – contrast stimuli for simple repetition. Kinematic and perceptual data revealed an improvement on nonspeech oral motor tasks and, to a lesser degree, speech motor tasks in the visually guided biofeedback condition. In the foil condition, the treated phonetic contrast showed only marginal improvement during treatment. Moreover, performance dropped back to baseline 10 weeks after the completion of therapy. Howard and Varley (1995) used EPG to treat severe AOS in a 47-year-old man. Therapy focused initially on front and back closures and on alternation between them. Single words were used to train the contrast between /d/ and /l/ word initially. Although this client was able to produce auditorily acceptable tokens of /l/ within a single session, the auditory impression of /d/ targets was that they were still variable and often unacceptable. To address this, EPG was used to model the dynamic pattern of the complete lingual gesture of /d/. The client was able to assimilate this information and translate it into his own productions within a single session.

When apraxia of speech is severe and the prospect of a client attaining functional speech appears remote, an AAC system should be adopted. Many apraxic clients develop, and use to good effect, their own system of naturalistic gesture. This is often achieved in the first days and weeks following a stroke or other cerebral injury and can be used to communicate basic needs or wants (e.g. tipping hand in front of one's mouth to request a drink). The advantage of naturalistic gestures is that many are immediately meaningful to people in the client's environment: namely, friends, family members and medical staff. More formal systems of sign language may be used to augment verbal communication in the apraxic client. The presence of additional disorders can have a negative impact on the apraxic client's ability to use naturalistic gesture and sign language. These disorders include aphasia, hemiparesis or hemiplegia and limb apraxia. Each should be assessed for its potential adverse effect on signing and on the use of AAC in general. AMERIND, a sign system based on American Indian sign language, can be used by hemiplegic clients. In this system, signs have been modified for performance with one hand (Yorkston et al. 1999).

5.4 Acquired Aphasia

The acquired communication disorders discussed in sections 5.2 and 5.3 are disorders of speech. However, many of the same cerebral diseases and injuries that cause dysarthria and apraxia of speech in adults can also give rise to a language disorder called aphasia. Aphasia can disrupt a range of language levels, including phonology, morphology, syntax, semantics and pragmatics. It is a multi-modal disorder, as all modes of language processing can be impaired. As well as being unable to produce and comprehend spoken language, the aphasic adult may also be unable to read (acquired dyslexia) and write (acquired dysgraphia). The implications of aphasia for the wider communication skills of an affected individual are thus very great indeed. In this section, we examine the (rather limited) prevalence and incidence data that exist for aphasia. Aphasia is a language disorder that arises through damage to the left hemisphere of the brain. We discuss the many diseases and injuries that can cause this damage within the aetiology of the disorder. As a result of extensive research, much is now known about the linguistic features of aphasia. In section 5.4.2, we examine these features within a wider discussion of aphasia syndromes. Aphasiologists have realised for some time that any assessment of aphasia must take in more than structural language testing. Specifically, assessment must consider how an aphasic client's language deficits and remaining language skills contribute to his or her overall communication effectiveness. In section 5.4.3, we consider these so-called pragmatic approaches to assessment of aphasia alongside more traditional techniques of language assessment. Methods of intervention will be discussed in section 5.4.4.

5.4.1 Epidemiology and Aetiology

To date, few studies have investigated the incidence and prevalence of aphasia. Engelter et al. (2006) assessed the incidence of aphasia attributable to first ever ischaemic stroke (FEIS) in a geographically defined population of 188,015 inhabitants. These investigators report an overall incidence rate of aphasia attributable to FEIS of 43 per 100,000 inhabitants. They also found that the risk of aphasia attributable to FEIS increased by 4 per cent with each year of patient's age. Kauhanen et al. (2000) examined 106 consecutive patients (mean age 65.8 years) with first ever ischaemic brain infarction. During the acute phase (first week after stroke), aphasia was diagnosed in 34 per cent of patients. Two-thirds of these patients were still aphasic 12 months later. Yavuzer et al. (2001) found aphasia in 70 patients (40 per cent) of 178 stroke patients who were admitted to a comprehensive rehabilitation programme for the first time between January 1998 and April 2000. Global and Broca's aphasia were the most common types of aphasia and were present in 20 patients each. The least common types of aphasia were subcortical and conduction aphasia, which were each present in five patients. Twenty-eight patients (49 per cent) changed their aphasia classification to a milder form at discharge.

Aphasia is a common sequela of damage to the brain's language centres. For most right-handed individuals,[25] these centres are located in the left hemisphere and consist of Broca's area (inferior frontal gyrus) and Wernicke's area (planum temporale).[26] A wide range of cerebral diseases, events and injuries can cause damage to these anatomical areas. CVAs are the most common cause of aphasia in adults, with cerebral infarctions that result in Wernicke's aphasia and global aphasia without hemiparesis frequently due to cardiac embolism (Delcker and Diener 1991). Gender differences have been observed in the incidence of aphasia following stroke. Using information from the Stroke Data Bank,[27] Hier et al. (1994) found that aphasia was present in 19.4 per cent of men and 22.5 per cent of women. Although no gender differences in aphasia incidence were observed among intracerebral haemorrhages, aphasia was more frequent in women with infarcts (37 per cent) than in men with infarcts (28.3 per cent). Hier et al. also found that Wernicke's, global and anomic aphasias were more common in women and that Broca's aphasia was somewhat more common in men.

The brain's language centres may also be damaged as a result of a head injury, brain tumours and infections such as encephalitis and meningitis, and by neurodegenerative disorders like Alzheimer's disease. Demir et al. (2006) examined 103 patients with TBI, 51 of whom had aphasia. These investigators report that the most frequent type of aphasia in these patients was Broca's aphasia (26.49 per cent), followed by anomic aphasia (19.6 per cent) and transcortical motor aphasia (15.6 per cent). Wacker et al. (2002) used the Aachen Aphasia Test to determine the incidence of aphasic symptoms in patients with brain tumours. Aphasic disturbances were detected in 50 per cent of patients with left-sided tumours and 36 per cent of patients with right-sided tumours. Khan and Ramsay (2006) describe the case of a 59-year-old woman who developed encephalitis caused by herpes simplex virus type 1. This woman's main presenting symptom was mild aphasia, for which she required longer-term speech therapy. Van de Beek et al. (2004) studied all Dutch adults with community-acquired acute bacterial meningitis from October 1998 to April 2002. On admission, aphasia was present in 121 episodes of meningitis (23 per cent). At discharge, aphasia occurred in 11 episodes of meningitis (2 per cent).

A range of neurodegenerative diseases can result in damage to the brain's language centres. Chief amongst them is Alzheimer's disease. Because the underlying neuropathology in a disorder such as Alzheimer's disease affects many brain regions and systems, impaired language is only one of a number of disrupted functions. Others include memory deficits and emotional disturbances, both typical symptoms of dementia. These additional, nonlinguistic impairments have made some clinicians reluctant to apply the label 'aphasia' to the language impairment in Alzheimer's disease and other neurodegenerative disorders – traditionally, this term has been taken to apply only to language impairment in the absence of any wider cognitive deterioration. In this section, we leave aside the question of the status of the language impairment in disorders such as Alzheimer's disease. Where the term 'aphasia' is applied to these language impairments, it is done so in the mundane sense of 'acquired language disorder'.

Alzheimer's disease (AD) is the most common neurodegenerative disease (see note 6). It is also the most frequent cause of dementia, accounting for some 55 per cent of all cases (Alzheimer's Society 2005). Amyloid plaques and neurofibrillary tangles develop in the brains of AD sufferers. Many other diseases may also cause dementia. Problems with the blood supply to the brain may lead to vascular dementia.[28] Some people with vascular dementia may also have AD (so-called mixed dementia). Vascular and mixed dementia account for some 20 per cent of dementia cases (Alzheimer's Society 2005). Abnormal protein deposits called Lewy bodies have been found in the brains of people with Parkinson's disease. However, when these deposits occur in the cerebral cortex, dementia with Lewy bodies results. Accounting for 15 per cent of dementia cases, dementia with Lewy bodies is increasingly being recognised as one of the more common forms of degenerative dementia after AD. Originally called Pick's disease, frontotemporal dementia is associated with degeneration of the frontal and temporal anterior lobes of the brain. This form of dementia is less common than other types of dementia, affecting some 5 per cent of cases. Due to the predominance of frontal lobe pathology, frontotemporal dementia has more personality and behaviour involvement and fewer memory deficits at first than other forms of dementia. Rarer causes of dementia include HIV infection, Creutzfeldt–Jakob disease and Korsakoff's syndrome (alcohol-related dementia). It should also be noted that people with multiple sclerosis, motor neurone disease, Parkinson's disease and Huntington's disease can also develop dementia.

5.4.2 Clinical Presentation

There are several systems of classification of aphasia. The traditional dominance of the medical model in language pathology has encouraged classifications based on the neuroanatomical site of lesion. In this way, nomenclature such as Broca's and Wernicke's aphasia and anterior and posterior aphasia reflect the presumed site of the causative lesion, namely, Broca's and Wernicke's areas which are located near the front (anterior) and back (posterior) of the brain, respectively. Similarly, the terms 'motor aphasia' and 'sensory aphasia' are intended to reflect the movement of nervous signals around the body. Typically, this movement occurs away from the centre (the central nervous system) towards the peripheral organs (the muscles) or from the periphery to the centre. The former nervous signals are motor or efferent signals (hence, motor aphasia), while the latter signals are sensory or afferent signals (sensory aphasia).

The neurological model that motivated the above nomenclature has declined in prominence in recent years. This decline has been brought about by the recognition that, while knowledge of lesion sites has an important role to play in the diagnosis of aphasia, the linguistic features of this disorder are of greater relevance to the assessment and treatment of aphasia. Terms such as 'fluent' and 'nonfluent' are now widely used[29] to characterise the effortless language output (fluent aphasia) and dysfluent output (nonfluent aphasia) of different forms of aphasia. Similarly, the terms 'receptive aphasia' and 'expressive aphasia' locate the principal linguistic impairment in the disorder in a breakdown of the comprehension and production of language, respectively. It should be emphasised that neither a language-based nor a lesion-based system of classification is mutually exclusive. In at least one major diagnostic test – the Boston Diagnostic Aphasia Examination (Goodglass et al. 2001) – both systems of classification are used.[30] As we review the findings of studies of aphasic subjects in the rest of this section, the reader will see that different classification systems are used across studies.

In fluent aphasia, language comprehension is often severely impaired in the presence of effortless, fluent speech. Fluent aphasics produce long, incoherent, well-articulated utterances that have the intonational and other suprasegmental features of normal speech. (These features often give a listener the impression that the fluent aphasic has greater language competence than is actually the case.) The lack of sense and incoherence of the fluent aphasic's language is related to his or her use of jargon (hence, the use of the term 'jargon aphasia' to describe this type of aphasia). In some types of jargon, English words are linked together to produce meaningless utterances (for example, the jargon speaker who described Interflora as 'a stage of firms that arrange the nation of children', or another jargon aphasic who described his/her daughter's holiday as 'She's got a rainbow, you know, three monthly rainbow going to Alaska').[31] In other types of jargon, new words are created ('neologisms'). For example, a jargon speaker, who was wanting to go for a walk in the park, uttered 'We have to go to the pargoney.' In still other forms of jargon, so many neologisms are used that utterances are entirely meaningless. For example, when asked what he had done during the week, one jargon speaker replied 'Oh I kegde trey-choinge and cortlidge, oh erm partlie chulz, potiler crediss my children ringer.' The poor language comprehension of fluent aphasics makes it difficult for these subjects to monitor and correct their own incoherent output. Other features of fluent aphasia include echolalia, the use of circumlocution (talking around a target word that the subject cannot produce), perseveration (continued use of a linguistic form beyond what is appropriate) and lexical retrieval problems.

These generic linguistic features of fluent aphasia receive support from recent research studies. Kim and Leach (2004) examined verb retrieval in four fluent aphasic subjects in single-word and narrative contexts. All aphasic subjects displayed impaired verb naming. Moreover, there was a syntactic effect in verb retrieval – two-place (transitive) verbs were more poorly retrieved than one-place (intransitive) verbs. The semantic complexity of verbs (i.e. their number of argument places) only had an effect on retrieval in a narrative context. Murray et al. (1998) examined the spoken language of subjects with mild fluent aphasia under three conditions: isolation, focused attention and divided attention. Under all three conditions, aphasic subjects performed more poorly than controls on most morphosyntactic, lexical and pragmatic measures of spoken language. While control subjects exhibited little qualitative or quantitative change in spoken language across conditions, aphasic subjects produced fewer syntactically complete and complex utterances, fewer words and had poorer word-finding accuracy in the transition from isolation to divided-attention conditions. The communication of aphasic subjects was considered to be pragmatically less successful and efficient. Murray et al. conclude that 'decrements of attentional capacity or its allocation may negatively affect the quantity and quality of the spoken language of individuals with mild aphasia' (1998:213).

As Murray et al.'s study demonstrates, pragmatic language skills may also be impaired in fluent aphasia. Recently, researchers have begun to examine the nature and extent of pragmatic and discourse impairments in this clinical population. Chapman et al. (1997) examined proverb processing in three groups of subjects: fluent aphasic patients, patients with Alzheimer's disease (AD) and normal controls. Subjects indicated their understanding of proverbs in two presentation conditions. In the spontaneous condition, subjects were required to express verbally their interpretation of proverbs that were presented in written and verbal form. In the multiple-choice condition, subjects were required to select from four proverb interpretations the one that most accurately reflected the proverb's meaning. Familiar and unfamiliar proverbs were presented in both conditions. Compared to normal controls, aphasic subjects had difficulty formulating an interpretation of both familiar and unfamiliar proverbs in the spontaneous condition. AD subjects, on the other hand, only displayed lower performance than normal controls on unfamiliar spontaneous proverbs. A very different pattern was observed in the multiple-choice condition, with aphasic subjects having little difficulty on this task and AD subjects failing to select the correct abstract interpretation of proverbs. These results are explained in terms of the linguistic and cognitive deficits in aphasic and AD subjects. Coelho and Flewellyn (2003) examined coherence in the story narratives of a subject with anomic aphasia over a 12-month period. These researchers found that, although microlinguistic skills improved over this period, local and global coherence failed to improve appreciably. Global coherence was more impaired than local coherence in this subject. Coelho and Flewellyn conclude that '[t]his pattern of impaired macrolinguistic abilities is consistent with that of individuals with Alzheimer's disease and closed head injuries, and suggests that difficulty with discourse organisation may result from focal as well as diffuse brain pathology' (2003:173). For further discussion of pragmatic deficits in aphasia, see Cummings (2007a).

In nonfluent aphasia, language production problems exist in the presence of relatively intact comprehension. Nonfluent aphasics struggle to produce utterances. Unlike their fluent counterparts, they are acutely aware of and frustrated by their often severe expressive difficulties. Articulation and suprasegmental features of speech are disrupted – intonation units are typically short. Syntax can be severely affected. Sentence structure is reduced and incomplete. The loss of function words (e.g. determiners, prepositions, pronouns) and verbs – two characteristics of Broca's spoken output – confers a telegrammatic quality on the expressive language of these subjects (hence, the use of the term 'agrammatic speech' in relation to nonfluent aphasics). For example, instead of saying 'I will take the dog for a walk,' the nonfluent aphasic will struggle to utter 'Walk dog.' Stereotypical forms are often used to maintain interaction when problems of expression are particularly acute. There are considerable lexical-semantic disturbances in nonfluent aphasia. Subjects may mis-select vocabulary, with chosen and target lexemes often semantically related (e.g. use of 'eye' instead of 'ear'). These errors are called semantic paraphasias. (A sound equivalent of these errors – phonemic (literal) paraphasias – occurs in fluent aphasia, e.g. use of 'stowcan' instead of 'snowman'.)

Studies of nonfluent aphasics have confirmed the linguistic features described above. Brookshire and Nicholas (1995) examined the connected speech of 40 adults with no brain damage, 10 adults with nonfluent aphasia and 10 adults with fluent aphasia. Speech samples from the nonfluent aphasic group contained significantly greater percentages of the word 'and' and nonword fillers than those of the non-brain-damaged subjects. Nonfluent aphasic subjects also produced significantly more nonword fillers than fluent aphasics. Ruigendijk and Bastiaanse (2002) examined the free speech production of 10 German agrammatic speakers. Each of these speakers omitted determiners and verbs in free speech. However, when presented with lexical verbs during an experimental task, production of determiners increased significantly. These investigators concluded that 'the impaired use of determiners is not caused by poor production of function words in general, but by problems with the production of verbs' (2002:383).

Verb production in agrammatic speakers has also been examined by Thompson et al. (1997). These investigators assessed verb argument structure production in 10 agrammatic aphasic speakers and 10 non-brain-damaged subjects. A consistent hierarchy of verb difficulty was observed, with aphasic subjects correctly producing obligatory one-place verbs significantly more often than three-place or complement verbs. The ability of agrammatic aphasic subjects to produce argument structures of the verb correctly depended on the type of argument required by the verb in a particular context and on the number of participant roles (e.g. agent) required by the verb. The complexity of the verb (i.e. the number of possible argument structure arrangements) influenced sentence production in the aphasic subjects. Finally, obligatory arguments were more often produced correctly than optional arguments. Thompson et al. claim that these results 'indicate that the argument structure properties of verbs . . . influence both verb retrieval and sentence production in agrammatic aphasic subjects' (1997:473). Cannito et al. (1992) examined the ability of 23 nonfluent aphasic subjects to use context to facilitate comprehension of auditorily presented reversible passive sentences. Aphasic subjects were assigned to one of three time post-onset groupings: acute (0–4 weeks), post-acute (six weeks to six months) and chronic (greater than six months). Sentences were presented in isolation or they were preceded by paragraphs that either predicted or did not predict the outcome of the target sentences. Predictive and nonpredictive contexts facilitated comprehension in the aphasic subjects. However, only predictive contexts facilitated comprehension early in the course of recovery – nonpredictive contexts had a facilitative effect later in the chronic stage of recovery. The facilitative effect of predictive contexts increased over time. Even some severely impaired aphasics benefitted from predictive contexts soon after onset.

Studies of fluent and nonfluent aphasia have tended to dominate the clinical literature. However, aphasia syndromes, such as conduction aphasia and transcortical motor aphasia, have also been investigated. Bartha and Benke (2003) investigated the linguistic performance of 20 patients with acute conduction aphasia. These subjects displayed a severe impairment of repetition and fluent expressive language functions with frequent phonemic paraphasias, word-finding difficulties, repetitive self-corrections and paraphasing. Tests of auditory and reading comprehension revealed a mild impairment of language comprehension. However, performance on the Token Test (a test of verbal comprehension of commands of increasing complexity) was poor in most subjects. In all but one patient, verbal-auditory short-term memory was reduced and appeared to be related to impaired syntactic comprehension. Follow-up of 12 patients revealed that conduction aphasia often results in a chronic language impairment. The posterior temporal and inferior parietal lobes were the location of lesions. Takemura et al. (2002) report the case of an 81-year-old woman with a left medial frontal lobe haematoma. Spontaneous speech was sparse and not fluent. However, repetition was good and articulation and auditory comprehension were normal. Although she had difficulty recalling words from a given category in a word fluency task, her performance in a confrontation naming task was excellent. These clinical features were used to diagnose her language disorder as transcortical motor aphasia.

Language impairment in Alzheimer's disease has been extensively investigated. The standard view of language breakdown in this clinical population is one of relatively preserved morphosyntax with impairments in lexical and semantic aspects of language and in pragmatic and discourse skills. Kavé and Levy (2003) collected speech samples from 14 patients with Alzheimer's disease and 48 elderly control subjects. These samples were assessed for semantic, syntactic and morphological knowledge or difficulties. AD subjects conveyed less information and made more semantic errors than control subjects. However, their language contained very few structural errors and used the same syntactic structures and morphological forms as control subjects. (For an alternative view of morphosyntax in AD, see Altmann et al. (2001).) Cuerva et al. (2001) examined pragmatic abilities in a consecutive series of 34 patients with probable AD. A test of pragmatic abilities that assessed indirect requests and conversational implicatures was conducted. AD patients had significantly more severe pragmatic deficits than age-comparable healthy controls. Moreover, there was a significant association in the AD subjects between pragmatic deficits and theory of mind skills. Feyereisen et al. (2007) examined referential communication in 13 subjects who were in the minimal or mild stage of senile dementia of Alzheimer's type. Compared to 13 healthy elderly adults, these subjects were less able to take previously shared information into account during a referential communication task, used more idiosyncratic descriptions of the referent and used no definite referential expressions. Moreover, the decline in communicative effectiveness in these subjects was not found to relate closely to executive deficits. (For further discussion of pragmatic deficits in Alzheimer's disease, see Cummings (2007a).)

Language impairments in a number of less common neurodegenerative conditions are now being increasingly investigated. Friend et al. (1999) examined naming, comprehension and verbal fluency in MS patients. These investigators found that patients with chronic-progressive and relapsing-remitting MS performed significantly more poorly than healthy controls on aural comprehension, naming, category fluency, letter fluency and other language-based cognitive measures. On tests of aural comprehension, letter and category fluency, chronic-progressive patients obtained significantly lower scores than relapsing-remitting patients. Rakowicz and Hodges (1998) found language impairment in 5 of 18 patients (28 per cent) with sporadic MND. Of these five patients, three had impaired language function in the presence of dementia. The remaining two patients, who did not have dementia, had an aphasic syndrome that was characterised by word-finding difficulties and anomia. Murray (2000) examined spoken language deficits in patients with Huntington's disease (HD) or Parkinson's disease (PD). HD patients produced shorter utterances, a larger proportion of simple sentences, a smaller proportion of grammatical utterances and fewer embeddings per utterance than non-brain-damaged peers. Their utterances were also shorter and syntactically simpler than those of PD patients. PD patients produced a smaller proportion of grammatical sentences than normal controls. Correlations between language measures and results on a battery of cognitive and motor speech tests indicate that spoken language abilities in HD and PD are related to neuropsychological and motor speech changes.

5.4.3 Aphasia Assessment

We described in section 5.4 how aphasia is a multi-modal disorder with potential impairments in a number of language levels. These impairments, we claimed, had an adverse effect not just on the linguistic abilities of affected individuals, but also on their wider communicative skills. The wide-ranging nature of any aphasic language disorder has implications for assessment. Clinicians must not only have a clear sense of the particular impairments of phonology, morphology, syntax and semantics that are part of the disorder, but they must also understand how these linguistic deficits impact on the aphasic client's ability to converse with a range of communicative partners in different social situations. Narrow linguistic deficits have traditionally been the focus of aphasia assessment and an abundance of language tests exists for this purpose. In recent years, there has been a growing recognition that assessment must also examine how these deficits impact on an individual's communicative skills. As a result, pragmatic and discourse approaches are now an integral part of aphasia assessment. In this section, we consider how clinicians assess linguistic and communicative skills in aphasia. As part of this discussion, we examine particular techniques of assessment as well as consider the clinical utility of these techniques.

Regardless of the aetiology of aphasia, it is generally agreed that early assessment and diagnosis is essential for achieving a successful outcome. Assessment can begin as soon as the patient is medically stable. This may be days or weeks, depending on the severity of a stroke or head injury. An initial assessment is normally undertaken at the patient's bedside. It must be quickly performed – fatigue and possible cognitive problems preclude a lengthy assessment – and should indicate those patients who require more thorough investigation of their language skills. Several screening tools have been developed for this purpose. In a review of aphasia screening tools, Salter et al. (2006) report that the Frenchay Aphasia Screening Test (Enderby et al. 2006) is the most widely used and thoroughly evaluated tool in the stroke research literature. This test takes between 3 and 10 minutes to complete and is suitable for use by general practitioners, junior medical staff and other nonspecialists (Enderby et al. 1987). Another screening tool – the Mississippi Aphasia Screening Test (MAST) – includes nine subscales that measure expressive and receptive language abilities and takes between 5 and 10 minutes to administer. Nakase-Thompson et al. (2005) recently used MAST to evaluate patients admitted to neurology, neurosurgery or rehabilitation units at two local hospitals. All patients were within 60 days of onset of a unilateral ischaemic or haemorrhagic stroke. These investigators found that the MAST had good criterion validity in differentiating communication impairments among clinical and control samples.

For a more comprehensive assessment of aphasia, language batteries such as the Boston Diagnostic Aphasia Examination (BADE) (Goodglass et al. 2001) and the Western Aphasia Battery – Revised (WAB-R) (Kertesz 2006) are available. The BDAE evaluates perceptual modalities (e.g. auditory, visual and gestural), processing functions (e.g. comprehension, analysis, problem-solving) and response modalities (e.g. writing, articulation and manipulation). The third edition of the assessment includes extended tools that test syntax comprehension, locate category-specific difficulties in word comprehension and word production and assess grapho–phonemic processing. The Boston Naming Test, which examines visual confrontation naming abilities, has also been incorporated into the third edition. The standard form of the assessment takes 90 minutes to complete, although a short form which takes 30–45 minutes is also available. The WAB-R is a battery of eight subtests (32 short tasks). These tests examine content, fluency, auditory comprehension, repetition, naming, reading, writing and calculation. Two new supplementary tasks – reading and writing of irregular words and nonwords – assist the clinician in distinguishing between surface, deep (phonological) and visual dyslexia. The full battery takes between 30 and 45 minutes to complete. However, a bedside version of the WAB-R can be carried out in 15 minutes.

Language batteries such as the BDAE and WAB-R provide clinicians with an overview of language skills. They can also be used to diagnose particular aphasia syndromes based on the surface symptoms of language impairment. However, these batteries cannot be used to elucidate the underlying nature of an aphasic language disorder. A cognitive neuropsychological approach to aphasia assessment has such elucidation at its centre. This approach systematically assesses the component processes in a cognitive task in order to establish which are intact and which are impaired. An aphasia assessment that is constructed on cognitive neuropsychological principles is Kay et al.'s Psycholinguistic Assessments of Language Processing in Aphasia (PALPA). PALPA consists of 60 tests that examine components of language structure, such as orthography and phonology, word and picture semantics and morphology and syntax. Spoken and written input and output modalities are assessed. Tests require subjects to perform simple procedures such as lexical decision, repetition and picture naming. Comprehensive guides help clinicians select the tests to use to investigate an individual client's impaired and intact abilities. Other cognitive neuropsychological assessments include Pyramids and Palm Trees (Howard and Patterson 1992), the Sentence Processing Resource Pack (Marshall et al. 1998) and the Comprehensive Aphasia Test (Swinburn et al. 2005).[32]

The assessments that have been discussed thus far examine linguistic deficits in the aphasic client. While these assessments can tell clinicians if a client is able to name pictures or perform a lexical decision task, these findings are, by themselves, relatively unrevealing about a client's use of language in a range of communicative situations.[33] To examine communicative performance, pragmatic and discourse analytic assessment techniques have been developed. These techniques include conversation analysis, the use of story retell procedures, story generation based on pictures and topic-elicited personal narratives. Conversation analysis has been used to examine collaborative repair in aphasic conversation (Perkins et al. 1999), aphasic grammar within the context of turns at talk in conversation (Beeke 2003; Beeke et al. 2003), word search strategies in aphasia (Oelschlaeger and Damico 2000) and the distribution of turns at talk in aphasic participants' conversations with a relative (Perkins 1995). The versatility and reliability[34] of conversation analysis as an assessment method has led to its widespread use amongst clients with acquired language disorder. While many such assessments are conducted informally according to procedures that are devised by clinicians, there are now a number of published resources that employ the methodology of conversation analysis to assess aphasia. One such resource is the Conversation Analysis Profile for People with Aphasia (CAPPA; Whitworth et al. 1997). A related profile – the Conversation Analysis Profile for People with Cognitive Impairment (CAPPCI; Whitworth et al. 1997) – is designed for use with clients who have generalised cognitive impairment, such as occurs in dementia or head injury.[35]

Studies have confirmed the clinical utility of discourse-based procedures in the assessment of aphasia and other acquired language disorders. Hula et al. (2003) examined the use of the story retell procedure (SRP) as a means of assessing discourse in adults with aphasia. Audio-recorded language samples from four aphasic and 11 normal subjects were assessed by four judges for percentage information units per minute. None of these judges had previously used the SRP. High inter-rater reliability was found. Reliability coefficients ranged from 0.89 to 0.995. The scoring of individual information units produced point-to-point reliability percentages ranging from 85 to 95 per cent, with an average of 91 per cent for both groups. The standard error of measurement associated with inter-rater scoring error ranged from 0.59 to 1.42 per cent information units per minute. Hula et al. conclude that '[t]he SRP is a potentially useful tool for quantifying connected language behaviour' (2003:523). Coelho et al. (2003) assessed the clinical utility of several commonly used measures of discourse performance. In order to establish if these measures could distinguish subjects with closed head injuries (CHI) from non-brain-injured (NBI) controls, these investigators elicited discourse samples from 32 CHI adults and 43 NBI adults. Samples consisted of two story narratives (generation and retelling) and 15 minutes of conversation. Discourse analyses included story narrative measures of grammatical complexity, cohesive adequacy and story grammar. Conversation measures included appropriateness and topic initiation. Discriminant function analyses revealed that the story narrative measures did not reliably discriminate CHI and NBI subjects. Only 70 per cent of cases were accurately classified by these measures (64.5 per cent of the CHI group and 74.4 per cent of the NBI group). However, the conversational measures classified over 77 per cent of cases correctly (78.1 per cent of the CHI group and 72.1 per cent of the NBI group). Coelho et al. conclude that the interactive nature of conversation as well as social factors may make this genre more difficult for CHI subjects. As a result, conversation may be a more sensitive index of the cognitive-communicative impairments of these subjects. For further discussion of pragmatic and discourse analytic assessment techniques, see Cummings (2007a).

5.4.4 Aphasia Intervention

The assessment process should indicate to clinicians key areas of language and communicative functioning that require intervention. Typically, intervention will seek to address specific linguistic deficits. These deficits can involve different language levels (e.g. syntax, semantics) and a range of language modalities (e.g. auditory comprehension, writing). However, to effect long-term communicative gains, the clinician must also consider how specific impairments of language structure relate to the wider communicative skills of the aphasic client. These skills are at the centre of pragmatic and functional approaches to intervention. The emphasis on communicative effectiveness in these approaches has seen the scope of aphasia intervention expand to include the use of group therapy with aphasic clients, the development of training programmes for the conversational partners of aphasic individuals and the use of AAC by severely impaired aphasic adults. This same emphasis on communicative effectiveness has also forced clinicians to reconsider how they assess the efficacy of particular interventions. For an intervention to be judged to have had a successful outcome, improved performance on formal language assessments must now also be accompanied by observations and reports of increased communicative effectiveness. In this section, we consider pragmatic and functional approaches to intervention, as well as techniques that target specific linguistic deficits. The efficacy of some of these techniques will also be examined.

Amongst the many linguistic deficits that occur in aphasia, impairments in syntax and semantics are two of the most common. Interventions for specific deficits in syntax include the attempt to train comprehension and production of structures involving wh- or NP-movement. Thompson et al. (2003) trained four subjects with agrammatic aphasia to comprehend and produce filler-gap sentences with wh-movement. The syntactic structures that were targeted in this intervention included object-extracted who-questions, object clefts, and sentences with object-relative clausal embedding. As well as treating structures that require wh-movement, Jacobs and Thompson (2000) and Thompson et al. (1997) trained passive sentences (NP-movement) in agrammatic aphasic subjects. Specific semantic-level deficits are also routinely targeted in aphasia intervention. Drew and Thompson (1999) used a semantic-based treatment to train naming of nouns in two semantic categories. The subjects in this intervention were four Broca's aphasic subjects who had severe naming deficits.

Testing of the lexical systems of these subjects revealed that their severe naming deficits were attributable in part to a semantic impairment. Kiran and Thompson (2003) used a semantic feature treatment to improve naming of either typical or atypical items within semantic categories in four subjects with fluent aphasia. Throughout training, naming errors evolved from those with no apparent relationship to the target to semantic and phonemic paraphasias.

Many aphasic clients experience written as well as spoken language impairments. Yet, written language interventions are altogether less common than interventions that focus on spoken language comprehension and production. Robson et al. (2001) treated written language output in six clients with jargon aphasia. For each client, a personally useful vocabulary was chosen and used in copying, word completion and written picture-naming tasks. Although these clients made progress in written naming, they were still unable to use these written words to convey messages. In a further stage of treatment, three clients received therapy that encouraged them to relate treated words to functional messages which were communicated to a partner. A message assessment and observation of communication and reports from relatives indicated that these clients made functional use of writing in a range of communication settings. Mortley et al. (2001) describe a written language intervention in a client with severe dysgraphia. A compensatory strategy was developed using the client's residual ability to spell words orally. A computer was used to facilitate intensive repetitive practice. Where a client has failed to respond to an intervention based on auditory/verbal stimuli, a written language intervention may be used to effect language gains. In this case, written language is not the target of therapy; rather, it is the modality through which therapy is conducted. Hough (1993) used visual/written information and visual word and sentence comprehension tasks to treat an adult with Wernicke's aphasia. This client had failed to make linguistic or communicative gains in the eight months following a stroke. All auditory/verbal stimulus presentation was excluded from the intervention. After two months of treatment, improvement was observed in naming abilities and in a general ability to communicate in conversation. Neologistic jargon decreased and semantic jargon increased. However, there was no improvement in the client's severe auditory comprehension deficit.

Group therapy is now used extensively in the management of aphasic clients. Its benefits in this clinical population are numerous. It provides an important opportunity for the generalisation of language skills to occur. Aphasic adults derive much needed psychological support[36] from engaging with other people who are experiencing similar communication problems. Also, group therapy more closely resembles everyday communication in both its number of participants and social dimensions than do individual sessions between a client and clinician. These benefits of group therapy and other gains are well supported by studies in this area. Brumfitt and Sheeran (1997) evaluated a group therapy intervention in six aphasic adults. Therapy consisted of 10 sessions, each of which was 90 minutes in duration. Therapy included communication activities that encouraged the sharing of personal experiences, videotaping of role-play activities for self- and group evaluation and practice tasks that were conducted outside the group. Functional communicative ability, attitudes to communication and psychological adjustment were assessed before and after intervention. Significant improvements were observed in communicative competence and attitudes to communication by the end of the group therapy. Improved attitudes to communication, greater attendance and completion of assignments were also predictive of reduced levels of depression. Ross et al. (2006) examined outcomes of a group intervention in seven individuals with chronic moderate aphasia. The specific outcomes investigated were communication, life participation and psychological well-being. Group intervention was based on a social model approach and involved the use of Total Communication to support conversation. Results showed evidence of statistically significant beneficial change in conversation experiences (many related to life participation) and, to a lesser degree, conversation abilities in these aphasic subjects. Some participants also displayed beneficial changes on measures of psychological well-being.

For some years, clinicians have recognised the vital role that conversational partners can play in facilitating communication in aphasic adults. This role is now addressed directly through the inclusion of training programmes for conversational partners in most interventions for aphasia. Booth and Swabey (1999) report a communication skills group programme for four carers of aphasic adults. The group took place once a week for six consecutive weeks and used conversation analysis to guide individualised advice to carers. Carer perceptions and strategies that facilitated interaction were encouraged, while those that impeded conversation were discouraged. The Conversation Analysis Profile for People with Aphasia (CAPPA) and a quantitative and qualitative analysis of repair management were conducted pre- and post-intervention to test if this approach was beneficial to carers. The use of individualised advice and targeting conversation management in a group setting was shown to be a useful way of providing advice to carers. Booth and Perkins (1999) also used conversation analysis to guide individualised advice to the brother of a man with aphasia. As well as motivating this advice, conversation analysis was used to evaluate the outcome of carer intervention. Kagan et al. (2001) evaluated an intervention called Supported Conversation for Adults with Aphasia (SCA). Twenty volunteers received SCA training and 20 control subjects merely interacted with aphasic clients. On ratings of acknowledging competence and revealing competence in their partners with aphasia, trained volunteers scored significantly higher than untrained volunteers. Even though aphasic adults did not receive training, there was nevertheless a positive change in ratings of social skills and message exchange skills in these clients as a result of their partners' training. Cunningham and Ward (2003) report four case studies in which the partners of aphasic adults participated in a training programme that ran for five weeks (1.5 hours/week). Training included education, video feedback and role play. On completion of training, conversation analysis and frequency counts of nonverbal behaviours were performed. The use of gesture increased in three of the four conversational dyads. The proportion of successful repair sequences also increased following intervention.

Where a language disorder is severe or is likely to deteriorate, an AAC system may be a client's only means of achieving functional communication. The choice of system is influenced by a range of factors, including residual language skills, the presence of cognitive deficits, visual and hearing impairments and the severity of any physical disability (e.g. hemiplegia). Pattee et al. (2006) report the case of a nonverbal adult who presented with a primary progressive aphasia[37] and AOS. The effects of two approaches on the communicative output of this individual were examined. This subject was trained to use a text-to-speech alternative communication device and American sign language. Communicative effectiveness was assessed in terms of number of words, correct information units and percentage correct information units. Increases occurred across all three of these measures for both the alternative communication device and American sign language. Koul et al. (2005) introduced a graphic symbol system to nine individuals with severe Broca's aphasia or global aphasia. A software program that turns a computer into a speech output communication device was used. Graphic symbol sentences ranged in complexity from two-word phrases to sentences that contained morphological inflections, transformations and relative clauses. The results of this intervention indicated that aphasic subjects are able to access and manipulate graphic symbols and combine them in sentences of increasing syntactical complexity. Waller et al. (1998) evaluated the use of a computer-based communication system called TalksBac. This system is designed specifically for use with nonfluent adults with aphasia. TalksBac is a word-based system that exploits the ability of some nonfluent aphasics to recognise familiar words and sentences. This system was used for a period of nine months by four nonfluent clients. A battery of tests was used to provide pre- and post-intervention data on the comprehension, expression and communication skills of subjects. To compare conversation skills in the presence and absence of the TalksBac system, conversations between aphasic subjects and their partners were videotaped. Although the results of formal assessments revealed little change in the underlying comprehension and expressive abilities of the aphasic subjects, conversational gains were observed in two of the subjects. A third subject's conversational abilities were not enhanced by the system, as he had developed nonverbal strategies which he considered to be more effective.

5.5 Acquired Dysphagia

The various neurological diseases and injuries that we have examined in this chapter can also cause a disorder of swallowing in adults. Known as dysphagia, this disorder can have potentially life-threatening consequences for the individuals whom it affects. These consequences include malnutrition, dehydration, aspiration, suffocation, pneumonia and death.[38] The diagnosis and management of dysphagia is an increasingly important part of the professional remit of speech and language therapists. In practice, however, the speech and language therapist is only one of several medical and health professionals who assess and treat dysphagia. This multidisciplinary team includes, in addition to speech and language therapists, gastroenterologists, neurologists, otolaryngologists, dieticians, radiographers and radiologists. In this section, we examine the disorders in which dysphagia occurs. We consider how common swallowing and related difficulties are in these disorders. The techniques that are used by therapists to assess and treat dysphagia in adults will also be discussed.

5.5.1 Epidemiology and Aetiology

The most common cause of dysphagia in adults is a stroke or CVA. Broadley et al. (2005) studied 104 patients admitted to an acute stroke unit and found that 55 (53 per cent) had dysphagia. Twenty patients (19 per cent) had dysphagia that required nonoral feeding/hydration for 14 days or more, or died while dysphagic prior to 14 days. Dysphagia in adults may also be caused by brain tumours. Newton et al. (1994) examined 17 patients with primary brain tumours who complained of dysphagia. On a bedside swallowing assessment, 11 of these patients had a moderate impairment that required supervision. Videofluoroscopic evaluation revealed a moderate to moderately severe abnormality and trace or frequent aspiration in 6 of 7 patients. Dysphagia is a common disorder in individuals with neurodegenerative diseases. Klugman and Ross (2002) studied 30 subjects with MS, 50 per cent of whom reported swallowing problems in a questionnaire. Hartelius and Svensson (1994) surveyed 460 patients with PD or MS. Forty one per cent of PD patients and 33 per cent of MS subjects indicated that they experienced impairment of chewing and swallowing abilities.

Savvopoulos et al. (1990) examined 17 cases of Huntington's chorea. These investigators reported dysphagia in 50 per cent of cases. Hadjikoutis et al. (2000) studied 37 subjects with MND. MND patients coughed and choked significantly more often and to a greater degree than healthy volunteers (26 of 37 MND patients compared to 2 of 23 volunteers). However, chest infections were only rarely reported among the MND patients. Dysphagia is also associated with myasthenia gravis, an acquired autoimmune disorder of neuromuscular transmission (see section 5.2.1). Kluin et al. (1996) examined eight elderly men with myasthenia gravis and found greater than expected pharyngeal phase dysphagia on videofluoroscopy in each of them. All eight subjects had decreased pharyngeal motility, which was indicated by residual material in the valleculae and pyriform sinuses bilaterally. Episodes of laryngeal penetration secondary to overflow of residual material occurred in seven subjects. Even though gag reflexes were present and subjects were able to cough on command, five subjects experienced silent aspiration. Feeding tubes were needed in five subjects because their dysphagia showed a poor response to treatment. Finally, dysphagia can sometimes be caused by medical interventions (iatrogenic dysphagia). Goguen et al. (2006) assessed the impact of sequential chemoradiation therapy for advanced head and neck cancer on swallowing in 59 patients. Of 23 patients who underwent modified barium swallow, 18 demonstrated aspiration. None of these subjects developed pneumonia and dysphagia generally slowly recovered 6–12 months after treatment.[39]

5.5.2 Clinical Presentation

The manifestations of dysphagia are numerous and can vary with the different aetiologies of the disorder. Zhang et al. (2006a) identified approximately 20 abnormal manifestations of dysphagia after stroke. Swallowing organ dysfunction included abnormal lip closure, decreased tongue motility, weakness of palate, decreased or absent gag reflex, abnormal lift of larynx and insufficient opening of the cricopharyngeal muscle. Oral phase dysfunction is the primary dysphagic symptom in the early stage of ALS. Kawai et al. (2003) examined 11 patients with ALS. Abnormal movements of the anterior and/or posterior tongue were recognised in eight cases. The severity of dysphagia was particularly influenced by dysfunction of the posterior tongue. The pattern of dysphagic symptoms is different in MS, with the pharyngeal phase principally compromised. Abraham and Yun (2002) examined 13 patients with MS. Eleven patients had primary pharyngeal dysphagia, one had primary laryngeal dysphagia and one had primary oral dysphagia. The predominant anterior pharyngeal segment dysfunction – laryngeal dysmotility – was present in all 13 patients. The predominant posterior pharyngeal segment dysfunction – pharyngeal constrictor dysmotility – was found in 11 of 13 patients. The severity of the MS patients' functional swallowing impairment was significantly related to posterior pharyngeal segment dysfunction.

5.5.3 Dysphagia Assessment

In order to assess dysphagia, clinicians must be aware of the wide range of symptoms associated with the disorder. They should also be aware that while symptoms such as pneumonia are often indicative of dysphagia, their absence should not be taken as a sign that dysphagia is not present. Goguen et al.'s (2006) study revealed that even when pneumonia does not occur, aspiration can still be present in patients who have received chemoradiation therapy for head and neck cancer. Cough may be an indicator of aspiration due to oral-pharyngeal dysphagia (Smith Hammond and Goldstein 2006). However, silent aspiration typically occurs in patients who lack a protective cough reflex. With these considerations in mind, the process of assessment generally begins with a bedside evaluation of the client. An oral peripheral examination is conducted in which the strength, range of motion and symmetry of structures are noted. Any drooling and noteworthy features of the client's dentition should be recorded. Loose-fitting dentures are a considerable obstacle to safe oral feeding. Voice quality has particular significance in a swallowing assessment. Hoarse voice quality indicates incomplete vocal fold adduction, while a 'wet' or 'gurgly' voice suggests that saliva and liquid may be pooling in the larynx. A weak voluntary cough also indicates poor vocal fold adduction. The palatal reflex can be triggered by stimulating the anterior surface of the velum. Chewing can be assessed by encouraging the client to chew on a roll of gauze that has been dipped in liquid. This should be carried out on both sides of the mouth. It is important to check tactile sensation, as the client with poor sensation will have difficulty locating food and liquid in his or her oral cavity. Laryngeal excursion[40] can be checked by placing fingers on the hyoid bone and larynx. Care must be taken when examining the gag reflex.[41] If vomiting occurs, the client may aspirate regurgitated food. Finally, it is important to note the client's overall cognitive state, as attention and cooperation will be required for further, more invasive investigations of swallowing and for intervention, if this is required.

Bedside assessments of swallowing are an important early screening tool for dysphagia and aspiration risk. However, the accuracy of these techniques is an ongoing concern for practitioners and researchers. In a recent review of assessment methods that are available to clinicians, Ramsey et al. (2003) concluded that bedside tests are safe, relatively straightforward and easily repeated. However, these same tests have variable sensitivity (42–92 per cent), specificity (59–91 per cent) and inter-rater reliability. Tohara et al. (2003) examined the accuracy of the water swallowing test and the food test for assessing risk of aspiration. In the water swallowing test, 3ml of water are placed under the tongue and the patient is asked to swallow. In the food test, 4g of pudding are placed on the dorsum of the tongue and the patient is asked to swallow. The summed scores of the water and food tests had a sensitivity of 90 per cent and specificity of 56 per cent. Tohara et al. conclude that these tests may be 'useful as screening procedures to determine which dysphagia patients need a videofluorographic swallowing study' (2003:126).

Instrumental and radiological techniques are now routinely used in the assessment of dysphagia. Chief amongst these techniques are videofluoroscopy (VF) and flexible endoscopic evaluation of swallowing (FEES).[42] Eisbruch et al. (2002) used VF and oesophagogram to assess swallowing function in 26 patients after intensive chemoradiation for locally advanced head and neck cancer. VF has also been used to assess the outcome of swallowing therapy. Robbins et al. (2005) used VF to assess the effects of an eight-week progressive lingual resistance exercise programme on swallowing in elderly subjects. Each subject underwent VF for kinematic and bolus flow assessment of swallowing at baseline and week eight. Prosiegel et al. (2005) used VF and/or FEES to examine the outcome of functional swallowing therapy in dysphagic patients with posterior fossa tumours, cerebellar haemorrhage or Wallenberg's syndrome.[43] Often described as the 'gold standard' in dysphagia assessment, VF has become the benchmark against which other assessment tools are evaluated. This can be seen in recent attempts to validate the technique of cervical auscultation. Leslie et al. (2004) compared the assessment of recorded swallow sounds obtained by cervical auscultation with videofluoroscopic evaluation of swallows in 10 patients with aspiration/penetration and 10 healthy controls. Stroud et al. (2002) compared the assessments of five speech and language therapists of recorded swallow sounds obtained by cervical auscultation on two occasions. The swallows of 16 patients were recorded simultaneously with VF.[44]

An alternative objective instrumental assessment to VF is FEES. This technique involves passing a fibreoptic nasendoscope transnasally which can then be used to visualise the hypopharynx and larynx during swallowing. Using FEES, clinicians can assess anatomical structures, secretion management and laryngopharyngeal sensation. The technique can also be used to examine trial swallows of food and liquids as well as the effects of postures, strategies and manoeuvres on swallowing. FEES is now in extensive use in clinical practice and research studies. Donzelli et al. (2005) used FEES to examine the incidence of laryngeal penetration and aspiration in 37 patients with known or suspected dysphagia and a tracheostomy tube.[45] Amin et al. (2006) used flexible endoscopic evaluation of swallowing with sensory testing (FEESST)[46] to evaluate laryngopharyngeal sensation in 22 patients with amyotrophic lateral sclerosis. Aviv et al. (2005) examined 1,340 consecutive FEESST evaluations that were performed over a period of 4.5 years in outpatient and inpatient settings. The most common reason for the performance of FEESST was stroke (343; 25.6 per cent). Other reasons included cardiac-related dysphagia (298; 22.3 per cent) following open heart surgery, heart attack, congestive heart failure or new arrhythmia, head and neck cancer (207; 15.4 per cent), pulmonary disease (141; 10.5 per cent), chronic neurologic disease (124; 9.3 per cent) and acid reflux disease (80; 6.0 per cent). There were no instances of airway compromise in these patients as a result of FEESST and only one patient (0.07 per cent) developed epistaxis (acute haemorrhage from the nostril, nasal cavity or nasopharynx). Aviv et al. conclude that 'FEESST is a relatively safe procedure for the sensory and motor assessment of dysphagia in a cohort of patients with a wide variety of underlying diagnoses' (2005:173).

5.5.4 Dysphagia Intervention

Clinicians who treat dysphagia in adults tend to draw upon a diverse range of techniques. Behavioural interventions are commonplace and include direct swallowing exercises (e.g. effortful swallowing, supraglottic swallow technique), swallowing compensation strategies (e.g. posture adjustment), safe swallowing advice and diet modification. Stimulation techniques, which aim to increase sensory stimuli to structures involved in swallowing, are also widely used in the treatment of dysphagic clients. These techniques include oral electrical stimulation and tactile-thermal stimulation. Biofeedback procedures, particularly surface electromyography (SEMG), are increasingly being used alongside other techniques in the treatment of dysphagia. Intra-oral prosthetics may be used to improve swallowing function. Where oral feeding is unsafe or is otherwise inadequate to support the nutritional needs of a client, nonoral methods of feeding must be introduced. Techniques such as nasogastric tube feeding and percutaneous endoscopic gastrostomy are central to the management of the nonoral dysphagic client. We discuss some of these techniques further in the following paragraphs.

Diet modification is an integral part of dysphagia intervention. Bolus size, temperature, texture, taste and viscosity must be considered when planning treatment. Thin liquids (e.g. water) often pose the greatest aspiration risk to the dysphagic adult. Hard, crisp foods that require chewing and foods with different textures (e.g. vegetable soup) are particularly problematic for the client with oral stage dysphagia. Postural changes must often be made to ensure safe and efficient swallowing. An aligned body position with normalised muscle tone can increase airway protection and pharyngeal clearance and reduce the effort of swallowing for the client. Specific postures (e.g. chin tuck, head back, head turn) can be used to compensate for a client's swallowing problem. The optimal position for a client can be confirmed by videofluoroscopic examination. Clients can also be instructed in the use of techniques such as effortful swallowing and the supraglottic swallow. In effortful swallowing, the client is encouraged to squeeze hard with his or her throat and neck muscles during a swallow. This technique increases the driving force of the tongue by exaggerating tongue retraction and helps to get food past the valleculae. In the supraglottic swallow, the client takes a breath and holds it while swallowing and then coughs after the swallow. This technique achieves the voluntary closure of the vocal folds before, during and after the swallow.

Recent studies have examined the use of these techniques to treat dysphagia in adult clients. Carnaby et al. (2006) studied 306 patients with dysphagia following a stroke. An equal number of patients was assigned to three treatment groups. In one treatment condition – usual care – physicians referred clients to the hospital speech pathology service where they received supervision for feeding, precautions for safe swallowing (e.g. positioning, slowed rate of feeding) and VF, if recommended by the referring physician. In a second treatment group – standard low-intensity swallowing therapy – patients received training in swallowing compensation strategies (e.g. upright positioning for feeding), safe swallowing advice and dietary modification three times a week for a month. In the third treatment group – standard high-intensity swallowing therapy – patients performed direct swallowing exercises (e.g. effortful swallowing, supraglottic swallow technique) and received diet modification every working day for a month. Standard swallowing therapy was associated with a significant reduction in swallowing-related medical complications, chest infection and death or institutionalisation. High-intensity therapy in particular was associated with an increased proportion of patients who returned to a normal diet and recovered swallowing by six months.

Dejaeger and Goeleven (2005) examined 400 patients who had had swallowing problems for at least several months. Half of these patients had problems swallowing solid food. More than 10 per cent were unable to take any food by mouth. Intervention comprised adjustments to diet and posture in 41 per cent of cases and logopaedic guidance in 36 per cent of cases. In 44 per cent of patients, the safety and comfort of swallowing improved. After intervention, 13 per cent were able to feed themselves orally again. In 11 per cent, there was still a need for a percutaneous endoscopic gastrostomy (PEG) catheter. Klor and Milianti (1999) enrolled 16 male nursing home patients who received PEG feedings in a treatment programme that was based on videofluoroscopic examination. Intervention consisted of dietary consistency modifications, compensatory techniques and direct swallow retraining. As a result of intervention, all patients returned to oral feeding. PEG tubes were removed in 10 out of 16 patients.

Stimulation techniques are frequently used alongside other methods in the treatment of dysphagia. Hägg and Larsson (2004) assessed the effect of motor and sensory stimulation on swallowing in stroke patients who had been dysphagic for more than six months. Seven patients received a treatment that comprised body regulation, manual oro-facial regulation (sensory and passive motor stimulation), palatal plate application (sensory and passive motor stimulation and active muscle exercises) and velopharyngeal closure training (active muscle exercise). Evaluation comprising a swallowing capacity test, a meal observation test, clinical examination of oral motor and sensory function, a velopharyngeal closure test and VF was conducted before and two weeks after treatment. Swallowing was also assessed by patients. On both objective and self-assessments of swallowing, all seven patients demonstrated swallowing improvement. Rosenbek et al. (1998) used tactile–thermal stimulation of varying intensities to treat dysphagia in 45 male stroke patients. An ice stick was used to rub each anterior faucial pillar three or more times. Clients were also encouraged to swallow hard. No single treatment intensity emerged as superior. However, there was significant change in some penetration–aspiration measures and improvement in some duration stage transition measures.

A treatment for dysphagia that is still largely experimental in nature is oral electrical stimulation. Four stroke patients with chronic dysphagia and a delayed swallow reflex were recruited into a study of oral electrical stimulation by Park et al. (1997). A palatal prosthesis was used to carry out oral electrical stimulation of swallowing. At the patients' maximum tolerance of stimulation, barium paste was introduced and a videofluoroscopic examination was used to confirm any effect of treatment on the clients' swallow function. Oral electrical stimulation led to improvements in swallow function in 2 of 4 patients. In all cases, the treatment was well tolerated and there were no adverse side effects. In a more recent study, Power et al. (2006) failed to find any beneficial effects of oral electrical stimulation on swallowing in poststroke dysphagic patients. The swallowing of 16 patients was assessed before and 60 minutes after 0.2Hz electrical or sham stimulation at the faucial pillar. VF was used to assess laryngeal closure and pharyngeal transit time. A validated penetration–aspiration scale was used to assess aspiration severity. Neither active nor sham stimulation produced any change in the speed of laryngeal elevation, pharyngeal transit time or aspiration severity in these dysphagic subjects.

Biofeedback techniques, particularly surface electromyography (SEMG), have been successfully used as an adjunct to other dysphagia treatments. Crary (1995) used SEMG in combination with swallowing instruction to treat six patients with dysphagia secondary to brainstem stroke. Gastrostomy feeding tubes were used to provide patients with total nutrition and hydration before treatment. At the onset of therapy, none could swallow their own saliva. Biofeedback from SEMG was used to provide patients with information about movement patterns (specifically, laryngeal elevation and pharyngeal contraction) in order that they may increase the strength of the pharyngeal component of swallowing. Three patients were able to resume consistent oral intake after three weeks of therapy. In five patients, positive results were maintained for up to two years post-therapy. Huckabee and Cannito (1999) examined physiological and functional outcomes of a SEMG-based intervention in 10 patients with chronic dysphagia subsequent to brainstem injury. Severity ratings of videofluoroscopic swallowing studies revealed physiological changes in swallowing in nine patients after one week or 10 treatment sessions. To establish functional change, diet level tolerance was assessed after one week of treatment and at six months and one year post-treatment. Eight patients returned to full oral intake (gastrostomy tube feedings were terminated) and two patients displayed no long-term change in functional swallowing. Crary et al. (2004) conducted a systematic therapy programme that was supplemented by SEMG biofeedback in 25 dysphagic stroke patients and 20 patients who were dysphagic following treatment for head and neck cancer. Overall, 39 patients (87 per cent) increased their functional oral intake of food and liquid. This included 92 per cent of stroke patients and 80 per cent of patients with head and neck cancer.

Most swallowing advice issued by speech and language therapists must be put into practice by nurses, carers and family members. It is therefore important that the dysphagia therapist work closely with other healthcare workers and family members to ensure compliance with this advice. Rosenvinge and Starke (2005) observed compliance with SLT recommendations on swallowing before and after the introduction of improved training and other measures. These measures included the establishment of a dysphagia link nurse programme, modification of an in-house training scheme and swallowing advice sheets. These investigators found improved compliance with the recommendations on consistency of fluids (48–64 per cent), amount given (35–69 per cent), adherence to safe swallow guidelines (51–90 per cent) and use of supervision (35–67 per cent). Improvements in compliance were evident on medical and geriatric wards and the stroke unit. Rosenvinge and Starke conclude that '[r]elatively simple and low-cost measures, including an educational programme tailored to the needs of individual disciplines, proved effective in improving the compliance with advice on swallowing in patients with dysphagia' (2005:587).

5.6 Schizophrenia

Many individuals with mental illness experience significant language problems. The language disorder that occurs in schizophrenia has been extensively discussed in the clinical literature. In this section, we examine this disorder and describe the diverse array of linguistic deficits that are associated with it. These deficits have been likened to the structural language impairments that are typical of aphasia. Yet, they are not caused by a focal lesion of the left hemisphere, as is the case in aphasia. We leave questions of the neuropathological basis of schizophrenic language disorder for another context.[47] We begin our discussion of schizophrenia with some general comments about the disorder's epidemiology and symptomatology.

Schizophrenia is a common mental illness. The Royal College of Psychiatrists in the UK reports that 1 person in 100 develops schizophrenia at some time in their life. Wu et al. (2006) used several administrative claims databases to calculate the annual prevalence of diagnosed schizophrenia in the US.

These investigators report that in 2002, the 12-month prevalence of diagnosed schizophrenia was estimated at 5.1 per 1,000 lives. The incidence of schizophrenia is considerably higher in men than in women. McGrath (2006) reports a male:female ratio of 1.4. The incidence of schizophrenia is also higher in migrants and in those living in urban areas (McGrath 2006). The age at onset also varies between men and women, with men tyically developing schizophrenia earlier than women. Gorwood et al. (1995) examined a population of 663 schizophrenic patients and found that the mean age at onset in males and females was 27.8 years and 31.5 years, respectively.

A diagnosis of schizophrenia is based on the identification of several symptoms. Chief amongst these characteristics are positive and negative symptoms. Positive symptoms include thought disorder (disorganised and illogical thought), delusions (the holding of false and bizarre beliefs) and hallucinations (perception of things that do not exist). Auditory hallucinations, in which the schizophrenic individual hears voices, are the most common type of hallucinatory symptom. Negative symptoms involve the absence of normal behaviours. They include affective flattening, alogia (poverty of speech), apathy, avolition (absence of initiative or motivation) and social withdrawal. Cognitive deficits are also common in schizophrenia and include problems with attention, memory and executive functions. Some theorists have argued that the language disorder in schizophrenia is the result of deficits in attention and the executive functions of the brain (Chaika 1997).

There is now evidence that all levels of language are disrupted in schizophrenia. These levels include phonology,[48] morphology, syntax, semantics and pragmatics. Walder et al. (2006) examined phonology, semantics and grammar in 31 schizophrenic outpatients and 27 healthy controls. Male schizophrenic patients performed significantly worse than their healthy counterparts on all three language domains.[49] Covington et al. (2005) identify two (perhaps not fully distinct) types of language impairment in schizophrenia. Thought disorder is characterised by a failure to maintain a discourse plan. Executive function and pragmatics are primarily disrupted and there is a possible impairment of the syntax-semantics interface. The language characteristics of schizophrenia include aphasia-like impairments such as clanging (glossomania[50]), neologism (related to a lexical access deficit) and unintelligible utterances. Speakers exhibit flat intonation or unusual voice quality, while phonology, morphology and syntax are relatively intact. (Some syntactic deficits have been reported.) We examine several of these language impairments further below.

Morphemic disturbances in schizophrenia are evident in the loss of word endings, like -ed and -ion in 'I am being help with the food and the medicate . . .' (Chaika 1990:24). Covington et al. (2005) argue that what appear to be morphemic errors in schizophrenia might equally be related to disruptions of syntax or lexical retrieval. In this way, the schizophrenic patient in the above example may have committed a syntactic error by selecting the wrong part of speech (the infinitive form *help* rather than the past participle *helped*) or a lexical retrieval error by selecting a word with the correct semantic meaning but from the wrong syntactic category (the verb *medicate* as opposed to the noun *medication*). In any event, Covington et al. state that '[a]bnormal morphology in schizophrenia is quite rare' (2005:90).

Syntactic errors are relatively common in schizophrenia. Schizophrenic subjects have been observed to use incomplete prepositional phrases and verb phrases. Chaika describes how one subject omitted the object of the preposition *for* in 'he was blamed for and I didn't think that was fair . . .' (1990:221). Ribeiro's schizophrenic subject routinely omitted the direct object of the verb *have*, as in 'No, only if you have. Do you have?' (1994:263). Clauses are started but not completed. In response to the interviewer's question 'Why do you think people believe in God?', a schizophrenic patient replied 'Um, *because* making a do in life. Isn't none of that stuff about evolution guiding isn't true any more now . . .' (Thomas 1997:40). The first sentence consists of a subordinate clause without a main clause. DeLisi (2001) found that sentence complexity was reduced in schizophrenia. The subjects with chronic schizophrenia in this study displayed reduced conjoined and embedded clauses.

Impairments in receptive syntax have been linked to cognitive deficits in schizophrenic speakers. Lelekov et al. (2000) investigated the hypothesis that syntactic comprehension impairment in schizophrenia reflects a deficit in cognitive sequence processing. Ten schizophrenic patients were tested using a standard measure of syntactic comprehension and a task that assessed nonlinguistic sequence processing. These investigators found that performance impairment on the two tasks was highly correlated. This finding, Lelekov et al. argue, suggests that 'syntactic comprehension deficits in schizophrenia reveal the dysfunction of cognitive sequence processing mechanisms' (2000:2145). Bagner et al. (2003) examined the hypothesis that language comprehension deficits in schizophrenia are associated with disturbances in working memory. Twenty-seven stable schizophrenic outpatients underwent a reading span task (a measure of working memory). Language comprehension was assessed by means of questions about auditorily presented sentences that varied in length and syntactic complexity. Working memory was found to be strongly correlated with language comprehension in these schizophrenic patients. Moreover, language comprehension deficits were significantly greater in these patients than in a group of 28 controls. Not all studies have conclusively demonstrated a link between receptive syntax impairments and cognitive deficits in schizophrenia. Condray et al. (2002) found that cognitive functions predicted but did not completely account for receptive syntax accuracy in 32 males diagnosed with schizophrenia.

Lexical semantics is disrupted in schizophrenia. Neologisms occur frequently in schizophrenic speech: for example, the use of *geshinker* in the following extract from Thomas: 'I got so angry I picked up a dish and threw it at the geshinker' (1997:38). Bizarre lexical choices are common. For example, Chaika's schizophrenic subject used 'the cash register man handled the financial matters' (1990:202) to refer to his ringing up money for an ice-cream cone. Sumiyoshi et al. (2001) used the ANIMAL category fluency test to examine semantic structure in 57 patients with schizophrenia. These investigators found that while normal controls demonstrated the domestic/size distinction in semantic structure, no such dimension was evident in the schizophrenic patients. Sumiyoshi et al. also found that age of onset and level of verbal intelligence, as indicated by vocabulary score, were closely related to the severity of degradation of semantic structure in schizophrenia. (Patients with later onset or high vocabulary score demonstrated relatively intact semantic structure.)

Semantic impairments have been linked to thought disorder in schizophrenia. Goldberg et al. (1998) performed a range of semantic processing and language comprehension tests on 23 schizophrenic patients and 23 normal controls. A series of multiple regression analyses revealed that two variables – the verbal fluency difference score and the Peabody Picture Vocabulary Test score – made significant contributions to the prediction of positive thought disorder. Goldberg et al. concluded that

> clinically rated thought disorder is associated with and may result from semantic processing abnormalities. In particular, patients with more severe thought disorder may have difficulty accessing semantic items because of disorganization of the semantic systems and, to a more limited degree, may also lack a semantic or conceptual knowledge base. (1998:1671)

Rodriguez-Ferrera et al. (2001) examined the relationship between language test performance and formal thought disorder in 40 schizophrenic patients. Significant correlations were obtained between three language test scores and formal thought disorder scores. Multiple regression analysis indicated particular associations of formal thought disorder with picture description and semantic comprehension.

Pragmatics is by far the most extensively investigated area of language impairment in schizophrenia. Behavioural evidence indicates that schizophrenic speakers perform poorly on tests of discourse planning/comprehension, understanding humour, sarcasm, metaphors, indirect requests and the generation/comprehension of emotional prosody (Mitchell and Crow 2005). These pragmatic aspects of language 'are essential to an accurate understanding of someone's communicative intent, and the deficits displayed by patients with schizophrenia may make a significant contribution to their social interaction deficits' (Mitchell and Crow 2005:963). In the rest of this section, we examine some of these deficits. We consider the findings of studies which demonstrate that schizophrenic speakers fail to process aspects of linguistic context. We also discuss the relationship between impaired pragmatics and cognitive deficits in schizophrenia. For further discussion of these issues, the reader is referred to Cummings (2007a).

Meilijson et al. (2004) examined the pragmatic skills of 43 subjects with chronic schizophrenia. To attain a general profile of pragmatic abilities in these subjects, Meilijson et al. used Prutting and Kirchner's (1987) pragmatic proto-col. Schizophrenic subjects displayed a high degree of inappropriate pragmatic abilities relative to a psychiatric control group (individuals with mixed anxiety-depression) and to subjects with hemispheric brain damage (data from Prutting and Kirchner 1987). Pragmatic parameters that were more than 50 per cent inappropriate included topic selection, introduction, maintenance and change; lexical specificity/accuracy; prosody; turn-taking quantity/conciseness and facial expressions. Among the 43 subjects with schizophrenia, three groups with different pragmatic profiles emerged. Almost half the subjects (21 subjects) displayed minimal impairment. A further 11 subjects had lexical impairment and 11 had interactional impairment. Subjects with lexical impairment had a low degree of inappropriateness in the nonverbal and turn-taking parameters and a high degree of inappropriateness in the lexical parameters. Subjects with minimal or interactional impairment displayed the same distribution of inappropriateness across parameters – increased inappropriateness in topic parameters with lower, but similar levels of inappropriateness in nonverbal, lexical, turn-taking and speech act parameters. However, inappropriateness was greater across all parameters for schizophrenic subjects with interaction impairment.

Experimental studies have repeatedly shown that schizophrenic subjects are unable to process aspects of linguistic context. Bazin et al. (2000) conducted an experiment in which 30 schizophrenic subjects and 30 control subjects were required to complete sentences using the first word(s) that come to mind. Each sentence contained an ambiguous word, the less frequent meaning of which was primed by a preceding sentence. Results showed that only control subjects were able to use the linguistic context provided by the preceding sentence to prime the less frequent meaning of the ambiguous word. Schizophrenic subjects, particularly those with thought disorder, used the most common meaning of the ambiguous word more frequently than controls. Sitnikova et al. (2002) used event-related potentials (ERPs) to examine deficits in language comprehension in schizophrenia. Sentences that contained two clauses were read by schizophrenic and control subjects. These investigators hypothesised that the processing of target words in the second clause would be influenced by preceding linguistic context in the control subjects only. Schizophrenic subjects, by contrast, were expected to be inappropriately affected by the dominant meaning of homographs in the first clause (e.g. the 'structure' meaning of 'bridge' in the sentence *The guests played bridge because the river had rocks in it*). This hypothesis was confirmed.

Many other pragmatic deficits have also been shown to occur in schizophrenia. Ténvi et al. (2002) examined the ability of schizophrenic subjects to recognise the intended meaning behind violations of Gricean implicatures. Twenty-six paranoid schizophrenic subjects and 26 normal controls were presented with four question and answer vignettes in which the maxim of relevance was violated. Subjects had to identify the speaker's intended meaning in each case. Ténvi et al. found that schizophrenic subjects made significantly more errors than controls in identifying the communicative intentions that lay behind violations of this maxim. Corcoran and Frith (1996) examined politeness and appreciation of the Gricean maxims of quantity, quality and relation in schizophrenic patients with different symptom profiles. Subjects had to select an appropriate final piece of speech for one of the characters in a series of stories. One piece of speech adhered to the rule under question, while the other flouted the rule. Control subjects, schizophrenic subjects with paranoid delusions and schizophrenic subjects with negative symptoms adhered to the maxim of relation. However, all other maxims were flouted by subjects with negative symptoms. Subjects with paranoid delusions often failed to respond in a polite fashion, but performed at a similar level to controls on stories involving the Gricean maxims. Much of the incoherence of schizophrenic language can be related to failures of reference, particularly reference to earlier parts of spoken discourse. Docherty et al. (2003) examined disturbances of referential communication in 48 schizophrenic patients. These patients scored significantly higher (more disordered) than controls on each of six types of referential disturbance. Five types of referential disturbance were stable over time in these subjects (confused reference, missing information reference, ambiguous word meaning, wrong word reference and structural unclarity). A sixth type of reference – vague reference – was not stable over time. Referential disturbances showed little or no association with the severity of positive or negative symptoms in these patients.

Finally, as with other language impairments in schizophrenia, pragmatic impairments have been linked to cognitive deficits. Linscott (2005) examined the relationship between pragmatic language impairment (PLI), thought disorder and generalised cognitive decline in 20 schizophrenic subjects. The Profile of Pragmatic Impairment in Communication (Hays et al. 2004; Linscott 1996) was used to score subjects for PLI. Significant PLI and generalised cognitive decline were found in the schizophrenic subjects. Furthermore, generalised cognitive decline predicted PLI. Linscott remarks that PLI in schizophrenia is secondary to generalised cognitive decline. Brüne and Bodenstein (2005) investigated the relation of proverb understanding in schizophrenia to the cognitive ability to engage in mindreading ('theory of mind'). Thirty-one schizophrenic patients completed a proverb test, a 'theory of mind' test battery and a variety of executive functioning and verbal intelligence tests. These patients' psychopathology was also assessed. 'Theory of mind', intelligence and executive functioning correlated strongly with the patients' ability to interpret proverbs correctly. Approximately 39 per cent of the variance of proverb comprehension in the schizophrenic patients was predicted by 'theory of mind' performance. Brüne and Bodenstein conclude that '[t]he ability to interpret such metaphorical speech that is typical of many proverbs crucially depends on schizophrenic patients' ability to infer mental states' (2005:233).

Notes

1. Fatality rates are greater for haemorrhagic than ischaemic (blood clot) strokes. Rosamond et al. (1999) report that the unadjusted 30-day case fatality rate for incident and recurrent hospitalised stroke combined was 7.6 per cent for ischaemic and 37.5 per cent for haemorrhagic events.

2. Using the National Hospital Discharge Survey from 1980 to 1998, Lynch et al. (2002) report that the rate of stroke for infants less than 30 days of age was 26.4/100,000 (6.7/100,000 for haemorrhagic stroke and 17.8/100,000 for ischaemic stroke). Based on these figures, neonatal stroke occurs in 1/4,000 live births per year. Earley et al. (1998) studied all children aged between 1 and 14 years who were discharged from 46 hospitals in central Maryland and Washington, DC, with a diagnosis of ischaemic stroke and intracerebral haemorrhage in the years 1988 and 1991. These investigators found that the overall incidence for childhood stroke was 1.29 per 100,000 per year (0.58 per 100,000 for ischaemic stroke and 0.71 per 100,000 for intracerebral haemorrhage).

3. Motor neurone diseases can also occur in children. They include spinal muscular atrophy (SMA), in which muscles weaken and atrophy due to degeneration of motor neurones in the spinal cord. There are three types of SMA in childhood which differ in age of onset and severity – infantile SMA (Werdnig–Hoffmann disease), intermediate SMA and juvenile SMA (Kugelberg–Welander disease).

4. Also called Lou Gehrig's disease after the baseball legend who died from ALS in 1941.

5. The Motor Neurone Disease Association in the UK states that ALS affects 65 per cent of MND individuals. Other forms of MND are less common – progressive bulbar palsy affects 25 per cent of MND sufferers, progressive muscular atrophy affects less than 10 per cent and primary lateral sclerosis affects approximately 2 per cent.

6. In 2005, 4,909 deaths in England and Wales were caused by Alzheimer's disease. PD was responsible for 4,165 deaths in the same year. MS and MND accounted for 962 and 1,568 deaths, respectively (National Statistics 2006).

7. *Borrelia burgdorferi* is a bacteria species that can cause acute meningitis in infected individuals.

8. At the beginning of section 5.2.2, I described how the results of objective techniques could sometimes conflict with the perceptual judgements of an assessor. This conflict may lead to the revision of those judgements. It is clear that McAuliffe et al. intend no such revision in this case. EPG did not confirm perceptual assessments of impaired speech rate, a fact that is explained by McAuliffe et al. as follows: 'It is . . . possible that EPG failed to detect lingual movement impairment as it does not measure the complete tongue movement towards and away from the hard palate' (2006:19).

9. Murdoch et al. (2000) state that '[i]n the past years, perceptual analysis of dysarthric speech has been the "gold standard" and preferred method by which clinicians made differential diagnoses and defined treatment programmes for their dysarthric clients' (138–9).

10. The authors of this review define non–progressive brain damage as damage that is acquired by means of stroke, TBI, meningitis, encephalitis and postsurgical meningioma and acoustic neuroma.

11. LSVT is included among the speech and language therapy recommendations in a recent report completed by the National Collaborating Centre for Chronic Conditions (NCC-CC). The four SLT recommendations in this report are (1) improvement of vocal loudness and pitch range, including speech therapy programmes such as LSVT, (2) teaching strategies to optimise speech intelligibility, (3) ensuring an effective means of communication is maintained throughout the course of the disease, including use of assistive technologies and (4) review and management to support the safety and efficiency of swallowing and to minimise the risk of aspiration.

12. The See-Scape is used to detect nasal emission of air during speech in clients who have velopharyngeal incompetence. The device consists of a nasal tip, which is inserted into one of the client's nares. This tip is connected to a rigid plastic tube, which contains a float, via a flexible plastic tube. The float rises in the tube in response to air emission. See-Scape provides clients with visual feedback of nasal air emission. As such, it is a valuable assessment and treatment tool in the management of clients with velopharyngeal incompetence.

13. In a point prevalence study of Canadian adults, aged 15 years and older, who survived TBI, Moscato et al. (1994) report that 84 per cent of their sample reported co-occurring disabilities. The median number of co-occurring disabilities was two, the most prevalent of which were disabilities of mobility and agility. (A prevalence rate for each of 42.8 per 100,000 was obtained.) Prevalence rates for self-reported disabilities of seeing and hearing were 15.9 per 100,000 and 19.6 per 100,000, respectively.

14. Encoding techniques include word prediction, alpha encoding and semantic compaction. Word prediction is where a device provides a list of possible words based

on the first one or two letters that an individual types. In alpha encoding, an individual recalls messages that have been pre-programmed into a device using letter codes. In semantic compaction, sequences of icons represent words, phrases or sentences.

15. A range of message formulation strategies is available. These include spelling letter by letter. Messages can be retrieved word by word, picture by picture, phrase by phrase, sentence by sentence or as full stories. Prepared speeches or talks can also be retrieved.

16. Yorkston and Beukelman (2000) state that '[s]taging of intervention is the sequencing of management so that current problems are addressed and future problems anticipated. Staging is important in dysarthria intervention because many of the conditions associated with dysarthria are not stable' (159). Yorkston and Beukelman describe the staging of treatment in three clinical populations with a varying clinical course: (1) TBI, which has a stable or recovering course, (2) PD, which has a slowly progressive course, and (3) ALS, which has a rapidly progressive course. AAC plays a prominent part in the management of each of these disorders. However, the timing of AAC intervention also varies with the course of the disorder. In TBI, dysarthria is most severe in the weeks and months postinjury. The development of augmentative communication in this postinjury period is needed to establish functional communication. Depending on the TBI patient's level of speech proficiency in the weeks and months following injury, augmentative techniques may be phased out or continued.

17 The patients in this study had the most severe degree of ALS impairment. These patients were dependent on invasive mechanical ventilation, required tube feeding and were confined to bed. They were all able to communicate effectively through physical motion.

18. Using figures from the Japan ALS Association, Hirano et al. state that invasive mechanical ventilation is initiated for approximately 36 per cent of Japanese ALS patients. These investigators emphasise that the decision to initiate ventilation is influenced by social, economic and cultural factors and that usage patterns vary between and within different cultures.

19. Hirano et al. emphasise that, as well as facilitating personal communication, computer-assisted communication also gives ALS patients access to support networks on the Internet.

20 In a review of the literature on voice onset time (VOT) in aphasia, AOS and dysarthria, Auzou et al. (2000) state that VOT perturbations in aphasia are characterised as phonemic or phonetic errors, while VOT abnormalities in AOS and dysarthria are taken to reflect a loss of motor control.

21 The PICA (Porch Index of Communicative Ability) permits an assessment of gestural, verbal and graphic performance. A PICA profile in which inordinately low verbal performance coexists with better graphic and gestural performance may signal AOS (Wertz et al. 1984).

22. The 15 articulation characteristics included in the Apraxia Battery for Adults are (1) exhibits phonemic anticipatory errors ('gleen glass' for 'green grass'), (2) exhibits phonemic perseverative errors ('pep' for 'pet'), (3) exhibits phonemic transposition errors ('Arifca' for 'Africa'), (4) exhibits phonemic voicing errors ('ben' for 'pen'), (5) exhibits phonemic vowel errors ('moan' for 'man'), (6) exhibits visible/audible searching, (7) exhibits numerous off-target attempts at the word, (8) errors are highly inconsistent, (9) errors increase as phonemic sequence increases, (10) exhibits fewer errors with automatic speech than volitional speech, (11) exhibits marked difficulty initiating speech, (12) intrudes schwa sound between syllables or in consonant clusters, (13) exhibits abnormal prosodic features, (14) exhibits awareness of errors and inability to correct them and (15) exhibits expressive-receptive gap.

23. In a recent review of interventions for AOS following stroke, West et al. (2005) conclude that '[t]here is no evidence from randomised trials to support or refute the effectiveness of therapeutic interventions for apraxia of speech. There is a need for high quality randomised trials to be undertaken in this area' (1).

24. Integral stimulation is a commonly used technique for the modelling of target sounds. The client is encouraged to watch the clinician and listen to his or her production of the target sound and then imitate it. Yorkston et al. (1999) state that

> [i]ntegral stimulation works well as a motor approach to treatment, because the focus is on the movement patterns and the goal is an adequate speech signal. The clinician's models of stimuli are both auditory and visual because the clinician is producing speech while the client watches. (554)

25 Springer et al. (1999) investigated language dominance in 100 right-handed, neurologically normal subjects using functional MRI. These researchers report that 94 per cent of subjects were considered left hemisphere-dominant for language. The remaining 6 per cent of subjects had bilateral, roughly symmetric language representation.

26 These anatomical areas have been confirmed as the loci of Broca's and Wernicke's aphasia. Zhang et al. (2006b) examined 12 patients with Broca's aphasia and 21 patients with Wernicke's aphasia. Magnetic resonance spectroscopy and perfusion-weighted imaging were used to examine cerebral blood flow and metabolism changes. Hypoperfusion and hypometabolism were found in Broca's and Wernicke's areas in the aphasic patients, indicating that these areas might be the mechanisms responsible for Broca's and Wernicke's aphasia.

27 The Stroke Data Bank is a cooperative effort involving four teaching hospitals and the National Institute for Neurological Disorders and Stroke in the US. Between July 1983 and June 1986, the Stroke Data Bank enrolled 1,805 patients with acute stroke. Of these patients, 237 had sustained an intracerebral haemorrhage, 936 ischaemic infarction (not-lacune), 337 lacunar infarction, 243 a subarachnoid haemorrhage and 52 a stroke due to other aetiology.

28. There are different types of vascular dementia. When single ischaemic or thromboembolic infarcts occur in strategic areas of the dominant hemisphere (e.g. angular gyri), they can cause the symptoms of dementia (single-infarct dementia). Multiple, small cerebral infarcts that are temporally staggered can cause cumulative damage and progressive cognitive deficits and dementia (multi-infarct dementia). Not all forms of vascular dementia are caused by stroke. In subcortical vascular dementia, there is damage to the small blood vessels supplying the deep white matter of the brain. This damage occurs in patients with poorly controlled hypertension, diabetes mellitus, or both. Pohjasvaara et al. (1997) examined the frequency of cognitive decline and dementia three months after ischaemic stroke in a large stroke cohort. Using the criteria for dementia in DSM-III, these investigators found that the frequency of dementia in this cohort was 25.5 per cent.

29. The National Aphasia Association in the US uses a system in which aphasia is broadly classified as fluent or nonfluent.

30. In the Boston Diagnostic Aphasia Examination, aphasics are first classified as fluent or nonfluent. Fluent aphasics are subdivided into Wernicke's, anomic, conduction and transcortical sensory aphasia. Nonfluent aphasics are subdivided into Broca's and transcortical motor aphasia. A further nonfluent aphasia and the seventh type of aphasia in the 'traditional classification' – global aphasia – is characterised by a severe impairment of all language functions.

31. See Marshall et al. (2001). Also, see Marshall et al. (1996a and 1996b) for the source of 'a stage of firms . . .'. The two examples of neologism in the main text are taken from Robson et al. (2003).

32. This test is unlike other language batteries that are commercially available. The Comprehensive Aphasia Test (CAT) (Swinburn et al. 2005) contains a total of 34 subtests arranged in three sections: cognitive screen, language battery and disability questionnaire. The language battery forms the main body of the test and assesses language comprehension, repetition, spoken language production, reading aloud and writing. The CAT is based on models of language processing from cognitive neuropsychology. As such, it is fully compatible with PALPA. In fact, clinicians are encouraged to use the CAT to find out where to focus larger assessments such as PALPA.

33. There is evidence to suggest that performance on tasks used in aphasia tests fails to reflect a client's skills at a conversational level. Mayer and Murray (2003) examined lexical retrieval in 14 individuals with aphasia. Word retrieval was assessed in three contexts: single-word confrontation naming (a typical method of assessing word retrieval in aphasia tests), composite description and conversational speech. These investigators found superior lexical retrieval and self-correction or errors in connected speech versus single-word naming tasks. Although confrontation naming scores were strongly related to the severity of aphasia (mild versus moderate), they were not significantly correlated with naming abilities in connected speaking tasks. Mayer and Murray conclude that '[t]hese findings endorse the incorporation of

discourse-level tasks into aphasia assessment and treatment protocols' (2003:481). Other studies have found evidence of a strong correlation between performance on language assessments and communicative performance. In a study of 67 aphasic acute stroke patients, Bakheit et al. (2005) found a statistically significant correlation between performance on the Western Aphasia Battery and the Communicative Effectiveness Index on study entry and at 4, 8, 12 and 24 weeks after the start of speech and language therapy. See also Ulatowska et al. (2003).

34. Perkins et al. (1999) examined the temporal reliability of analyses of collaborative repair in aphasic conversation. These investigators compared quantitative and qualitative analyses of collaborative repair undertaken during conversations between aphasic individuals and their relatives on four different occasions. Quantitative analysis revealed significant within-subject variation in the amount of collaborative repair that occurred in the conversations and even greater between-subject variation. Qualitative analysis indicated reliability in the interactional challenges that occurred as a result of aphasia (the trouble sources that triggered collaborative repair were consistent across the four conversations) and in the interactional mechanisms that were used to deal with trouble areas (there was consistency across conversations in the resolution of collaborative repair).

35. The CAPPA and CAPPCI consist of three components. The first component is a structured interview that is to be undertaken with the key conversational partner of the aphasic/cognitively impaired client. The second feature of this profile is a method for the analysis of a 10-minute sample of unscripted conversation between the client and his or her conversational partner. The third component, a summary profile, combines information from the interview and conversational sampler.

36. Muller (1999) argues for incorporating psychosocial adjustment into treatment plans for people with aphasia.

37. Primary progressive aphasia is a form of dementia that is characterised by isolated language impairment for at least two years. The most common variants of the disorder are progressive nonfluent aphasia, semantic dementia and logopenic progressive aphasia (Amici et al. 2006).

38. Apart from these more serious consequences of dysphagia for an individual's health, studies have also revealed an adverse impact of this disorder on clients' quality of life. Klugman and Ross (2002) conducted a questionnaire on 30 respondents with multiple sclerosis. Fifty three per cent of MS respondents who reported swallowing problems perceived that it had an adverse influence on quality of life.

39. Kulbersh et al. (2006) examined the effect of pretreatment swallowing exercises on dysphagia in 37 patients who underwent primary radiation or combined chemoradiation treatment for newly diagnosed hypopharyngeal, laryngeal or oropharyngeal primary tumours. Patients who performed these exercises showed improvement in overall score on a dysphagia inventory compared to control subjects who received post-treatment therapy.

40. The timing and range of laryngeal excursion are frequently disrupted in dysphagia. Kwon et al. (2005) examined laryngeal excursion (hyolaryngeal excursion) in 46 patients with unilateral medullary infarction. Seven patients (54 per cent) with lateral medullary infarction had problems with the range of hyolaryngeal excursion, five (38 per cent) had problems with the timing of excursion and one patient (8 per cent) had both. For patients with medial medullary infarction, problems with the timing of excursion were frequent (86 per cent), while problems with the range of excursion were present in only one patient (14 per cent).

41. The clinical significance of an absent gag reflex is uncertain. While some investigators believe that it is predictive of aspiration in patients, other studies suggest that it may have little significance for aspiration or dysphagia in general. Davies et al. (1995), for example, found that up to 30 per cent of healthy younger adults and 44 per cent of healthy older adults may have unilateral or bilateral absent gag reflexes.

42. Other techniques include electromyography, manometry, scintigraphy and respiratory inductance plethysmography. Shaw et al. (2004) used a scintigraphic technique to quantify the efficiency of bolus clearance during the oral-pharyngeal swallow in subjects with dysphagia. Moreau-Gaudry et al. (2005) propose the use of respiratory inductance plethysmography to investigate swallowing and swallowing disorders in elderly patients.

43. Wallenberg's syndrome is a neurological condition that is caused by a stroke in the brainstem's vertebral or posterior inferior cerebellar artery. Symptoms include problems with swallowing, nausea and vomiting, dizziness, hoarseness, nystagmus (rapid involuntary movements of the eyes), balance and gait coordination.

44. Leslie et al. (2004) found that the reliability of individual judges varied widely and that agreement between judges was poor. Moreover, comparison with videofluoroscopic findings yielded 66 per cent specificity and 62 per cent sensitivity. Stroud et al. (2002) found high agreement between raters when aspiration occurred. However, there was significant overdetection of aspiration in nonaspirating swallows. On the basis of these findings at least, cervical auscultation has some way to go before it can be considered a reliable and valid tool for the detection of aspiration.

45. The modified Evan's blue dye test (MEBDT) is an inexpensive, relatively simple bedside technique for the assessment of aspiration in the tracheotomised patient. Food and liquid are mixed with blue dye. If blue dye is found in the patient's suctioned secretions, aspiration is presumed to have occurred. Belafsky et al. (2003) examined the accuracy of the MEBDT in predicting aspiration in tracheotomised patients. Thirty patients (mean age = 65 years) with a tracheostomy tube, who underwent a bedside swallowing evaluation between October 2001 and March 2002 in a long-term acute care hospital, were assessed using the MEBDT and FEES. The MEBDT had sensitivity of 82 per cent and specificity of 38 per cent. Sensitivity was 100 per cent for patients receiving mechanical ventilation and 76 per cent for those who did not receive ventilation. Regardless of ventilator status,

the specificity of the MEBDT was low (33–40 per cent). Belafsky et al. conclude that these results support the use of the MEBDT as a screening tool for patients with a tracheostomy tube.

46. Sensory testing is a relatively recent adjunct to the FEES procedure. During sensory testing, air pulse stimuli are delivered to the mucosa innervated by the superior laryngeal nerve via a flexible endoscope. This technique permits an objective determination of laryngopharyngeal sensory discrimination thresholds. Setzen et al. (2003) found that laryngopharyngeal sensory deficits were more likely to be associated with aspiration in the presence of impaired pharyngeal motor function. Specifically, the prevalence of aspiration in patients with a moderate or severe decrease in laryngopharyngeal sensation was 0 per cent and 15 per cent, respectively, in persons with intact pharyngeal function and 67 per cent and 100 per cent, respectively, in persons with impaired pharyngeal function.

47. See Kuperberg and Caplan (2003) for discussion of the neural correlates of language abnormalities in schizophrenia.

48. The standard view is that phonology is intact in schizophrenia. Covington et al. (2005) state that '[a]ccording to all reports, segmental phonology in schizophrenia is obstinately normal' (90). However, findings such as those of Walder et al. (2006), discussed in the main text, suggest that this view may be in need of some revision. Also see note 49.

49. The aim of Walder et al.'s study was to examine sex differences in language dysfunction in schizophrenia. While the language performance of male schizophrenic patients was depressed relative to controls, language function was found to be relatively preserved in female patients. Phonology was the least affected language domain in male patients and the most affected domain in female patients.

50. Schizophrenic subjects are known to produce long sequences of utterances in which sound or meaning associations between words are developed. The phenomenon of glossomania is demonstrated by the following examples from Cohen (1978:29):

> (Subject is asked the colour of an object. It is salmon pink)
> A fish swims. You call it a salmon. You cook it. You put it in a can. You open the can. You look at it in this colour.
> Looks like clay. Sounds like gray. Take you for a roll in the hay. Hay-day. Mayday. Help. I need help.

Covington et al. (2005) describe glossomania as a form of derailment that is driven by self-monitoring.

6

Disorders of Fluency

6.1 Introduction

Stuttering (or stammering) has been one of the most extensively examined communication disorders in the clinical literature. It is also one of the few communication disorders that holds a position of prominence amongst members of the public. Notwithstanding the intense professional and public scrutiny that this disorder has received, stuttering remains to this day an elusive disorder that has evaded most attempts to capture its nature. It is unsurprising, therefore, that Wingate (2002) should remark that the three 'most thoroughly supportable and significant facts about stuttering' are that 'its cause is unknown, its essential nature is not understood and there is no known cure' (11). In this chapter, we leave aside perennial questions about cures for stuttering and turn our attention instead to a number of other concerns relating to the characterisation and management of this disorder. Specifically, we will examine the prevalence of stuttering and current thinking about the aetiology of this disorder. Many different techniques are used to assess and treat stuttering. We examine several of these techniques with particular emphasis on the methods that are used to treat stuttering. A question of particular concern to clinicians is the efficacy of the techniques that are used to treat child and adult stutterers. We examine the findings of several efficacy studies. Despite being the most prominent and extensively investigated disorder of fluency, stuttering is not the only fluency disorder that is assessed and treated by clinicians. The less well known disorder of cluttering will also be examined in this chapter.

6.2 Stuttering

While there is little clinical consensus on issues such as the cause of stuttering or the most effective methods of treatment for this disorder, clinicians are largely in agreement on the presenting features of stuttering. Wingate defines stuttering as a speech disorder in which there is 'a unique anomaly in the flow of speech characterized by iterative and/or perseverative speech elements involving word/syllable-initial position' (2002:9). The 'speech elements' that are involved in iterations are single speech sounds or two speech sounds. For example, in attempting to say 'spoke', the stutterer may engage in iteration of /s/ or /sp/. A vowel sound, typically a schwa, may also be involved in the iteration, e.g. /spə/ for 'spoke'. The 'speech elements' that are involved in perseverations or protractions are always single speech sounds. The protracted sound may be unreleased, as in /sːːː/ for 'soap'. Both iterations and protractions may be silent or audible and occur only in word- and syllable-initial position. This initial-position feature is frequently overlooked in discussions of stuttering (Wingate 2002). Yet, along with the features of iteration and protraction of speech sounds, it is important in distinguishing the dysfluencies of stammering from nonfluencies that occur in normal speech.[1] As well as speech features, stutterers may present with one or more accessory or secondary features. These behaviours are diverse in nature and include eye blinking, grimace and lip tremor. We will examine the speech and accessory features of stuttering further in section 6.2.2.

6.2.1 Epidemiology and Aetiology

The prevalence of stuttering varies considerably with the age and sex of speakers in a population. Craig et al. (2002) report that the prevalence of stuttering over a whole population in the state of New South Wales in Australia was 0.72 per cent. Prevalence rates were higher in younger children (1.4–1.44) and lowest in adolescence (0.53). Across all ages, the male-to-female ratio was 2.3:1. This increased to 4:1 in adolescence. The incidence or risk of stuttering was 2.1 per cent in adults aged 21–50 years, 2.8 per cent in children aged 2–5 years and 3.4 per cent in children aged 6–10 years. Van Borsel et al. (2006) studied 21,027 school pupils aged 6–20 years in Flanders, Belgium, and obtained a prevalence figure for stuttering of 0.58 per cent. Ardila et al. (1994) examined 1,879 Spanish-speaking university students and obtained a prevalence rate of 2 per cent of self-reported stuttering. Månsson (2000) studied the entire population of children born within a two-year period on the Danish island of Bornholm. The incidence of stuttering in this population reached 5.19 per cent.

Investigators have reported higher prevalence rates for stuttering in several special populations. Van Borsel et al. (2006) report a prevalence of stuttering of

2.28 per cent in a special school population of 1,272 pupils aged between 6 and 15 years. (Compare with an overall prevalence of 0.58 per cent in a regular school population examined in the same study.) Devenny and Silverman (1990) examined 31 adults with Down's syndrome and found that 42 per cent were stutterers. Stansfield (1990) studied 793 adults with learning disabilities and found that 6.3 per cent of this population had idiopathic dysfluencies. In other special populations, there is evidence that the prevalence of stuttering is lower than that of the general population. For example, Montgomery and Fitch (1988) surveyed 9,930 students in 77 regional, private and state schools for the hearing-impaired. Dysfluency was examined in both oral and manual modes of communication. Across both modes, the prevalence of stuttering was 0.12 per cent. Dalston et al. (1987) studied 534 patients with structural abnormalities of the velopharyngeal complex. Only one subject's speech could be characterised as stuttering, giving a prevalence rate for this population of 1.87 per 1,000. These investigators concluded that this prevalence rate did not differ significantly from 7 per 1,000, the prevalence rate of stuttering that would be expected in the general population.

The aetiology of stuttering is likely to be multifactorial in nature. Genetic factors have been known for some time to play an important role in the development of this disorder. Felsenfeld et al. (2000) screened a large population-based twin sample from the Australian Twin Registry for stuttering. These investigators found that approximately 70 per cent of the variance in liability to stuttering was found to be attributable to additive genetic effects, with non-shared environmental effects accounting for the remaining variance. As every clinician knows, many stutterers have a positive family history for stuttering. Among a clinical population of 169 adult and adolescent stutterers, Poulos and Webster (1991) found that 112 subjects (66 per cent) reported a family history of stuttering. Viswanath et al. (2000) found that the biological relatives of stutterers have an approximately 10-fold higher risk of stuttering than that in the general population. Ambrose et al. (1993) found that 71 per cent of their sample had a positive family history of stuttering in their immediate or extended families. This decreased to 43 per cent when only first-degree relatives were considered. The frequency of stuttering was significantly higher amongst the male relatives of probands in this study than amongst the female relatives. For male probands, the male-to-female ratio of stuttering relatives was 3.49. This ratio decreased to 1.50 for relatives of female probands. Ambrose et al. concluded that the inheritance of liability for stuttering in the families in this study is most consistent with transmission of a single major genetic locus.

As well as genetic factors being linked to the development of stuttering, neurological factors have also been found to play a role in the aetiology of the disorder. This has been the case for an acquired form of stuttering called neurogenic stuttering[2] more than in developmental stuttering. Ward (2006) remarks that '[i]n contrast to the limited number of regions identified as associated with developmental stuttering, most cortical and subcortical areas, with the exception of the occipital lobe, have been implicated in neurogenic stuttering' (333). Alm (2004) argues that the basal ganglia–thalamocortical motor circuits through the putamen are likely to play a key role in stuttering.[3] Doi et al. (2003) examined a 60-year-old man who acquired stuttering after a brainstem infarction. These investigators claim that the midbrain and upper pons could be lesion sites responsible for acquired stuttering. Balasubramanian et al. (2003) examined a 57-year-old male who developed neurogenic stuttering following an ischaemic lesion to the orbital surface of the right frontal lobe and the pons. Helm-Estabrooks and Hotz (1998) report the case of a 30-year-old woman who developed stuttering following a head injury sustained in a road traffic accident.[4] One week after this accident, MRI revealed a right frontal/parietal lesion. Van Borsel et al. (2003) describe the case of a 38-year-old male who presented with neurogenic stuttering subsequent to an ischaemic lesion of the left thalamus. Sakai et al. (2002) studied a 57-year-old man who developed stuttering as an early symptom of progressive supranuclear palsy. MRI revealed atrophy of the midbrain tegmentum and dilatation of the third ventricle with a few lacunar infarcts in the basal ganglia.[5]

Thus far, we have only considered organic factors in the aetiology of stuttering. However, psychological factors have also been credited with playing a significant role in the development of stuttering. In fact, notwithstanding our increasing knowledge of the role of organic factors in stuttering, it is still psychological frameworks that have the greatest influence on therapies for stuttering. Ward (2006) discusses these various frameworks, which include the view that stuttering is a habit, an operant disorder, a disorder arising due to anticipatory struggle behaviour or approach-avoidance conflict and a diagnosogenic disorder (stuttering arising due to parental misdiagnosis in early development). The diagnosogenic theory of stuttering is now discredited, although aspects of this theory still influence other approaches. Cognitive-behavioural therapies, such as Van Riper's (1973) speech modification approaches, draw on concepts relating to anticipatory struggle and approach-avoidance. The view that stuttering is an operant disorder is the basis of a number of therapies, including the Lidcombe Program. We examine this program in section 6.2.4, along with several other interventions that treat the aetiology of stuttering as psychological in nature.

6.2.2 Clinical Presentation

The main features of stuttering were introduced in section 6.2. In this section, we examine those features in more detail, as well as consider other characteristics of the disorder. We examine, for example, the effect of various linguistic factors on stuttering. Other communication disorders have been frequently reported to occur in stuttering. We discuss, in particular, the presence of phonological and language impairments in children who stutter. Auditory perceptual and auditory processing deficits have been reported to occur in stuttering. On account of the role of auditory processing in some treatment techniques, we conclude this section by considering these deficits in stuttering.

The iterations and protractions of stuttering have been the focus of several studies. Natke et al. (2006) examined dysfluencies in 24 German-speaking preschool children who stutter. Several stuttering dysfluencies – namely, prolongations, blocks and part- and one-syllable word repetitions – were significantly more frequent in these preschoolers (mean = 9.2 per cent) than in a control group of 24 children who did not stutter (mean = 1.2 per cent). There were no significant differences between these groups with regard to 'normal' dysfluencies. Children who stutter also produced significantly more iterations (mean = 1.28 iterations) than nonstuttering children (mean = 1.09 iterations). The dysfluencies of children who had been stuttering for 1–5 months did not differ from those of children who had stuttered for 8–22 months. Time since stuttering onset was a significant factor in the number and type of dysfluencies produced by 36 children who were studied by Pellowski and Conture (2002). The percentage of dysfluencies was significantly related to the time since stuttering onset in these children. Additionally, there was a moderate correlation between time since onset and the percentage of dysfluencies consisting of dysrhythmic phonations in four-year-old stutterers. (This same correlation was not found in three-year-old stutterers.) Children who stutter in this study differed from nonstuttering controls in the percentage of total dysfluencies, percentage of stuttering-like dysfluencies (SLD), weighted SLD measure and mean number of repetition units.

While several studies have examined the frequency and type of dysfluency in children who stutter, considerably fewer studies have undertaken to measure the duration of speech sound iterations and protractions in stuttering. A notable exception is a study by Zebrowski (1994), who measured the duration of sound prolongations and sound/syllable repetitions in the conversational speech of school-age children who stutter. The average duration of stuttering in these children was approximately three-quarters of a second and was not correlated significantly with age, frequency of speech dysfluency or length of postonset interval. Zebrowski (1991) examined the duration of within-word dysfluencies in 10 children who had been stuttering for one year or less and in 10 nonstuttering children. No significant group differences were found in the duration of acoustically measured sound/syllable repetitions and sound prolongations. Zebrowski concludes that these results 'support findings from previous perceptual work that type and frequency of speech dysfluency, not duration, are the principal characteristics listeners use in distinguishing these two talker groups' (1991:483).

Several studies have reported dysfluencies in word-final position in children. Van Borsel et al. (2005) studied word-final dysfluencies in a 12-year-old boy. Word-final dysfluencies were the major type of dysfluency in this child and most often involved repetition of a linguistic unit larger than a single consonant. These dysfluenices occurred more frequently on multisyllabic than on monosyllabic words, on content than on function words and at the end of a phrase rather than in initial or medial position. McAllister and Kingston (2005) examined final part-word repetitions in the speech of two school-age boys. Repetitions occurred in spontaneous conversation and during reading and sentence repetition. The majority of repetitions were observed in spontaneous speech. Dysfluencies were produced on both content and function words. In neither boy was there apparent awareness of the dysfluencies, abnormal muscle tension or accessory behaviours. Wingate and others place emphasis on word- and syllable-initial position in stuttering (see section 6.2). The relationship of word-final dysfluencies to stuttering is thus unclear.

The literature on stuttering contains numerous reports of verbal and nonverbal behaviours occurring as secondary or accessory features of the disorder.[6] Vanryckeghem et al. (2004) examined the behaviours employed secondary to the anticipation or occurrence of speech disruption by 42 adults who stutter. The top 10 behaviours used by these adults included substitution of one word for another, pausing, avoidance of eye contact, silent rehearsal and looking away. The total number of these behaviours used by adults who stutter ranged from a low of 6 to a high of 59. (Compare to a range of 0–28 in adults who do not stutter.) While none of the adults who stutter used less than six different behaviours, nine nonstuttering adults (12 per cent) used none of these behaviours. The difference in the mean number of behaviours used by adults who do and do not stutter – 20.79 and 5.38, respectively – was found to be statistically significant. As well as a difference in the number of behaviours used, adults who do and do not stutter differ in the types of behaviour used. Five behaviours that were most reported by adults who stutter were not among the top 10 behaviours used by adults who do not stutter. These behaviours were pausing before a feared word, silently rehearsing a sound, word or phrase, pretending not to know an answer, taking a deep breath before speaking and omitting particular words. Vanryckeghem et al. conclude that

> the findings that have resulted from this investigation highlight the importance of responses secondary to stuttering . . . Though these responses are secondary to stuttering, rather than a constituent element of it, the frequency with which they occur, their often aberrant and attention getting nature and the fact that they can interfere

with communication all point to the need for a better understanding of their nature and use. (2004:246)

Several linguistic factors have been linked to stuttering in children and adults. Dayalu et al. (2002) examined the frequency of stuttering in 10 adults as a function of grammatical word type (i.e. content and function words). A list of 126 words, which were matched for initial sound and approximate number of syllables, was read aloud by the adults in this study. Stuttering frequency was significantly greater for content words in isolation than for function words. Dayalu et al. use word frequency to explain this finding. Specifically, the greater frequency with which function words are used may lead to a 'generalised adaptation effect' for these words and a concomitant reduction in stuttering frequency. Dworzynski et al. (2003) studied German-speaking adults who stutter and found that stuttering rate increased significantly on content words. Word length also increased stuttering rate significantly in these adults. As well as observing an effect of increasing word length on stuttering, investigators have also observed an effect of increasing utterance length and syntactic complexity on stuttering. Zackheim and Conture (2003) studied six children who stutter and found that both stuttering and nonstuttering dysfluencies are most likely to occur on utterances that are long and complex. Also, utterances that exceeded these children's mean length of utterance were more apt to be stuttered or dysfluent. Kleinow and Smith (2000) found that the speech motor stability of eight adults who stutter decreased with increasing syntactic complexity of utterances.

Children and adults who stutter often present with other communication disorders. Blood et al. (2003) surveyed 2,628 children who stutter and found that 62.8 per cent had co-occurring speech disorders, language disorders or non–speech-language disorders.[7] The most frequently reported speech disorders were articulation disorders (33.5 per cent) and phonology disorders (12.7 per cent), both of which occurred more commonly in males than in females. Arndt and Healey (2001) recorded concomitant disorders that occurred in 467 children who stutter. Amongst these children, 262 (56 per cent) had a fluency disorder only, while 205 (44 per cent) had a verified phonological and/or language disorder. Ryan (1992) administered a series of articulation, language and fluency tests to 20 stuttering and 20 nonstuttering preschool children. Stuttering children attained lower scores than nonstuttering children on 7 out of 8 language measures. Moreover, their language performance was also slightly lower than the average score for their age group according to the tests' normative samples. Although 25 per cent of the stuttering group (all boys) required treatment for articulation problems, these groups did not differ in terms of articulation proficiency. Bajaj et al. (2004) found that children who do not stutter were significantly better than children who do stutter in judging syntactically and semantically anomalous sentences. Several studies have failed to find evidence of a relationship between stuttering and language and phonology disorders. Gregg and Yairi (2007) found no relationship between phonological skills and stuttering severity in 28 preschool children who were near the onset of their stuttering. Anderson and Conture (2000) found that the difference between receptive/expressive language and receptive vocabulary scores was not significantly correlated with overall stuttering frequency in 20 children who stutter. Nippold (2004) found that stuttering children who have at least one additional disorder are more likely to be recommended for treatment than children who have stuttering alone. Studies that attempt to establish the number of concomitant communication disorders in children who stutter by performing caseload surveys, Nippold argues, are thus overestimating the rate of these disorders. See also Nippold (2001, 2002).

Several treatment techniques for stuttering (e.g. delayed auditory feedback) function by modifying the auditory signal to the stutterer. For this reason, we conclude this section by examining studies that have found evidence of auditory processing deficits in stuttering. Foundas et al. (2004) found that left-handed male stutterers and right-handed female stutterers have atypical auditory processing. Dietrich (1997) found evidence of central auditory processing problems in 11 males who stuttered. Howell et al. (2000) used a backward masking task to investigate central auditory processing in children who stutter. These children had deficits in backward masking compared with a group of fluent children. Moreover, backward-masking thresholds were positively correlated with stuttering frequency. Howell et al. (2006) examined the performance of 30 children who stutter in a backward-masking task. These children were judged to be stuttering at least one year before their 12th birthday. They were assessed again at age 12 plus to determine if their stutter had persisted or recovered. Twelve speakers persisted in their stuttering, while 18 recovered from stuttering. Howell et al. found that thresholds on this backward-masking task were significantly higher for persistent than for recovered stutterers. Corbera et al. (2005) found evidence that adults with persistent developmental stuttering have auditory perceptual deficits. These individuals had abnormal permanent traces for speech sounds. This abnormal speech sound representation, Corbera et al. argue, may underlie their speech disorder. Howell and Williams (2004) found that children who stutter, like fluent children, continue to develop auditory sensitivity for sounds in noise through to teenage years. However, children who stutter have a different pattern of auditory development compared with participants who do not stutter.

6.2.3 Clinical Assessment

It is now widely recognised that assessment of stuttering must be multidimensional in nature. Susca (2002), for example, argues that assessment of the child who stutters in the school environment from multiple perspectives reveals motor, linguistic, social, affective and cognitive issues. Ward (2006) describes 'two basic strands of the disorder' that are normally examined during assessment: motor speech activity and the cognitive perspective of the disorder. The former strand, Ward argues, is assessed by means of speech rate data and fluency counts. The latter strand is assessed using attitudinal questionnaires. In this section, we examine both these dimensions of stuttering. The information that is gleaned from a multidimensional assessment of stuttering is integral to treatment planning. In section 6.2.4, we examine different approaches to the treatment of stuttering as well as consider the efficacy of these approaches.

The most commonly used method of assessing stuttering severity is the stuttering frequency count. This measure is expressed as a percentage of stuttered syllables or words and is calculated by dividing the total number of stuttered syllables (words) in a speech sample by the total number of syllables (words) spoken. Alongside the stuttering frequency count, clinicians often report various measures of speech rate. Expressed as either the number of syllables or the number of words spoken per minute, these measures are calculated by dividing the total number of all syllables spoken (speaking rate) or the total number of nonstuttered syllables spoken (articulatory rate) by the total length of time taken (in seconds), which is then multiplied by 60. These various calculations are only useful to the extent that resulting figures can be compared to normative data. Andrews and Ingham (1971), for example, have obtained normative data for speaking rate that have been universally accepted. These investigators have calculated a mean figure of 196 syllables per minute and a standard deviation of 34 (in other words, 162–230 syllables per minute) for conversational speech of nonstuttering adult speakers. Similarly, Ambrose and Yairi (1999) state that a child who produces three or more stuttering-like dysfluencies per 100 syllables should be suspected of exhibiting stuttering. On the average, children who are normally fluent present with less than 1.5 stuttering-like dysfluencies per 100 syllables.[8]

The measurements of speech rate and fluency described above have been extensively used by clinicians and researchers to assess the severity of stuttering in clients. In this way, Brundage et al. (2006) calculated the percentage of stuttered syllables for 2–3 adults in a study that examined the frequency of stuttering in challenging and supportive virtual reality job interview conditions. Dayalu et al. (2001) calculated stuttering frequency counts in a study of the effects of producing and listening to the vowel /a/ on the overt stuttering moments of eight subjects. Stuttering frequency counts are included in the Stuttering Severity Instrument (Riley 1972, 1994), an established, standardised test of stuttering that has been validated for use with both children and adults.[9] Hall et al. (1999) compared two metrics of articulatory rate – syllables per second and phones per second – in a study of developmental changes in speaking rate in preschool children who stutter. Notwithstanding the widespread use of these measurements, they are not without various problems. The sample upon which these measurements are based has been the subject of much controversy. Ward (2006) states that most clinicians advocate using a speech sample that contains two minutes of the client's speech, excluding pauses. Other researchers collect samples that contain a certain number of syllables. For example, De Andrade et al. (2003) collected speech samples that contained at least 200 fluent syllables in a study of speech rate in adults who stutter. The significance of sample size is clearly demonstrated in a study by Sawyer and Yairi (2006). These investigators found a statistically significant difference in the number of SLDs per 100 syllables between the early and later sections of speech samples that were obtained from 20 stuttering children of varying dysfluency levels. In general, group means for SLDs grew larger as the sample size increased. Further problems with fluency measures include which speech features to count as stuttered dysfluencies (and which to treat as normal nonfluencies), issues relating to reliability[10] and whether to include moments of secondary stuttering in fluency counts. For further discussion of these problems and other issues relating to fluency measurements, the reader is referred to chapter 9 in Ward (2006).

Assessments which examine the client's attitude to stuttering began to emerge in the late 1960s. These so-called cognitive assessments go beyond the overt stuttering behaviours that are assessed by means of the fluency and rate measures just examined to consider cognitive and affective aspects of the disorder. One of the first cognitive assessments was the Perceptions of Stuttering Inventory (PSI) (Woolf 1967). The PSI contains a list of 60 questions, 20 of which address issues of struggle, avoidance and expectancy in stuttering. Questions require the respondent either to agree or to disagree that the statement is characteristic of him or her. This assessment is still in use today. Blomgren et al. (2005) used the PSI as part of a multidimensional evaluation of the outcomes of a three-week intensive stuttering modification treatment programme. Immediately post-treatment, statistically significant improvements were observed on scores for the struggle, avoidance and expectancy subscales of the PSI. At six months post-treatment, statistically significant improvements were still observed on the avoidance and expectancy subscales. A second cognitive assessment used by Blomgren et al. was the Locus of Control of Behaviour Scale (LCBS) (Craig et al. 1984). This scale consists of 17 questions which probe the extent to which the person with a stutter views his or her speech behaviour as the product of events that are internally or externally controlled.

A recent cognitive assessment that is based on the World Health Organization's International Classification of Functioning, Disability and

Health is the Overall Assessment of the Speaker's Experience of Stuttering (OASES) (Yaruss and Quesal 2004). This assessment examines all aspects of the stuttering disorder under four headings: (1) general perspectives about stuttering, (2) affective, behavioural and cognitive reactions to stuttering, (3) functional communication difficulties and (4) impact of stuttering on the speaker's quality of life. The OASES questionnaire probes these areas by having respondents circle a number on a five-point scale. Scale development, reliability and validity assessment and scoring procedures have recently been summarised by Yaruss and Quesal (2006), who argue that OASES can help document treatment outcomes in adults who stutter. While most cognitive assessments are devised for use with adolescents and adults, a growing number are being used with child clients. Vanryckeghem et al. (2005) used a self-report measure called the KiddyCAT to compare the speech-associated attitude of 45 children aged between 3 and 6 years who stutter with that of 63 nonstuttering children. These investigators found that the children who stutter had a significantly more negative attitude towards their speech than did their nonstuttering peers. Vanryckeghem et al. state that this finding 'suggests the need to measure, by standardized means, the speech-associated attitude of incipient stutterers and, when appropriate, to make the assessment and treatment of negative attitude toward speech a meaningful aspect of therapy' (2005:307). For further discussion of instruments that are used to measure cognitive and affective aspects of stuttering, see Susca (2006).

In general, cognitive assessments are conducted by means of self-report measures. These measures, it is argued, are able to reflect covert aspects of stuttering and are more ecologically valid than assessments that examine clinic-based fluency. These attributes have made self-report measures a popular choice amongst clinicians and researchers who are concerned to evaluate interventions for stuttering. Guntupalli et al. (2006) argue that

> [a]ny efficient and effective means of evaluating intervention methods over the long term should include a form of self-report as a primary tool as it best accesses the experiential sense of 'loss of control' and other covert behaviours. Overt measures should be used to supplement or complement the self-report data. (1)

As well as measuring behaviours that are lost to assessments of overt stuttering, self-report measures have been found to have good inter- and intra-rater reliability. O'Brian et al. (2004) found that self-ratings of stuttering severity made by adults immediately after speaking showed good agreement with the ratings of a speech-language pathologist in 9 out of 10 cases studied. Also, in eight of these cases there was good agreement between ratings made initially and those undertaken six months later from recordings.[11]

Measures of social anxiety are often included in assessments of stuttering. Kraaimaat et al. (2002) administered the Inventory of Interpersonal Situations (IIS) (Van Dam-Baggen and Kraaimaat 1999) to 89 people who stutter and 131 nonstuttering subjects. These investigators found that subjects who stutter experienced significantly higher levels of emotional tension or discomfort in social situations and made significantly fewer social responses than subjects who do not stutter. Also, when the scores of the adults on the IIS were examined, it was found that approximately 50 per cent fell within the range of a group of highly socially anxious psychiatric patients. Messenger et al. (2004) examined the role of expectancies of social harm in anxiety in 34 subjects who stutter. These subjects and 34 individuals who do not stutter completed the Fear of Negative Evaluation (FNE) Scale (Watson and Friend 1969) and the Endler Multi-dimensional Anxiety Scales – Trait (EMAS-T) (Endler et al. 1991). There was a significant difference between stuttering and nonstuttering subjects on the FNE scale, with people who stutter exhibiting anxiety that is restricted to the social domain. On the EMAS-T, there were significant differences between these two groups of subjects on subtests that address people and social interactions in which social evaluation might occur. Cabel et al. (2002) examined self-reported anxiety in people who do and do not stutter. During a speech evaluation session, each stuttering and nonstuttering participant was stopped and asked to rate his or her anxiety at that particular moment. Ratings were obtained during a baseline period, during a period in which subjects were thinking about their speech and during three different speaking tasks. Subjects who stutter reported significantly more anxiety throughout the entire session than nonstuttering subjects. Conditions during the session had no significant effect on reports of anxiety.

6.2.4 Clinical Intervention

Extensive clinical and research effort has been directed towards the treatment of stuttering. Numerous treatment programmes are now in use with preschool, school-age and adult clients who stutter. Treatment approaches variously aim to modify the client's speaking environment (in the case of the preschool and school-age child), address attitudes related to speaking and stuttering (cognitive approach), train clients in the use of techniques designed to enhance fluency (fluency-shaping approach) or encourage clients to produce less effortful stuttering (stuttering modification approach). In reality, two or more of these approaches may be integrated within a single treatment programme. In this section, we discuss each of these approaches and examine some of the techniques that clinicians use to treat children and adults who stutter. An issue of central significance in stuttering research and practice is the efficacy of treatment. This issue has once again been brought into sharp focus by a recent study by Kalinowski et al. (2005), which found that therapy for stuttering in children may not contribute any improvement beyond that which comes about through natural spontaneous remission.[12] This rather depressing finding is a stark reminder that we still have some way to go in terms of our understanding and treatment of this speech disorder. At a minimum, it indicates that a key component of any future research agenda in stuttering must be the development of new techniques and/or revision of current techniques with a view to improving the efficacy of treatment methods.

Having assessed the child client, the clinician may decide that an indirect approach to therapy is the best course of action. Such an approach may be indicated if the child is showing signs of a marginal stutter. Alternatively, some clinicians prefer to use an indirect approach initially and will later adopt more direct techniques if this is found not to be successful. Whatever clinical judgements motivate the decision to use an indirect approach, the common element in all indirect treatments is the emphasis placed on manipulating the child's environment. Such manipulation may involve instructing parents in new conversation and interaction styles. For example, parents may be taught to slow their rate of speech and to ask fewer closed questions of their child. Also, they may be encouraged to spend more one-to-one time with their child or to introduce more consistent home routines. Therapy that focuses on parent–child interaction has both its supporters and detractors. Since 1993, specialist therapists have been developing a parent–child interaction approach at the Michael Palin Centre for Stammering Children in London. Opponents of this approach point to studies that demonstrate little or no relationship between parental interaction styles and fluency in children who stutter.[13] Yaruss et al. (2006) used a parent–child training programme to treat 17 children, aged 31–62 months, who stutter. Parents were taught strategies that were designed to help them reduce their concerns about stuttering and modify their communication behaviours. Children were also taught strategies to improve communication and develop healthy, appropriate communication attitudes. (This approach therefore goes beyond merely manipulating the parents' interaction style.) This treatment programme achieved a significant reduction in the children's dysfluency rates. (Mean stuttering frequency before and after treatment was 16.4 per cent and 3.2 per cent, respectively.) By the stage of follow-up evaluation (average period = 2.3 years), all 17 children had been dismissed from formal therapy for stuttering. Matthews et al. (1997) found a significant improvement in a four-year-old boy's dysfluency as a result of parent–child interaction therapy. Moreover, there was stabilisation of this new, lower rate of dysfluencies during the maintenance period.

Direct approaches to stuttering therapy in children target the act of stuttering itself. These approaches may be used on their own or in combination with indirect treatments. A relatively recent direct approach that has been found to be a particularly effective treatment for stuttering in preschool children is the Lidcombe Program. Developed as a joint project of the Faculty of Health Sciences, University of Sydney and the Stuttering Unit, Bankstown Health Service, Sydney, the Lidcombe Program is a parent-administered intervention that is based on operant methodology. The parent reinforces stutter-free speech and discourages stuttering through a number of verbal contingencies that are given as soon as possible after fluent or stuttered speech has occurred. After stutter-free speech, the parent may acknowledge the child's response (e.g. 'That was smooth'), praise the response (e.g. 'That was good talking') or request that the child evaluate the response (e.g. 'Were there any bumpy words then?'). Unambiguous stuttering is followed by the parent acknowledging the response in a nonpunitive tone of voice (e.g. 'That was a bit bumpy') or requesting that the child correct the response (e.g. 'Can you try that again?'). Verbal contingencies for stutter-free speech and stuttering should occur in a ratio of at least 5:1. At the start of treatment (stage 1), verbal contingencies are given during one or more structured conversations each day of between 10 and 15 minutes' duration. As treatment progresses, verbal contingencies are given during unstructured, naturalistic conversations that take place at various times during the day. During the maintenance phase (stage 2), verbal contingencies are gradually withdrawn. Clinic visits also become less frequent during this stage. The clinician also trains the parent in how to conduct daily ratings of the severity of the child's stuttering. A 10-point severity rating scale is used, where 1 indicates no stuttering and 10 indicates extremely severe stuttering. Ratings may be made for the whole day or for a particular speaking situation that took place on a certain day. To ensure agreement between parental ratings and ratings made by the clinician, severity ratings are discussed and compared during weekly clinic visits until scores differ by no more than one scale value.

Several studies have evaluated the efficacy of the Lidcombe Program. In one study, Jones et al. (2005) recruited 54 children from two public schools in New Zealand. All children were aged between 3 and 6 years and had a frequency of stuttering of at least 2 per cent syllables stuttered. Twenty-nine children received Lidcombe intervention and 25 children were assigned to a control group. The proportion of syllables stuttered was calculated from audio recordings of conversational speech made by parents outside the clinic. Speech samples were collected in three different speaking situations before subjects were assigned to groups and at 3, 6 and 9 months after assignment. At nine months after assignment, there was a highly significant difference in the mean proportion of syllables stuttered by subjects who received the Lidcombe treatment (1.5 per cent) and those in the control group (3.9 per cent). The resulting effect size of 2.3 per cent of syllables stuttered was more than double the minimum clinically worthwhile difference specified in the trial protocol. The Lidcombe Program, Jones et al. conclude, is an efficacious treatment for stuttering in preschool-age children. Moreover, these fluency gains are not achieved at the expense of children's language skills. Lattermann et al. (2005) found that four preschool boys who received Lidcombe treatment achieved an increase in stutter-free speech alongside increases in mean length of utterance, percentage of complex sentences and number of different words used. Harrison et al. (2004) investigated the clinical value of two components of the Lidcombe Program. The components in question were parental verbal contingencies and severity ratings. Thirty-eight preschool children who stutter were randomly assigned to one of four treatment conditions in which verbal contingencies and severity ratings were either present or absent. While there were some preliminary indications that verbal contingencies contributed to treatment outcomes, there was no evidence of a contribution to outcomes of parent severity ratings.

The school-age child who stutters must deal with a number of issues that are not so immediately pressing for his preschool counterpart. The school-age child is confronted with new and challenging speaking situations which may serve to reveal the inadequacy of his or her speaking skills. This increased awareness of communication failure may lead the child to develop avoidance strategies as well as negative attitudes about speaking and stuttering. Group therapy is an effective means of addressing these strategies and attitudes. Children who may normally be unwilling to discuss their stutter with others can often be encouraged to do so in a group setting. Many clinicians have reported that children who work in groups can share their experiences of stuttering. For example, Ward (2006) describes how during a group session with teenagers a rather reserved participant reported that he would sometimes give himself a different name on the telephone rather than stutter on the production of his own name. This was the first time this information had ever been disclosed to anyone. Much to his surprise, he discovered that two other group members employed the same avoidance strategy on the telephone. As well as facilitating revelations of this nature, group therapy can also provide children with many opportunities to use their emerging fluent speech in a range of natural speaking situations (Druce et al. 1997).

Fluency-shaping techniques and stuttering modification are typically integrated within treatment programmes for school-age children. Fluency-shaping procedures aim to modify specific speech production subsystems (respiration, phonation and articulation) with a view to achieving greater fluency. Many people who stutter employ a shallow, tense type of breathing. So-called clavicular breathing is a significant impediment to fluency and is the target of breathing techniques that aim to establish a smooth, continuous airflow for speech. With guidance and practice, the person who stutters can be taught to use the more speech-efficient pattern of diaphragmatic breathing. Abnormal patterns of phonation are also common in people who stutter. Blocking on vowels can be associated with spasmodic laryngeal closure, in which the vocal folds adduct abruptly and involuntarily. Having established smooth airflow for speech, the clinician sets about modelling soft initiation of vocal fold vibration. Hard and soft glottal onsets – e.g. [ʔa] and [ha] – are first demonstrated by the clinician and identified by the client. He or she will be encouraged to extend the time between the onset of airflow and the initiation of phonation. Initially at least, it may sound as if a [h] has been placed before the initial vowel of a word, e.g. *hhaaaample* for 'ample'. With practice, the person who stutters can learn to build soft glottal onsets into a steady but inaudible airflow. Contact between articulators is often excessively forceful in people who stutter. The technique of soft consonant contact aims to reduce the tension and force of articulatory contact, particularly in word-initial consonants and semivowels. Simple nonwords with varying phonetic categories in word-initial position are commonly used to teach this technique. The clinician can first demonstrate the difference between hard and soft articulatory contacts. This is more easily achieved for visible articulators such as the lips and teeth. The client can then attempt his or her own soft contact productions. As with other techniques, the person who stutters must become sensitive to different levels of articulatory tension if he or she is to monitor speech production and make necessary adjustments.[14]

The fluency techniques described above can also form the basis of stuttering modification approaches with school-age children.[15] However, the use of fluency skills in these approaches is more selective than in a fluency-shaping approach. Also, stuttering modification approaches address the child's perceptions and attitudes about stuttering. Ward (2006) describes how he integrates stuttering modification techniques such as cancellations and pull-outs[16] within an integrated fluency programme used to treat primary school children at the Apple House Centre for Stammering in Oxford. Baumeister et al. (2003) used elements of a fluency-shaping approach and a stuttering modification approach in a stuttering therapy summer camp for children and adolescents organised under the auspices of Austria-Self-Aid-Initiative Stuttering. Participants, who were aged between 9 and 19 years, were assessed before and after treatment and at follow-up. There was a significant reduction in stuttering frequency from 22.2 per cent to 9.5 per cent (effect size 1.29). Questionnaires completed by participants and their parents and goal attainment scalings also indicated clear improvements as a result of intervention. Healey and Scott (1995) describe a model of service delivery for school-age children who stutter that emphasises the integration of fluency-shaping and stuttering modification approaches. Guitar (1998) and Kully and Langevin (1999) advocate integrated approaches to the treatment of adolescent stuttering.

Approaches that integrate stuttering modification and fluency-shaping techniques alongside consideration of cognitive and affective factors are commonplace in the treatment of adult stuttering. Over 30 years on from the publication of his book, *The Treatment of Stuttering*, Van Riper's block modification therapy is still one of the most widely used and influential stuttering modification approaches to the treatment of stuttering.[17] Treatment involves a series of stages which can overlap. During identification, the client learns to recognise the motoric aspects of his or her stutter and identifies reactions towards it. Behaviours that are described and examined during the identification stage include core behaviours such as prolongations and repetitions, avoidance strategies that are used by the client (e.g. avoidance of particular words and speaking situations), areas of bodily tension (e.g. neck, shoulders), reactions to moments of stuttering (e.g. embarrassment) and negative attitudes towards speaking and stuttering. In the desensitisation phase of treatment, the clinician and client jointly address the various negative reactions that have built up around stuttering. The client is taught how to deal with his or her own negative reactions to stuttering, as well as the negative reactions of others. The aim of this phase is to lessen the client's fear of stuttering. Techniques that facilitate desensitisation include open stuttering, in which the client is asked to use words or engage in speaking situations that he or she habitually avoids, pseudo-stuttering or voluntary stuttering (the deliberate use of stuttering on words, for example, that would normally not induce stuttering) and freezing (in the middle of a moment of stuttering, the client holds the vocal tract in its posture until told to release it).

In the modification phase of treatment, the aim is to encourage controlled stuttering. The less effortful type of stuttering that is instituted in this phase is desirable because it is not accompanied by negative speaker and listener reactions. The client is encouraged to learn more appropriate stuttering behaviour, dispense with previously learned stuttering behaviours and develop proprioceptive awareness of motor speech activity.[18] The modification of stuttering is achieved through the techniques of cancellation, pull–outs (see note 16) and preparatory sets (the repositioning of articulators before a difficult word). Before embarking on stuttering modification, the client must be prepared to tackle feared words and stop using postponing devices, such as the insertion of words in the approach to a problematic word or sound. These desensitisation activities may require further work in the modification phase. During stabilisation, controlled or fluent stuttering is consolidated and used in a range of speaking situations. Less time is spent in direct contact with the clinician. The client continues to develop his or her ability to deal with difficult speech situations by using stuttering modification techniques. For example, where preparatory sets or pull–outs fail to prevent an episode of stuttering, cancellation may be used to 'cancel' this episode. This can prevent frustration and other negative emotions that may be triggered by the client's perceived inability to use preparatory sets and pull–outs. Similarly, pseudostuttering may be used to gain further practice in employing pull-outs and cancellation. The reader is referred to Ward (2006) for a more detailed account of Van Riper's approach.

Fluency-shaping approaches are also used extensively in the treatment of adults who stutter. These approaches have in common their use of techniques to control respiration, phonation and articulation. On the most popular fluency-shaping approach – slowed speech or prolonged speech – the fluency skills outlined previously (e.g. soft articulatory contact) are used to attain fluency alongside a much-reduced speech rate (60 syllables per minute or slower, initially). Progression to the next speech rate is conditional on the client's successful use of fluency techniques and the maintenance of fluency at the slower speech rate. Rate increments vary between programmes. Neilson and Andrews (1993) increase speech rate by 10 syllables per minute until a final rate of 200 syllables per minute is achieved. In Boberg and Kully's (1985) comprehensive stuttering programme, increments of 30 syllables per minute occur until a final speech rate of around 180 syllables per minute is obtained. Neilson and Andrews attain a slow speech rate by extending all phonemes, while vowels are extended more than consonants in Boberg and Kully's programme. Both of these programmes require a considerable commitment of time on the part of clients and clinicians – five days a week for three weeks, with the addition of some evenings in Boberg and Kully's programme. Other interventions have been able to achieve favourable fluency results with considerably less client–clinician contact time (e.g. Ward (1992) and Harrison et al. (1998)).

Through the use of prolonged speech (PS), adults can attain high levels of fluency in a relatively short period of time. However, even when normal speech rates are attained, the speech that is produced with PS can sound unnatural. In a study of the experiences of 10 adults who use PS to control stuttering, Cream et al. (2003) reported that PS users found themselves having to make a choice between being dysfluent when they did not use PS and sounding unnatural when they did use PS. One adult, Rick, explains the dilemma that PS users face as follows:

> I realise now that I can't always sound perfectly natural and be perfectly fluent. That's the price I sometimes have to pay to be fluent, to sound very unnatural, using a heavy version of smooth speech. (387)

There are two sources of speech unnaturalness in PS. First, the fluency techniques may make speech sound abnormal. For example, techniques that are designed to regulate respiration, such as smooth airflow, can give speech an unnaturally breathy quality. Second, even when speech rates are near normal, the prolongation of vowels in this approach can still be heard as the stretching of syllables. These distortions in speech naturalness have been shown to discourage speakers from using PS, even when significant improvements in fluency have been achieved. In a study of a PS treatment called the Camperdown Program, O'Brian et al. (2003) found minimal or no stuttering in everyday speaking situations and speech rates in the normal range in 16 participants up to 12 months after entering the maintenance programme. However, 55 per cent of these participants also reported that they would prefer to stutter rather than use an unnatural speech pattern at least some of the time. Investigators are now attempting to establish variables that can be used to predict responsiveness to PS treatments (Block et al. 2006). For further discussion of the experience of adults with PS, see Cream et al. (2004).

As well as stuttering modification and fluency-shaping approaches, many other techniques are used to treat stuttering in adults. An approach that is strongly cognitive in orientation is Sheehan's approach–avoidance conflict therapy (see chapter 12 in Ward (2006) for further discussion). Sheehan's model is used extensively to treat a subgroup of stutterers for whom covert or interiorised stuttering is a significant problem. Counselling approaches are increasingly being used to treat adults who stutter, particularly in the UK. One such approach is George Kelly's (1955) personal construct psychology, which has been adapted for use in stuttering treatment by Fay Fransella (1972) – for a review of the contribution of personal construct psychology to stuttering therapy, see Stewart and Birdsall (2001) and Hayhow and Stewart (2006). Altered feedback therapies can confer immediate fluency on individuals who stutter. These therapies involve the use of devices that variously deliver delayed auditory feedback, frequency altered feedback and masked auditory feedback to the speaker (see below). Finally, interest in drug treatments for stuttering has increased in the last 15 years. Several drugs (e.g. olanzapine, risperidone) have now been tested in people who stutter and positive speech results have been reported (Maguire et al. 2004a, 2004b; Stager et al. 2005). As more becomes known about the neurological correlates of stuttering, it is likely that further drug treatments will be developed.

Recent technological developments have led to a resurgence of interest in the use of delayed auditory feedback (DAF) in the treatment of stuttering. In-the-ear devices have permitted clients to harness continuously the fluency-enhancing effects of DAF, effects that were once confined to the clinic. Kalinowski (2003) describes the effect of an all-in-the-ear canal prosthetic device on his own stuttering behaviour. The device, which delivered DAF and frequency altered feedback (FAF), resulted in speech that was relatively free from stuttering after 10 months of use. Speech was also natural-sounding and relatively spontaneous and unlaboured. Subsequent studies have served to replicate these findings across other speakers. Kalinowski et al. (2004) examined questionnaires that were completed by 105 subjects (aged 7–81 years) who wore an ear-level prosthetic device. The questionnaire assessed seven parameters of stuttering behaviour before the device was worn and after subjects had used the device for an average of six months with minimal clinical intervention. Subjects recorded a significant improvement across each parameter after wearing the device, as well as high overall satisfaction ratings. Stuart et al. (2006) examined the effect of an altered auditory feedback in-the-ear device on stuttering in nine subjects. Objective and subjective measures were taken at 12 months following fitting of the device. Relative to prefitting, the proportions of stuttering events and self-reported perception of struggle, avoidance and expectancy were significantly reduced. Speech samples that were produced by these subjects while wearing the device were judged by naive listeners to be significantly more natural-sounding than those produced in the absence of the device. Armson et al. (2006) examined the effect of SpeechEasy[19] on stuttering frequency during speech produced in a laboratory setting. When the device was fitted according to the manufacturer's protocol, stuttering was reduced by 74, 36 and 49 per cent in reading, monologue and conversation, respectively. Stuart et al. (2004) examined the effect of an ear-level device fitted monaurally on stuttering during reading and monologue in two adolescents and five adults. The device delivered a frequency shift of +500Hz and delayed auditory feedback of 60ms to its user. With the device in place, the proportion of stuttered syllables was significantly reduced by 90 and 67 per cent during reading and monologue, respectively. Saltuklaroglu and Kalinowski (2005) argue that '[i]n order to induce natural sounding, fluent speech [in children who stutter], it is suggested that one uses primarily derivations of choral speech such as altered auditory feedback' (360).

6.3 Cluttering

A second, less extensively investigated disorder of fluency is cluttering. Daly and Burnett (1996) define cluttering as

> a disorder of speech and language processing, resulting in rapid, dysrhythmic, sporadic, unorganized, and frequently unintelligible speech. Accelerated speech is not always present, but an impairment in formulating language almost always is. (239)

This definition captures what Ward (2006) has described as the 'two basic strands to the disorder', that cluttering has both 'a language component and a motor one' (141). In this section, we discuss what is known about the epidemiology and aetiology of cluttering. While anomalies of speech rate and language are frequently discussed in relation to cluttering, many other symptoms have also been associated with this disorder. We examine the large number of symptoms that clinicians and researchers have identified as part of the disorder of cluttering. As investigations of cluttering gather pace, clinicians and researchers are learning more about how to assess and treat this disorder. We examine some of the assessment and treatment techniques that are used with this clinical population.

While the prevalence of stuttering is well attested to, prevalence data for cluttering do not yet exist. The disorder is considerably more common in males than in females. From a survey of speech-language pathologists (SLPs) and educators, St Louis and Hinzman (1986) obtained sex ratios of 75.1 per cent male versus 24.9 per cent female (for SLPs) and 75.4 per cent male versus 24.6 per cent female (for educators). As with stuttering, genetic and neurological factors have been implicated in the aetiology of cluttering. Cluttering has been reported to occur in several syndromes, including Tourette's syndrome (Van Borsel and Vanryckeghem 2000) and fragile X syndrome (Hanson et al. 1986). Cluttering has also been linked to brain damage in adults. Lebrun (1996) describes cluttering in two adult patients with idiopathic parkinsonism. Thacker and De Nil (1996) report the case of a 61-year-old woman with cortical, subcortical, cerebellar and medulla lesions who acquired cluttering. Hashimoto et al. (1999) describe the case of a 57-year-old woman with dementia related to frontal pathology who developed cluttering-like speech.

Several features set cluttering apart from stuttering.[20] St Louis and Myers (1995) state that the person who clutters does not display evidence of physiological struggle at the within-word level of speech production. Sound prolongations and tense pauses, which are common in stuttering, are almost nonexistent in cluttering. Units larger than the sound or syllable are involved in fluency breakdowns (e.g. repetition of words and phrases, incomplete phrases and revisions). The person who clutters has a fast and/or spurty speaking rate. There is poor cohesion and coherence of discourse on account of linguistic encoding difficulties. Articulatory anomalies, which are secondary to a fast rate, result in reduced speech intelligibility. Also, unlike the person who stutters, the clutterer has poor self-monitoring skills. Consensus on the core features or symptoms of cluttering is vital if a differential diagnosis of the disorder is to be achieved.[21] In a survey of 29 clutterers in 12 articles, St Louis (1996) identified 53 symptoms that were used by the authors of these articles to characterise cluttering. The three most commonly reported symptoms were excessive dysfluencies, rate of speech too fast and rate of speech too irregular. Myers and St Louis (1996) studied two youths who clutter. These subjects shared the traits of rate anomalies, dysfluencies, poor speech intelligibility and linguistic maze behaviours.[22] Both these subjects were recently studied by St Louis et al. (2004), who found that the rate and speech naturalness of these speakers were perceptually least acceptable to listeners (speech-language pathology students), while dysfluency and language were most acceptable. (Articulation was judged by these listeners to have intermediate acceptability.)

For a differential diagnosis of cluttering to be made, the clinician must be prepared to undertake a comprehensive assessment of the client. St Louis and Myers (1995) argue that an evaluation protocol for cluttering should contain measures of fluency, rate (average and peak values), articulation, language, psychoeducational and academic skills (e.g. reading and spelling), hearing, auditory and visual perception, fine motor coordination (including handwriting) and cognitive/intellectual function. Preus (1996) states that '[o]ne of the most important gains to the understanding and management of cluttering in the last few years has been the publication of diagnostic material' (352). Preus identifies an assessment instrument developed by Daly and Burnett-Stolnack (1995) as particularly promising. Daly's Checklist for Possible Cluttering and a Profile Analysis for Planning Treatment with Cluttering Clients are still popular assessment instruments today. The checklist contains 33 criteria and is completed by the client, who ranks a number of statements between 0 and 4, depending on how applicable each is to him or her. The planning profile is completed by the clinician who scores on a six-point scale ranging from 'undesirably different from normal' to 'desirably different from normal'. Ward (2006) uses a checklist of cluttering behaviour that is based on several sources and his own clinical experience. The checklist contains 43 criteria that are arranged according to seven categories – speech rate and speech fluency; articulation; language and linguistic fluency; disorganised thinking; writing; attention; and other nonverbal attributes. Each criterion is ranked according to whether it is within normal limits, is somewhat abnormal or is markedly abnormal.

Treatment for cluttering employs many of the same techniques that are used to treat stuttering. St Louis et al. (1996) used DAF to treat two male clutterers who were aged 12 and 16 years. Although fluency criteria were met during treatment, both subjects had difficulty transferring gains to probe sessions during which no therapeutic suggestions of procedures were given. Ward (2006) describes an intervention for cluttering that he has developed at the Apple House. Therapy begins with the identification of cluttering. This can be a difficult stage for clutterers, many of whom do not perceive themselves to have a problem and are often in treatment at the request of someone like an employer. During this phase of treatment, work also begins on improving the client's monitoring of his or her speech and increasing his or her self-awareness of speech difficulties. The modification phase of treatment targets specific areas that are contributing to cluttering. The most significant of these areas is typically the client's excessively fast speech rate. However, speech rhythm, intonation, articulation, language, narrative structure and pragmatics may also be targeted. The maintenance phase of treatment depends on the client's ability to continue self-monitoring speech and implementing the techniques and procedures acquired during therapy. While Ward reports that fewer clutterers than stutterers return for 'top-up' therapy, he acknowledges that this may simply reflect a lapse into a pretherapy state of dysfluency in a group of speakers who are less inclined than stutterers to seek out additional help.

Although most cluttering occurs in the presence of stuttering, studies of treatment in persons who clutter and stutter are relatively few in number. Craig (1996) examined the effects of an intensive smooth speech treatment programme on speech and psychological status in a 21-year-old man who both stuttered and cluttered. Initial speech rate was estimated to be between 260 and 300 syllables per minute (SPM). Before intervention, the frequency of stuttering was 7 per cent syllables stuttered. Immediately after a three-week intervention using smooth speech, speech rate and stuttering frequency were both significantly reduced (233 SPM and 0.4 per cent syllables stuttered). At 10-month follow-up, speech rate and stuttering frequency were still lower than pretreatment levels (228 SPM and 2.8 per cent syllables stuttered). After the 10-month assessment, cluttering symptoms were almost nonexistent. Scores for locus of control and negative communication attitudes showed improvement immediately after treatment with gains maintained at 10-month follow-up. Langevin and Boberg (1996) used the Comprehensive Stuttering Program (Boberg and Kully 1985) to treat four adult male subjects who clutter and stutter. These subjects substantially decreased their post-treatment percentage of syllables stuttered in all speech samples. One-year follow-up data, which were available for only one of these subjects, revealed that this subject appeared to be maintaining fluency control, despite a small increase in percentage of syllables stuttered. Post-treatment syllables per minute data decreased for all subjects in conversation and reading conditions and increased in a telephone condition. These cluttering-stuttering subjects made modest improvements in attitudes and confidence as a result of treatment, but little improvement in perceptions.

Notes

1. Repetition of monosyllabic words, repetition of phrases and extension of sounds in word-final position are all normal nonfluencies. This is because both types of repetition involve units greater than single speech sounds and the extended sound in the third nonfluency does not occur in word-initial position.

2. Neurogenic stuttering is most commonly caused by brain damage associated with stroke (Doi et al. 2003; Balasubramanian et al. 2003; Rao 1991; Van Borsel et al. 2003). However, other causes of neurogenic stuttering have also reported including closed head injury (Yeoh et al. 2006), medical procedures such as myelography (Hayashi et al. 2005), brain dysfunction secondary to anorexia nervosa (Byrne et al. 1993), Parkinson's disease (Burghaus et al. 2006; Benke et al. 2000), drugs (Movsessian 2005), seizure (Chung et al. 2004), progressive supranuclear palsy

(Sakai et al. 2002; Kluin et al. 1993) and cerebral dysfunction secondary to infection (Tsao et al. 2004).

3. Burghaus et al. (2006) also support the role of the basal ganglia in the development of stuttering. In their study of a patient with Parkinson's disease, they argue that '[c]linical and imaging findings in this patient support the hypothesis that the basal ganglia circuitry plays an important role in the pathophysiology of stuttering' (625).

4. These investigators address the diagnostic question of whether this woman's stuttering is a result of her brain injury (neurogenic stuttering) or is a psychological reaction to physical trauma (psychogenic stuttering). Bijleveld et al. (1994) examined a case of acquired stuttering which, they argue, confirms the reality of neurogenic stuttering: 'the syndrome can exist in its own right. It is not simply a secondary psychological consequence of brain damage but a direct result of the cerebral lesion' (250). In a significant number of cases, however, psychological and neurological factors are not so easily disentangled. Eighty two per cent of the cases diagnosed by Baumgartner and Duffy (1997) as psychogenic also had complaints or a history that raised the possibility of neurological disease.

5. Some studies have investigated neuroanatomical anomalies in adults with persistent developmental stuttering. Foundas et al. (2001) found anomalous anatomy in perisylvian speech and language areas in a study of 16 adults with persistent developmental stuttering. In a study of 10 adults with persistent developmental stuttering, Jancke et al. (2004) found evidence of anomalous anatomy in perisylvian speech and language areas and prefrontal and sensorimotor areas.

6. Although these reports are numerous, Wingate (2002) states that the actual occurrence of these behaviours is not that common in practice: 'It is important to emphasize that such acts are not regularly observed to accompany stutters, which is the principal reason for their designation as "accessory"' (44).

7. Non-speech-language disorders occurred in 34.3 per cent of these children. The most frequently reported disorders were learning disabilities (15.2 per cent), literacy disorders (8.2 per cent) and attention deficit disorders (5.9 per cent).

8. Conture (1997) claims that if a child exhibits three or more within-word (stuttered) speech dysfluencies per 100 words of conversational speech, then he or she is at risk for continuing to stutter.

9. The Stuttering Severity Instrument (SSI) does not include an assessment of speech rate. However, De Andrade et al. (2003) recently attempted to correlate this instrument with speech rate in a study of 70 adults who stutter. Results indicated that the severity of stuttering as measured on the SSI, and speech rate present significant variation. That is, the more severe a subject's stuttering, the lower is his or her speech rate in words and syllables per minute.

10. Einarsdottir and Ingham (2005) state that

   because disfluency-type measures show poor reliability and conflate stuttered and nonstuttered speech, they have only limited heuristic value for research and provide no obvious benefits for clinicians. At best, they should be regarded as imprecise descriptors of observable stuttering and not a fundamental measure of stuttering. (260)

11. Finn and Ingham (1994) examined the reliability and validity of two types of self-rating made by adults who stutter: the naturalness of their speech and the naturalness of their speech monitoring. Results indicated that, with some qualifications, these subjects were consistent and valid self-raters of the naturalness of speech and of speech monitoring.

12. Kalinowski et al. (2005) surveyed 290 speech and language therapists who provide stuttering therapy to children in schools in North Carolina, USA. Amongst the 101 therapists who responded, a total of 2,036 children who stutter were surveyed. These investigators found that the median reported recovery rate among respondents was 13.9 per cent. No recoveries were reported by 28 therapists and five recoveries or fewer were reported by 81 therapists. The median time spent by a child in therapy was three years. Saltuklaroglu and Kalinowski (2005) state that this recovery rate 'is an indicator of therapeutic inefficiency and ineffectiveness' (359). See also Pothier et al. (2006) and Saltuklaroglu and Kalinowski (2006).

13. Nippold and Rudzinski (1995) conducted a critical review of the literature on the relation between parents' speech behaviours and children's stuttering. These investigators concluded that 'there is little convincing evidence to support the view that parents of children who stutter differ from parents of children who do not stutter in the way they talk with their children' (978). Nippold and Rudzinski also remark that 'there is little objective support for the argument that parents' speech behaviours contribute to children's stuttering or that modifying parents' speech behaviours facilitates children's fluency' (1995:978). Guitar et al. (1992) conducted a single-case study of indirect stuttering treatment. The relationship between parents' speech rates and percentages of nonaccepting statements, interruptions, questions, nonaccepting questions and talk time on the one hand and the child's per cent syllables stuttered on the other hand was examined. The mother's speech rate was the only parent variable significantly correlated with the child's stuttering.

14. For a review of fluency-shaping techniques for use with school age children, see Bothe (2002).

15. For discussion of how stuttering modification techniques can be used in the school setting, see Williams and Dugan (2002).

16. These stuttering modification techniques were devised by Van Riper (1973). Cancellation (or post-block modification) involves repeating a stuttered word using controlling strategies and then resuming speech. Pull-outs (or within-block modification) involve a smooth withdrawal from an ongoing stuttering moment.

17. Van Riper's approach is evident in several treatment programmes, one of which is the Successful Stuttering Management Program (SSMP) (Breitenfeldt and Lorenz 1989). The SSMP is designed for group use with adolescents and adults who

stutter. However, it can also be adapted for use with individuals. The programme combines avoidance reduction therapy and the stuttering modification techniques advocated by Van Riper. The three phases of the programme include confrontation of stuttering, modification of stuttering and transfer and maintenance.

18. These first two goals of the modification phase of treatment reflect Van Riper's belief that stuttering is in large part a learned behaviour. Van Riper also believed that stuttering was related to disturbed auditory feedback. In order to monitor the motor aspects of speech more closely, techniques should be used that could block auditory feedback. One such technique, delayed auditory feedback (DAF), is now used extensively to treat stuttering in adults. We return to the use of DAF later in the main text.

19. SpeechEasy is a fluency device that delivers DAF and FAF to its users. It was introduced in 2001.

20. Although cluttering can occur in pure form, it is more likely to coexist with stuttering. Of the fluency clients seen by Daly (1986) since the mid-1970s, less than 5 per cent were pure clutterers. Pure stutterers accounted for 55 per cent of these clients and 40 per cent were combined clutterers and stutterers. Williams and Wener (1996) describe the case of a young adult professional who presented with deficits that were consistent with both stuttering and cluttering. Langevin and Boberg (1996) report on the response to a stuttering therapy programme of four adults who stutter and clutter.

21. In 1996, Curlee remarked that 'widespread agreement on the signs and symptoms that are necessary or sufficient for the diagnosis of cluttering are lacking and may, in fact, vary from one study or clinician to another' (368). The question of core features continues to dominate the literature. Daly and Cantrell (2006) asked 60 fluency experts to rate 50 statements from the literature describing the characteristics of cluttering. Fifteen items were rated as characteristic of cluttering 66 per cent or more of the time. Interestingly, 'repetition of multisyllabic words' and 'rapid rate with intact articulation' were not included in the top 15 items.

22. The expression 'maze behaviours' describes sequences of, or parts of, words that sound out of place, superfluous or meaningless. It was originally used by Loban (1976).

7

Disorders of Voice

7.1 Introduction

For a significant number of children and adults the production of voice is so deviant that it poses a considerable barrier to effective communication. In this chapter, we examine the large range of diseases, injuries and other events that can compromise voice production throughout the human lifespan. The medically fragile baby may sustain laryngeal trauma as a result of early endotracheal intubation. The school-age child may develop vocal nodules as a consequence of sustained vocal abuse (e.g. shouting in the playground). The adolescent male may continue to experience a prepubescent voice beyond the time during which voice mutation occurs. The adult who uses his or her voice for professional purposes (e.g. singers, teachers) may develop maladaptive vocal patterns that damage laryngeal structures. Neurological disorders caused by stroke and Parkinson's disease may compromise voice production in later years, as may the development of laryngeal carcinomas.

As well as examining the aetiologies of voice disorders, we consider what is known about the prevalence of these disorders. Knowledge of the prevalence of these disorders, particularly within specific populations (e.g. occupational groups), is essential if preventive programmes that emphasise healthy vocal habits and patterns of voice use are to be developed. The assessment and treatment of voice disorders involves a range of medical and health professionals, most notably the otolaryngologist and speech and language therapist. We examine the perceptual and instrumental techniques of voice assessment that are used by these professionals. Speech and language therapy also plays a key role in decisions regarding the surgical management of voice disorders. In some cases, speech and language therapy may eliminate the need for surgical voice intervention. In other cases, it forms an integral part of a client's postsurgical intervention (e.g. in laryngectomy). We consider the various techniques used by therapists in the treatment of voice disorders.

7.2 Voice Disorders

The phonatory activity of the larynx is the basis of all voice production. Voice is produced when subglottal air pressure forces the vocal folds (cords) apart. As pulmonary air passes through the glottis, the resulting decrease in subglottal air pressure causes the vocal folds to close. The folds remain closed until the build-up of subglottal air pressure once again forces them apart. This entire glottal cycle is repeated several hundred times per second. When it is disrupted by the presence, for example, of nodules on the speaker's vocal folds, the resulting perceptually deviant voice is described as a voice disorder of phonation. The voice that is produced by the vibratory action of the vocal folds in the larynx is itself altered as it passes through the oral, nasal and pharyngeal resonatory chambers. Defects of or obstructions in any part of this supraglottic resonator (e.g. nasal polyps) can adversely affect the voice that is produced and that is perceived by the listener. So-called voice disorders of resonance have been addressed in several earlier contexts (e.g. cleft lip and palate in chapter 2) and will be examined less directly in the present chapter.

7.2.1 Epidemiology and Aetiology

Several recent studies have obtained figures for the prevalence of voice disorders in the general population. Duff et al. (2004) examined the presence of voice disorders in 2,445 African-American and European-American preschool children aged between 2 and 6 years. Of these children, 1,246 were males and 1,199 were females. Voice disorders, which were identified by two speech-language pathologists, were found in 95 children or 3.9 per cent of the sample. There were no significant differences for age, gender or race. Carding et al. (2006) examined the prevalence of dysphonia in a cohort of 7,389 children who were eight years of age. Research speech and language therapists reported a dysphonia prevalence of 6 per cent in these children. (This compares with a prevalence rate of 11 per cent based on parental report.) Older siblings and sex (male) were significant risk factors for dysphonia. Roy et al. (2005) conducted a telephone questionnaire on a random sample of 1,326 adults in Iowa and Utah. These investigators obtained a lifetime prevalence rate of voice disorder of 29.9 per cent and a prevalence rate of current voice disorder of 6.6 per cent. Factors that contributed to increased odds of reporting a chronic voice disorder included sex (female), age (40–59 years), voice use patterns and demands, oesophageal reflux, chemical exposures and frequent colds and sinus infections. Perhaps surprisingly, alcohol and tobacco use did not independently increase the odds of reporting a chronic voice disorder.

The prevalence of voice disorders in certain occupational and clinical groups is greater than in the population in general. It is well known that occupations which place a high vocal load on speakers result in increased levels of voice disorder. Roy et al. (2004) found that the prevalence of current voice problems in a sample of 1,243 teachers was 11 per cent. This figure is significantly greater than a prevalence of 6.2 per cent in a sample of 1,288 nonteachers examined in the same study. There was also a significantly greater prevalence of voice disorders during the lifetime in teachers than in nonteachers (57.7 and 28.8 per cent, respectively). A significantly greater number of teachers than nonteachers had consulted a physician or speech–language pathologist about a voice disorder (14.3 versus 5.5 per cent). Women had both a higher lifetime prevalence of voice disorder than men (46.3 versus 36.9 per cent) and a higher prevalence of chronic voice disorders than acute voice disorders (20.9 versus 13.3 per cent). Sliwinska-Kowalska et al. (2006) examined the prevalence of voice problems in 425 female Polish teachers aged 23–61 years. Overall lifetime vocal symptoms were more common in teachers than in a control group of 83 female nonteachers (69 versus 36 per cent). In teachers and controls, the mean number of voice symptoms was 3.21 and 1.98, respectively. Occupational voice disorders and hyperfunctional dysphonia were more common in teachers than in nonteachers (32.7 and 9.6 per cent, respectively).

As well as an increased prevalence of voice disorders in certain occupational groups, particular age groups and clinical populations also have more voice problems than the general population. Golub et al. (2006) found that the prevalence of dysphonia in a population of geriatric subjects was 20 per cent. Akif Kiliç et al. (2004) examined the prevalence of vocal nodules in 617 children aged from 7 to 16 years. Larynogoscopic examination revealed that 187 children (30.3 per cent) had minimal lesion, an immature nodule, a mature nodule or a vocal polyp. Speyer et al. (2008) examined the prevalence of dysphonia in 166 subjects with rheumatoid arthritis and 148 healthy controls. Subjects completed two questionnaires that assessed the quality of the individual's voice and the extent of impairment related to dysphonia in social and occupational settings. The subjects with rheumatoid arthritis had a statistically significant higher prevalence and relative risk of dysphonia than the control subjects. Prevalence of dysphonia in arthritic subjects ranged from 12 to 27 per cent, depending on the questionnaire used. (Compare with a prevalence of 3–8 per cent in control subjects.) The relative risk of dysphonia in subjects with rheumatoid arthritis varied from about 3 to 4 when compared to healthy subjects.

Voice disorders can be caused by structural abnormalities of the larynx, neurological disorders, traumatic injuries to the larynx, infections, endocrine disorders, a range of surgical and medical interventions, vocal abuse and misuse and gastro-oesophageal reflux. Benign lesions of the larynx are a common cause of dysphonia. These growths include viral papilloma, laryngeal mucous gland retention cysts, epidermoid cysts and vocal process granulomas. Vocal nodules are a further type of benign growth that are the result of vocal abuse and misuse (Williams and Carding 2005). Gallivan et al. (2008) report the case of a 52-year-old male who described a 40-year history of severe hoarseness with recent progressive dysphonia. Two intracordal lesions in the left vocal fold were observed during strobovideolaryngoscopy. One lesion was a benign epi-dermoid malformation cyst, while the other was a retention cyst. Papilloma is a benign growth that frequently occurs in the trachea or larynx of children. It is caused by the human papilloma virus (types HPV6 and HPV11). As well as causing dysphonia, these growths can obstruct the airway. Papillomas tend to proliferate and often require surgical excisions (Harvey 1996). Vocal nodules are the most common cause of voice disorders in school-age children. They are small benign swellings that occur along the margins of the vocal folds mostly at the junction of the anterior and middle third of the vocal fold. Sapienza et al. (2004) remark that

> [t]he general consensus of opinions points to vocal nodules as an edema or hemorrhage of some part of the mucosal layer resulting from persistent trauma at the anterior third and posterior two thirds of the vocal fold, the area of greatest mechanical stress. (303)[1]

Malignant growths of the larynx are less common than benign lesions. However, these growths are ultimately more destructive of the larynx and its surrounding tissues than benign lesions. An estimated 11,700 new cases of laryngeal cancer occur every year in the US (Nwiloh and Fortson 2001). A sig-nificant percentage of these cases require laryngectomy and stoma care (see section 7.2.4.1). Laryngeal cancer is largely a disease of more advanced years. Luna-Ortiz et al. (2006) reviewed the clinical records of 500 patients with laryngeal cancer in the period 1989–2004. These investigators found that only 15 patients (4.4 per cent) were less than 40 years of age. There are signs that, in the US at least, the number of people developing laryngeal cancer is declin-ing. Davies and Welch (2006) recorded a reduction in the incidence of laryn-geal cancer of 26 per cent in the US in 2001. The large majority of laryngeal cancers are squamous cell carcinomas. However, several other types of cancer can also occur. Pignataro et al. (2006) describe a rare cartilaginous tumour called a chondrosarcoma in a patient who presented with homolateral vocal fold paralysis. The tumour arose from the posterior plate of the cricoid carti-lage and was treated by means of a total laryngectomy and right hemithy-roidectomy.[2]

Other organic disorders that compromise the structure and function of the larynx include laryngomalacia and subglottic stenosis. Laryngomalacia is a common congenital anomaly in which the cartilage of the larynx is soft or abnormally flaccid. The disorder is diagnosed in infancy and normally resolves without intervention by one year of age. Laryngomalacia is characterised by stridor (a harsh, high-pitched sound on inhalation). Subglottic stenosis is a congenital or acquired condition in which there is a narrowing of the subglottic airway. It is the most common abnormality requiring tracheotomy in children under a year. It can be treated by a procedure called laryngotracheal reconstruction (LTR). Harvey (1996) describes the case of HR, an eight-year-old girl with a diagnosis of congenital subglottic stenosis. At three years of age, HR had a tracheotomy. By the stage of initial voice evaluation she had also undergone LTR and LTR revision.

Neurological disorders are a common cause of dysphonia. Sewall et al. (2006) report that nearly one-third of patients with idiopathic Parkinson's disease (PD) cite dysphonia as their most debilitating deficit. Dysphonia can be the first presenting sign of PD (Merati et al. 2005). Dogan et al. (2007) conducted a stroboscopic examination of 27 female patients with multiple sclerosis (MS). These investigators found that 16 of these patients (59 per cent) had a 'posterior chink' as their glottic closure pattern. Several acoustic and perceptual anomalies of voice in MS were also identified. Montero–Odasso (2006) describes the presence of fluctuating dysphonia as the first symptom of late-onset myasthenia gravis in an elderly man. Stroke or cerebrovascular accident may also cause dysphonia. Isolated vocal fold paralysis is an uncommon manifestation of stroke (Merati et al. 2005). However, when paralysis occurs, it is most commonly associated with brainstem stroke, lateral medullary syndrome, Claude Bernard–Horner syndrome and Wallenberg's syndrome. Rigueiro-Veloso et al. (1997) found that dysphonia was the commonest symptom in 25 patients with Wallenberg's syndrome.

Bacterial, viral and fungal infections of the larynx can cause voice disorders. Nalini and Vinayak (2006) report two cases of laryngeal tuberculosis (TB) in a retrospective study of 117 patients with head and neck TB. The vocal cords were the commonest site affected by laryngeal TB. Ozudogru et al. (2005) describe a case of laryngeal and pulmonary TB in a 28-year-old female. These investigators state that although laryngeal TB can be successfully treated, TB of the larynx can cause 'irreversible changes in voice quality' (374). Lacy et al. (1994) report the case of a 73-year-old woman with late congenital pharyngo-laryngeal syphilis. There are reports of mycobacterial infection of the larynx (McEwan et al. 2001). The larynx may also be infected by anthrax (Leblebicioglu et al. 2006). Marelli et al. (1992) report a case of cytomegalovirus infection of the larynx in a patient with AIDS. McGregor et al. (2003) describe an unusual case of laryngitis caused by *Cryptococcus neoformans* (an encapsulated yeast) in an immunocompetent patient. Subramaniam et al. (2005) report the case of a 52-year-old man in whom biopsy of the laryngeal mucosa confirmed a diagnosis of histoplasmosis (a disease caused by the fungus *Histoplasma capsulatum*). Finally, the larynx is also susceptible to infection by parasites. Fontes Rezende et al. (2006) produce the first report of a case of *Trypanosoma cruzi* infection (Chagas' disease) in which there is involvement of the larynx.

Other causes of voice disorders include laryngeal trauma. Kim et al. (2006) report two cases in which laryngeal injuries were sustained from a full-face helmet. Irwin and Lonnee (2006) state that blunt laryngeal trauma, although uncommon, has a mortality that can be as high as 40 per cent. Surgical and medical interventions may damage the larynx and associated structures. The recurrent laryngeal nerve may be damaged during thoracic surgery (Krasna and Forti 2006). Lee et al. (2006) describe a case of cardiovocal syndrome[3] in an 81-year-old man, which was caused by aortic dissection. Inhaled corticosteroids, that are used in the treatment of asthma,[4] have adverse effects on voice (Gallivan et al. 2006). Hormones have long been linked to voice changes in adolescents and adults. Premenstrual and menopausal voice syndromes are now well documented (Abitbol et al. 1999). Sex hormones are also believed to play a role in mutational dysphonia, voice changes during pregnancy and voice changes in bodybuilders who use anabolic androgenic steroids. In section 7.2.4.3, we will see how sex hormones can be used to induce voice changes in transsexual clients. Further hormone-related voice changes can be observed in hypo- and hyperthyroidism. Altman et al. (2003) state that 'alterations in the voice may occur even in cases of mild thyroid failure, suggesting that the larynx is a target tissue for thyroid hormone' (1931).

Each of the causes of voice disorder that have been discussed thus far is organic in nature. However, voice disorders may also have a nonorganic aetiology. So-called functional voice disorders have been defined as those in which 'significant voice abnormalities are noted in the presence of an apparently normal larynx' (Peppard 1996:257). The disorder is usually attributed to psychological factors (hence, the term 'psychogenic' voice disorder). Conversion aphonia and persistent falsetto (puberphonia) are two functional voice disorders. In conversion or functional aphonia, there may be a lack of vocal fold adduction during attempted phonation. However, vocal fold adduction is normal, as evidenced during coughing. The aphonia is usually a reaction to a psychologically traumatic event. In puberphonia, the male adolescent's voice has a higher pitch than is typical of other males of the same age. This voice disorder is related to emotional stress, which results from the psychosocial changes that occur during puberty. Recently, Seifert and Kollbrunner (2006) examined psychosocial factors in nonorganic voice disorders. Compared to a group of control subjects with organic voice disorders (vocal cord paralysis), these investigators found that subjects with nonorganic voice disorders sought a quick solution in conflict situations or expected other people to provide one. This prevented them from understanding the underlying causes of the conflict.

7.2.2 Clinical Presentation

Voice disorders have accompanying physical symptoms and acoustic features. Physical symptoms may include bleeding, pain, dysphagia and coughing. Acoustic features are highly variable and reflect changes in the following parameters: habitual pitch (speaking fundamental frequency), pitch range, loudness, vocal note quality, vocal flexibility and vocal stamina. In this way, a disordered voice may have a rough or breathy quality, may be too loud or too quiet or may have an excessively high or low habitual pitch. Other acoustic features may arise in an attempt to compensate for these primary phonatory features.[5] So-called secondary phonatory features may include a rough quality that is produced by the adduction of the false vocal folds during phonation or a rise in speaking fundamental frequency with increased hyperfunction (Mathieson 2001). In this section, we examine some of the physical symptoms and acoustic features of voice disorder.

The physical symptoms that accompany voice disorders are often valuable diagnostic indicators of the cause of a disorder. Dysphagia, earache, weight loss, blood-stained saliva or neck swellings are suggestive of pharyngeal or laryngeal cancer (Ng 2000). Dyspepsia and heartburn suggest that gastro-oesophageal reflux may be the cause of a voice disorder. Ollivere et al. (2006) studied 30 patients with unilateral vocal fold palsy and found that 56 per cent had associated dysphagia. Coope and Connett (2006) state that children with laryngeal papillomatosis may present with cough, pneumonia, dysphagia or stridor, as well as hoarseness. Respiratory distress and stridor are common presenting symptoms in laryngomalacia (Leung and Cho 1999), subglottic stenosis and bilateral vocal cord palsy (Kaushal et al. 2005).

A range of acoustic parameters and perceptual features may be deviant in a voice disorder. Tavares and Martins (2007) conducted a perceptual vocal assessment of 40 teachers without vocal symptoms or with sporadic symptoms, and 40 teachers with frequent vocal symptoms. Hard glottal attack, excessive laryngeal resonance, inadequate coordination of breathing and voicing, low pitch and decreased loudness were most frequent in the latter teachers. These teachers also had the highest GIRBAS scores, particularly for grade (degree of voice abnormality), roughness and breathiness (see section 7.2.3 below for explanation of scale). Pribuisiene et al. (2006) performed perceptual voice assessment of 108 patients with reflux laryngitis using the GRB (grade, roughness, breathiness) scale. These investigators found a slight hoarseness reliably prevailed in these patients. There was no statistically significant difference between the mean fundamental frequency of the voice in the reflux laryngitis

patients and healthy controls. However, the mean jitter, shimmer and normalised noise energy of the voice of laryngitis patients were significantly
increased compared to the mean values of controls. Ettema et al. (2006) conducted a perceptual voice analysis using the GRBAS scale of 31 patients with
subglottic stenosis. Grade, breathiness and asthenia assessments were significantly worse in patients with multilevel stenosis. Overall grade was also
impacted by vocal fold motion impairment. In patients with prior airway
surgery, grade, roughness and breathiness were significantly worse.

7.2.3 Clinical Assessment

Voice disorders are assessed by means of a range of instrumental, acoustic and
perceptual techniques. The otolaryngologist uses instruments to observe the
larynx, either directly or indirectly, and examine its function during phonation.
The longest-established method of indirectly viewing the interior of the larynx
is mirror laryngoscopy. In this procedure, the otolaryngologist places a laryngeal mirror against the patient's elevated soft palate as he or she says 'ee' at a
relatively high pitch. The patient's tongue is wrapped in gauze and held by the
examiner. A mirror worn on the examiner's head reflects light from an external source on to the laryngeal mirror, which then reflects it into the pharynx
and larynx. Although this technique enables the larynx to be viewed at rest and
during phonation, it does not permit an assessment of the larynx during connected speech. (The presence of the laryngeal mirror in the oral cavity prevents
speech.) It is also a procedure that is not tolerated by some patients, for whom
the presence of a laryngeal mirror may elicit gagging. For these patients, fibreoptic laryngoscopy may be a more appropriate technique. In this procedure, a
flexible endoscope is passed transnasally into a position above the larynx. The
insertion of the endoscope is made more tolerable by the use of a local anaesthetic spray. This procedure also allows the clinician to assess the velopharyngeal port – the optic is positioned in this case just above the soft palate.
Phonation during connected speech can be assessed using fibreoptic laryngoscopy. Rigid endoscopy is another form of indirect laryngoscopy. Both rigid
endoscopy and fibreoptic laryngoscopy permit the larynx to be viewed on a TV
monitor and recorded for subsequent analysis.

A technique that has become 'the definitive tool in differential diagnoses of
laryngeal pathology' is videostrobolaryngoscopy (Mathieson 2001:433). In this
procedure, intermittent flashes of light, which are delivered by means of a rigid
or flexible endoscope, have the effect of simulating slow motion of the vocal
folds. This enables the otolaryngologist to examine different stages of the vibratory cycle. Unlike mirror and fibreoptic laryngoscopy, which only permit
detection of gross disorders of vocal fold motion, videostrobolaryngoscopy
allows even minute lesions and their effect on the mucosal wave to be examined.

This technique has been linked to the revision of diagnoses in a number of studies. Remacle (1996) found that videostroboscopy modified the initial diagnosis in 17 per cent of dysfunctional dysphonias, 20 per cent of nodules, 23 per cent of Reinke's oedemas and 17 per cent of granulomas.

Acoustic assessments of voice provide objective data that can be compared to normative values and used as a baseline for treatment. Sound spectrography analyses the periodic waveform of the vocal signal into sine waves, each with a different frequency and amplitude (Mathieson 2001). The resulting spectrogram displays the interrelationship of amplitude, frequency and time, with frequency typically represented on the vertical axis of the graph, time on the horizontal axis and intensity by the degree of blackening of the trace. The standard spectrogram presents a graphic representation of the harmonics-to-noise ratio. The Voice Range Profile (formerly known as a phonetogram) provides a display of vocal intensity range versus fundamental frequency. Commercially available techniques of acoustic assessment include the Kay Computerised Speech Lab: Multi-Dimensional Voice Program (see section 5.2.3 in chapter 5), VisiSpeech and Kay Visi-Pitch. Niebudek-Bogusz et al. (2006) conducted an acoustic analysis of 66 female teachers using IRIS software. These investigators found lowered fundamental frequency and incorrect values of shimmer and noise to harmonic ratio after a 30-minute vocal loading test in these teachers.

Objective data that describe various acoustic parameters of the voice are still no substitute for how a voice sounds to a listener. A perceptual evaluation of voice is thus a central component of the assessment process. Such evaluation can be conducted formally and informally and requires considerable experience on the part of the assessing clinician. Informal perceptual evaluation begins as soon as the clinician first meets a client. The clinician can observe the client's habitual breathing patterns both at rest and during connected speech. Anomalies such as breathlessness, a 'noisy' chest, effortful and rapid breathing, inspiratory stridor, noisy air intake and the use of residual air towards the end of phrases and sentences should be noted. Phonatory features can also be informally observed during the initial interview. The clinician should note any anomalies in fundamental vocal note quality (e.g. rough, breathy voice), habitual pitch, pitch range, loudness, resonance, voice onset (e.g. hard glottal attack), vocal habits (e.g. throat-clearing), extrinsic laryngeal muscles, vocal stamina/ fatigue and the effect of posture on phonation. Remarkable articulatory features should also be recorded, as they may provide important clues about the aetiology of a voice disorder. For example, the presence of dysarthria may indicate that the voice disorder has a neurogenic aetiology. Also, over-articulation or marked mouth closure during speech may suggest a muscle tension dysphonia.

Formal perceptual evaluation employs many of the same categories that are used to assess a voice informally. Additionally, however, formal assessments permit the various dimensions of a voice disorder to be quantified. Typically, this is achieved by means of scales. One of the most widely used scales in the UK and internationally is the GRBAS scale of the Japan Society of Logopaedics and Phoniatrics, which was given its introduction in Hirano (1981). This perceptual rating system contains five parameters: G (overall grade of hoarseness), R (roughness), B (breathiness), A (asthenic) and S (strained quality). Each parameter is given a rating on a four-point scale between 0 and 3, where '0' indicates nonhoarse or normal, '1' slight, '2' moderate and '3' severe. The GRBAS scale is not fully comprehensive – it does not include parameters for vocal pitch, for example (Freeman and Fawcus 2000). Nevertheless, this scale is a reliable method of perceptual assessment that has also been shown to correlate with voice-related quality of life (Karnell et al. 2007; Jones et al. 2006).

The perceptual scheme that is most often used by British speech and language therapists is Laver et al.'s (1981) Vocal Profile Analysis Scheme (Shewell 1998). The scheme assesses supralaryngeal features, tension features, phonation type and prosodic features within a series of specific subcategories. For example, prosodic features include pitch (mean, range, variability), tremor and loudness (mean, range, variability). Clary et al. (1996) used the Vocal Profile Analysis Scheme to assess long–term voice function in 33 children who underwent augmentation procedures for laryngotracheal stenosis. Eight children were judged to have normal voices on this scheme. Amongst the remaining 25 children, abnormalities were found in the following parameters: harshness (52 per cent), whisper (36 per cent), ventricular band phonation (21 per cent), continuity (27 per cent), mean pitch (27 per cent) and falsetto voice (12 per cent). Another commonly used perceptual voice evaluation is the Buffalo III Voice Screening Profile (Wilson 1987). It rates the following parameters on a five-point scale: laryngeal tone, loudness, pitch, nasal resonance, oral resonance, breath supply, muscles, voice abuse, rate, speech anxiety, speech intelligibility and overall voice efficiency. Munoz et al. (2002) report good reliability values using this screening profile in the evaluation of two voice samples by expert listeners. For further discussion of perceptual voice evaluation, see Carding et al. (2000).

7.2.4 Clinical Intervention

Ideally, voice disorders should be treated by a multidisciplinary team consisting of the laryngologist, speech and language therapist, gastroenterologist, psychologist (counsellor or psychotherapist), psychiatrist, radiologist and occupational health worker. Voice treatments include surgery, drugs, radiotherapy and voice therapy, which are typically undertaken in combination rather than in isolation. For example, in the case of serious laryngeal pathologies such as carcinomas, radiotherapy and/or surgery (partial or total laryngectomy) may be the primary modes of treatment. However, postsurgical voice restoration requires intervention by a speech and language therapist. Similarly, phono-surgery to remove vocal nodules must be accompanied by a programme of voice therapy and vocal hygiene if the client is to adopt less damaging patterns of phonation and vocal habits in the future. In this section, we examine some of the techniques that are available to specialists who treat voice disorders.

7.2.4.1 Surgery

A wide range of voice disorders, including those caused by vocal fold paralysis and benign and malignant lesions, can be successfully treated by surgical tech-niques. In the past seven years, preferred treatment methods for unilateral vocal fold paralysis have included Bioplastique injection and lipoaugmentation of the vocal cords, as well as medialisation thyroplasty using a titanium implant (Bihari et al. 2006). Varices and ectasias – both vascular abnormalities of the vocal folds – can be successfully treated using pulsed angiolytic lasers (Zeitels et al. 2006). Knott et al. (2006) used endoscopic carbon dioxide laser resection in conjunction with cryoablation – the application of extreme cold to destroy cancer cells – to treat patients with early-stage glottic cancer. Autologous trans-plantation of fascia into the vocal fold has been used to treat sulcus vocalis (Tsunoda et al. 2005). Surgical procedures are increasingly being used to help the transsexual client attain the voice of his or her newly assigned sex. Cricothyroid approximation may be undertaken to raise the fundamental fre-quency of clients who are unable to achieve desired pitch changes through non-surgical means (McNeil 2006). Other surgical techniques that are used to raise the pitch of the male-to-female transsexual voice are anterior commissure advancement, scarification, injection of triamcinolone into the vocal folds and endolaryngeal shortening of the vocal folds (Gross 1999).

Recurrent early-stage laryngeal cancer often requires total laryngectomy. Although total laryngectomy may also be used as primary treatment in cases of advanced laryngeal carcinoma, it is more often used as a salvage procedure in centres that treat patients initially using larynx preservation protocols (Genden et al. 2007). The removal of the larynx during laryngectomy necessitates the establishment of an alternative route for respiration. The surgeon must direct the trachea on to the patient's neck, where a permanent tracheal stoma will be formed for respiration and expectoration (see Figure 7.1). This stoma can become infected in the postoperative period and may also close over (tracheal stomal stenosis). It will require ongoing cleaning and protection by the patient after surgery. Other surgical complications include the development of pharyn-gocutaneous fistula (Makitie et al. 2006). Depending on the extent of the laryn-geal tumour, further surgical procedures may be required, including neck

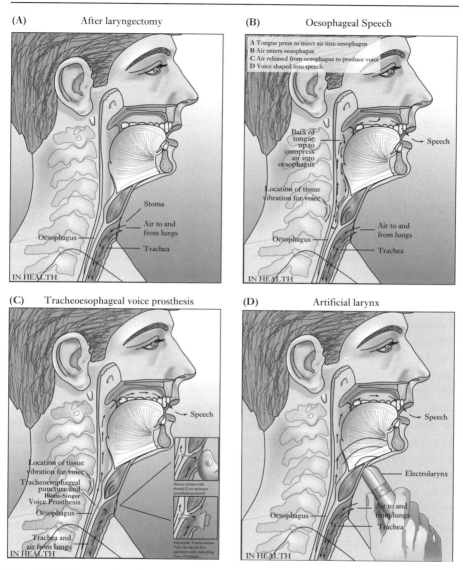

(A) After laryngectomy

Stoma

Air to and from lungs

Oesophagus

Trachea

IN HEALTH

(B) Oesophageal Speech

A Tongue press to inject air into oesophagus
B Air enters oesophagus
C Air released from oesophagus to produce voice
D Voice shaped into speech

Back of tongue up to compress air into oesophagus

Speech

Location of tissue vibration for voice

Oesophagus

Air to and from lungs

Trachea

IN HEALTH

(C) Tracheoesophageal voice prosthesis

Speech

Location of tissue vibration for voice

Tracheoesophageal puncture and Blom-Singer Voice Prosthesis

Oesophagus

Trachea and air from lungs

IN HEALTH

Stoma closure with thumb (Low pressure prosthesis pictured)

Adjustable Tracheostoma Valve for hands-free operation with indwelling Voice Prosthesis

(D) Artificial larynx

Speech

Electrolarynx

Air to and from lungs

Trachea

Oesophagus

IN HEALTH

Figure 7.1: Diagrams showing anatomical structures after laryngectomy (A) and various means of postlaryngectomy voice production: oesophageal voice (B), tracheo–oesophageal voice prosthesis (C) and artificial larynx (D) (Illustrations provided by courtesy of InHealth Technologies, www.Inhealth.com)

dissection, pharyngolaryngectomy and pharyngo–laryngo–oesophagectomy. The last two procedures are necessary when there is extensive involvement of the pharynx and oesophagus. Surgery is now playing an increasing role in restoring voice to the laryngectomy client.[6] A tracheoesophageal voice prosthesis provides a route for pulmonary air to enter the oesophagus, where it vibrates the pharyngo–oesophageal segment. The resulting voice is more easily produced than oesophageal voice. It is also of higher pitch and greater fluency than oesophageal voice (Mathieson 2001). When this technique was first developed, occlusion of the tracheostoma with a finger was necessary to direct pulmonary air into the oesophagus (Rudert 1979). Tracheostoma valves (e.g. Provox tracheostoma valve) are now available which eliminate the need for manual occlusion (Lorenz et al. 2006).

7.2.4.2 Radiotherapy

While surgery is used for salvage in the case of recurrence of a laryngeal tumour, radiotherapy tends to be the primary form of treatment in Britain for laryngeal tumours at stages T1 and T2[7] (Freeman and Fawcus 2000). Radiotherapy has implications for the medical recovery of patients, as well as implications for the post-treatment production of voice. Preoperative radiotherapy has been linked to the development of postlaryngectomy pharyngocutaneous fistula (Paydarfar and Birkmeyer 2006). Wu et al. (2005) found that postoperative radiotherapy was one of several factors that correlated with laryngeal stenosis. Even in the absence of medical complications, voice problems can be caused by radiotherapy. In a study of 54 patients who were using valved speech following total laryngectomy, Kazi et al. (2007) found that functional aspects of voice were significantly affected by radiotherapy. Radiation was also seen to influence voice handicap scores. Van Gogh et al. (2005) studied 177 patients after radiotherapy or laser surgery for early glottic cancer. Voice impairment was reported by 44 per cent of the patients who received radiotherapy. Twenty-nine per cent of patients who received endoscopic laser surgery reported voice impairment. Roh et al. (2005) reported subjective vocal dysfunction and stroboscopic abnormality in a group of 20 patients who received wide-field radiotherapy for glottic cancer. There were no significant differences between the acoustic or aerodynamic profiles of these patients and the profiles of 20 patients who had received limited radiotherapy of the larynx. Salivary gland hypofunction was found to be significantly correlated with vocal dysfunction.[8]

7.2.4.3 Drugs

Drugs may also be used to treat voice disorders and conditions that cause voice disorders. Harris (1992) discusses the pharmacological treatment of symptoms such as cough and vocal fatigue, of allergy and other causes of vocal tract inflammation and the treatment of dysphonia in dyskinetic and dystonic conditions. It is now widely accepted that botulinum toxin is an effective treatment for adductor spasmodic dysphonia (Woodson et al. 2006). Voice disorders that are caused by gastro–oesophageal reflux may be treated by proton pump inhibitors. Issing et al. (2004) used a proton pump inhibitor (esomeprazole) to treat reflux-related otolaryngological disorders in 22 patients. Sixty-eight per cent of patients had no laryngopharyngeal symptoms within four weeks of treatment. Within eight weeks, 95 per cent were free of symptoms. Intralesional injection of the antiviral drug cidofovir has been found to be efficacious in treating recurrent respiratory papillomatosis (Lee and Rosen 2004).

Watts et al. (2001) report the use of an oral corticosteroid (methyl prednisolone) to treat a 32-year-old male professional singer with vocal oedema. Following treatment, improvements were observed in acoustic parameters and perceptual evaluation of the voice. Also, endoscopic examination revealed reduced oedema. Sulica (2005) reported a good response to oral fluconazole (an antifungal medication) in eight patients with thrush isolated to the larynx. The drugs that are used to achieve feminisation in male-to-female transsexuals can also produce voice changes. A wide range of oestrogens may be used for this purpose, although oral 17 beta-oestradiol valerate or transdermal 17 beta-oestradiol is the treatment of choice (Gooren 2005). Similarly, the testosterone preparations that are used to induce virilisation in female-to-male transsexuals can also bring about voice change.

7.2.4.4 Voice Therapy

Voice therapy is integral to the treatment of voice disorders. The range of techniques used by speech and language therapists to treat voice disorders is extensive and a full treatment of them is beyond the scope of the current chapter. The reader is referred to other volumes for a detailed examination of specific voice treatment techniques (Mathieson 2001; Freeman and Fawcus 2000). These texts also discuss the use of voice therapy techniques in the treatment of particular client groups. For our present purposes, we examine studies in which different techniques have been used to treat child and adult clients with voice disorders. Techniques may be used which target the phonatory and respiratory mechanisms that are the basis of voice production. Where psychological issues and anxiety may be contributing to a voice disorder, relaxation and counselling techniques may be employed. As well as using direct and indirect treatment techniques, therapists also have an important role to play in advising clients in voice care. We examine the nature of this advice and the clients for whom it is appropriate. Finally, in an era of evidence-based practice in healthcare, the question of the efficacy of voice therapy is of paramount concern to clinicians and medical professionals who are charged with the delivery of services to clients with voice disorders. We conclude this section and chapter by examining the findings of what is still a relatively small body of literature on the efficacy of voice therapy.

Direct techniques of voice treatment are amply demonstrated in a recent study by Schindler et al. (2008). These investigators studied the use of a range of such techniques to treat 40 patients with unilateral vocal fold paralysis of different aetiologies. The aim of voice therapy in these patients was to improve glottal closure and at the same time avoid undesirable compensatory behaviours (e.g. tongue backing to aid glottal closure). Progressive development of optimal breathing, abdominal support and gentle improvement of intrinsic muscle strength and agility were the focus of therapy. To maintain appropriate subglottal air pressure, abdominal breathing was practised. Shallow, upper chest breathing and phonation on residual air were both actively discouraged. To reach appropriate tone focus without tension of the oral and pharyngeal musculature, humming and resonant voice were used. When an improvement in glottal competence was perceived by the treating clinician, patients were encouraged to sustain vowels and glide from the lowest to the highest note, and vice versa. On account of the risk of causing hyperfunctional compensation, hard glottal attacks, pushing and half-swallow boom were used in only a few cases.

The techniques employed by Schindler et al. are designed to encourage more effective laryngeal valving of the pulmonary airstream in the patient with unilateral vocal fold paralysis. A quite different set of techniques is employed when a voice disorder has been caused by hyperfunctional voice use.[9] Glaze (1996) states that '[c]hildren with hyperfunctional voice disorders may respond readily to behavioral voice therapy based on education, voice conservation strategies, direct vocal function exercises, family and peer support, and relaxation' (244). Three 'direct vocal function exercises' described by Glaze include easy onset of voice plus resonant tone, the accent method of phonation and physiological exercises. During easy onset of voice, children are made aware of their sharp glottal attack or tense voice onset. By touching his or her thyroid cartilage, the child can feel the difference between rapid, forced vowel onset in words and slower, more relaxed onsets that occur in /h/ + vowel sequences. Gentle onset must be accompanied by good, resonant tone in order to avoid breathy phonation. The accent method of phonation involves the coordination of phonation and respiratory support in specific accented patterns and rhythms. Breathing exercises are taught initially. They are then combined with voice exercises. A stream of sounds is produced in varied rhythms and pitch changes as breath is expressed. This technique is suitable for use with children and adults (Mathieson 2001).

Psychological factors may be prominent in the aetiology of a voice disorder.[10] Two voice disorders in which psychological factors play a significant role are puberphonia in adolescent males and conversion aphonia. Even when psychological factors have not played a causal role in the development of a voice disorder, the presence of dysphonia may produce considerable anxiety and distress in the affected individual. Whether psychological problems are the cause or consequence of a voice disorder, their presence is likely to frustrate attempts at voice remediation, if they are not adequately addressed. Andersson and Schalén (1998) studied 30 patients with psychogenic voice disorder. These researchers found that interpersonal conflicts related to family and work precipitated voice disorder in these subjects. Treatment consisted of traditional vocal exercises. In addition, one of the researchers, who was trained in psychosomatic disorders and behavioural techniques, used interactive therapeutic discourse with the aim of mapping the patterns of the patients' social networks and focusing on conflicts. Baker (2003) reports the cases of two women who developed psychogenic voice disorders following earlier traumatic stress experiences. One of these women had suffered a sexual assault some months earlier. The other woman, who was 52 years old, had experienced a drowning episode at the age of 15 and was nearly sexually assaulted at the age of 12. These earlier traumatic experiences were awakened by a recent event – a second, modified thyroplasty for a unilateral vocal fold paresis – that had caused this woman considerable anxiety. Treatment of this second woman was conducted by the investigator, who had dual credentials in psychotherapy and family therapy. Symptomatic therapy was integrated with psychotherapeutic work.

The voice therapist has an important role to play in educating clients in a wide range of issues relating to voice care. This may include advice to clients on what type of voice use is appropriate following various surgical procedures (e.g. phonosurgery to remove vocal nodules). It may also include information and advice on different aspects of vocal hygiene.[11] While clients are generally aware of the adverse effects of smoking on the voice – even if they do not use this knowledge to alter their smoking behaviour – they are less aware of the dehydrating effects of alcohol, tea, coffee and low ambient humidity on the voice. They also require information on the damaging effects of gastric reflux, allergens and environmental pollutants on the laryngeal mucosa. Where there is high vocal demand in a client, for example, in the case of a professional voice user, the voice therapist must educate the client in how to avoid adverse vocal consequences of sustained voice use. Unfortunately, by the time most professional voice users come into contact with a voice therapist, it is because their vocal mechanism is already beginning to show the adverse effects of vocally abusive patterns of voice use. This has led to the greater involvement of therapists in preventive voice work. Bovo et al. (2007) evaluated the effectiveness of a preventive voice programme that was implemented with kindergarten and primary school female teachers. A total of 264 teachers participated in the programme, which included two lectures on voice care, a short voice therapy group, home-controlled voice exercises and vocal hygiene. Evaluation at three months revealed that programme participants displayed improvement in global dysphonia rates, jitter, shimmer, maximum phonation time and voice handicap index scores. Positive effects remained at 12 months after the course, although they were slightly reduced.

Research studies are now increasingly beginning to investigate the efficacy of voice therapy in different clinical groups. Berg et al. (2008) examined the medical records of 54 patients aged over 60 years who had been diagnosed with age-related dysphonia. Of these patients, 19 agreed to undergo voice therapy and complete voice-related quality of life questionnaires (VRQOL) before and after treatment. Six subjects with age-related dysphonia did not receive treatment and served as controls. Patients who received therapy experienced a mean improvement in VRQOL scores of 19.21. This was achieved after a mean of 4.1 voice therapy sessions and 5.1 months. After a mean of 3.3 months, control subjects experienced a mean change in VRQOL score of 0.42. Berg et al. conclude that '[v]oice therapy leads to statistically significant improvement in the VRQOL in elderly patients with age-related dysphonia'. Schindler et al. (2008) examined the efficacy of voice therapy in patients with unilateral vocal fold paralysis. Where only eight patients were able to achieve complete glottal closure before voice therapy, complete glottal closure occurred in 14 patients after therapy. Significant improvements were also observed in mean maximum phonation time, perceptual voice parameters, spectrographic analysis, perturbation analysis and voice handicap index scores following therapy. Schindler et al. state that '[a] significant improvement of voice quality and quality of life after voice therapy is an often reached and reasonable goal in patients with unilateral vocal fold paralysis'. Andersson and Schalén (1998) performed voice therapy in 30 patients with psychogenic voice disorder. These investigators found no evidence of relapse in 88 per cent of patients during the follow-up period of 1.9–8.4 years. Researchers have also conducted efficacy studies into voice therapy for vocal nodules (Holmberg et al. 2001) and into specific treatment schemes such as the accent method of voice therapy (Bassiouny 1998).

Notes

1. Bamboo nodes are a rare type of vocal fold lesion that is related to autoimmune disease. Schwemmle and Ptok (2007) report the case of a 43-year-old woman with Sharp syndrome and dysphonia. Laryngoscopy revealed transverse deposits on both vocal folds that were diagnosed as bamboo nodes. Murano et al. (2001) report the cases of two patients with autoimmune disease and bamboo nodes. One patient had Sjögren's syndrome, while the other had systemic lupus erythematosus.

2. Dysphonia may also be caused by malignant tumours that occur outside the larynx. Molina Garrido et al. (2006) describe the case of a woman with dysphonia and dysphagia as a result of a thyroid mass. This mass was the first manifestation of a metastatic breast cancer.

3. Cardiovocal syndrome, or Ortner's syndrome, is characterised by left recurrent laryngeal nerve palsy. It is normally caused by cardiovascular disease, but can be caused by aortic dissection in rare cases (Lee et al. 2006).

4. A disorder that is often mistaken for asthma is paradoxical vocal fold motion (PVFM). Once thought to affect adults only, PVFM has been increasingly reported and treated in the child and adolescent population (Sandage and Zelazny 2004). PVFM involves the inappropriate closure or adduction of the true vocal folds during inspiration and/or expiration. It may result in upper airway obstruction and stridor. The co-occurrence of asthma and reflux makes a diagnosis of PVFM difficult. Doshi and Weinberger (2006) examined 49 patients, aged 8–25 years, who were diagnosed as having PVFM from 1989 to 2002. Although 41 of these patients had been treated previously for asthma, that diagnosis was confirmed as a comorbidity in only 12 patients.

5. Mathieson (2001) states that primary phonatory features are those that are 'the direct result of the initial disordered function of the vocal tract' (121).

6. Seinsch (2001) examined more than 7,000 laryngectomy patients in stationary rehabilitation between 1980 and 1999. Until 1992, oesophageal speech was more common than voice prosthesis surgery, which was performed in less than 1 per cent of patients. However, since 1994 the number of voice-prosthesis procedures has been increasing at about 10 per cent a year to 60 per cent in 1998 and 1999.

7. In a T1 glottic carcinoma, the tumour is limited to the vocal folds, which have normal mobility. A T2 tumour extends to the subglottic and/or supraglottic region with impairment of vocal fold mobility.

8. It should be emphasised that several studies have also found no link between pre-operative and postoperative radiotherapy on the one hand and medical complications and voice problems on the other hand. Diaz et al. (2000) found that preoperative and postoperative radiotherapy was not statistically related to the risk of immediate laryngeal stenosis in 376 patients who underwent supracricoid partial laryngectomy. Calder et al. (2006) found that radiotherapy was not statistically significant in predicting complications in patients fitted with tracheo-oesophageal fistula speech valves. Chone et al. (2005) found that the use of radiotherapy did not influence the successful use of indwelling Blom–Singer voice prosthesis in patients who underwent either primary or secondary tracheo-oesophageal puncture. Cheng et al. (2006) found that neither preoperative nor postoperative radiotherapy had any effect on complication rates or voice restoration in 68 patients who underwent tracheo-oesophageal puncture.

9. Andrews (1996) states that vocal hyperfunction 'is an overarching descriptive term that includes patterns of vocal abuse, misuse, and musculoskeletal tension' (254).

10. Willinger et al. (2005) screened 61 patients with functional dysphonia for additional psychiatric disorders. When compared with healthy controls, dysphonic subjects had significantly higher scores in depressive symptoms, in symptoms of nonspecific and general anxiety and in symptoms of specific anxiety concerning

health. DSM-IV criteria for a mood disorder, an anxiety disorder or an adjustment disorder were fulfilled by 57 per cent of patients.

11. There is clear evidence that even professional voice users do not appreciate the implications of bad vocal hygiene. Timmermans et al. (2003) questioned 27 future professional voice users (radio students) and 53 professional voice users (radio professionals) on their vocal hygiene. These investigators found that radio professionals did not have superior vocal hygiene compared to radio students. In radio professionals, intake of coffee was significantly higher than in radio students. Moreover, professionals indicated significantly more vocal fatigue than students. However, radio students experienced more acid reflux problems and hoarseness than radio professionals. Also, smoking was more common than one would expect in future and current professional voice users – 33 per cent and 28 per cent, respectively.

Bibliography

Abitbol, J., Abitbol, P. and Abitbol, B. (1999), 'Sex Hormones and the Female Voice', *Journal of Voice*, 13:3, 424–46.

Abkarian, G. G. (1992), 'Communication Effects of Prenatal Alcohol Exposure', *Journal of Communication Disorders*, 25:4, 221–40.

Abraham, S. S. and Yun, P. T. (2002), 'Laryngopharyngeal Dysmotility in Multiple Sclerosis', *Dysphagia*, 17:1, 69–74.

Ackermann, H., Hertrich, I. and Hehr, T. (1995), 'Oral Diadochokinesis in Neurological Dysarthrias', *Folia Phoniatrica et Logopaedica*, 47:1, 15–23.

Adams, C. (2002), 'Practitioner Review: The Assessment of Language Pragmatics', *Journal of Child Psychology and Psychiatry*, 43:8, 973–87.

Adams, C., Green, J., Gilchrist, A. and Cox, A. (2002), 'Conversational Behaviour of Children with Asperger Syndrome and Conduct Disorder', *Journal of Child Psychology and Psychiatry*, 43:5, 679–90.

Aguilar-Mediavilla, E. M., Sanz-Torrent, M. and Serra-Raventos, M. (2002), 'A Comparative Study of the Phonology of Pre-School Children with Specific Language Impairment (SLI), Language Delay (LD) and Normal Acquisition', *Clinical Linguistics and Phonetics*, 16:8, 573–96.

Akif Kiliç, M., Okur, E., Yildirim, I. and Güzelsoy, S. (2004), 'The Prevalence of Vocal Fold Nodules in School Age Children', *International Journal of Pediatric Otorhinolaryngology*, 68:4, 409–12.

Albert, M. L., Sparks, R. W. and Helm, N. A. (1973), 'Melodic Intonation Therapy for Aphasia', *Archives of Neurology*, 29:2, 130–1.

Albery, E. H., Bennett, J. A., Pigott, R. W. and Simmons, R. M. (1982), 'The Results of 100 Operations for Velopharyngeal Incompetence – Selected on the Findings of Endoscopic and Radiological Examination', *British Journal of Plastic Surgery*, 35:2, 118–26.

Albery, L. (1993), 'Approaches to the Treatment of Speech Problems', in J. Stengelhofen (ed.), *Cleft Palate: The Nature and Remediation of Communication Problems*, London: Whurr, pp. 97–110.

Albery, L. and Russell, J. (1994), *Cleft Palate Sourcebook*, Oxon: Winslow.

Allen, D. A. and Rapin, I. (1992), 'Autistic Children are Also Dysphasic', in H. Naruse and E. M. Ornitz (eds), *Neurobiology of Infantile Autism*, Amsterdam: Elsevier Science, pp. 157–68.

Alm, P. A. (2004), 'Stuttering and the Basal Ganglia Circuits: A Critical Review of Possible Relations', *Journal of Communication Disorders*, 37:4, 325–69.

ALS Association (2004), *Epidemiology of ALS and Suspected Clusters*, Calabasas Hills, CA: ALS Association.

Alt, M., Plante, E. and Creusere, M. (2004), 'Semantic Features in Fast-Mapping: Performance of Preschoolers with Specific Language Impairment Versus Preschoolers with Normal Language', *Journal of Speech, Language, and Hearing Research*, 47:2, 407–20.

Altman, K. W., Haines, G. K., Vakkalanka, S. K., Keni, S. P., Kopp, P. A. and Radosevich, J. A. (2003), 'Identification of Thyroid Hormone Receptors in the Human Larynx', *Laryngoscope*, 113:11, 1931–4.

Altmann, L. J. P., Kempler, D. and Andersen, E. S. (2001), 'Speech Errors in Alzheimer's Disease', *Journal of Speech, Language, and Hearing Research*, 44:5, 1069–82.

Alzheimer's Society (2005), *Understanding Vascular Dementia*, London: Alzheimer's Society.

Ambrose, N. G. and Yairi, E. (1999), 'Normative Disfluency Data for Early Childhood Stuttering', *Journal of Speech, Language, and Hearing Research*, 42:4, 895–909.

Ambrose, N. G., Yairi, E. and Cox, N. (1993), 'Genetic Aspects of Early Childhood Stuttering', *Journal of Speech and Hearing Research*, 36:4, 701–6.

American Cleft Palate-Craniofacial Association (2000), *Parameters for Evaluation and Treatment of Patients with Cleft Lip/Palate or Other Craniofacial Anomalies*, Chapel Hill, NC: American Cleft Palate-Craniofacial Association.

American Heart Association (2006), *Heart Disease and Stroke Statistics – 2006 Update*, Dallas, TX: American Heart Association.

American Psychiatric Association (2000), *Diagnostic and Statistical Manual of Mental Disorders*, Washington: American Psychiatric Association.

American Speech-Language-Hearing Association (2001), *Scope of Practice in Speech-Language Pathology*, Rockville, MD: Author.

Amici, S., Gorno-Tempini, M. L., Ogar, J. M., Dronkers, N. F. and Miller, B. L. (2006), 'An Overview on Primary Progressive Aphasia and its Variants', *Behavioural Neurology*, 17:2, 77–87.

Amin, M. R., Harris, D., Cassel, S. G., Grimes, E. and Heiman-Patterson, T. (2006), 'Sensory Testing in the Assessment of Laryngeal Sensation in Patients With Amyotrophic Lateral Sclerosis', *Annals of Otology, Rhinology and Laryngology*, 115:7, 528–34.

424

Anderson, J. D. and Conture, E. G. (2000), 'Language Abilities of Children Who Stutter: A Preliminary Study', *Journal of Fluency Disorders*, 25:4, 283–304.

Andersson, K. and Schalén, L. (1998), 'Etiology and Treatment of Psychogenic Voice Disorder: Results of a Follow-Up Study of Thirty Patients', *Journal of Voice*, 12:1, 96–106.

Andrews, G. and Ingham, R. J. (1971), 'Stuttering: Considerations in the Evaluation of Treatment', *British Journal of Disorders of Communication*, 6:2, 129–38.

Andrews, M. L. (1996), 'Treatment of Vocal Hyperfunction in Adolescents', *Language, Speech, and Hearing Services in Schools*, 27:3, 251–6.

Anthony, A., Bogle, D., Ingram, T. T. S. and McIsaac, M. W. (1971), *The Edinburgh Articulation Test*, Edinburgh and London: E&S Livingstone.

Ardila, A., Bateman, J. R., Nino, C. R., Pulido, E., Rivera, D. B. and Vanegas, C. J. (1994), 'An Epidemiologic Study of Stuttering', *Journal of Communication Disorders*, 27:1, 37–48.

Armson, J., Kiefte, M., Mason, J. and De Croos, D. (2006), 'The Effect of SpeechEasy on Stuttering Frequency in Laboratory Conditions', *Journal of Fluency Disorders*, 31:2, 137–52.

Arndt, J. and Healey, E. C. (2001), 'Concomitant Disorders in School-Age Children Who Stutter', *Language, Speech, and Hearing Services in Schools*, 32:2, 68–78.

Arvedson, J. C. (1998), 'Management of Pediatric Dysphagia', *Otolaryngologic Clinics of North America*, 31:3, 453–76.

Arvedson, J. C. and Brodsky, L. (2002), *Pediatric Swallowing and Feeding: Assessment and Management*, Albany, NY: Singular.

Ashwal, S., Russman, B. S., Blasco, P. A., Miller, G., Sandler, A., Shevell, M. and Stevenson, R. (2004), 'Practice Parameter: Diagnostic Assessment of the Child with Cerebral Palsy', *Neurology*, 62:6, 851–63.

Auzou, P., Ozsancak, C., Jan, M., Leonardon, S., Menard, J. F., Gaillard, M. J., Eustache, F. and Hannequin, D. (1998), 'Clinical Assessment of Dysarthria: Presentation and Validation of a Method', *Revue Neurologique*, 154:6–7, 523–30.

Auzou, P., Ozsancak, C., Morris, R. J., Jan, M., Eustache, F. and Hannequin, D. (2000), 'Voice Onset Time in Aphasia, Apraxia of Speech and Dysarthria: A Review', *Clinical Linguistics and Phonetics*, 14:2, 131–50.

Aviv, J. E., Murry, T., Zschommler, A., Cohen, M. and Gartner, C. (2005), 'Flexible Endoscopic Evaluation of Swallowing with Sensory Testing: Patient Characteristics and Analysis of Safety in 1,340 Consecutive Examinations', *Annals of Otology, Rhinology and Laryngology*, 114:3, 173–6.

Baddeley, A. D. (1986), *Working Memory*, Oxford: Oxford University Press.

Baddeley, A. D. (2000), 'The Episodic Buffer: A New Component of Working Memory?', *Trends in Cognitive Sciences*, 4:11, 417–23.

Baddeley, A. D. and Hitch, G. (1974), 'Working Memory', in G. Bower (ed.), *The Psychology of Learning and Motivation*, New York: Academic, pp. 47–90.

Bagner, D. M., Melinder, M. R. D. and Barch, D. M. (2003), 'Language Comprehension and Working Memory Deficits in Patients With Schizophrenia', *Schizophrenia Research*, 60:2–3, 299–309.

Bailey, A., Le Couteur, A., Gottesman, I., Bolton, P., Simonoff, E., Yuzda, E. and Rutter, M. (1995), 'Autism as a Strongly Genetic Disorder: Evidence from a British Twin Study', *Psychological Medicine*, 25:1, 63–77.

Bailey, A., Palferman, S., Heavey, L. and Le Couteur, A. (1998), 'Autism: The Phenotype in Relatives', *Journal of Autism and Developmental Disorders*, 28:5, 369–92.

Bajaj, A., Hodson, B. and Schommer-Aikins, M. (2004), 'Performance on Phonological and Grammatical Awareness Metalinguistic Tasks by Children Who Stutter and Their Fluent Peers', *Journal of Fluency Disorders*, 29:1, 63–77.

Baker, J. (2003), 'Psychogenic Voice Disorders and Traumatic Stress Experience: A Discussion Paper with Two Case Reports', *Journal of Voice*, 17:3, 308–18.

Bakheit, A. M., Carrington, S., Griffiths, S. and Searle, K. (2005), 'High Scores on the Western Aphasia Battery Correlate with Good Functional Communication Skills (as Measured with the Communicative Effectiveness Index) in Aphasic Stroke Patients', *Disability and Rehabilitation*, 27:6, 287–91.

Balasubramanian, V., Max, L., Van Borsel, J., Rayca, K. O. and Richardson, D. (2003), 'Acquired Stuttering Following Right Frontal and Bilateral Pontine Lesion: A Case Study', *Brain and Cognition*, 53:2, 185–9.

Ball, L. J., Beukelman, D. R. and Pattee, G. L. (2004), 'Communication Effectiveness of Individuals with Amyotrophic Lateral Sclerosis', *Journal of Communication Disorders*, 37:3, 197–215.

Ballard, K. J. (2001), 'Response Generalization in Apraxia of Speech Treatments: Taking Another Look', *Journal of Communication Disorders*, 34:1–2, 3–20.

Bankson, N. W. and Bernthal, J. E. (1990), *Bankson-Bernthal Test of Phonology*, Chicago, IL: Riverside.

Baraff, L. J., Lee, S. I. and Schriger, D. L. (1993), 'Outcomes of Bacterial Meningitis in Children: A Meta-Analysis', *Pediatric Infectious Disease Journal*, 12:5, 389–94.

Baranek, G. T., Barnett, C. R., Adams, E. M., Wolcott, N. A., Watson, L. R. and Crais, E. R. (2005), 'Object Play in Infants with Autism: Methodological Issues in Retrospective Video Analysis', *American Journal of Occupational Therapy*, 59:1, 20–30.

Bartak, L., Rutter, M. and Cox, A. (1975), 'A Comparative Study of Infantile Autism and Specific Developmental Receptive Language Disorder: I. The Children', *British Journal of Psychiatry*, 126:2, 127–45.

Bartha, L. and Benke, T. (2003), 'Acute Conduction Aphasia: An Analysis of 20 Cases', *Brain and Language*, 85:1, 93–108.

Bartle, C. J., Goozee, J. V., Scott, D., Murdoch, B. E. and Kuruvilla, M. (2006), 'EMA Assessment of Tongue-Jaw Co-ordination During Speech in Dysarthria Following Traumatic Brain Injury', *Brain Injury*, 20:5, 529–45.

Bartlett, C. W., Flax, J. F., Logue, M. W., Vieland, V. J., Bassett, A. S., Tallal, P. and Brzustowicz, L. M. (2002), 'A Major Susceptability Locus for Specific Language Impairment is Located on 13q21', *American Journal of Human Genetics*, 71:1, 45–55.

Bartlett, S. C., Armstrong, E. and Roberts, J. (2005), 'Linguistic Resources of Individuals with Asperger Syndrome', *Clinical Linguistics and Phonetics*, 19:3, 203–13.

Barton, M. and Volkmar, F. (1998), 'How Commonly are Known Medical Conditions Associated with Autism?', *Journal of Autism and Developmental Disorders*, 28:4, 273–8.

Bassiouny, S. (1998), 'Efficacy of the Accent Method of Voice Therapy', *Folia Phoniatrica et Logopaedica*, 50:3, 146–64.

Bauman, M. L. and Kemper, T. L. (1994), 'Neuroanatomic Observations of the Brain in Autism', in M. L. Bauman and T. L. Kemper (eds), *The Neurobiology of Autism*, Baltimore, MD: Johns Hopkins University Press, pp. 119–45.

Bauman, M. L. and Kemper, T. L. (2005), 'Neuroanatomic Observations of the Brain in Autism: A Review and Future Directions', *International Journal of Developmental Neuroscience*, 23:2–3, 183–7.

Baumeister, H., Caspar, F. and Herziger, F. (2003), 'Treatment Outcome Study of the Stuttering Therapy Summer Camp 2000 for Children and Adolescents', *Psychotherapie, Psychosomatik, Medizinische Psychologie*, 53:11, 455–63.

Baumgartner, J. and Duffy, J. R. (1997), 'Psychogenic Stuttering in Adults with and without Neurologic Disease', *Journal of Medical Speech-Language Pathology*, 5:2, 75–95.

Baynes, K., Kegl, J. A., Brentari, D., Kussmaul, C. and Poizner, H. (1998), 'Chronic Auditory Agnosia Following Landau-Kleffner Syndrome: A 23 Year Outcome Study', *Brain and Language*, 63:3, 381–425.

Bazin, N., Perruchet, P., Hardy-Bayle, M. C. and Feline, A. (2000), 'Context-Dependent Information Processing in Patients with Schizophrenia', *Schizophrenia Research*, 45:1–2, 93–101.

Becker, M., Warr-Leeper, G. A. and Leeper, H. A. (1990), 'Fetal Alcohol Syndrome: A Description of Oral Motor, Articulatory, Short-Term Memory, Grammatical, and Semantic Abilities', *Journal of Communication Disorders*, 23:2, 97–124.

Bedore, L. M. and Leonard, L. B. (1998), 'Specific Language Impairment and Grammatical Morphology: A Discriminant Function Analysis', *Journal of Speech, Language, and Hearing Research*, 41:5, 1185–92.

Beeke, S. (2003), ' "I suppose" as a Resource for the Construction of Turns at Talk in Agrammatic Aphasia', *Clinical Linguistics and Phonetics*, 17:4–5, 291–8.

Beeke, S., Wilkinson, R. and Maxim, J. (2003), 'Exploring Aphasic Grammar. 1: A Single Case Analysis of Conversation', *Clinical Linguistics and Phonetics*, 17:2, 81–107.

Belafsky, P. C., Blumenfeld, L., LePage, A. and Nahrstedt, K. (2003), 'The Accuracy of the Modified Evan's Blue Dye Test in Predicting Aspiration', *Laryngoscope*, 113:11, 1969–72.

Belmonte, M. and Carper, R. (1998), 'Neuroanatomical and Neurophysiological Clues to the Nature of Autism', in B. Garreau (ed.), *Neuroimaging in Child Neuropsychiatric Disorders*, Paris: Springer-Verlag, pp. 157–71.

Belton, E., Salmond, C. H., Watkins, K. E., Vargha-Khadem, F. and Gadian, D. G. (2003), 'Bilateral Brain Abnormalities Associated with Dominantly Inherited Verbal and Orofacial Dyspraxia', *Human Brain Mapping*, 18:3, 194–200.

Benke, T., Hohenstein, C., Poewe, W. and Butterworth, B. (2000), 'Repetitive Speech Phenomena in Parkinson's Disease', *Journal of Neurology, Neurosurgery and Psychiatry*, 69:3, 319–24.

Berg, E. E., Hapner, E., Klein, A. and Johns, M. M. (2008), 'Voice Therapy Improves Quality of Life in Age-Related Dysphonia: A Case-Control Study', *Journal of Voice*.

Bernard-Opitz, V., Ing, S. and Kong, T. Y. (2004), 'Comparison of Behavioural and Natural Play Interventions for Young Children with Autism', *Autism*, 8:3, 319–33.

Bernhardt, B. and Major, E. (2005), 'Speech, Language and Literacy Skills 3 Years Later: A Follow-Up Study of Early Phonological and Metaphonological Intervention', *International Journal of Language and Communication Disorders*, 40:1, 1–27.

Bernhardt, B. H. and Holdgrafer, G. (2001), 'Beyond the Basics I: The Need for Strategic Sampling for In-Depth Phonological Analysis', *Language, Speech, and Hearing Services in Schools*, 32:1, 18–27.

Bess, F. H., Dodd-Murphy, J. and Parker, R. A. (1998), 'Children with Minimal Sensorineural Hearing Loss: Prevalence, Educational Performance, and Functional Status', *Ear and Hearing*, 19:5, 339–54.

Betz, S. K. and Stoel-Gammon, C. (2005), 'Measuring Articulatory Error Consistency in Children with Developmental Apraxia of Speech', *Clinical Linguistics and Phonetics*, 19:1, 53–66.

Beverly, B. L. and Williams, C. C. (2004), 'Present Tense *Be* Use in Young Children with Specific Language Impairment: Less is More', *Journal of Speech, Language, and Hearing Research*, 47:4, 944–56.

Bihari, A., Meszaros, K., Remenyi, A. and Lichtenberger, G. (2006), 'Voice Quality Improvement after Management of Unilateral Vocal Cord Paralysis with Different Techniques', *European Archives of Oto-Rhino-Laryngology*, 263:12, 1115–20.

Bijleveld, H., Lebrun, Y. and van Dongen, H. (1994), 'A Case of Acquired Stuttering', *Folia Phoniatrica et Logopaedica*, 46:5, 250–3.

Bird, J., Bishop, D. V. M. and Freeman, N. H. (1995), 'Phonological Awareness and Literacy Development in Children with Expressive Phonological Impairments', *Journal of Speech and Hearing Research*, 38:2, 446–62.

Bishop, D. V. and Baird, G. (2001), 'Parent and Teacher Report of Pragmatic Aspects of Communication: Use of the Children's Communication Checklist in a Clinical Setting', *Developmental Medicine and Child Neurology*, 43:12, 809–18.

Bishop, D. V., North, T. and Donlan, C. (1995), 'Genetic Basis of Specific Language Impairment: Evidence from a Twin Study', *Developmental Medicine and Child Neurology*, 37:1, 56–71.

Bishop, D. V. M. (1983), *The Test for Reception of Grammar*, Manchester: University of Manchester.

Bishop, D. V. M. (1998), 'Development of the Children's Communication Checklist (CCC): A Method for Assessing Qualitative Aspects of Communicative Impairment in Children', *Journal of Child Psychology and Psychiatry*, 39:6, 879–91.

Bishop, D. V. M. (2000a), 'Pragmatic Language Impairment: A Correlate of SLI, a Distinct Subgroup, or Part of the Autistic Continuum?', in D. V. M. Bishop and L. B. Leonard (eds), *Speech and Language Impairments in Children: Causes, Characteristics, Intervention and Outcome*, Hove: Psychology Press, pp. 99–113.

Bishop, D. V. M. (2000b), 'What's So Special about Asperger Syndrome? The Need for Further Exploration of the Borderlands of Autism', in A. Klin, F. R. Volkmar and S. S. Sparrow (eds), *Asperger Syndrome*, New York: Guilford, pp. 254–77.

Bishop, D. V. M. (2003), *The Children's Communication Checklist, version 2 (CCC-2)*, London: Psychological Corporation.

Bishop, D. V. M., Byers Brown, B. and Robson, J. (1990), 'The Relationship between Phoneme Discrimination, Speech Production, and Language Comprehension in Cerebral-Palsied Individuals', *Journal of Speech and Hearing Research*, 33:2, 210–19.

Bishop, D. V. M., Chan, J., Adams, C., Hartley, J. and Weir, F. (2000), 'Conversational Responsiveness in Specific Language Impairment: Evidence of Disproportionate Pragmatic Difficulties in a Subset of Children', *Development and Psychopathology*, 12:2, 177–99.

Bishop, D. V. M. and Rosenbloom, L. (1987), 'Classification of Childhood Language Disorders', in W. Yule and M. Rutter (eds), *Language Development and Disorders*, London: MacKeith, pp. 16–41.

Blanc, R., Adrien, J. L., Roux, S. and Barthelemy, C. (2005), 'Dysregulation of Pretend Play and Communication Development in Children with Autism', *Autism*, 9:3, 229–45.

Blasco, P. A. (2002), 'Management of Drooling: 10 Years after the Consortium on Drooling, 1990', *Developmental Medicine and Child Neurology*, 44:11, 778–81.

Bleile, K. (2002), 'Evaluating Articulation and Phonological Disorders when the Clock is Running', *American Journal of Speech-Language Pathology*, 11:3, 243–9.

Bliss, C. (1965), *Semantography (Blissymbolics)*, Sydney: Semantography.

Block, S., Onslow, M., Packman, A. and Dacakis, G. (2006), 'Connecting Stuttering Management and Measurement: IV. Predictors of Outcome for a Behavioural Treatment for Stuttering', *International Journal of Language and Communication Disorders*, 41:4, 395–406.

Blomgren, M., Roy, N., Callister, T. and Merrill, R. M. (2005), 'Intensive Stuttering Modification Therapy: A Multidimensional Assessment of Treatment Outcomes', *Journal of Speech, Language, and Hearing Research*, 48:3, 509–23.

Blood, G. W., Ridenour, V. J., Qualls, C. D. and Hammer, C. S. (2003), 'Co-occurring Disorders in Children Who Stutter', *Journal of Communication Disorders*, 36:6, 427–48.

Bloodstein, O. (1979), *Speech Pathology: An Introduction*, Boston, MA: Houghton Mifflin.

Bluestone, C. D., Paradise, J. L., Beery, Q. C. and Wittel, R. (1972), 'Certain Effects of Cleft Palate Repair on Eustachian Tube Function', *Cleft Palate Journal*, 9:3, 183–93.

Boberg, E. and Kully, D. (1985), *Comprehensive Stuttering Program*, San Diego, CA: College Hill.

Bondy, A. S. and Frost, L. A. (1998), 'The Picture Exchange Communication System', *Seminars in Speech and Language*, 19:4, 373–88.

Booth, S. and Perkins, L. (1999), 'The Use of Conversation Analysis to Guide Individualized Advice to Carers and Evaluate Change in Aphasia: A Case Study', *Aphasiology*, 13:4–5, 283–303.

Booth, S. and Swabey, D. (1999), 'Group Training in Communication Skills for Carers of Adults with Aphasia', *International Journal of Language and Communication Disorders*, 34:3, 291–309.

Boring, C. C., Squires, T. S. and Tong, T. (1991), 'Cancer Statistics, 1991', *CA-A Cancer Journal for Clinicians*, 41:1, 19–36.

Bornman, J., Alant, E. and Meiring, E. (2001), 'The Use of a Digital Voice Output Device to Facilitate Language Development in a Child with Developmental Apraxia of Speech: A Case Study', *Disability and Rehabilitation*, 23:14, 623–34.

Boscolo, B., Ratner, N. B. and Rescorla, L. (2002), 'Fluency of School-Aged Children with a History of Specific Expressive Language Impairment: An Exploratory Study', *American Journal of Speech-Language Pathology*, 11:1, 41–9.

Bose, A., Square, P. A., Schlosser, R. and van Lieshout, P. (2001), 'Effects of PROMPT Therapy on Speech Motor Function in a Person with Aphasia and Apraxia of Speech', *Aphasiology*, 15:8, 767–85.

Bothe, A. K. (2002), 'Speech Modification Approaches to Stuttering Treatment in Schools', *Seminars in Speech and Language*, 23:3, 181–6.

Botting, N. and Adams, C. (2005), 'Semantic and Inferencing Abilities in Children with Communication Disorders', *International Journal of Language and Communication Disorders*, 40:1, 49–66.

Boudreau, D. M. and Hedberg, N. L. (1999), 'A Comparison of Early Literacy Skills in Children with Specific Language Impairment and their Typically Developing Peers', *American Journal of Speech-Language Pathology*, 8:3, 249–60.

Bovo, R., Galceran, M., Petruccelli, J. and Hatzopoulos, S. (2007), 'Vocal Problems Among Teachers: Evaluation of a Preventive Voice Program', *Journal of Voice*, 21:6, 705–22.

Bowens, A. and Smith, I. (1999), *Childhood Dyspraxia: Some Issues for the NHS*. Nuffield Portfolio Programme Report No. 2, Leeds: Nuffield Institute for Health.

Boyle, C. A., Yeargin-Allsopp, M., Doernberg, N. S., Holmgreen, P., Murphy, C. C. and Schendel, D. E. (1996), 'Prevalence of Selected Developmental Disabilities in Children 3–10 Years of Age: The Metropolitan Atlanta Developmental Disabilities Surveillance Program, 1991', *Morbidity and Mortality Weekly Report*, 45 (SS-2), 1–14.

Breitenfeldt, D. H. and Lorenz, D. R. (1989), *Successful Stuttering Management Program*, Cheney, WA: Eastern Washington University.

Briscoe, J., Bishop, D. V. M. and Norbury, C. F. (2001), 'Phonological Processing, Language and Literacy: A Comparison of Children with Mild-to-Moderate Sensorineural Hearing Loss and Those with Specific Language Impairment', *Journal of Child Psychology and Psychiatry*, 42:3, 329–40.

Bristol, M. M., Cohen, D. J., Costello, E. J., Denckla, M., Eckberg, T. J., Kallen, R., Kraemer, H. C., Lord, C., Maurer, R., McIlvane, W. J., Minshew, N., Sigman, M. and Spence, M. A. (1996), 'State of the Science in Autism: Report to the National Institutes of Health', *Journal of Autism and Developmental Disorders*, 26:2, 121–54.

Broadley, S., Cheek, A., Salonikis, S., Whitham, E., Chong, V., Cardone, D., Alexander, B., Taylor, J. and Thompson, P. (2005), 'Predicting Prolonged Dysphagia in Acute Stroke: The Royal Adelaide Prognostic Index for Dysphagic Stroke (RAPIDS)', *Dysphagia*, 20:4, 303–10.

Broen, P. A., Devers, M. C., Doyle, S. S., Prouty, J. M. and Moller, K. T. (1998), 'Acquisition of Linguistic and Cognitive Skills by Children with Cleft Palate', *Journal of Speech, Language, and Hearing Research*, 41:3, 676–87.

Brookes, M., MacMillan, R., Cully, S., Anderson, E., Murray, S., Mendelow, A. D. and Jennett, B. (1990), 'Head Injuries in Accident and Emergency Departments. How Different are Children from Adults?', *Journal of Epidemiology and Community Health*, 44:2, 147–51.

Brookshire, R. H. and Nicholas, L. E. (1995), 'Performance Deviations in the Connected Speech of Adults with no Brain Damage and Adults with Aphasia', *American Journal of Speech-Language Pathology*, 4:4, 118–23.

Brumfitt, S. M. and Sheeran, P. (1997), 'An Evaluation of Short-Term Group Therapy for People with Aphasia', *Disability and Rehabilitation*, 19:6, 221–30.

Brundage, S. B., Graap, K., Gibbons, K. F., Ferrer, M. and Brooks, J. (2006), 'Frequency of Stuttering During Challenging and Supportive Virtual Reality Job Interviews', *Journal of Fluency Disorders*, 31:4, 325–39.

Brüne, M. and Bodenstein, L. (2005), 'Proverb Comprehension Reconsidered – 'Theory of Mind' and the Pragmatic Use of Language in Schizophrenia', *Schizophrenia Research*, 75:2–3, 233–9.

Buckley, S. (1995a), 'Improving the Expressive Language Skills of Teenagers with Down's Syndrome', *Down Syndrome Research and Practice*, 3:3, 110–15.

Buckley, S. (1995b), 'Teaching Children with Down Syndrome to Read and Write', in L. Nadel and D. Rosenthal (eds), *Down Syndrome: Living and Learning in the Community*, New York: Wiley-Liss, pp. 158–69.

Buckley, S. (1999), 'Improving the Speech and Language Skills of Children and Teenagers with Down Syndrome', *Down Syndrome News and Update*, 1:3, 111–28.

Buckley, S. (2002), 'The Significance of Early Reading for Children with Down Syndrome', *Down Syndrome News and Update*, 2:1, 1.

Buckley, S. and Le Prevost, P. (2002), 'Speech and Language Therapy for Children with Down Syndrome', *Down Syndrome News and Update*, 2:2, 70–6.

Burghaus, L., Hilker, R., Thiel, A., Galldiks, N., Lehnhardt, F. G., Zaro-Weber, O., Sturm, V. and Heiss, W. D. (2006), 'Deep Brain Stimulation of the Subthalamic Nucleus Reversibly Deteriorates Stuttering in Advanced Parkinson's Disease', *Journal of Neural Transmission*, 113:5, 625–31.

Byrne, A., Byrne, M. K. and Zibin, T. O. (1993), 'Transient Neurogenic Stuttering', *International Journal of Eating Disorders*, 14:4, 511–14.

Cabel, R. M., Colcord, R. D. and Petrosino, L. (2002), 'Self-Reported Anxiety of Adults Who Do and Do Not Stutter', *Perceptual and Motor Skills*, 94:3:1, 775–84.

Cahill, L. M., Turner, A. B., Stabler, P. A., Addis, P. E., Theodoros, D. G. and Murdoch, B. E. (2004), 'An Evaluation of Continuous Positive Airway Pressure (CPAP) Therapy in the Treatment of Hypernasality Following Traumatic Brain Injury: A Report of 3 Cases', *Journal of Head Trauma Rehabilitation*, 19:3, 241–53.

Cajavec, B., Herzel, H. and Bernard, S. (2006), 'Death of Neuronal Clusters Contributes to Variance of Age at Onset in Huntington's Disease', *Neurogenetics*, 7:1, 21–5.

Calandrella, A. M. and Wilcox, M. J. (2000), 'Predicting Language Outcomes for Young Prelinguistic Children with Developmental Delay', *Journal of Speech, Language and Hearing Research*, 43:5, 1061–71.

Calculator, S. and Dollaghan, C. (1982), 'The Use of Communication Boards in a Residential Setting: An Evaluation', *Journal of Speech and Hearing Disorders*, 47:3, 281–7.

Calder, N., MacAndie, C. and MacGregor, F. (2006), 'Tracheoesophageal Voice Prostheses Complications in North Glasgow', *Journal of Laryngology and Otology*, 120:6, 487–91.

California Health and Human Services Agency (1999), *Changes in the Population of Persons with Autism and Pervasive Developmental Disorders in California's Developmental Services System: 1987 Through 1998*, California: California Health and Human Services Agency.

Campbell, T. F. (1998), *Department of Audiology and Communication Disorders General Communication Outcome Questionnaire*, Pittsburgh, PA: Children's Hospital of Pittsburgh.

Campbell, T. F. (1999), 'Functional Treatment Outcomes in Young Children with Motor Speech Disorders', in A. J. Caruso and E. A. Strand (eds), *Clinical Management of Motor Speech Disorders in Children*, New York: Thieme Medical, pp. 385–96.

Campbell, T. F. and Dollaghan, C. A. (1995), 'Speaking Rate, Articulatory Speed, and Linguistic Processing in Children and Adolescents with Severe Traumatic Brain Injury', *Journal of Speech and Hearing*, 38:4, 864–75.

Cannito, M. P., Vogel, D., Pierce, R. S. and Hough, M. (1992), 'Time Post Onset and Contextualised Sentence Comprehension in Nonfluent Aphasia', *Clinical Aphasiology*, 21, 225–33.

Carding, P., Carlson, E., Epstein, R., Mathieson, L. and Shewell, C. (2000), 'Formal Perceptual Evaluation of Voice Quality in the United Kingdom', *Logopedics Phoniatrics Vocology*, 25:3, 133–8.

Carding, P. N., Roulstone, S., Northstone, K. and the ALSPAC Study Team (2006), 'The Prevalence of Childhood Dysphonia: A Cross-Sectional Study', *Journal of Voice*, 20:4, 623–30.

Carnaby, G., Hankey, G. J. and Pizzi, J. (2006), 'Behavioural Intervention for Dysphagia in Acute Stroke: A Randomised Controlled Trial', *Lancet Neurology*, 5:1, 31–7.

Carper, R. A. and Courchesne, E. (2000), 'Inverse Correlation between Frontal Lobe and Cerebellum Sizes in Children with Autism', *Brain*, 123:4, 836–44.

Carper, R. A., Moses, P., Tigue, Z. D. and Courchesne, E. (2002), 'Cerebral Lobes in Autism: Early Hyperplasia and Abnormal Age Effects', *NeuroImage*, 16:4, 1038–51.

Carroll, K., Murad, S., Eliahoo, J. and Majeed, A. (2001), 'Stroke Incidence and Risk Factors in a Population-Based Prospective Cohort Study', *Health Statistics Quarterly*, 12, 18–26.

Caruso, A. J. and Strand, E. A. (1999), 'Motor Speech Disorders in Children: Definitions, Background, and a Theoretical Framework', in A. J. Caruso and E. A. Strand (eds), *Clinical Management of Motor Speech Disorders in Children*, New York: Thieme Medical, pp. 1–27.

Carvill, S. (2001), 'Sensory Impairments, Intellectual Disability and Psychiatry', *Journal of Intellectual Disability Research*, 45:6, 467–83.

Catts, H. W. (1986), 'Speech Production/Phonological Deficits in Reading-Disordered Children', *Journal of Learning Disabilities*, 19:8, 504–8.

Catts, H. W., Adlof, S. M., Hogan, T. P. and Weismer, S. E. (2005), 'Are Specific Language Impairment and Dyslexia Distinct Disorders?', *Journal of Speech, Language, and Hearing Research*, 48:6, 1378–96.

Chaika, E. (1990), *Understanding Psychotic Speech: Beyond Freud and Chomsky*, Springfield, IL: Charles C. Thomas.

Chaika, E. (1997), 'Intention, Attention, and Deviant Schizophrenic Speech', in J. France and N. Muir (eds), *Communication and the Mentally Ill Patient: Developmental and Linguistic Approaches to Schizophrenia*, London: Jessica Kingsley, pp. 18–29.

Chapman, K. L. (2004), 'Is Presurgery and Early Postsurgery Performance Related to Speech and Language Outcomes at 3 Years of Age for Children with Cleft Palate?', *Clinical Linguistics and Phonetics*, 18:4–5, 235–57.

Chapman, K. L., Hardin-Jones, M. and Halter, K. A. (2003), 'The Relationship between Early Speech and Later Speech and Language Performance for Children with Cleft Lip and Palate', *Clinical Linguistics and Phonetics*, 17:3, 173–97.

Chapman, R. S. (1999), 'Language Development in Children and Adolescents with Down Syndrome', in J. F. Miller, M. Leddy and L. A. Leavitt (eds), *Improving the Communication of People with Down Syndrome*, Baltimore, MD: Paul H. Brookes, pp. 41–60.

Chapman, R. S., Hesketh, L. J. and Kistler, D. J. (2002), 'Predicting Longitudinal Change in Language Production and Comprehension in Individuals with Down Syndrome: Hierarchical Linear Modeling', *Journal of Speech, Language, and Hearing Research*, 45:5, 902–15.

Chapman, R. S., Seung, H-K., Schwartz, S. E. and Bird, E. K-R. (2000), 'Predicting Language Production in Children and Adolescents with Down Syndrome: The Role of Comprehension', *Journal of Speech, Language, and Hearing Research*, 43:2, 340–50.

Chapman, S. B., Ulatowska, H. K., Franklin, L. R., Shobe, A. E., Thompson, J. L. and McIntire, D. D. (1997), 'Proverb Interpretation in Fluent Aphasia and Alzheimer's Disease: Implications Beyond Abstract Thinking', *Aphasiology*, 11:4–5, 337–50.

Charlop-Christy, M. H., Carpenter, M., Le, L., Le Blanc, L. A. and Kellet, K. (2002), 'Using the Picture Exchange Communication System (PECS) with Children with Autism: Assessment of PECS Acquisition, Speech, Social-Communicative Behavior, and Problem Behavior', *Journal of Applied Behavior Analysis*, 35:3, 213–31.

Cheng, E., Ho, M., Ganz, C., Shaha, A., Boyle, J. O., Singh, B., Wong, R. J., Patel, S., Shah, J., Branski, R. C. and Kraus, D. H. (2006), 'Outcomes of Primary and Secondary Tracheoesophageal Puncture: A 16-Year Retrospective Analysis', *Ear, Nose, and Throat Journal*, 85:4, 262, 264–7.

Chess, S. (1977), 'Follow-Up Report on Autism in Congenital Rubella', *Journal of Autism and Childhood Schizophrenia*, 7:1, 69–81.

Cheuk, D. K., Wong, V. and Leung, G. M. (2005), 'Multilingual Home Environment and Specific Language Impairment: A Case-Control Study in Chinese Children', *Paediatric and Perinatal Epidemiology*, 19:4, 303–14.

Chiou, C. C., Groll, A. H., Gonzalez, C. E., Callender, D., Venzon, D., Pizzo, P. A., Wood, L. and Walsh, T. J. (2000), 'Esophageal Candidiasis in Pediatric Acquired Immunodeficiency Syndrome: Clinical Manifestations and Risk Factors', *Pediatric Infectious Disease Journal*, 19:8, 729–34.

Chone, C. T., Spina, A. L., Crespo, A. N. and Gripp, F. M. (2005), 'Speech Rehabilitation after Total Laryngectomy: Long-Term Results with Indwelling Voice Prosthesis Blom-Singer', *Revista Brasileira de Otorrinolaringologia*, 71:4, 504–9.

Chumpelik, D. (1984), 'The PROMPT System of Therapy: Theoretical Framework and Applications for Developmental Apraxia of Speech', *Seminars in Speech and Language*, 5:2, 139–56.

Chung, S. J., Im, J. H., Lee, J. H. and Lee, M. C. (2004), 'Stuttering and Gait Disturbance after Supplementary Motor Area Seizure', *Movement Disorders*, 19:9, 1106–9.

Church, M. W. and Kaltenbach, J. A. (1997), 'Hearing, Speech, Language, and Vestibular Disorders in the Fetal Alcohol Syndrome: A Literature Review', *Alcoholism: Clinical and Experimental Research*, 21:3, 495–512.

Church, M. W., Eldis, F., Blakley, B. W. and Bawle, E. V. (1997), 'Hearing, Language, Speech, Vestibular, and Dentofacial Disorders in Fetal Alcohol Syndrome', *Alcoholism: Clinical and Experimental Research*, 21:2, 227–37.

Clary, R. A., Pengilly, A., Bailey, M., Jones, N., Albert, D., Comins, J. and Appleton, J. (1996), 'Analysis of Voice Outcomes in Pediatric Patients Following Surgical Procedures for Laryngotracheal Stenosis', *Archives of Otolaryngology – Head and Neck Surgery*, 122:11, 1189–94.

Clem, K. and Morgenlander, J. C. (2006), *Amyotrophic Lateral Sclerosis*, USA: eMedicine.com (website: http://www.emedicine.com/emerg/topic24.htm).

Clevens, R. A., Esclamado, R. M., Hartshorn, D. O. and Lewin J. S. (1993), 'Voice Rehabilitation after Total Laryngectomy and Tracheoesophageal Puncture Using Nonmuscle Closure', *Annals of Otology, Rhinology and Laryngology*, 102:10, 792–6.

Clibbens, J. (2001), 'Signing and Lexical Development in Children with Down Syndrome', *Down Syndrome Research and Practice*, 7:3, 101–5.

Clough, C. G., Chaudhuri, K. R. and Sethi, K. D. (2003), *Parkinson's Disease*, Oxford: Health Press.

Coelho, C. A. and Flewellyn, L. (2003), 'Longitudinal Assessment of Coherence in an Adult with Fluent Aphasia', *Aphasiology*, 17:2, 173–82.

Coelho, C. A., Youse, K. M., Le, K. N. and Feinn, R. (2003), 'Narrative and Conversational Discourse of Adults with Closed Head Injuries and Non-Brain-Injured Adults: A Discriminant Analysis', *Aphasiology*, 17:5, 499–510.

Cohen, B. D. (1978), 'Referent Communication Disturbances in Schizophrenia', in S. Schwartz (ed.), *Language and Cognition in Schizophrenia*, Hillsdale, NJ: Lawrence Erlbaum, pp. 1–34.

Condray, R., Steinhauer, S. R., van Kammen, D. P. and Kasparek, A. (2002), 'The Language System in Schizophrenia: Effects of Capacity and Linguistic Structure', *Schizophrenia Bulletin*, 28:3, 475–90.

Conti-Ramsden, G., Hutcheson, G. D. and Grove, J. (1995), 'Contingency and Breakdown: Children with SLI and their Conversations with Mothers and Fathers', *Journal of Speech and Hearing Research*, 38:8, 1290–302.

Conti-Ramsden, G., Simkin, Z. and Pickles, A. (2006), 'Estimating Familial Loading in SLI: A Comparison of Direct Assessment Versus Parental Interview', *Journal of Speech, Language, and Hearing Research*, 49:1, 88–101.

Conture, E. G. (1997), 'Evaluating Childhood Stuttering', in R. F. Curlee and G. M. Siegal (eds), *Nature and Treatment of Stuttering: New Directions*, Boston, MA: Allyn & Bacon, pp. 239–56.

Coope, G. and Connett, G. (2006), 'Juvenile Laryngeal Papillomatosis', *Primary Care Respiratory Journal*, 15:2, 125–7.

Corbera, S., Corral, M. J., Escera, C. and Idiazabal, M. A. (2005), 'Abnormal Speech Sound Representation in Persistent Developmental Stuttering', *Neurology*, 65:8, 1246–52.

Corcoran, R. and Frith, C. D. (1996), 'Conversational Conduct and the Symptoms of Schizophrenia', *Cognitive Neuropsychiatry*, 1:4, 305–18.

Cornwell, P. L., Murdoch, B. E., Ward, E. C. and Kellie, S. (2003a), 'Perceptual Evaluation of Motor Speech Following Treatment for Childhood Cerebellar Tumour', *Clinical Linguistics and Phonetics*, 17:8, 597–615.

Cornwell, P. L., Murdoch, B. E., Ward, E. C. and Morgan, A. (2003b), 'Dysarthria and Dysphagia as Long-Term Sequelae in a Child Treated for a Posterior Fossa Tumour', *Pediatric Rehabilitation*, 6:2, 67–75.

Covington, M. A., He, C., Brown, C., Naçi, L., McClain, J. T., Fjordbak, B. S., Semple, J. and Brown, J. (2005), 'Schizophrenia and the Structure of Language: The Linguist's View', *Schizophrenia Research*, 77:1, 85–98.

Craig, A. (1996), 'Long-Term Effects of Intensive Treatment for a Client with both a Cluttering and Stuttering Disorder', *Journal of Fluency Disorders*, 21:3–4, 329–35.

Craig, A., Hancock, K., Tran, Y., Craig, M. and Peters, K. (2002), 'Epidemiology of Stuttering in the Community Across the Entire Life Span', *Journal of Speech, Language, and Hearing Research*, 45:6, 1097–105.

Craig, A. R., Franklin, J. A. and Andrews, G. (1984), 'A Scale to Measure Locus of Control of Behaviour', *British Journal of Medical Psychology*, 57:2, 173–80.

Crary, M. A. (1995), 'A Direct Intervention Program for Chronic Neurogenic Dysphagia Secondary to Brainstem Stroke', *Dysphagia*, 10:1, 6–18.

Crary, M. A., Carnaby, G. D., Groher, M. E. and Helseth, E. (2004), 'Functional Benefits of Dysphagia Therapy using Adjunctive sEMG Biofeedback', *Dysphagia*, 19:3, 160–4.

Crawford, D. C., Acuña, J. M. and Sherman, S. L. (2001), 'FMR1 and the Fragile X Syndrome: Human Genome Epidemiology Review', *Genetics in Medicine*, 3:5, 359–71.

Cream, A., Onslow, M., Packman, A. and Llewellyn, G. (2003), 'Protection from Harm: The Experience of Adults after Therapy with Prolonged-Speech', *International Journal of Language and Communication Disorders*, 38:4, 379–95.

Cream, A., Packman, A. and Llewellyn, G. (2004), 'The Playground Rocker: A Metaphor for Communication after Treatment for Adults who Stutter', *Advances in Speech-Language Pathology*, 6:3, 182–7.

Crystal, D. (1997), *The Cambridge Encyclopedia of Language*, Cambridge: Cambridge University Press.

Cuerva, A. G., Sabe, L., Kuzis, G., Tiberti, C., Dorrego, F. and Starkstein, S. E. (2001), 'Theory of Mind and Pragmatic Abilities in Dementia', *Neuropsychiatry, Neuropsychology and Behavioral Neurology*, 14:3, 153–8.

Cumley, G. D. and Swanson, S. (1999), 'Augmentative and Alternative Communication Options for Children with Developmental Apraxia of Speech: Three Case Studies', *Augmentative and Alternative Communication*, 15:2, 110–25.

Cummings, L. (2005), *Pragmatics: A Multidisciplinary Perspective*, Edinburgh: Edinburgh University Press.

Cummings, L. (2007a), 'Pragmatics and Adult Language Disorders: Past Achievements and Future Directions', *Seminars in Speech and Language*, 28:2, 98–112.

Cummings, L. (2007b), 'Clinical Pragmatics: A Field in Search of Phenomena?', *Language and Communication*, 27:4, 396–432.

Cummins, S. K., Nelson, K. B., Grether, J. K. and Velie, E. M. (1993), 'Cerebral Palsy in Four Northern California Counties, Births 1983 Through 1985', *Journal of Pediatrics*, 123:2, 230–7.

Cunningham, R. and Ward, C. D. (2003), 'Evaluation of a Training Programme to Facilitate Conversation between People with Aphasia and their Partners', *Aphasiology*, 17:8, 687–707.

Curlee, R. F. (1996), 'Cluttering: Data in Search of Understanding', *Journal of Fluency Disorders*, 21:3–4, 367–71.

D'Antonio, L. L. and Scherer, N. J. (1995), 'The Evaluation of Speech Disorders Associated with Clefting', in R. J. Shprintzen and J. Bardach (eds), *Cleft Palate Speech Management: A Multidisciplinary Approach*, St Louis, MO: Mosby, pp. 176–220.

Dabul, B. (2000), *Apraxia Battery for Adults*, 2nd edn, Austin, TX: Pro-Ed.

Dagenais, P. A., Brown, G. R. and Moore, R. E. (2006), 'Speech Rate Effects upon Intelligibility and Acceptability of Dysarthric Speech', *Clinical Linguistics and Phonetics*, 20:2–3, 141–8.

Dalston, R. M. (1992), 'Timing of Cleft Palate Repair: A Speech Pathologist's Viewpoint', *Problems in Plastic and Reconstructive Surgery*, 2:1, 30–8.

Dalston, R. M., Martinkosky, S. J. and Hinton, V. A. (1987), 'Stuttering Prevalence among Patients at Risk for Velopharyngeal Inadequacy: A Preliminary Investigation', *Cleft Palate Journal*, 24:3, 233–9.

Daly, D. A. (1986), 'The Clutterer', in K. O. St Louis (ed.), *The Atypical Stutterer: Principles and Practices of Rehabilitation*, Orlando, FL: Academic, pp. 155–92.

Daly, D. A. and Burnett, M. L. (1996), 'Cluttering: Assessment, Treatment Planning, and Case Study Illustration', *Journal of Fluency Disorders*, 21:3–4, 239–48.

Daly, D. A. and Burnett-Stolnack, M. (1995), 'Identification of and Treatment Planning for Cluttering Clients: Two Practical Tools', *Clinical Connection*, 8, 1–5.

Daly, D. A. and Cantrell, R. P. (2006), Cluttering: Characteristics Identified as Diagnostically Significant by Fluency Experts, Paper Presented at the Fifth World Congress on Fluency Disorders, Dublin, Ireland, July 2006.

Darley, F. L., Aronson, A. E. and Brown, J. R. (1969a), 'Clusters of Deviant Speech Dimensions in the Dysarthrias', *Journal of Speech and Hearing Research*, 12:3, 462–96.

Darley, F. L., Aronson, A. E. and Brown, J. R. (1969b), 'Differential Diagnostic Patterns of Dysarthria', *Journal of Speech and Hearing Research*, 12:2, 246–69.

Darley, F. L., Aronson, A. E. and Brown, J. R. (1975), *Motor Speech Disorders*, Philadelphia, PA: Saunders.

Davies, A. E., Stone, S. P., Kidd, D. and MacMahon, J. (1995), 'Pharyngeal Sensation and Gag Reflex in Healthy Subjects', *Lancet*, 345:8948, 487–8.

Davies, L. and Welch, H. G. (2006), 'Epidemiology of Head and Neck Cancer in the United States', *Otolaryngology – Head and Neck Surgery*, 135:3, 451–7.

Davis, B. L., Jacks, A. and Marquardt, T. P. (2005), 'Vowel Patterns in Developmental Apraxia of Speech: Three Longitudinal Case Studies', *Clinical Linguistics and Phonetics*, 19:4, 249–74.

Davis, B. L., Jakielski, K. J. and Marquardt, T. P. (1998), 'Developmental Apraxia of Speech: Determiners of Differential Diagnosis', *Clinical Linguistics and Phonetics*, 12:1, 25–45.

Dayalu, V. N., Kalinowski, J., Stuart, A., Holbert, D. and Rastatter, M. P. (2002), 'Stuttering Frequency on Content and Function Words in Adults who Stutter: A Concept Revisited', *Journal of Speech, Language, and Hearing Research*, 45:5, 871–8.

Dayalu, V. N., Saltuklaroglu, T., Kalinowski, J., Stuart, A. and Rastatter, M. P. (2001), 'Producing the Vowel /a/ Prior to Speaking Inhibits Stuttering in Adults in the English Language', *Neuroscience Letters*, 306:1–2, 111–15.

De Andrade, C. R., Cervone, L. M. and Sassi, F. C. (2003), 'Relationship Between the Stuttering Severity Index and Speech Rate', *Sao Paulo Medical Journal*, 121:2, 81–4.

De Lau, L. M. L. and Breteler, M. M. B. (2006), 'Epidemiology of Parkinson's Disease', *Lancet Neurology*, 5:6, 525–35.

Deevy, P. and Leonard, L. B. (2004), 'The Comprehension of *Wh*-Questions in Children with Specific Language Impairment', *Journal of Speech, Language, and Hearing Research*, 47:4, 802–15.

Defloor, T., Van Borsel, J. and Curfs, L. (2002), 'Articulation in Prader-Willi Syndrome', *Journal of Communication Disorders*, 35:3, 261–82.

Dejaeger, E. and Goeleven, A. (2005), 'Multidisciplinary Approach to Patients with Persistent Swallowing Problems; The First Experiences, 1996/'02 in Louvain', *Nederlands Tijdschrift Voor Geneeskunde*, 149:5, 251–6.

Delcker, A. and Diener, H. C. (1991), 'Neurological Diagnosis and Therapeutic Measures in Cerebral Embolism', *Herz*, 16:6, 434–43.

DeLisi, L. E. (2001), 'Speech Disorder in Schizophrenia: Review of the Literature and Exploration of its Relation to the Uniquely Human Capacity for Language', *Schizophrenia Bulletin*, 27:3, 481–96.

Demir, S. O., Görgülü, G. and Köseoglu, F. (2006), 'Comparison of Rehabilitation Outcome in Patients with Aphasic and Non-Aphasic Traumatic Brain Injury', *Journal of Rehabilitation Medicine*, 38:1, 68–71.

Deonna, T. (2000), 'Acquired Epileptic Aphasia (AEA) or Landau-Kleffner Syndrome: From Childhood to Adulthood', in D. V. M. Bishop and L. B. Leonard (eds), *Speech and Language Impairments in Children: Causes, Characteristics, Intervention and Outcome*, Hove: Psychology Press, pp. 261–72.

Department of Health (2001), *Valuing People: A New Strategy for Learning Disability for the 21st Century*, London: Department of Health.

Department of Health (2004), *Children in Need and Blood-Borne Viruses: HIV and Hepatitis*, London: Department of Health.

Devenny, D. A. and Silverman, W. P. (1990), 'Speech Dysfluency and Manual Specialization in Down's Syndrome', *Journal of Mental Deficiency Research*, 34:3, 253–60.

Dewart, H. and Summers, S. (1988), *The Pragmatics Profile of Early Communication Skills*, Windsor: NFER-Nelson.

Diaz, E. M., Laccourreye, L., Veivers, D., Garcia, D., Brasnu, D. and Laccourreye, O. (2000), 'Laryngeal Stenosis after Supracricoid Partial Laryngectomy', *Annals of Otology, Rhinology and Laryngology*, 109:11, 1077–81.

Dietrich, S. (1997), 'Central Auditory Processing in People Who Stutter', *Journal of Fluency Disorders*, 22:2, 148.

Docherty, N. M., Cohen, A. S., Nienow, T. M., Dinzeo, T. J. and Dangelmaier, R. E. (2003), 'Stability of Formal Thought Disorder and Referential Communication Disturbances in Schizophrenia', *Journal of Abnormal Psychology*, 112:3, 469–75.

Dogan, M., Midi, I., Yazici, M. A., Kocak, I., Gunal, D. and Sehitoglu, M. A. (2007), 'Objective and Subjective Evaluation of Voice Quality in Multiple Sclerosis', *Journal of Voice*, 21:6, 735–40.

Doherty, C. P., Fitzsimons, M., Asenbauer, B., McMackin, D., Bradley, R., King, M. and Staunton, H. (1999), 'Prosodic Preservation in Landau-Kleffner Syndrome: A Case Report', *European Journal of Neurology*, 6:2, 227–34.

Doi, M., Nakayasu, H., Soda, T., Shimoda, K., Ito, A. and Nakashima, K. (2003), 'Brainstem Infarction Presenting with Neurogenic Stuttering', *Internal Medicine*, 42:9, 884–7.

Donkervoort, M., Dekker, J., van den Ende, E., Stehmann-Saris, J. C. and Deelman, B. G. (2000), 'Prevalence of Apraxia among Patients with a First Left Hemisphere Stroke in Rehabilitation Centres and Nursing Homes', *Clinical Rehabilitation*, 14:2, 130–6.

Donnelly, M. J. (1994), 'Hypernasality following Adenoid Removal', *Irish Journal of Medical Science*, 163:5, 225–7.

Donzelli, J., Brady, S., Wesling, M. and Theisen, M. (2005), 'Effects of the Removal of the Tracheotomy Tube on Swallowing During the Fiberoptic Endoscopic Exam of the Swallow (FEES)', *Dysphagia*, 20:4, 283–9.

Dorf, D. S. and Curtin, J. W. (1982), 'Early Cleft Palate Repair and Speech Outcome', *Plastic and Reconstructive Surgery*, 70:1, 74–9.

Doshi, D. R. and Weinberger, M. M. (2006), 'Long-Term Outcome of Vocal Cord Dysfunction', *Annals of Allergy, Asthma and Immunology*, 96:6, 794–9.

Doyle, W. J., Reilly, J. S., Jardini, L. and Rovnak, S. (1986), 'Effect of Palatoplasty on the Function of the Eustachian Tube in Children with Cleft Palate', *Cleft Palate Journal*, 23:1, 63–8.

Drew, R. L. and Thompson, C. K. (1999), 'Model-Based Semantic Treatment for Naming Deficits in Aphasia', *Journal of Speech, Language, and Hearing Research*, 42:4, 972–89.

Druce, T., Debney, S. and Byrt, T. (1997), 'Evaluation of an Intensive Treatment Program for Stuttering in Young Children', *Journal of Fluency Disorders*, 22:3, 169–86.

Duff, M. C., Proctor, A. and Yairi, E. (2004), 'Prevalence of Voice Disorders in African American and European American Preschoolers', *Journal of Voice*, 18:3, 348–53.

Duffy, J. R. (1995), *Motor Speech Disorders: Substrates, Differential Diagnosis, and Management*, St Louis, MO: Mosby.

Dunn, L. M. and Dunn, L. M. (1997), *Peabody Picture Vocabulary Test*, 3rd edn, Circle Pines, MN: American Guidance Service.

Dunn, L. M., Dunn, L. M. and Whetton, C. (1982), *British Picture Vocabulary Scale*, Windsor: NFER-Nelson.

Dworkin, J. P. and Culatta, R. A. (1980), *Dworkin-Culatta Oral Mechanism Examination*, Nicholasville, KY: Edgewood.

Dworzynski, K., Howell, P. and Natke, U. (2003), 'Predicting Stuttering from Linguistic Factors for German Speakers in Two Age Groups', *Journal of Fluency Disorders*, 28:2, 95–112.

Eadie, P. A., Fey, M. E., Douglas, J. M. and Parsons, C. L. (2002), 'Profiles of Grammatical Morphology and Sentence Imitation in Children with Specific Language Impairment and Down Syndrome', *Journal of Speech, Language, and Hearing Research*, 45:4, 720–32.

Earley, C. J., Kittner, S. J., Feeser, B. R., Gardner, J., Epstein, A., Wozniak, M. A., Wityk, R., Stern, B. J., Price, T. R., Macko, R. F., Johnson, C., Sloan, M. A. and Buchholz, D. (1998), 'Stroke in Children and Sickle-Cell Disease: Baltimore-Washington Cooperative Young Stroke Study', *Neurology*, 51:1, 169–76.

Edwards, J. and Lahey, M. (1996), 'Auditory Lexical Decisions of Children with Specific Language Impairment', *Journal of Speech and Hearing Research*, 39:6, 1263–73.

Einarsdottir, J. and Ingham, R. J. (2005), 'Have Disfluency-Type Measures Contributed to the Understanding and Treatment of Developmental Stuttering?', *American Journal of Speech-Language Pathology*, 14:4, 260–73.

Eisbruch, A., Lyden, T., Bradford, C. R., Dawson, L. A., Haxer, M. J., Miller, A. E., Teknos, T. N., Chepeha, D. B., Hogikyan, N. D., Terrell, J. E. and Wolf, G. T. (2002), 'Objective Assessment of Swallowing Dysfunction and Aspiration after Radiation Concurrent with Chemotherapy for Head-and-Neck Cancer', *International Journal of Radiation Oncology, Biology, Physics*, 53:1, 23–8.

Eisenmajer, R., Prior, M., Leekam, S., Wing, L., Gould, J., Welham, M. and Ong, B. (1996), 'Comparison of Clinical Symptoms in Autism and Asperger's

Disorder', *Journal of the American Academy of Child and Adolescent Psychiatry*, 35:11, 1523–31.

Elbert, M. and Gierut, J. A. (1986), *Handbook of Clinical Phonology: Approaches to Assessment and Treatment*, London: Taylor & Francis.

Elliott, C. D. (1996), *British Abilities Scales II*, London: NFER-Nelson.

Emerich, D. M., Creaghead, N. A., Grether, S. M., Murray, D. and Grasha, C. (2003), 'The Comprehension of Humorous Materials by Adolescents with High-Functioning Autism and Asperger's Syndrome', *Journal of Autism and Developmental Disorders*, 33:3, 253–7.

Enderby, P., Wood, V. and Wade, D. (2006), *Frenchay Aphasia Screening Test*, Chichester: John Wiley.

Enderby, P. M., Wood, V. A., Wade, D. T. and Hewer, R. L. (1987), 'The Frenchay Aphasia Screening Test: A Short, Simple Test for Aphasia Appropriate for Non-Specialists', *International Rehabilitation Medicine*, 8:4, 166–70.

Endler, N. S., Edwards, J. M. and Vitelli, R. (1991), *Endler Multidimensional Anxiety Scales (EMAS): Manual*, Los Angeles, CA: Western Psychological Services.

Enemark, H., Bolund, S. and Jørgensen, I. (1990), 'Evaluation of Unilateral Cleft Lip and Palate Treatment: Long Term Results', *Cleft Palate Journal*, 27:4, 354–61.

Engelter, S. T., Gostynski, M., Papa, S., Frei, M., Born, C., Ajdacic-Gross, V., Gutzwiller, F. and Lyrer, P. A. (2006), 'Epidemiology of Aphasia Attributable to First Ischemic Stroke: Incidence, Severity, Fluency, Etiology, and Thrombolysis', *Stroke*, 37:6, 1379–84.

Epstein, L. G., Sharer, L. R., Oleske, J. M., Connor, E. M., Goudsmit, J., Bagdon, L., Robert-Guroff, M. and Koenigsberger, M. R. (1986), 'Neurologic Manifestations of Human Immunodeficiency Virus Infection in Children', *Pediatrics*, 78:4, 678–87.

Esposito, S. J., Mitsumoto, H. and Shanks, M. (2000), 'Use of Palatal Lift and Palatal Augmentation Prostheses to Improve Dysarthria in Patients with Amyotrophic Lateral Sclerosis: A Case Series', *Journal of Prosthetic Dentistry*, 83:1, 90–8.

Estrem, T. and Broen, P. A. (1989), 'Early Speech Production of Children with Cleft Palate', *Journal of Speech and Hearing Research*, 32:1, 12–23.

Ettema, S. L., Tolejano, C. J., Thielke, R. J., Toohill, R. J. and Merati, A. L. (2006), 'Perceptual Voice Analysis of Patients with Subglottic Stenosis', *Otolaryngology – Head and Neck Surgery*, 135:5, 730–5.

Fager, S., Hux, K., Beukelman, D. R. and Karantounis, R. (2006), 'Augmentative and Alternative Communication Use and Acceptance by Adults with Traumatic Brain Injury', *Augmentative and Alternative Communication*, 22:1, 37–47.

Falkman, K. W., Sandberg, A. D. and Hjelmquist, E. (2002), 'Preferred Communication Modes: Prelinguistic and Linguistic Communication in Non-Speaking Preschool Children with Cerebral Palsy', *International Journal of Language and Communication Disorders*, 37:1, 59–68.

441

Fall, P-A., Axelson, O., Fredriksson, M., Hansson, G., Lindvall, B., Olsson, J- E. and Granérus, A- K. (1996), 'Age-Standardized Incidence and Prevalence of Parkinson's Disease in a Swedish Community', *Journal of Clinical Epidemiology*, 49:6, 637–41.

Fazio, B. B. (1998), 'The Effect of Presentation Rate on Serial Memory in Young Children with Specific Language Impairment', *Journal of Speech, Language, and Hearing Research*, 41:6, 1375–83.

Feijo, A. V., Parente, M. A., Behlau, M., Haussen, S., de Veccino, M. C. and Martignago, B. C. (2004), 'Acoustic Analysis of Voice in Multiple Sclerosis Patients', *Journal of Voice*, 18:3, 341–7.

Felsenfeld, S., Broen, P. A. and McGue, M. (1992), 'A 28-Year Follow-Up of Adults with a History of Moderate Phonological Disorder: Linguistic and Personality Results', *Journal of Speech and Hearing Research*, 35:5, 1114–25.

Felsenfeld, S., Kirk, K. M., Zhu, G., Statham, D. J., Neale, M. C. and Martin, N. G. (2000), 'A Study of the Genetic and Environmental Etiology of Stuttering in a Selected Twin Sample', *Behavior Genetics*, 30:5, 359–66.

Felsenfeld, S., McGue, M. and Broen, P. A. (1995), 'Familial Aggregation of Phonological Disorders: Results from a 28-Year Follow-Up', *Journal of Speech and Hearing Research*, 38:5, 1091–107.

Fenson, L., Dale, P. S., Reznick, J. S., Thal, D. A., Bates, E., Hartung, J. P., Pethick, S. and Reilly, J. S. (1993), *MacArthur Communicative Development Inventories*, San Diego, CA: Singular.

Fey, M. E., Krulik, T. E., Loeb, D. F. and Proctor-Williams, K. (1999), 'Sentence Recast Use by Parents of Children with Typical Language and Children with Specific Language Impairment', *American Journal of Speech-Language Pathology*, 8:3, 273–86.

Fey, M. E., Long, S. H., Finestack, L. H. (2003), 'Ten Principles of Grammar Facilitation for Children with Specific Language Impairments', *American Journal of Speech-Language Pathology*, 12:1, 3–15.

Feyereisen, P., Berrewaerts, J. and Hupet, M. (2007), 'Pragmatic Skills in the Early Stages of Alzheimer's Disease: An Analysis by Means of a Referential Communication Task', *International Journal of Language and Communication Disorders*, 42:1, 1–17.

Filipek, P. A. et al. (1999), 'The Screening and Diagnosis of Autistic Spectrum Disorders', *Journal of Autism and Developmental Disorders*, 29:6, 439–84.

Finn, P. and Ingham, R. J. (1994), 'Stutterers' Self-Ratings of How Natural Speech Sounds and Feels', *Journal of Speech and Hearing Research*, 37:2, 326–40.

Fisher, S. E., Vargha-Khadem, F., Watkins, K. E., Monaco, A. P. and Pembrey, M. E. (1998), 'Localisation of a Gene Implicated in a Severe Speech and Language Disorder', *Nature Genetics*, 18:2, 168–70.

Flax, J. F., Realpe-Bonilla, T., Hirsch, L. S., Brzustowicz, L. M., Bartlett, C. W. and Tallal, P. (2003), 'Specific Language Impairment in Families: Evidence for

Co-Occurrence with Reading Impairments', *Journal of Speech, Language, and Hearing Research*, 46:3, 530–43.

Fletcher, S. G. (1978), *The Fletcher Time-by-Count Test of Diadochokinetic Syllable Rate*, Tigard, OR: C.B.

Fokes, J. (1982), 'Problems Confronting the Theorist and Practitioner in Child Phonology', in M. Crary (ed.), *Phonological Intervention: Concepts and Procedures*, San Diego, CA: College Hill, pp. 13–34.

Foley, B. E. and Pollatsek, A. (1999), 'Phonological Processing and Reading Abilities in Adolescents and Adults with Severe Congenital Speech Impairments', *Augmentative and Alternative Communication*, 15:3, 156–73.

Fombonne, E. (2002), 'Prevalence of Childhood Disintegrative Disorder', *Autism*, 6:2, 149–57.

Fombonne, E. (2003), 'Epidemiology of Pervasive Developmental Disorders', *Trends in Evidence-Based Neuropsychiatry*, 5:1, 29–36.

Fombonne, E., Du Mazaubrun, C., Cans, C. and Grandjean, H. (1997), 'Autism and Associated Medical Disorders in a French Epidemiological Survey', *Journal of the American Academy of Child and Adolescent Psychiatry*, 36:11, 1561–9.

Fong, G. C., Cheng, T. S., Lam, K., Cheng, W. K., Mok, K. Y., Cheung, C. M., Chim, C. S., Mak, W., Chan, K. H., Tsang, K. L., Kwan, M. C., Tsoi, T. H., Cheung, R. T. and Ho, S. L. (2005), 'An Epidemiological Study of Motor Neuron Disease in Hong Kong', *Amyotrophic Lateral Sclerosis and Other Motor Neuron Disorders*, 6:3, 164–8.

Fontes Rezende, R. E., Lescano, M. A., Zambelli Ramalho, L. N., de Castro Fiqueiredo, J. F., Oliveira Dantas, R., Garzella Meneghelli, U. and Pimenta Modena, J. L. (2006), 'Reactivation of Chagas' Disease in a Patient with Non-Hodgkin's Lymphoma: Gastric, Oesophageal and Laryngeal Involvement', *Transactions of the Royal Society of Tropical Medicine and Hygiene*, 100:1, 74–8.

Foreman, P. and Crews, G. (1998), 'Using Augmentative Communication with Infants and Young Children with Down Syndrome', *Down Syndrome Research and Practice*, 5:1, 16–25.

Forrest, K. (2003), 'Diagnostic Criteria of Developmental Apraxia of Speech used by Clinical Speech–Language Pathologists', *American Journal of Speech-Language Pathology*, 12:3, 376–80.

Forrest, K. and Morrisette, M. L. (1999), 'Feature Analysis of Segmental Errors in Children with Phonological Disorders', *Journal of Speech, Language, and Hearing Research*, 42:1, 187–94.

Foundas, A. L., Bollich, A. M., Corey, D. M., Hurley, M. and Heilman, K. M. (2001), 'Anomalous Anatomy of Speech-Language Areas in Adults with Persistent Developmental Stuttering', *Neurology*, 57:2, 207–15.

Foundas, A. L., Corey, D. M., Hurley, M. M. and Heilman, K. M. (2004), 'Verbal Dichotic Listening in Developmental Stuttering: Subgroups with Atypical Auditory Processing', *Cognitive and Behavioral Neurology*, 17:4, 224–32.

Fowler, A. E. (1990), 'Language Abilities in Children with Down Syndrome: Evidence for a Specific Syntactic Delay', in D. Cicchetti and M. Beeghley (eds), *Children with Down Syndrome: A Developmental Perspective*, New York: Cambridge University Press, pp. 302–28.

Fransella, F. (1972), *Personal Change and Reconstruction*, New York: Academic Press.

Freed, D. B., Marshall, R. C. and Frazier, K. E. (1997), 'Long-Term Effectiveness of PROMPT Treatment in a Severely Apractic-Aphasic Speaker', *Aphasiology*, 11:4–5, 365–72.

Freeman, M. and Fawcus, M. (2000), *Voice Disorders and Their Management*, London: Whurr.

Friel-Patti, S. and Finitzo, T. (1990), 'Language Learning in a Prospective Study of Otitis Media with Effusion in the First Two Years of Life', *Journal of Speech and Hearing Research*, 33:1, 188–94.

Friend, K. B., Rabin, B. M., Groninger, L., Deluty, R. H., Bever, C. and Grattan, L. (1999), 'Language Functions in Patients with Multiple Sclerosis', *Clinical Neuropsychologist*, 13:1, 78–94.

Fukae, J., Kubo, S., Hattori, N., Komatsu, K., Kato, M., Aoki, M. and Mizuno, Y. (2005), 'Hoarseness Due to Bilateral Vocal Cord Paralysis as an Initial Manifestation of Familial Amyotrophic Lateral Sclerosis', *Amyotrophic Lateral Sclerosis and Other Motor Neuron Disorders*, 6:2, 122–4.

Gagnon, L., Mottron, L. and Joanette, Y. (1997), 'Questioning the Validity of the Semantic-Pragmatic Syndrome Diagnosis', *Autism*, 1:1, 37–55.

Gallivan, G. J., Gallivan, H. K. and Eitnier, C. M. (2008), 'Dual Intracordal Unilateral Vocal Fold Cysts: A Perplexing Diagnostic and Therapeutic Challenge', *Journal of Voice*.

Gallivan, G. J., Gallivan, K. H. and Gallivan, H. K. (2006), 'Inhaled Corticosteroids: Hazardous Effects on Voice – An Update', *Journal of Voice*, 21:1, 101–11.

Ganz, J. B. and Simpson, R. L. (2004), 'Effects on Communicative Requesting and Speech Development of the Picture Exchange Communication System in Children with Characteristics of Autism', *Journal of Autism and Developmental Disorders*, 34:4, 395–409.

Gauger, L. M., Lombardino, L. J. and Leonard, C. M. (1997), 'Brain Morphology in Children with Specific Language Impairment', *Journal of Speech, Language, and Hearing Research*, 40:6, 1272–84.

Gaulin, C. and Campbell, T. (1994), 'Procedure for Assessing Verbal Working Memory in Normal School-Age Children: Some Preliminary Data', *Perceptual and Motor Skills*, 79:1, 55–64.

Genden, E. M., Ferlito, A., Silver, C. E., Jacobson, A. S., Werner, J. A., Suárez, C., Leemans, R., Bradley, P. J. and Rinaldo, A. (2007), 'Evolution of the Management of Laryngeal Cancer', *Oral Oncology*, 43:5, 431–9.

Gerber, S. E. (1998), *Etiology and Prevention of Communication Disorders*, San Diego, CA: Singular.

Gernsbacher, M. A. and Goldsmith, H. H., 'Toward a Dyspraxic Subtype of Autism Spectrum Disorder: A Research Hypothesis', Unpublished manuscript.

Gernsbacher, M. A., Goldsmith, H. H., O'Reilly, M. C., Sauer, E. A., DeRuyter, J. L. and Blanc, M. (2002), *Infant Motor Dyspraxia as a Predictor of Speech in Childhood Autism*. Poster Presented at the 13th Biennial Meeting of the International Conference on Infant Studies, Toronto, Canada, April 2002.

Geurts, H. M., Verté, S., Oosterlaan, J., Roeyers, H., Hartman, C. A., Mulder, E. J., van Berckelaer-Onnes, I. A. and Sergeant, J. A. (2004), 'Can the Children's Communication Checklist Differentiate Between Children with Autism, Children with ADHD, and Normal Controls?', *Journal of Child Psychology and Psychiatry*, 45:8, 1437–53.

Ghaziuddin, M. and Butler, E. (1998), 'Clumsiness in Autism and Asperger Syndrome: A Further Report', *Journal of Intellectual Disability Research*, 42:1, 43–8.

Ghaziuddin, M. and Mountain-Kimchi, K. (2004), 'Defining the Intellectual Profile of Asperger Syndrome: Comparison with High-Functioning Autism', *Journal of Autism and Developmental Disorders*, 34:3, 279–84.

Ghaziuddin, M., Al-Khouri, I. and Ghaziuddin, N. (2002), 'Autistic Symptoms Following Herpes Encephalitis', *European Child and Adolescent Psychiatry*, 11:3, 142–6.

Gibbon, F., McCann, J., Peppé, S., O'Hare, A. and Rutherford, M. (2004), 'Articulation Abilities of Children with High-Functioning Autism', in B. Murdoch, J. Goozee, B. Whelan and K. Docking (eds), Proceedings of the 26th World Congress of the International Association of Logopedics and Phoniatrics, Brisbane, Australia: IALP.

Gibbon, F., Stewart, F., Hardcastle, W. J. and Crampin, L. (1999), 'Widening Access to Electropalatography for Children with Persistent Sound System Disorders', *American Journal of Speech-Language Pathology*, 8:4, 319–34.

Gibbon, F. E. (2004), 'Abnormal Patterns of Tongue-Palate Contact in the Speech of Individuals with Cleft Palate', *Clinical Linguistics and Phonetics*, 18:4–5, 285–311.

Gibbon, F. E., McNeill, A. M., Wood, S. E. and Watson, J. M. M. (2003), 'Changes in Linguapalatal Contact Patterns During Therapy for Velar Fronting in a 10-Year-Old with Down's Syndrome', *International Journal of Language and Communication Disorders*, 38:1, 47–64.

Gibbon, F. E. and Wood, S. E. (2003), 'Using Electropalatography (EPG) to Diagnose and Treat Articulation Disorders Associated with Mild Cerebral Palsy: A Case Study', *Clinical Linguistics and Phonetics*, 17:4–5, 365–74.

Gierut, J. A. (2001), 'Complexity in Phonological Treatment: Clinical Factors', *Language, Speech, and Hearing Services in Schools*, 32:4, 229–41.

Gilbertson, M. and Kamhi, A. G. (1995), 'Novel Word Learning in Children with Hearing Impairment', *Journal of Speech and Hearing Research*, 38:3, 630–42.

Gillam, R. B., Cowan, N. and Marler, J. A. (1998), 'Information Processing by School-Age Children with Specific Language Impairment: Evidence from a Modality Effect Paradigm', *Journal of Speech, Language, and Hearing Research*, 41:4, 913–26.

Gillberg, C. (1989), 'Asperger's Syndrome in 23 Swedish Children', *Developmental Medicine and Child Neurology*, 31:4, 520–31.

Gillon, G. T. (2000), 'The Efficacy of Phonological Awareness Intervention for Children with Spoken Language Impairment', *Language, Speech, and Hearing Services in Schools*, 31:2, 126–41.

Gisel, E. G. (1988), 'Chewing Cycles in 2- to 8-Year-Old Normal Children: A Developmental Profile', *American Journal of Occupational Therapy*, 42:1, 40–6.

Glaze, L. E. (1996), 'Treatment of Voice Hyperfunction in the Pre-Adolescent', *Language, Speech, and Hearing Services in Schools*, 27:3, 244–50.

Glennen, S. L. and Calculator, S. N. (1985), 'Training Functional Communication Board Use: A Pragmatic Approach', *Augmentative and Alternative Communication*, 1:4, 134–42.

Goberman, A. M. and Elmer, L. W. (2005), 'Acoustic Analysis of Clear Versus Conversational Speech in Individuals with Parkinson Disease', *Journal of Communication Disorders*, 38:3, 215–30.

Goffman, L. and Leonard, J. (2000), 'Growth of Language Skills in Preschool Children with Specific Language Impairment: Implications for Assessment and Intervention', *American Journal of Speech-Language Pathology*, 9:2, 151–61.

Goguen, L. A., Posner, M. R., Norris, C. M., Tishler, R. B., Wirth, L. J., Annino, D. J., Gagne, A., Sullivan, C. A., Sammartino, D. E. and Haddad, R. I. (2006), 'Dysphagia after Sequential Chemoradiation Therapy for Advanced Head and Neck Cancer', *Otolaryngology – Head and Neck Surgery*, 134:6, 916–22.

Goldberg, T. E., Aloia, M. S., Gourovitch, M. L., Missar, D., Pickar, D. and Weinberger, D. R. (1998), 'Cognitive Substrates of Thought Disorder, I: The Semantic System', *American Journal of Psychiatry*, 155:12, 1671–6.

Golding-Kushner, K. J. (1995), 'Treatment of Articulation and Resonance Disorders Associated with Cleft Palate and VPI', in R. J. Shprintzen and J. Bardach (eds), *Cleft Palate Speech Management: A Multidisciplinary Approach*, St Louis, MO: Mosby, pp. 327–51.

Goldman, R. and Fristoe, M. (1986), *Goldman-Fristoe Test of Articulation*, Circle Pines, MN: American Guidance Service.

Goldman, S. M., Tanner, C. M., Oakes, D., Bhudhikanok, G. S., Gupta, A. and Langston, J. W. (2006), 'Head Injury and Parkinson's Disease Risk in Twins', *Annals of Neurology*, 60:1, 65–72.

Golub, J. S., Chen, P. H., Otto, K. J., Hapner, E. and Johns, M. M. (2006), 'Prevalence of Perceived Dysphonia in a Geriatric Population', *Journal of the American Geriatrics Society*, 54:11, 1736–9.

Goodglass, H., Kaplan, E. and Barresi, B. (2001), *Boston Diagnostic Aphasia Examination*, 3rd edn, Baltimore, MD: Lippincott Williams & Wilkins.

Goodrich, J. M. (2004), *Cytomegalovirus*, USA: eMedicine.com (website: http://www.emedicine.com/med/topic504.htm).

Gooren, L. (2005), 'Hormone Treatment of the Adult Transsexual Patient', *Hormone Research*, 64:S2, 31–6.

Goozee, J. V., Murdoch, B. E. and Theodoros, D. G. (2001), 'Physiological Assessment of Tongue Function in Dysarthria Following Traumatic Brain Injury', *Logopedics, Phoniatrics, Vocology*, 26:2, 51–65.

Gordon, N. (1990), 'Acquired Aphasia in Childhood: The Landau–Kleffner Syndrome', *Developmental Medicine and Child Neurology*, 32:3, 270–4.

Gordon, N. (1997), 'The Landau-Kleffner Syndrome: Increased Understanding', *Brain and Development*, 19:5, 311–16.

Gorlin, R. J., Cohen, M. M. and Hennekam, R. C. M. (2001), *Syndromes of the Head and Neck*, New York: Oxford University Press.

Gorwood, P., Leboyer, M., Jay, M., Payan, C. and Feingold, J. (1995), 'Gender and Age at Onset in Schizophrenia: Impact of Family History', *American Journal of Psychiatry*, 152:2, 208–12.

Gould, J. B., Benitz, W. E. and Liu, H. (2000), 'Mortality and Time to Death in Very Low Birth Weight Infants: California, 1987 and 1993', *Pediatrics*, 105:3, p. e37.

Grant, H. R., Quiney, R. E., Mercer, D. M. and Lodge, S. (1988), 'Cleft Palate and Glue Ear', *Archives of Disease in Childhood*, 63:2, 176–9.

Grant, J., Karmiloff-Smith, A., Berthoud, J. and Christophe, A. (1996), 'Is the Language of People with Williams Syndrome Mere Mimicry? Phonological Short-Term Memory in a Foreign Language', *Cahiers de Psychologie Cognitive*, 15:6, 615–28.

Gray, S. (2003), 'Word-Learning by Preschoolers with Specific Language Impairment: What Predicts Success?', *Journal of Speech, Language, and Hearing Research*, 46:1, 56–67.

Gray, S. (2004), 'Word Learning by Preschoolers with Specific Language Impairment: Predictors and Poor Learners', *Journal of Speech, Language, and Hearing Research*, 47:5, 1117–32.

Gray, S. (2005), 'Word Learning by Preschoolers with Specific Language Impairment: Effect of Phonological or Semantic Cues', *Journal of Speech, Language, and Hearing Research*, 48:6, 1452–67.

Gregg, B. A. and Yairi, E. (2007), 'Phonological Skills and Disfluency Levels in Preschool Children Who Stutter', *Journal of Communication Disorders*, 40:2, 97–115.

Grela, B. G. (2003), 'Do Children with Down Syndrome Have Difficulty with Argument Structure', *Journal of Communication Disorders*, 36:4, 263–79.

Grela, B. G. and Leonard, L. B. (2000), 'The Influence of Argument-Structure Complexity on the Use of Auxiliary Verbs by Children with SLI', *Journal of Speech, Language, and Hearing Research*, 43:5, 1115–25.

Grelotti, D. J., Gauthier, I. and Schultz, R. T. (2002), 'Social Interest and the Development of Cortical Face Specialization: What Autism Teaches Us About Face Processing, *Developmental Psychobiology*, 40:3, 213–25.

Grether, J. K., Nelson, K. B. and Cummins, S. K. (1993), 'Twinning and Cerebral Palsy: Experience in Four Northern California Counties, Births 1983 Through 1985', *Pediatrics*, 92:6, 854–8.

Grether, J. K., Nelson, K. B., Walsh, E., Willoughby, R. E. and Redline, R. W. (2003), 'Intrauterine Exposure to Infection and Risk of Cerebral Palsy in Very Preterm Infants', *Archives of Pediatrics and Adolescent Medicine*, 157:1, 26–32.

Grice, H. P. (1957), 'Meaning', *Philosophical Review*, 67, 377–87.

Gross, M. (1999), 'Pitch-Raising Surgery in Male-to-Female Transsexuals', *Journal of Voice*, 13:2, 246–50.

Grote, C. L., Van Slyke, P. and Hoeppner, J. B. (1999), 'Language Outcome Following Multiple Subpial Transection for Landau–Kleffner Syndrome', *Brain*, 122:3, 561–6.

Grove, N., Dockrell, J. and Woll, B. (1996), 'The Two-Word Stage in Manual Signs: Language Development in Signers with Intellectual Impairments', in S. von Tetzchner and M. H. Jensen (eds), *Augmentative and Alternative Communication: European Perspectives*, London: Whurr, pp. 101–18.

Grove, N. and McDougall, S. (1991), 'Exploring Sign Use in Two Settings', *British Journal of Special Education*, 18:4, 149–56.

Grunwell, P. (1981), *The Nature of Phonological Disability in Children*, New York: Academic.

Grunwell, P. (1985), *Phonological Assessment of Child Speech*, Windsor: NFER-Nelson.

Grunwell, P. (1987), *Clinical Phonology*, London: Croom Helm.

Grunwell, P. and Harding, A. (1995), *PACS TOYS: A Screening Assessment of Phonological Development*, Windsor: NFER-Nelson.

Grytten, N., Glad, S. B., Aarseth, J. H., Nyland, H., Midgard, R. and Myhr, K. M. (2006), 'A 50-Year Follow-Up of the Incidence of Multiple Sclerosis in Hordaland County, Norway', *Neurology*, 66:2, 182–6.

Guitar, B. (1998), *Stuttering: An Integrated Approach to its Nature and Treatment*, Philadelphia, PA: Lippincott Williams & Wilkins.

Guitar, B., Schaefer, H. K., Donahue-Kilburg, G. and Bond, L. (1992), 'Parent Verbal Interactions and Speech Rate: A Case Study in Stuttering', *Journal of Speech and Hearing Research*, 35:4, 742–54.

Guntupalli, V. K., Kalinowski, J. and Saltuklaroglu, T. (2006), 'The Need for Self-Report Data in the Assessment of Stuttering Therapy Efficacy: Repetitions and Prolongations of Speech. The Stuttering Syndrome', *International Journal of Language and Communication Disorders*, 41:1, 1–18.

Gustaw, K. and Mirecka, U. (2001), 'Dysarthria as the Isolated Clinical Symptom of Borreliosis. A Case Report', *Annals of Agricultural and Environmental Medicine*, 8:1, 95–7.

Hadjikoutis, S., Eccles, R. and Wiles, C. M. (2000), 'Coughing and Choking in Motor Neuron Disease', *Journal of Neurology, Neurosurgery and Psychiatry*, 68:5, 601–4.

Hagberg, B., Hagberg, G., Beckung, E. and Uvebrant, P. (2001), 'Changing Panorama of Cerebral Palsy in Sweden. VIII. Prevalence and Origin in the Birth Year Period 1991–94', *Acta Paediatrica*, 90:3, 271–7.

Hägg, M. and Larsson, B. (2004), 'Effects of Motor and Surgery Stimulation in Stroke Patients with Long-Lasting Dysphagia', *Dysphagia*, 19:4, 219–30.

Haley, K. L., Ohde, R. N. and Wertz, R. T. (2000), 'Precision of Fricative Production in Aphasia and Apraxia of Speech: A Perceptual and Acoustic Study', *Aphasiology*, 14:5–6, 619–34.

Hall, C. D., Golding-Kushner, K. J., Argamaso, R. V. and Strauch, B. (1991), 'Pharyngeal Flap Surgery in Adults', *Cleft Palate-Craniofacial Journal*, 28:2, 179–82.

Hall, K. D., Amir, O. and Yairi, E. (1999), 'A Longitudinal Investigation of Speaking Rate in Preschool Children who Stutter', *Journal of Speech, Language, and Hearing Research*, 42:6, 1367–77.

Hall, P. K., Hardy, J. C. and LaVelle, W. E. (1990), 'A Child with Signs of Developmental Apraxia of Speech with whom a Palatal Lift Prosthesis was used to Manage Palatal Dysfunction', *Journal of Speech and Hearing Disorders*, 55:3, 454–60.

Hall, P. K., Jordan, L. S. and Robin, D. A. (1993), *Developmental Apraxia of Speech: Theory and Clinical Practice*, Austin, TX: Pro-Ed.

Hamilton, C. (1993), 'Investigation of the Articulatory Patterns of Young Adults with Down's Syndrome Using Electropalatography', *Down Syndrome Research and Practice*, 1:1, 15–28.

Hansen, T. W., Henrichsen, B., Rasmussen, R. K., Carling, A., Andressen, A. B. and Skjeldal, O. (1996), 'Neuropsychological and Linguistic Follow-Up Studies of Children with Galactosaemia from an Unscreened Population', *Acta Paediatrica*, 85:10, 1197–201.

Hanson, D. M., Jackson, A. W. and Hagerman, R. J. (1986), 'Speech Disturbances (Cluttering) in Mildly Impaired Males with the Martin-Bell/Fragile X Syndrome', *American Journal of Medical Genetics*, 23:1–2, 195–206.

Hardcastle, W. J., Jones, W., Knight, C., Trudgeon, A. and Calder, A. (1989), 'New Developments in Electropalatography: A State-of-the-Art Report', *Clinical Linguistics and Phonetics*, 3:1, 1–38.

Hardcastle, W. J., Morgan Barry, R. A. and Clark, C. J. (1985), 'Articulatory and Voicing Characteristics of Adult Dysarthric and Verbal Dyspraxic Speakers: An Instrumental Study', *British Journal of Disorders of Communication*, 20:3, 249–70.

Hardcastle, W. J., Morgan Barry, R. A. and Clark, C. J. (1987), 'An Instrumental Phonetic Study of Lingual Activity in Articulation-Disordered Children', *Journal of Speech and Hearing Research*, 30:2, 171–84.

Harding, A., Harland, K. and Razzell, R. (1997), *Cleft Audit Protocol for Speech (CAPS)*, Essex: Speech/Language Therapy Department, St Andrew's Plastic Surgery Centre.

Hardin-Jones, M. A. and Jones, D. L. (2005), 'Speech Production of Preschoolers with Cleft Palate', *Cleft Palate-Craniofacial Journal*, 42:1, 7–13.

Hardy, J. C., Netsell, R., Schweiger, J. W. and Morris, H. L. (1969), 'Management of Velopharyngeal Dysfunction in Cerebral Palsy', *Journal of Speech and Hearing Disorders*, 34:2, 123–37.

Hardy, J. C., Rembolt, R. R., Spriestersbach, D. C. and Jayapathy, B. (1961), 'Surgical Management of Palatal Paresis and Speech Problems in Cerebral Palsy: A Preliminary Report', *Journal of Speech and Hearing Disorders*, 26:4, 320–5.

Harris, T. M. (1992), 'The Pharmacological Treatment of Voice Disorders', *Folia Phoniatrica et Logopaedica*, 44:3–4, 143–54.

Harrison, E., Onslow, M., Andrews, C., Packman, A. and Webber, M. (1998), 'Control of Stuttering with Prolonged Speech: Development of a One-Day Instatement Program', in A. C. Kordes and R. I. Ingham (eds), *Treatment Efficacy for Stuttering: A Search for Empirical Bases*, San Diego, CA: Singular, pp. 191–212.

Harrison, E., Onslow, M. and Menzies, R. (2004), 'Dismantling the Lidcombe Program of Early Stuttering Intervention: Verbal Contingencies for Stuttering and Clinical Measurement', *International Journal of Language and Communication Disorders*, 39:2, 257–67.

Hartelius, L., Buder, E. H. and Strand, E. A. (1997), 'Long-Term Phonatory Instability in Individuals with Multiple Sclerosis', *Journal of Speech, Language and Hearing Research*, 40:5, 1056–72.

Hartelius, L. and Lillvik, M. (2003), 'Lip and Tongue Function Differently Affected in Individuals with Multiple Sclerosis', *Folia Phoniatrica et Logopaedica*, 55:1, 1–9.

Hartelius, L., Runmarker, B. and Andersen, O. (2000), 'Prevalence and Characteristics of Dysarthria in a Multiple-Sclerosis Incidence Cohort: Relation to Neurological Data', *Folia Phoniatrica et Logopaedica*, 52:4, 160–77.

Hartelius, L. and Svensson, P. (1994), 'Speech and Swallowing Symptoms Associated with Parkinson's Disease and Multiple Sclerosis: A Survey', *Folia Phoniatrica et Logopaedica*, 46:1, 9–17.

Harvey, G. L. (1996), 'Treatment of Voice Disorders in Medically Complex Children', *Language, Speech, and Hearing Services in Schools*, 27:3, 282–91.

Hashimoto, R., Taguchi, T., Kano, M., Hanyu, S., Tanaka, Y., Nishizawa, M. and Nakano, I. (1999), 'A Case Report of Dementia with Cluttering-Like Speech Disorder and Apraxia of Gait', *Rinsho Shinkeigaku*, 39:5, 520–6.

Hawley, C. A., Ward, A. B., Magnay, A. R. and Long, J. (2004), 'Outcomes Following Childhood Head Injury: A Population Study', *Journal of Neurology, Neurosurgery and Psychiatry*, 75:5, 737–42.

Hayashi, T., Miyazaki, H., Toda, Y., Ishiyama, N. and Harada, T. (2005), 'Speech Disturbance Following Myelography with Iohexol: A Case Report', *No To Shinkei*, 57:9, 796–9.

Hayden, D. A. (1994), 'Differential Diagnosis of Motor Speech Dysfunction in Children', *Clinics in Communication Disorders*, 4:2, 119–41.

Hayhow, R. and Stewart, T. (2006), 'Introduction to Qualitative Research and its Application to Stuttering', *International Journal of Language and Communication Disorders*, 41:5, 475–93.

Hays, S. J., Niven, B. E., Godfrey, H. P. D. and Linscott, R. J. (2004), 'Clinical Assessment of Pragmatic Language Impairment: A Generalisability Study of Older People with Alzheimer's Disease', *Aphasiology*, 18:8, 693–714.

Healey, E. C. and Scott, L. A. (1995), 'Strategies for Treating Elementary School-Age Children who Stutter: An Integrative Approach', *Language, Speech, and Hearing Services in Schools*, 26:2, 151–61.

Hedrick, D., Prather, E. and Tobin, A. (1984), *Sequenced Inventory of Communication Development – Revised*, Seattle, WA: University of Washington Press.

Helfrich-Miller, K. (1994), 'A Clinical Perspective: Melodic Intonation Therapy for Developmental Apraxia', *Clinics in Communication Disorders*, 4:3, 175–82.

Helm-Estabrooks, N. and Hotz, G. (1998), 'Sudden Onset of "Stuttering" in an Adult: Neurogenic or Psychogenic?', *Seminars in Speech and Language*, 19:1, 23–9.

Heerey, E. A., Capps, L. M., Keltner, D. and Kring, A. M. (2005), 'Understanding Teasing: Lessons from Children with Autism', *Journal of Abnormal Child Psychology*, 33:1, 55–68.

Hertrich, I. and Ackermann, H. (1994), 'Acoustic Analysis of Speech Timing in Huntington's Disease', *Brain and Language*, 47:2, 182–96.

Hier, D. B., Yoon, W. B., Mohr, J. P., Price, T. R. and Wolf, P. A. (1994), 'Gender and Aphasia in the Stroke Data Bank', *Brain and Language*, 47:1, 155–67.

Hirano, M. (1981), *Clinical Examination of Voice*, New York: Springer-Verlag.

Hirano, Y. M., Yamazaki, Y., Shimizu, J., Togari, T. and Bryce, T. J. (2006), 'Ventilator Dependence and Expressions of Need: A Study of Patients with Amyotrophic Lateral Sclerosis in Japan', *Social Science and Medicine*, 62:6, 1403–13.

Ho, A. K., Iansek, R., Marigliani, C., Bradshaw, J. L. and Gates, S. (1998), 'Speech Impairment in a Large Sample of Patients with Parkinson's Disease', *Behavioural Neurology*, 11:3, 131–7.

Hodgdon, L. (1995), 'Solving Social-Behavioral Problems Through the Use of Visually Supported Communication', in K. A. Quill (ed.), *Teaching Children with Autism: Strategies to Enhance Communication and Socialization*, New York: Delmar, pp. 265–86.

Hodgdon, L. (1996), *Visual Strategies for Improving Communication. Volume 1: Practical Supports for School and Home*, Troy, MI: Quirk Roberts.

Hodge, M. M. and Hancock, H. R. (1994), 'Assessment of Children with Developmental Apraxia of Speech: A Procedure', *Clinics in Communication Disorders*, 4:2, 102–18.

Hodge, M. M. and Wellman, L. (1999), 'Management of Children with Dysarthria', in A. Caruso and E. Strand (eds), *Clinical Management of Motor Speech Disorders in Children*, New York: Thieme Medical, pp. 209–80.

Hodson, B. W. (1986), *The Assessment of Phonological Processes-Revised*, Austin, TX: Pro-Ed.

Hodson, B. W. (1995), *Assessment of Metaphonological Skills – Preschool*, Unpublished Manuscript, Wichita, KS: Wichita State University.

Hodson, B. W. (2004), *Hodson Assessment of Phonological Patterns*, 3rd edn, Austin, TX: Pro-Ed.

Hodson, B. W. and Paden, E. E. (1991), *Targeting Intelligible Speech: A Phonological Approach to Remediation*, Austin, TX: Pro-Ed.

Hodson, B. W., Scherz, J. A. and Strattman, K. H. (2002), 'Evaluating Communicative Abilities of a Highly Unintelligible Preschooler', *American Journal of Speech-Language Pathology*, 11:3, 236–42.

Hoffman, L. M. and Gillam, R. B. (2004), 'Verbal and Spatial Information Processing Constraints in Children with Specific Language Impairment', *Journal of Speech, Language, and Hearing Research*, 47:1, 114–25.

Hoffman, P. R. and Norris, J. A. (2002), 'Phonological Assessment as an Integral Part of Language Assessment', *American Journal of Speech-Language Pathology*, 11:3, 230–5.

Holmberg, E. B., Hillman, R. E., Hammarberg, B., Sodersten, M. and Doyle, P. (2001), 'Efficacy of a Behaviorally Based Voice Therapy Protocol for Vocal Nodules', *Journal of Voice*, 15:3, 395–412.

Homer, C. J. and Kleinman, L. (1999), 'Technical Report: Minor Head Injury in Children', *Pediatrics*, 104:6, p. e 78.

Honbolygó, F., Csépe, V., Fekésházy, A., Emri, M., Márián, T., Sárközy, G. and Kálmánchey, R. (2006), 'Converging Evidences on Language Impairment in Landau-Kleffner Syndrome Revealed by Behavioral and Brain Activity Measures: A Case Study', *Clinical Neurophysiology*, 117:2, 295–305.

Horii, Y. (1980), 'An Accelerometric Approach to Nasality Measurement: A Preliminary Report', *Cleft Palate Journal*, 17:3, 254–61.

Hough, M. S. (1993), 'Treatment of Wernicke's Aphasia with Jargon: A Case Study', *Journal of Communication Disorders*, 26:2, 101–11.

Hough, M. S. and Klich, R. J. (1998), 'Lip EMG Activity During Vowel Production in Apraxia of Speech', *Journal of Speech, Language, and Hearing Research*, 41:4, 786–801.

Howard, D. and Patterson, K. E. (1992), *Pyramids and Palm Trees: A Test of Semantic Access From Pictures and Words*, Bury St Edmunds: Thames Valley Test Company.

Howard, S. and Varley, R. (1995), 'Using Electropalatography to Treat Severe Acquired Apraxia of Speech', *European Journal of Disorders of Communication*, 30:2, 246–55.

Howell, P. and Williams, S. M. (2004), 'Development of Auditory Sensitivity in Children who Stutter and Fluent Children', *Ear and Hearing*, 25:3, 265–74.

Howell, P., Davis, S. and Williams, S. M. (2006), 'Auditory Abilities of Speakers who Persisted, or Recovered, from Stuttering', *Journal of Fluency Disorders*, 31:4, 257–70.

Howell, P., Rosen, S., Hannigan, G. and Rustin, L. (2000), 'Auditory Backward-Masking Performance by Children who Stutter and its Relation to Dysfluency Rate', *Perceptual and Motor Skills*, 90:2, 355–63.

Howlin, P. (2003), 'Outcome in High-Functioning Adults with Autism with and without Early Language Delays: Implications for the Differentiation between Autism and Asperger Syndrome', *Journal of Autism and Developmental Disorders*, 33:1, 3–13.

Howlin, P. and Moore, A. (1997), 'Diagnosis in Autism', *Autism*, 1:2, 135–62.

Huckabee, M. L. and Cannito, M. P. (1999), 'Outcomes of Swallowing Rehabilitation in Chronic Brainstem Dysphagia: A Retrospective Evaluation', *Dysphagia*, 14:2, 93–109.

Hula, W. D., McNeil, M. R., Doyle, P. J., Rubinsky, H. J. and Fossett, T. R. D. (2003), 'The Inter-Rater Reliability of the Story Retell Procedure', *Aphasiology*, 17:5, 523–8.

Huskie, C. F. (1993), 'Assessment of Speech and Language Status: Subjective and Objective Approaches to Appraisal of Vocal Tract Structure and Function', in J. Stengelhofen (ed.), *Cleft Palate: The Nature and Remediation of Communication Problems*, London: Whurr, pp. 64–96.

Ingram, D. (1976), *Phonological Disability in Children*, London: Arnold.

Ingram, D. and Ingram, K. D. (2001), 'A Whole-Word Approach to Phonological Analysis and Intervention', *Language, Speech, and Hearing Services in Schools*, 32:4, 271–83.

Irwin, E. and Lonnee, H. (2006), 'Management of Near Fatal Blunt Laryngeal Trauma', *Acta Anaesthesiologica Scandinavica*, 50:6, 766–7.

Irwin, K., Birch, V., Lees, J., Polkey, C., Alarcon, G., Binnie, C., Smedley, M., Baird, G. and Robinson, R. O. (2001), 'Multiple Subpial Transection in Landau-Kleffner Syndrome', *Developmental Medicine and Child Neurology*, 43:4, 248–52.

Issing, W. J., Karkos, P. D., Perreas, K., Folwaczny, C. and Reichel, O. (2004), 'Dual-Probe 24-Hour Ambulatory pH Monitoring for Diagnosis of Laryngopharyngeal Reflux', *Journal of Laryngology and Otology*, 118:11, 845–8.

Jacks, A., Marquardt, T. P. and Davis, B. L. (2006), 'Consonant and Syllable Structure Patterns in Childhood Apraxia of Speech: Developmental Change in Three Children', *Journal of Communication Disorders*, 39:6, 424–41.

Jacobs, B. J. and Thompson, C. K. (2000), 'Cross-Modal Generalization Effects of Training Noncanonical Sentence Comprehension and Production in Agrammatic Aphasia', *Journal of Speech, Language, and Hearing Research*, 43:1, 5–20.

Jancke, L., Hanggi, J. and Steinmetz, H. (2004), 'Morphological Brain Differences Between Adult Stutterers and Non-Stutterers', *BMC Neurology*, 4, 23.

Jarrold, C. and Baddeley, A. D. (2001), 'Short-Term Memory in Down Syndrome: Applying the Working Memory Model', *Down Syndrome Research and Practice*, 7:1, 17–23.

Jeanes, A. C. and Owens, C. M. (2002), 'Imaging of HIV Disease in Children', *Imaging*, 14:1, 8–23.

Jenkin, D. (1996), 'Long-Term Survival of Children with Brain Tumors', *Oncology*, 10:5, 715–19.

Johnson, R. K., Goran, M. I., Ferrara, M. S. and Poehlman, E. T. (1995), 'Athetosis Increases Resting Metabolic Rate in Adults with Cerebral Palsy', *Journal of the American Dietetic Association*, 96:2, 145–8.

Jones, M., Onslow, M., Packman, A., Williams, S., Ormond, T., Schwarz, I. and Gebski, V. (2005), 'Randomised Controlled Trial of the Lidcombe Programme of Early Stuttering Intervention', *British Medical Journal*, 331:7518, 659–61.

Jones, S. M., Carding, P. N. and Drinnan, M. J. (2006), 'Exploring the Relationship Between Severity of Dysphonia and Voice-Related Quality of Life', *Clinical Otolaryngology*, 31:5, 411–17.

Jordan, R., Jones, G. and Morgan, H. (2001), *A Guide to Services for Children with Autistic Spectrum Disorders for Commissioners and Providers*, London: Mental Health Foundation.

Josephs, K. A., Boeve, B. F., Duffy, J. R., Smith, G. E., Knopman, D. S., Parisi, J. E., Petersen, R. C. and Dickson, D. W. (2005), 'Atypical Progressive Supranuclear Palsy Underlying Progressive Apraxia of Speech and Nonfluent Aphasia', *Neurocase*, 11:4, 283–96.

Josephs, K. A., Duffy, J. R., Strand, E. A., Whitwell, J. L., Layton, K. F., Parisi, J. E., Hauser, M. F., Witte, R. J., Boeve, B. F., Knopman, D. S., Dickson, D. W., Jack, C. R. and Petersen, R. C. (2006), 'Clinicopathological and Imaging Correlates of Progressive Aphasia and Apraxia of Speech', *Brain*, 129:6, 1385–98.

Kagan, A., Black, S. E., Duchan, F. J., Simmons-Mackie, N. and Square, P. (2001), 'Training Volunteers as Conversation Partners Using "Supported Conversation for Adults With Aphasia" (SCA): A Controlled Trial', *Journal of Speech, Language, and Hearing Research*, 44:3, 624–38.

Kalinowski, J. (2003), 'Self-Reported Efficacy of an All-in-the-Ear-Canal Prosthetic Device to Inhibit Stuttering during One Hundred Hours of University Teaching: An Autobiographical Clinical Commentary', *Disability and Rehabilitation*, 25:2, 107–11.

Kalinowski, J., Guntupalli, V. K., Stuart, A. and Saltuklaroglu, T. (2004), 'Self-Reported Efficacy of an Ear-Level Prosthetic Device that Delivers Altered Auditory Feedback for the Management of Stuttering', *International Journal of Rehabilitation Research*, 27:2, 167–70.

Kalinowski, J., Saltuklaroglu, T., Dayalu, V. N. and Guntupalli, V. (2005), 'Is it Possible for Speech Therapy to Improve upon Natural Recovery Rates in Children who Stutter?', *International Journal of Language and Communication Disorders*, 40:3, 349–58.

Kamhi, A. G. and Catts, H. W. (1986), 'Toward an Understanding of Developmental Language and Reading Disorders', *Journal of Speech and Hearing Disorders*, 51:4, 337–47.

Karmiloff-Smith, A., Grant, J., Berthoud, J., Davies, M., Howlin, P. and Udwin, O. (1997), 'Language and Williams Syndrome: How Intact is "Intact"?', *Child Development*, 68:2, 246–62.

Karmiloff-Smith, A., Klima, E., Bellugi, U., Grant, J. and Baron-Cohen, S. (1995), 'Is There a Social Module? Language, Face Processing, and Theory of Mind in Individuals with Williams Syndrome', *Journal of Cognitive Neuroscience*, 7:2, 196–208.

Karmiloff-Smith, A., Tyler, L. K., Voice, K., Sims, K., Udwin, O., Howlin, P. and Davies, M. (1998), 'Linguistic Dissociations in Williams Syndrome: Evaluating Receptive Syntax in On-Line and Off-Line Tasks', *Neuropsychologia*, 36:4, 343–51.

Karnell, M. P., Melton, S. D., Childes, J. M., Coleman, T. C., Dailey, S. A. and Hoffman, H. T. (2007), 'Reliability of Clinician-Based (GRBAS and CAPE-V) and Patient-Based (V-RQOL and IPVI) Documentation of Voice Disorders, *Journal of Voice*, 21:5, 576–90.

Katz, W. F., Bharadwaj, S. V. and Carstens, B. (1999), 'Electromagnetic Articulography Treatment for an Adult with Broca's Aphasia and Apraxia of Speech', *Journal of Speech, Language, and Hearing Research*, 42:6, 1355–66.

Kauhanen, M. -L., Korpelainen, J. T., Hiltunen, P., Määttä, R., Mononen, H., Brusin, E., Sotaniemi, K. A. and Myllylä, V. V. (2000), 'Aphasia, Depression, and Non-Verbal Cognitive Impairment in Ischaemic Stroke', *Cerebrovascular Diseases*, 10:6, 455–61.

Kaushal, M., Upadhyay, A., Aggarwal, R. and Deorari, A. K. (2005), 'Congenital Stridor Due to Bilateral Vocal Cord Palsy', *Indian Journal of Pediatrics*, 72:5, 443–4.

Kavé, G. and Levy, Y. (2003), 'Morphology in Picture Descriptions Provided by Persons With Alzheimer's Disease', *Journal of Speech, Language, and Hearing Research*, 46:2, 341–52.

Kawai, S., Tsukuda, M., Mochimatsu, I., Enomoto, H., Kagesato, Y., Hirose, H., Kuroiwa, Y. and Suzuki, Y. (2003), 'A Study of the Early Stage of Dysphagia in Amyotrophic Lateral Sclerosis', *Dysphagia*, 18:1, 1–8.

Kay Elemetrics (1993), *Multi-Dimensional Voice Program (MDVP) – Computer Program*, Pine Brook, NJ: Author.

Kay, J., Lesser, R. and Coltheart, M. (1992), *Psycholinguistic Assessments of Language Processing in Aphasia*, Hove: Lawrence Erlbaum.

Kaye, J. A., Del Mar Melero-Montes, M. and Jick, H. (2001), 'Mumps, Measles and Rubella Vaccine and the Incidence of Autism Recorded by General Practitioners: A Time Trend Analysis', *British Medical Journal*, 322:7284, 460–3.

Kazi, R., De Cordova, J., Singh, A., Venkitaraman, R., Nutting, C. M., Clarke, P., Rhys-Evans, P. and Harrington, K. J. (2007), 'Voice-Related Quality of Life in Laryngectomees: Assessment Using the VHI and V-RQOL Symptom Scales', *Journal of Voice*, 21:6, 728–34.

Kelly, G. (1955), *The Psychology of Personal Constructs*, New York: Norton.

Kemper, T. L. and Bauman, M. L. (1993), 'The Contribution of Neuropathologic Studies to the Understanding of Autism', *Behavioral Neurology*, 11:1, 175–87.

Kent, L., Evans, J., Paul, M. and Sharp, M. (1999), 'Comorbidity of Autistic Spectrum Disorders in Children with Down Syndrome', *Developmental Medicine and Child Neurology*, 41:3, 153–8.

Kent, R. D., Vorperian, H. K., Kent, J. F. and Duffy, J. R. (2003), 'Voice Dysfunction in Dysarthria: Application of the Multi-Dimensional Voice Program', *Journal of Communication Disorders*, 36:4, 281–306.

Kernahan, D. A. and Stark, R. B. (1958), 'A New Classification for Cleft Lip and Cleft Palate', *Plastic and Reconstructive Surgery*, 22:5, 435–41.

Kertesz, A. (2006), *Western Aphasia Battery – Revised*, San Antonio, TX: Harcourt Assessment.

Khan, O. A. and Ramsay, A. (2006), 'Herpes Encephalitis Presenting as Mild Aphasia: Case Report', *BMC Family Practice*, 7:22.

Kiernan, B. J. and Snow, D. P. (1999), 'Bound-Morpheme Generalization by Children with SLI: Is There a Functional Relationship with Accuracy of Response to Training Targets?', *Journal of Speech, Language, and Hearing Research*, 42:3, 649–62.

Kim, M. and Leach, T. (2004), 'Verb Retrieval in Fluent Aphasia in Two Elicitation Contexts', *34th Clinical Aphasiology Conference*, Park City, UT, May 2004.

Kim, P. T., Van Heest, R., Anderson, D. W. and Simons, R. K. (2006), 'Laryngeal Injuries from a Full Face Helmet: A Report of Two Cases', *Journal of Trauma Injury, Infection, and Critical Care*, 61:4, 998–1000.

Kim, Y. T. and Lombardino, L. J. (1991), 'The Efficacy of Script Contexts in Language Comprehension Intervention with Children who have Mental Retardation', *Journal of Speech and Hearing Research*, 34:4, 845–57.

King, A. D., Leung, S. F., Teo, P., Lam, W. W., Chan, Y. L. and Metreweli, C. (1999), 'Hypoglossal Nerve Palsy in Nasopharyngeal Carcinoma', *Head and Neck*, 21:7, 614–19.

Kiran, S. and Thompson, C. K. (2003), 'The Role of Semantic Complexity in Treatment of Naming Deficits', *Journal of Speech, Language, and Hearing Research*, 46:3, 773–87.

Kirk, S. J., McCarthy, J. and Kirk, W. D. (1968), *Illinois Test of Psycholinguistic Abilities*, Urbana, IL: University of Illinois Press.

Kjelgaard, M. M. and Tager-Flusberg, H. (2001), 'An Investigation of Language Impairment in Autism: Implications for Genetic Subgroups', *Language and Cognitive Processes*, 16:2–3, 287–308.

Klasner, E. R. and Yorkston, K. M. (2000), 'AAC for Huntington Disease and Parkinson's Disease: Planning for Change', in D. R. Beukelman, K. M. Yorkston and J. Reichle (eds), *Augmentative and Alternative Communication for Adults with Acquired Neurologic Disorders*, Baltimore, MD: Paul H. Brookes, pp. 233–70.

Klebanoff, M. A., Regan, J. A., Rao, A. V., Nugent, R. P., Blackwelder, W. C., Eschenbach, D. A., Pastorek, J. G., Williams, S., Gibbs, R. S. and Carey, J. C. (1995), 'Outcome of the Vaginal Infections and Prematurity Study: Results of a Clinical Trial of Erythromycin among Pregnant Women Colonized with Group B Streptococci', *American Journal of Obstetrics and Gynecology*, 172:5, 1540–5.

Kleinow, J. and Smith, A. (2000), 'Influences of Length and Syntactic Complexity on the Speech Motor Stability of the Fluent Speech of Adults who Stutter', *Journal of Speech, Language, and Hearing Research*, 43:2, 548–59.

Klick, S. L. (1985), 'Adapted Cuing Technique for Use in Treatment of Dyspraxia', *Language, Speech, and Hearing Services in Schools*, 16:4, 256–9.

Klick, S. L. (1994), 'Adapted Cuing Technique: Facilitating Sequential Phoneme Production', *Clinics in Communication Disorders*, 4:3, 183–9.

Klin, A., Jones, W., Schultz, R., Volkmar, F. and Cohen, D. (2002), 'Visual Fixation Patterns During Viewing of Naturalistic Social Situations as Predictors of Social Competence in Individuals with Autism', *Archives of General Psychiatry*, 59:9, 809–16.

Klin, A., Sparrow, S. S., Marans, W. D., Carter, A. and Volkmar, F. R. (2000), 'Assessment Issues in Children and Adolescents with Asperger Syndrome', in A. Klin, F. R. Volkmar and S. S. Sparrow (eds), *Asperger Syndrome*, New York: Guilford, pp. 309–39.

Klin, A. and Volkmar, F. R. (1995), *Asperger's Syndrome: Guidelines for Assessment and Diagnosis*, Pittsburgh, PA: Learning Disabilities Association of America.

Klin, A. and Volkmar, F. R. (2000), 'Treatment and Intervention Guidelines for Individuals with Asperger Syndrome', in A. Klin, F. R. Volkmar and S. S. Sparrow (eds), *Asperger Syndrome*, New York: Guilford, pp. 340–66.

Klin, A., Volkmar, F. R., Sparrow, S. S., Cicchetti, D. V. and Rourke, B. P. (1995), 'Validity and Neuropsychological Characterization of Asperger Syndrome: Convergence with Nonverbal Learning Disabilities Syndrome', *Journal of Child Psychology and Psychiatry*, 36:7, 1127–40.

Kline, A. D., Stanley, C., Belevich, J., Brodsky, K., Barr, M. and Jackson, L. G. (1993), 'Developmental Data on Individuals with the Brachmann-de Lange Syndrome', *American Journal of Medical Genetics*, 47:7, 1053–8.

Klor, B. M. and Milianti, F. J. (1999), 'Rehabilitation of Neurogenic Dysphagia with Percutaneous Endoscopic Gastrostomy', *Dysphagia*, 14:3, 162–4.

Klugman, T. M. and Ross, E. (2002), 'Perceptions of the Impact of Speech, Language, Swallowing, and Hearing Difficulties on Quality of Life of a Group of South African Persons with Multiple Sclerosis', *Folia Phoniatrica et Logopaedica*, 54:4, 201–21.

Kluin, K. J., Bromberg, M. B., Feldman, E. L. and Simmons, Z. (1996), 'Dysphagia in Elderly Men with Myasthenia Gravis', *Journal of the Neurological Sciences*, 138:1–2, 49–52.

Kluin, K. J., Foster, N. L., Berent, S. and Gilman, S. (1993), 'Perceptual Analysis of Speech Disorders in Progressive Supranuclear Palsy', *Neurology*, 43:3, 563–6.

Knott, P. D., Milstein, C. F., Hicks, D. M., Abelson, T. I., Byrd, M. C. and Strome, M. (2006), 'Vocal Outcomes After Laser Resection of Early-Stage Glottic Cancer with Adjuvant Cryotherapy', *Archives of Otolaryngology – Head and Neck Surgery*, 132:11, 1226–30.

Kok, A. J., Kong, T. Y. and Bernard-Opitz, V. (2002), 'A Comparison of the Effects of Structured Play and Facilitated Play Approaches on Preschoolers with Autism', *Autism*, 6:2, 181–96.

Koning, C. and Magill-Evans, J. (2001), 'Social and Language Skills in Adolescent Boys with Asperger Syndrome', *Autism*, 5:1, 23–36.

Kono, D., Young, L. and Holtmann, B. (1981), 'The Association of Submucous Cleft Palate and Clefting of the Primary Palate', *Cleft Palate Journal*, 18:3, 207–9.

Kopp, S. and Gillberg, C. (1992), 'Girls with Social Deficits and Learning Problems: Autism, Atypical Asperger Syndrome or a Variant of These Conditions', *European Child and Adolescent Psychiatry*, 1:2, 89–99.

Korkman, M., Kirk, U. and Kemp, S. (1998), *NEPSY: A Developmental Neuropsychological Assessment*, San Antonio, TX: Psychological Corporation, Harcourt Brace.

Koul, R., Corwin, M. and Hayes, S. (2005), 'Production of Graphic Symbol Sentences by Individuals with Aphasia: Efficacy of a Computer-Based Augmentative and Alternative Communication Intervention', *Brain and Language*, 92:1, 58–77.

Kouri, T. A. (2005), 'Lexical Training Through Modeling and Elicitation Procedures with Late Talkers who Have Specific Language Impairment and Developmental Delays', *Journal of Speech, Language, and Hearing Research*, 48:1, 157–71.

Kozinetz, C. A., Skender, M. L., MacNaughton, N., Almes, M. J., Schultz, R. J., Percy, A. K. and Glaze, D. G. (1993), 'Epidemiology of Rett Syndrome: A Population-Based Registry', *Pediatrics*, 91:2, 445–50.

Kraaimaat, F. W., Vanryckeghem, M. and Van Dam-Baggen, R. (2002), 'Stuttering and Social Anxiety', *Journal of Fluency Disorders*, 27:4, 319–30.

Kraijer, D. (2000), 'Review of Adaptive Behavior Studies in Mentally Retarded Persons with Autism/Pervasive Developmental Disorder', *Journal of Autism and Developmental Disorders*, 30:1, 39–47.

Krasna, M. J. and Forti, G. (2006), 'Nerve Injury: Injury to the Recurrent Laryngeal, Phrenic, Vagus, Long Thoracic, and Sympathetic Nerves during Thoracic Surgery', *Thoracic Surgery Clinics*, 16:3, 267–75.

Krauss, T. and Galloway, H. (1982), 'Melodic Intonation Therapy with Language Delayed Apraxic Children', *Journal of Music Therapy*, 19:2, 102–13.

Kravits, T. R., Kamps, D. M., Kemmerer, K. and Potucek, J. (2002), 'Brief Report: Increasing Communication Skills for an Elementary-Aged Student with Autism Using the Picture Exchange Communication System', *Journal of Autism and Developmental Disorders*, 32:3, 225–30.

Kulbersh, B. D., Rosenthal, E. L., McGrew, B. M., Duncan, R. D., McColloch, N. L., Carroll, W. R. and Magnuson, J. S. (2006), 'Pretreatment, Preoperative Swallowing Exercises May Improve Dysphagia Quality of Life', *Laryngoscope*, 116:6, 883–6.

Kully, D. and Langevin, M. (1999), 'Intensive Treatment for Adults', in R. Curlee (ed.), *Stuttering and Related Disorders of Fluency*, New York: Thieme Medical, pp. 139–59.

Kumin, L. (1996), 'Speech and Language Skills in Children with Down Syndrome', *Mental Retardation and Developmental Disabilities Research Reviews*, 2:2, 109–15.

Kumin, L. (1999), 'Comprehensive Speech and Language Treatment for Infants, Toddlers, and Children with Down Syndrome', in T. J. Hassold and D. Patterson (eds), *Down Syndrome: A Promising Future, Together*, New York: Wiley-Liss, pp. 145–53.

Kumin, L., Councill, C. and Goodman, M. (1994), 'A Longitudinal Study of the Emergence of Phonemes in Children with Down Syndrome', *Journal of Communication Disorders*, 27:4, 293–303.

Kumin, L., Councill, C. and Goodman, M. (1995), 'The Pacing Board: A Technique to Assist the Transition from Single Word to Multiword Utterances', *Infant-Toddler Intervention*, 5:1, 23–30.

Kummer, A. W., Strife, J. L., Grau, W. H., Creaghead, N. A. and Lee, L. (1989), 'The Effects of Le Fort 1 Osteotomy with Maxillary Movement on Articulation, Resonance, and Velopharyngeal Function', *Cleft Palate Journal*, 26:3, 193–200.

Kuperberg, G. R. and Caplan, D. (2003), 'Language Dysfunction in Schizophrenia', in R. B. Schiffer, S. M. Rao and B. S. Fogel (eds), *Neuropsychiatry*, Philadelphia, PA: Lippincott Williams & Wilkins, pp. 444–66.

Kwon, M., Lee, J. H. and Kim, J. S. (2005), 'Dysphagia in Unilateral Medullary Infarction: Lateral vs Medial Lesions', *Neurology*, 65:5, 714–18.

La Malfa, G., Lassi, S., Bertelli, M., Salvini, R. and Placidi, G. F. (2004), 'Autism and Intellectual Disability: A Study of Prevalence on a Sample of the Italian Population', *Journal of Intellectual Disability Research*, 48:3, 262–7.

Lacy, P. D., Alderson, D. J. and Parker, A. J. (1994), 'Late Congenital Syphilis of the Larynx and Pharynx Presenting at Endotracheal Intubation', *Journal of Laryngology and Otology*, 108:8, 688–9.

Lahey, M. and Edwards, J. (1996), 'Why Do Children with Specific Language Impairment Name Pictures More Slowly Than Their Peers?', *Journal of Speech and Hearing Research*, 39:5, 1081–98.

Lahey, M. and Edwards, J. (1999), 'Naming Errors of Children with Specific Language Impairment', *Journal of Speech, Language, and Hearing Research*, 42:1, 195–205.

Landau, W. M. (1992), 'Landau-Kleffner Syndrome: An Eponymic Badge of Ignorance', *Archives of Neurology*, 49:4, 353.

Langevin, M. and Boberg, E. (1996), 'Results of Intensive Stuttering Therapy with Adults who Clutter and Stutter', *Journal of Fluency Disorders*, 21:3–4, 315–27.

Langmore, S. E. and Lehman, M. E. (1994), 'Physiologic Deficits in the Orofacial System Underlying Dysarthria in Amyotrophic Lateral Sclerosis', *Journal of Speech and Hearing Research*, 37:1, 28–37.

Larrivee, L. S. and Catts, H. W. (1999), 'Early Reading Achievement in Children with Expressive Phonological Disorders', *American Journal of Speech-Language Pathology*, 8:2, 118–28.

Larsen, S. C. and Hammill, D. D. (1994), *Test of Written Spelling – Third Edition*, Austin, TX: Pro-Ed.

Lattermann, C., Shenker, R. C. and Thordardottir, E. (2005), 'Progression of Language Complexity during Treatment with the Lidcombe Program for Early

Stuttering Intervention', *American Journal of Speech-Language Pathology*, 14:3, 242–53.

Launonen, K. (1996), 'Enhancing Communication Skills of Children with Down Syndrome: Early Use of Manual Signs', in S. von Tetzchner and M. H. Jensen (eds), *Augmentative and Alternative Communication: European Perspectives*, London: Whurr, pp. 213–31.

Lavås, J., Slotte, A., Jochym-Nygren, M., van Doorn, J. and Engerström, I. (2006), 'Communication and Eating Proficiency in 125 Females with Rett Syndrome: The Swedish Rett Center Survey', *Disability and Rehabilitation*, 28:20, 1267–79.

Laver, J. D., Wirz, S. L., Mackenzie, J. and Miller, S. (1981), 'A Perceptual Protocol for the Analysis of Vocal Profiles', *Edinburgh University Department of Linguistics Work in Progress*, 14, 139–55.

Law, J., Boyle, J., Harris, F., Harkness, A. and Nye, C. (2000), 'Prevalence and Natural History of Primary Speech and Language Delay: Findings from a Systematic Review of the Literature', *International Journal of Language and Communication Disorder*, 35:2, 165–88.

Laws, G. (2004), 'Contributions of Phonological Memory, Language Comprehension and Hearing to the Expressive Language of Adolescents and Young Adults with Down Syndrome', *Journal of Child Psychology and Psychiatry*, 45:6, 1085–95.

Laws, G. and Bishop, D. V. M. (2004), 'Pragmatic Language Impairment and Social Deficits in Williams Syndrome: A Comparison with Down's Syndrome and Specific Language Impairment', *International Journal of Language and Communication Disorders*, 39:1, 45–64.

Laws, G., Buckley, S., Bird, G., MacDonald, J. and Broadley, I. (1995), 'The Influence of Reading Instruction on Language and Memory Development in Children with Down's Syndrome', *Down Syndrome Research and Practice*, 3:2, 59–64.

Layton, T. L. and Savino, M. A. (1990), 'Acquiring a Communication System by Sign and Speech in a Child with Down Syndrome: A Longitudinal Investigation', *Child Language Teaching and Therapy*, 6, 59–76.

Leblebicioglu, H., Turan, D., Eroglu, C., Esen, S., Sunbul, M. and Bostanci, F. (2006), 'A Cluster of Anthrax Cases Including Meningitis', *Tropical Doctor*, 36:1, 51–3.

Lebrun, Y. (1996), 'Cluttering after Brain Damage', *Journal of Fluency Disorders*, 21:3–4, 289–95.

Leddy, M. and Gill, G. (1999), 'Enhancing the Speech and Language Skills of Adults with Down Syndrome', in J. F. Miller, M. Leddy and L. A. Leavitt (eds), *Improving the Communication of People with Down Syndrome*, Baltimore, MD: Paul H. Brookes, pp. 205–13.

Lee, A. S. and Rosen, C. A. (2004), 'Efficacy of Cidofovir Injection for the Treatment of Recurrent Respiratory Papillomatosis', *Journal of Voice*, 18:4, 551–6.

Lee, L. L. (1969), *Northwestern Syntax Screening Test*, Evanston, IL: Northwestern University Press.

Lee, S. I., Pyun, S. B. and Jang, D. H. (2006), 'Dysphagia and Hoarseness Associated with Painless Aortic Dissection: A Rare Case of Cardiovocal Syndrome', *Dysphagia*, 21:2, 129–32.

Lees, J. A. (2005), *Children with Acquired Aphasias*, London: Whurr.

Lelekov, T., Franck, N., Dominey, P. F. and Georgieff, N. (2000), 'Cognitive Sequence Processing and Syntactic Comprehension in Schizophrenia', *NeuroReport*, 11:10, 2145–9.

Lennon, N., Miller, F., Castagno, P., Richards, J. (1996), 'Variability of Energy Consumption Measures in Children with Cerebral Palsy', *Gait and Posture*, 4:2, 171–2.

Lennox, P. (2001), 'Hearing and ENT Management', in A. C. H. Watson, D. A. Sell and P. Grunwell (eds), *Management of Cleft Lip and Palate*, London: Whurr, pp. 210–23.

Leonard, L. B. (1995), 'Functional Categories in the Grammars of Children with Specific Language Impairment', *Journal of Speech and Hearing Research*, 38:6, 1270–83.

Leonard, L. B. (1998), *Children with Specific Language Impairment*, Cambridge, MA: MIT Press.

Leonard, L. B., Camarata, S. M., Brown, B. and Camarata, M. N. (2004), 'Tense and Agreement in the Speech of Children with Specific Language Impairment: Patterns of Generalization through Intervention', *Journal of Speech, Language, and Hearing Research*, 47:6, 1363–79.

Leonard, L. B., Deevy, P., Miller, C. A., Rauf, L., Charest, M. and Kurtz, R. (2003), 'Surface Forms and Grammatical Functions: Past Tense and Passive Participle Use by Children with Specific Language Impairment', *Journal of Speech, Language, and Hearing Research*, 46:1, 43–55.

Leslie, P., Drinnan, M. J., Finn, P., Ford, G. A. and Wilson, J. A. (2004), 'Reliability and Validity of Cervical Auscultation: A Controlled Comparison Using Videofluoroscopy', *Dysphagia*, 19:4, 231–40.

Leung, A. K. and Cho, H. (1999), 'Diagnosis of Stridor in Children', *American Family Physician*, 60:8, 2289–96.

Lewis, B. A., Freebairn, L. A., Hansen, A. J., Iyengar, S. K. and Taylor, H. G. (2004), 'School-Age Follow-Up of Children with Childhood Apraxia of Speech', *Language, Speech and Hearing Services in Schools*, 35:2, 122–40.

Lewis, B. A., Freebairn, L. A. and Taylor, H. G. (2000), 'Follow-Up of Children with Early Expressive Phonology Disorders', *Journal of Learning Disabilities*, 33:5, 433–44.

Lewis, M. B. and Pashayan, H. M. (1980), 'Management of Infants with Robin Anomaly', *Clinical Pediatrics*, 19:8, 519–21, 525–8.

Light, J. C. (1985), *The Communicative Interaction Patterns of Young Nonspeaking Physically Disabled Children and Their Primary Caregivers*, Toronto: Blissymbolics Communication Institute.

Light, J. C., Roberts, B., Dimarco, R. and Greiner, N. (1998), 'Augmentative and Alternative Communication to Support Receptive and Expressive Communication for People with Autism', *Journal of Communication Disorders*, 31:2, 153–80.

Link, D. T., Willging, J. P., Miller, C. K., Cotton, R. T. and Rudolph, C. D. (2000), 'Pediatric Laryngopharyngeal Sensory Testing during Flexible Endoscopic Evaluation of Swallowing: Feasible and Correlative', *Annals of Otology, Rhinology and Laryngology*, 109:10, 899–905.

Linscott, R. J. (1996), 'The Profile of Functional Impairment in Communication (PFIC): A Measure of Communication Impairment for Clinical Use', *Brain Injury*, 10:6, 397–412.

Linscott, R. J. (2005), 'Thought Disorder, Pragmatic Language Impairment, and Generalized Cognitive Decline in Schizophrenia', *Schizophrenia Research*, 75:2–3, 225–32.

Loban, W. (1976), *Language Development: Kindergarten Through Grade Twelve*, Urbana, IL: National Council of Teachers of English.

Logemann, J. A. (1983), *Evaluation and Treatment of Swallowing Disorders*, San Diego, CA: College Hill.

Lopez, A., Dietz, V. J., Wilson, M., Navin, T. R. and Jones, J. L. (2000), 'Preventing Congenital Toxoplasmosis', *Morbidity and Mortality Weekly Report*, 49, (RR02), 57–75.

Lopez, O. L., Becker, J. T., Dew, M. A., Banks, G., Dorst, S. K. and McNeil, M. (1994), 'Speech Motor Control Disorder after HIV Infection', *Neurology*, 44:11, 2001–5.

Lorenz, K. J., Groll, K., Ackerstaff, A. H., Hilgers, F. J. and Maier, H. (2006), 'Hands-Free Speech after Surgical Voice Rehabilitation with a Provox ((R)) Voice Prosthesis: Experience with the Provox Free Hands HME Tracheostoma Valve ((R)) System', *European Archives of Oto-Rhino-Laryngology*, 264:2, 151–7.

Lotz, W. K. and Netsell, R. (1989), 'Velopharyngeal Management for a Child with Dysarthria and Cerebral Palsy', in K. M. Yorkston and D. R. Beukelman (eds), *Recent Advances in Clinical Dysarthria*, Boston, MA: College Hill, pp. 139–43.

Love, R. J. and Webb, W. G. (2001), *Neurology for the Speech-Language Pathologist*, Boston, MA: Butterworth-Heinemann.

Loveland, K. A., Landry, S. H., Hughes, S. O., Hall, S. K. and McEvoy, R. E. (1988), 'Speech Acts and the Pragmatic Deficits of Autism', *Journal of Speech and Hearing Research*, 31:4, 593–604.

Luna-Ortiz, K., Villavicencio-Valencia, V., Saucedo-Ramirez, O. J. and Rascon-Ortiz, M. (2006), 'Laryngeal Cancer in Patients Younger than 40 Years', *Cirugia y Cirujanos*, 74:4, 225–9.

Lynch, J. K., Hirtz, D. G., De Veber, G. and Nelson, K. B. (2002), 'Report of the National Institute of Neurological Disorders and Stroke Workshop on Perinatal and Childhood Stroke', *Pediatrics*, 109:1, 116–23.

Maassen, B., Groenen, P. and Crul, T. (2003), 'Auditory and Phonetic Perception of Vowels in Children with Apraxic Speech Disorders', *Clinical Linguistics and Phonetics*, 17:6, 447–67.

McAllister, J. and Kingston, M. (2005), 'Final Part-Word Repetitions in School-Age Children: Two Case Studies', *Journal of Fluency Disorders*, 30:3, 255–67.

McAuliffe, M. J., Ward, E. C. and Murdoch, B. E. (2006), 'Speech Production in Parkinson's Disease: II. Acoustic and Electropalatographic Investigation of Sentence, Word and Segment Durations', *Clinical Linguistics and Phonetics*, 20:1, 19–33.

McCann, J. and Peppé, S. (2003), 'Prosody in Autism Spectrum Disorders: A Critical Review', *International Journal of Language and Communication Disorders*, 38:4, 325–50.

McCathren, R. B., Yoder, P. J. and Warren, S. F. (1999), 'Prelinguistic Pragmatic Functions as Predictors of Later Expressive Vocabulary', *Journal of Early Intervention*, 22:3, 205–16.

McEwan, J. A., Mohsen, A. H., Schmid, M. L. and McKendrick, M. W. (2001), 'A Hoarse Voice: Atypical Mycobacterial Infection of the Larynx', *Journal of Laryngology and Otology*, 115:11, 920–2.

McGrath, J. J. (2006), 'Variations in the Incidence of Schizophrenia: Data Versus Dogma', *Schizophrenia Bulletin*, 32:1, 195–7.

McGregor, D. K., Citron, D. and Shahab, I. (2003), 'Cryptococcal Infection of the Larynx Simulating Laryngeal Carcinoma', *Southern Medical Journal*, 96:1, 74–7.

McGregor, K. K., Newman, R. M., Reilly, R. M. and Capone, N. C. (2002), 'Semantic Representation and Naming in Children with Specific Language Impairment', *Journal of Speech, Language, and Hearing Research*, 45:5, 998–1014.

McKinlay, A., Dalrymple-Alford, J. C., Horwood, L. J. and Fergusson, D. M. (2002), 'Long Term Psychosocial Outcomes after Mild Head Injury in Early Childhood', *Journal of Neurology, Neurosurgery and Psychiatry*, 73:3, 281–8.

McKinstry, A. and Perry, A. (2003), 'Evaluation of Speech in People with Head and Neck Cancer: A Pilot Study', *International Journal of Language and Communication Disorders*, 38:1, 31–46.

McLaughlin, J. F. and Kriegsmann, E. (1980), 'Developmental Dyspraxia in a Family with X-Linked Mental Retardation (Renpenning Syndrome)', *Developmental Medicine and Child Neurology*, 22:1, 84–92.

McNeil, E. J. (2006), 'Management of the Transgender Voice', *Journal of Laryngology and Otology*, 120:7, 521–3.

McNeil, M. R., Weismer, G. and Adams, S. (1990), 'Oral Structure Nonspeech Motor Control in Normal, Dysarthric, Aphasic, and Apraxic Speakers', *Journal of Speech and Hearing Research*, 33:2, 255–68.

McRae, P. A., Tjaden, K. and Schoonings, B. (2002), 'Acoustic and Perceptual Consequences of Articulatory Rate Change in Parkinson Disease', *Journal of Speech, Language and Hearing Research*, 45:1, 35–50.

McWilliams, B. J. (1991), 'Submucous Clefts of the Palate: How Likely are They to be Symptomatic?', *Cleft Palate-Craniofacial Journal*, 28:3, 247–9.

MacDermot, K. D., Bonora, E., Sykes, N., Coupe, A. M., Lai, C. S., Vernes, S. C., Vargha-Khadem, F., McKenzie, F., Smith, R. L., Monaco, A. P. and Fisher, S. E.

(2005), 'Identification of FOXP2 Truncation as a Novel Cause of Developmental Speech and Language Deficits', *American Journal of Human Genetics*, 76:6, 1074–80.

Mackie, C. and Dockrell, J. E. (2004), 'The Nature of Written Language Deficits in Children With SLI', *Journal of Speech, Language, and Hearing Research*, 47:6, 1469–83.

Magiati, I. and Howlin, P. (2003), 'A Pilot Evaluation Study of the Picture Exchange Communication System (PECS) for Children with Autistic Spectrum Disorders', *Autism*, 7:3, 297–320.

Maguire, G. A., Riley, G. D., Franklin, D. L., Maguire, M. E., Nguyen, C. T. and Brojeni, P. H. (2004a), 'Olanzapine in the Treatment of Developmental Stuttering: A Double-Blind, Placebo-Controlled Trial', *Annals of Clinical Psychiatry*, 16:2, 63–7.

Maguire, G. A., Yu, B. P., Franklin, D. L. and Riley, G. D. (2004b), 'Alleviating Stuttering with Pharmacological Interventions', *Expert Opinion on Pharmacotherapy*, 5:7, 1565–71.

Maharaj, S. C. (1980), *Pictogram Ideogram Communication*, Regina, Canada: George Reed Foundation for the Handicapped.

Makitie, A. A., Niemensivu, R., Hero, M., Keski-Santti, H., Back, L., Kajanti, M., Lehtonen, H. and Atula, T. (2006), 'Pharyngocutaneous Fistula following Total Laryngectomy: A Single Institution's 10-Year Experience', *European Archives of Otorhinolaryngology*, 263:12, 1127–30.

Månsson, H. (2000), 'Childhood Stuttering: Incidence and Development', *Journal of Fluency Disorders*, 25:1, 47–57.

Marchman, V. A., Wulfeck, B. and Weismer, S. E. (1999), 'Morphological Productivity in Children with Normal Language and SLI: A Study of the English Past Tense', *Journal of Speech, Language, and Hearing Research*, 42:1, 206–19.

Marelli, R. A., Biddinger, P. W. and Gluckman, J. L. (1992), 'Cytomegalovirus Infection of the Larynx in the Acquired Immunodeficiency Syndrome', *Otolaryngology – Head and Neck Surgery*, 106:3, 296–301.

Marquardt, T. P., Duffy, G. and Cannito, M. P. (1995), 'Acoustic Analysis of Accurate Word Stress Patterning in Patients with Apraxia of Speech and Broca's Aphasia', *American Journal of Speech-Language Pathology*, 4:4, 180–5.

Marquardt, T. P., Jacks, A. and Davis, B. L. (2004), 'Token-to-Token Variability in Developmental Apraxia of Speech: Three Longitudinal Case Studies', *Clinical Linguistics and Phonetics*, 18:2, 127–44.

Marquardt, T. P., Sussman, H. M., Snow, T. and Jacks, A. (2002), 'The Integrity of the Syllable in Developmental Apraxia of Speech', *Journal of Communication Disorders*, 35:1, 31–49.

Mars, M. (2001), 'Alveolar Bone Grafting', in A. C. H. Watson, D. A. Sell and P. Grunwell (eds), *Management of Cleft Lip and Palate*, London: Whurr, pp. 326–37.

Mars, M., Asher-McDade, C., Brattström, V., Dahl, E., McWilliam, J., Mølsted, K., Plint, D. A., Prahl-Andersen, B., Semb, G., Shaw, W. C. and The, R. P. S. (1992), 'A Six-Center International Study of Treatment Outcome in Patients with Clefts of the Lip and Palate: Part 3. Dental Arch Relationships', *Cleft Palate-Craniofacial Journal*, 29:5, 405–8.

Marshall, J., Black, M. and Byng, S. (1998), *The Sentence Processing Resource Pack*, London: Winslow.

Marshall, J., Pring, T., Chiat, S. and Robson, J. (1996a), 'Calling a Salad a Federation: An Investigation of Semantic Jargon. Part 1 – Nouns', *Journal of Neurolinguistics*, 9:4, 237–50.

Marshall, J., Chiat, S., Robson, J. and Pring, T. (1996b), 'Calling a Salad a Federation: An Investigation of Semantic Jargon. Part 2 – Verbs', *Journal of Neurolinguistics*, 9:4, 251–60.

Marshall, J., Pring, T., Chiat, S. and Robson, J. (2001), 'When Ottoman is Easier Than Chair: An Inverse Frequency Effect in Jargon Aphasia', *Cortex*, 37:1, 33–53.

Martin, I. and McDonald, S. (2004), 'An Exploration of Causes of Non-Literal Language Problems in Individuals with Asperger Syndrome', *Journal of Autism and Developmental Disorders*, 34:3, 311–28.

Marton, K. and Schwartz, R. G. (2003), 'Working Memory Capacity and Language Processes in Children With Specific Language Impairment', *Journal of Speech, Language, and Hearing Research*, 46:5, 1138–53.

Massaro, D. W. (2001), 'Speech Perception', in N. M. Smelser and P. B. Baltes (eds), *International Encyclopedia of Social and Behavioral Sciences*, Amsterdam: Elsevier, pp. 14870–5.

Mathieson, L. (2001), *Greene and Mathieson's The Voice and Its Disorders*, London: Whurr.

Matthews, S., Williams, R. and Pring, T. (1997), 'Parent-Child Interaction Therapy and Dysfluency: A Single-Case Study', *European Journal of Disorders of Communication*, 32:3, 346–57.

Mayer, J. F. and Murray, L. L. (2003), 'Functional Measures of Naming in Aphasia: Word Retrieval in Confrontation Naming Versus Connected Speech', *Aphasiology*, 17:5, 481–97.

Mayes, S. D. and Calhoun, S. L. (2001), 'Non-Significance of Early Speech Delay in Children with Autism and Normal Intelligence and Implications for DSM-IV Asperger's Disorder', *Autism*, 5:1, 81–94.

Medical Research Council (2001), *MRC Review of Autism Research: Epidemiology and Causes*, London: Medical Research Council.

Meilijson, S. R., Kasher, A. and Elizur, A. (2004), 'Language Performance in Chronic Schizophrenia: A Pragmatic Approach', *Journal of Speech, Language, and Hearing Research*, 47:3, 695–713.

Mennella, J. A. and Beauchamp, G. K. (1991), 'The Transfer of Alcohol to Human Milk. Effects on Flavor and the Infant's Behavior', *New England Journal of Medicine*, 325:14, 981–5.

Mennella, J. A. and Beauchamp, G. K. (1993), 'Beer, Breast Feeding, and Folklore', *Developmental Psychobiology*, 26:8, 459–66.

Merati, A. L., Heman-Ackah, Y. D., Abaza, M., Altman, K. W., Sulica, L. and Belamowicz, S. (2005), 'Common Movement Disorders Affecting the Larynx: A Report from the Neurolaryngology Committee of the AAO-HNS', *Otolaryngology – Head and Neck Surgery*, 133:5, 654–5.

Merson, R. M. and Rolnick, M. I. (1998), 'Speech-Language Pathology and Dysphagia in Multiple Sclerosis', *Physical Medicine and Rehabilitation Clinics of North America*, 9:3, 631–41.

Messenger, M., Onslow, M., Packman, A. and Menzies, R. (2004), 'Social Anxiety in Stuttering: Measuring Negative Social Expectancies', *Journal of Fluency Disorders*, 29:3, 201–12.

Metz-Lutz, M- N., De Saint Martin, A., Hirsch, E., Maquet, P. and Marescaux, C. (1996), 'Auditory Verbal Processing Following Landau and Kleffner Syndrome', *Brain and Language*, 55:1, 147–50.

Miccio, A. W. (2002), 'Clinical Problem Solving: Assessment of Phonological Disorders', *American Journal of Speech-Language Pathology*, 11:3, 221–9.

Miccio, A. W., Elbert, M. and Forrest, K. (1999), 'The Relationship Between Stimulability and Phonological Acquisition in Children with Normally Developing and Disordered Phonologies', *American Journal of Speech-Language Pathology*, 8:4, 347–63.

Miccio, A. W. and Ingrisano, D. R. (2000), 'The Acquisition of Fricatives and Affricates: Evidence from a Disordered Phonological System', *American Journal of Speech-Language Pathology*, 9:3, 214–29.

Mikati, M. A. and Shamseddine, A. N. (2005), 'Management of Landau–Kleffner Syndrome', *Paediatric Drugs*, 7:6, 377–89.

Miller, C. A., Kail, R., Leonard, L. B. and Tomblin, J. B. (2001), 'Speed of Processing in Children with Specific Language Impairment', *Journal of Speech, Language, and Hearing Research*, 44:2, 416–33.

Miller, J. F. (1992), 'Development of Speech and Language in Children with Down Syndrome' in I. T. Lott and E. E. McCoy (eds), *Down Syndrome: Advances in Medical Care*, New York: Wiley–Liss, pp. 39–50.

Miller, J. F. and Chapman, R. S. (1981), 'The Relation Between Age and Mean Length of Utterance in Morphemes', *Journal of Speech and Hearing Research*, 24:2, 154–61.

Miller, N. (2000), 'Changing Ideas in Apraxia of Speech', in I. Papathanasiou (ed.), *Acquired Neurogenic Communication Disorders: A Clinical Perspective*, London: Whurr, pp. 173–202.

Miller, S. B. and Toca, J. M. (1979), 'Adapted Melodic Intonation Therapy: A Case Study of an Experimental Language Program for an Autistic Child', *Journal of Clinical Psychiatry*, 40:4, 201–3.

Milloy, N. and Morgan-Barry, R. (1990), 'Developmental Neurological Disorders', in P. Grunwell (ed.), *Developmental Speech Disorders: Clinical Issues and Practical Implications*, Edinburgh: Churchill Livingstone, pp. 109–32.

Mistry, M., Petralia, R., Simons, G., Wilkinson, Z. and Armitage, C. (2004), 'Summertime Learning', *RCSLT Bulletin*, 626, 8–9.

Mitchell, R. L. C. and Crow, T. J. (2005), 'Right Hemisphere Language Functions and Schizophrenia: The Forgotten Hemisphere', *Brain*, 128:5, 963–78.

Molina Garrido, M. J., Guillen Ponce, C., Macia Escalante, S., Martinez Y Sevila, C. and Carrato Mena, A. (2006), 'Dysphagia and Dysphonia in a Woman with a Previous Breast Cancer', *Clinical and Translational Oncology*, 8:7, 533–5.

Montero-Odasso, M. (2006), 'Dysphonia as First Symptom of Late-Onset Myasthenia Gravis', *Journal of General Internal Medicine*, 21:6, C4–6.

Montgomery, D. M. and Fitch, J. L. (1988), 'The Prevalence of Stuttering in the Hearing-Impaired School Age Population', *Journal of Speech and Hearing Disorders*, 53:2, 131–5.

Montgomery, J. W. (1995), 'Sentence Comprehension in Children with Specific Language Impairment: The Role of Phonological Working Memory', *Journal of Speech and Hearing Research*, 38:1, 187–99.

Montgomery, J. W. (2000), 'Verbal Working Memory and Sentence Comprehension in Children with Specific Language Impairment', *Journal of Speech, Language, and Hearing Research*, 43:2, 293–308.

Moreau-Gaudry, A., Sabil, A., Benchetrit, G. and Franco, A. (2005), 'Use of Respiratory Inductance Plethysmography for the Detection of Swallowing in the Elderly', *Dysphagia*, 20:4, 297–302.

Mortley, J., Enderby, P. and Petheram, B. (2001), 'Using a Computer to Improve Functional Writing in a Patient with Severe Dysgraphia', *Aphasiology*, 15:5, 443–61.

Morton, R. E., Bonas, R., Fourie, B. and Minford, J. (1993), 'Videofluoroscopy in the Assessment of Feeding Disorders of Children with Neurological Problems', *Developmental Medicine and Child Neurology*, 35:5, 388–95.

Moscato, B. S., Trevisan, M. and Willer, B. S. (1994), 'The Prevalence of Traumatic Brain Injury and Co-occurring Disabilities in a National Household Survey of Adults', *Journal of Neuropsychiatry and Clinical Neurosciences*, 6:2, 134–42.

Motor Neurone Disease Association (2005), *Motor Neurone Disease: A Problem Solving Approach*, Northampton: MND Association.

Movsessian, P. (2005), 'Neuropharmacology of Theophylline Induced Stuttering: The Role of Dopamine, Adenosine and GABA', *Medical Hypotheses*, 64:2, 290–7.

Mukand, J. A., Blackinton, D. D., Crincoli, M. G., Lee, J. J. and Santos, B. B. (2001), 'Incidence of Neurologic Deficits and Rehabilitation of Patients with Brain Tumors', *American Journal of Physical Medicine and Rehabilitation*, 80:5, 346–50.

Muller, D. (1999), 'Managing Psychosocial Adjustment to Aphasia', *Seminars in Speech and Language*, 20:1, 85–91.

Munoz, J., Mendoza, E., Fresneda, M. D., Carballo, G. and Ramirez, I. (2002), 'Perceptual Analysis in Different Voice Samples: Agreement and Reliability', *Perceptual and Motor Skills*, 94:2, 1187–95.

Munson, B., Bjorum, E. M. and Windsor, J. (2003), 'Acoustic and Perceptual Correlates of Stress in Nonwords Produced by Children with Suspected Developmental Apraxia of Speech and Children with Phonological Disorder', *Journal of Speech, Language and Hearing Research*, 46:1, 189–202.

Murano, E., Hosako-Naito, Y., Tayama, N., Oka, T., Miyaji, M., Kumada, M. and Niimi, S. (2001), 'Bamboo Node: Primary Vocal Fold Lesion as Evidence of Autoimmune Disease', *Journal of Voice*, 15:3, 441–50.

Murdoch, B. E., Hudson, L. J. and Boon, D. L. (1999), 'Effects of Treatment for Paediatric Cancer on Brain Structure and Function', in B. Murdoch (ed.), *Communication Disorders in Childhood Cancer*, London: Whurr, pp. 21–54.

Murdoch, B. E., Spencer, T. J., Theodoros, D. G. and Thompson, E. C. (1998), 'Lip and Tongue Function in Multiple Sclerosis: A Physiological Analysis', *Motor Control*, 2:2, 148–60.

Murdoch, B. E., Thompson, E. C. and Theodoros, D. G. (1997), 'Spastic Dysarthria', in M. R. McNeil (ed.), *Clinical Management of Sensorimotor Speech Disorders*, New York: Thieme Medical, pp. 287–310.

Murdoch, B. E., Ward, E. C. and Theodoros, D. G. (2000), 'Dysarthria: Clinical Features, Neuroanatomical Framework and Assessment', in I. Papathanasiou (ed.), *Acquired Neurogenic Communication Disorders: A Clinical Perspective*, London: Whurr, pp. 103–48.

Murphy, C. C., Yeargin-Allsopp, M., Decoufle, P. and Drews, C. D. (1993), 'Prevalence of Cerebral Palsy among Ten-Year-Old Children in Metropolitan Atlanta, 1985 Through 1987', *Journal of Pediatrics*, 123:5, S13–20.

Murphy, J. (2004), 'Communication Strategies of People with ALS and Their Partners', *Amyotrophic Lateral Sclerosis and Other Motor Neuron Disorders*, 5:2, 121–6.

Murray, L. L. (2000), 'Spoken Language Production in Huntington's and Parkinson's Diseases', *Journal of Speech, Language, and Hearing Research*, 43:6, 1350–66.

Murray, L. L., Holland, A. L. and Beeson, P. M. (1998), 'Spoken Language of Individuals with Mild Fluent Aphasia under Focused and Divided-Attention Conditions', *Journal of Speech, Language, and Hearing Research*, 41:1, 213–27.

Myers, F. L. and St Louis, K. O. (1996), 'Two Youths who Clutter, but is that the Only Similarity?', *Journal of Fluency Disorders*, 21:3–4, 297–304.

Nadol, J. B. and Eavey, R. D. (1995), 'Acute and Chronic Mastoiditis: Clinical Presentation, Diagnosis, and Management', *Current Clinical Topics in Infectious Diseases*, 15, 204–29.

Nakase-Thompson, R., Manning, E., Sherer, M., Yablon, S. A., Gontkovsky, S. L. and Vickery, C. (2005), 'Brief Assessment of Severe Language Impairments: Initial Validation of the Mississippi Aphasia Screening Test', *Brain Injury*, 19:9, 685–91.

Nalini, B. and Vinayak, S. (2006), 'Tuberculosis in Ear, Nose, and Throat Practice: Its Presentation and Diagnosis', *American Journal of Otolaryngology*, 27:1, 39–45.

Nation, K., Clarke, P., Marshall, C. M. and Durand, M. (2004), 'Hidden Language Impairments in Children: Parallels Between Poor Reading Comprehension and

Specific Language Impairment?', *Journal of Speech, Language, and Hearing Research*, 47:1, 199–211.

National Collaborating Centre for Chronic Conditions (2006), *Parkinson's Disease: National Clinical Guideline for Diagnosis and Management in Primary and Secondary Care*, London: Royal College of Physicians.

National Meningitis Trust (1996), *Meningitis Resource Pack*, Stroud: Meningitis Trust.

National Statistics (2006), 'Death Registrations in England and Wales, 2005: Causes', *Health Statistics Quarterly*, 30, 46–55.

Natke, U., Sandrieser, P., Pietrowsky, R. and Kalveram, K. T. (2006), 'Disfluency Data of German Preschool Children who Stutter and Comparison Children', *Journal of Fluency Disorders*, 31:3, 165–76.

Neilson, M. and Andrews, G. (1993), 'Intensive Fluency Training of Chronic Stutterers', in R. Curlee (ed.), *Stuttering and Related Disorders of Fluency*, New York: Thieme Stratton, pp. 139–65.

Nelson, C. D., Waggoner, D. D., Donnell, G. N., Tuerck, J. M. and Buist, N. R. (1991), 'Verbal Dyspraxia in Treated Galactosemia', *Paediatrics*, 88:2, 346–50.

Nelson, K. E., Camarata, S. M., Welsh, J., Butkovsky, L. and Camarata, M. (1996), 'Effects of Imitative and Conversational Recasting Treatment on the Acquisition of Grammar in Children with Specific Language Impairment and Younger Language-Normal Children', *Journal of Speech and Hearing Research*, 39:4, 850–9.

Newton, H. B., Newton, C., Pearl, D. and Davidson, T. (1994), 'Swallowing Assessment in Primary Brain Tumor Patients with Dysphagia', *Neurology*, 44:10, 1927–32.

Ng, T. Y. (2000), 'Adult Voice Disorders', *Hong Kong Practitioner*, 22, 71–9.

Niccols, G. A. (1994), 'Fetal Alcohol Syndrome: Implications for Psychologists', *Clinical Psychology Review*, 14:2, 91–111.

Niebudek-Bogusz, E., Fiszer, M., Kotylo, P. and Sliwinska-Kowalska, M. (2006), 'Diagnostic Value of Voice Acoustic Analysis in Assessment of Occupational Voice Pathologies in Teachers', *Logopedics Phoniatrics Vocology*, 31:3, 100–6.

Nijland, L., Maassen, B. and van der Meulen, S. (2003a), 'Evidence of Motor Programming Deficits in Children Diagnosed with DAS', *Journal of Speech, Language, and Hearing Research*, 46:2, 437–50.

Nijland, L., Maassen, B., Van der Meulen, S., Gabreels, F., Kraaimaat, F. W. and Schreuder, R. (2003b), 'Planning of Syllables in Children with Developmental Apraxia of Speech', *Clinical Linguistics and Phonetics*, 17:1, 1–24.

Nippold, M. A. (2001), 'Phonological Disorders and Stuttering in Children: What is the Frequency of Co-Occurrence?', *Clinical Linguistics and Phonetics*, 15:3, 219–28.

Nippold, M. A. (2002), 'Stuttering and Phonology: Is There an Interaction?', *American Journal of Speech-Language Pathology*, 11:2, 99–110.

Nippold, M. A. (2004), 'Phonological and Language Disorders in Children who Stutter: Impact on Treatment Recommendations', *Clinical Linguistics and Phonetics*, 18:2, 145–59.

Nippold, M. A. and Rudzinski, M. (1995), 'Parents' Speech and Children's Stuttering: A Critique of the Literature', *Journal of Speech and Hearing Research*, 38:5, 978–89.

Nishio, M. and Niimi, S. (2006), 'Comparison of Speaking Rate, Articulation Rate and Alternating Motion Rate in Dysarthric Speakers', *Folia Phoniatrica et Logopaedica*, 58:2, 114–31.

Noens, I. L. J. and van Berckelaer-Onnes, I. A. (2005), 'Captured by Details: Sense-Making, Language and Communication in Autism', *Journal of Communication Disorders*, 38:2, 123–41.

Norbury, C. F. and Bishop, D. V. M. (2002), 'Inferential Processing and Story Recall in Children with Communication Problems: A Comparison of Specific Language Impairment, Pragmatic Language Impairment and High-Functioning Autism', *International Journal of Language and Communication Disorders*, 37:3, 227–51.

Norbury, C. F., Bishop, D. V. M. and Briscoe, J. (2001), 'Production of English Finite Verb Morphology: A Comparison of SLI and Mild–Moderate Hearing Impairment', *Journal of Speech, Language, and Hearing Research*, 44:1 165–78.

Nordin, V. and Gillberg, C. (1996), 'Autism Spectrum Disorders in Children with Physical or Mental Disability or Both. I: Clinical and Epidemiological Aspects', *Developmental Medicine and Child Neurology*, 38:4, 297–313.

Northern, J. L. and Downs, M. P. (2002), *Hearing in Children*, Baltimore, MD: Lippincott Williams & Wilkins.

Nuffield Hearing & Speech Centre (2004), *The Nuffield Centre Dyspraxia Programme*, 3rd edn, Windsor: Miracle Factory.

Nwiloh, J. and Fortson, J. (2001), 'Aspirated Foreign Body in a Laryngectomized Patient: Case Report and Literature Review', *ENT Journal*, 80:10.

O'Brian, S., Onslow, M., Cream, A. and Packman, A. (2003), 'The Camperdown Program: Outcomes of a New Prolonged-Speech Treatment Model', *Journal of Speech, Language, and Hearing Research*, 46:4, 933–46.

O'Brian, S., Packman, A. and Onslow, M. (2004), 'Self-Rating of Stuttering Severity as a Clinical Tool', *American Journal of Speech-Language Pathology*, 13:3, 219–26.

O'Brien, E. K., Zhang, X., Nishimura, C., Tomblin, J. B. and Murray, J. C. (2003), 'Association of Specific Language Impairment (SLI) to the Region of 7q31', *American Journal of Human Genetics*, 72:6, 1536–43.

O'Brien, G. and Pearson, J. (2004), 'Autism and Learning Disability', *Autism*, 8:2, 125–40.

O'Dwyer, T. P. and Conlon, B. J. (1997), 'The Surgical Management of Drooling – A 15 Year Follow-Up', *Clinical Otolaryngology*, 22:3, 284–7.

Odell, K., McNeil, M. R. and Rosenbek, J. C. (1991), 'Perceptual Characteristics of Vowel and Prosody Production in Apraxic, Aphasic and Dysarthric Speakers', *Journal of Speech and Hearing Research*, 34:1, 67–80.

Odell, K. H. and Shriberg, L. D. (2001), 'Prosody-Voice Characteristics of Children and Adults with Apraxia of Speech', *Clinical Linguistics and Phonetics*, 15:4, 275–307.

470

Oelschlaeger, M. L. and Damico, J. S. (2000), 'Partnership in Conversation: A Study of Word Search Strategies', *Journal of Communication Disorders*, 33:3, 205–23.

Oetting, J. B. (1999), 'Children with SLI Use Argument Structure Cues to Learn Verbs', *Journal of Speech, Language, and Hearing Research*, 42:5, 1261–74.

Oetting, J. B. and Horohov, J. E. (1997), 'Past-Tense Marking by Children with and without Specific Language Impairment', *Journal of Speech, Language, and Hearing Research*, 40:1, 62–74.

Oetting, J. B., Rice, M. L. and Swank, L. K. (1995), 'Quick Incidental Learning (QUIL) of Words by School-Age Children with and without SLI', *Journal of Speech and Hearing Research*, 38:2, 434–45.

Ogar, J., Willock, S., Baldo, J., Wilkins, D., Ludy, C. and Dronkers, N. (2006), 'Clinical and Anatomical Correlates of Apraxia of Speech', *Brain and Language*, 97:3, 343–50.

Ollivere, B., Duce, K., Rowlands, G., Harrison, P. and O'Reilly, B. J. (2006), 'Swallowing Dysfunction in Patients with Unilateral Vocal Fold Paralysis: Aetiology and Outcomes', *Journal of Laryngology and Otology*, 120, 38–41.

Ono, T., Hamamura, M., Honda, K. and Nokubi, T. (2005), 'Collaboration of a Dentist and Speech–Language Pathologist in the Rehabilitation of a Stroke Patient with Dysarthria: A Case Study', *Gerodontology*, 22:2, 116–19.

Ozudogru, E., Cakli, H., Altuntas, E. E. and Gurbuz, M. K. (2005), 'Effects of Laryngeal Tuberculosis on Vocal Fold Functions: Case Report', *ACTA Otorhinolaryngologica Italica*, 25:6, 374–7.

Palmen, S. J. M. C., van Engeland, H., Hof, P. R. and Schmitz, C. (2004), 'Neuropathological Findings in Autism', *Brain*, 127:12, 2572–83.

Park, C. L., O'Neill, P. A. and Martin, D. F. (1997), 'A Pilot Exploratory Study of Oral Electrical Stimulation on Swallow Function Following Stroke: An Innovative Technique', *Dysphagia*, 12:3, 161–6.

Parkes, J., Donnelly, M. and Hill, N. (2001), *Focusing on Cerebral Palsy: Reviewing and Communicating Needs for Services*, London: Scope.

Parkinson's Disease Society (2002), *Facing the Future: An Introduction to Parkinson's Disease and the Parkinson's Disease Society*, London: Parkinson's Disease Society.

Parsons, C. L., Iacono, T. A. and Rozner, L. (1987), 'Effect of Tongue Reduction on Articulation in Children with Down Syndrome', *American Journal of Mental Deficiency*, 91:4, 328–32.

Patel, M. R. (2005), *Herpes Encephalitis*, USA: eMedicine.com (website: http://www.emedicine.com/radio/topic334.htm).

Paterson, S. (2001), 'Language and Number in Down Syndrome: The Complex Developmental Trajectory from Infancy to Adulthood', *Down Syndrome Research and Practice*, 7:2, 79–86.

Pattee, C., Von Berg, S. and Ghezzi, P. (2006), 'Effects of Alternative Communication on the Communicative Effectiveness of an Individual with a Progressive Language Disorder', *International Journal of Rehabilitation Research*, 29:2, 151–3.

Paul, R., Augustyn, A., Klin, A. and Volkmar, F. R. (2005), 'Perception and Production of Prosody by Speakers with Autism Spectrum Disorders', *Journal of Autism and Developmental Disorders*, 35:2, 205–20.

Paydarfar, J. A. and Birkmeyer, N. J. (2006), 'Complications in Head and Neck Surgery: A Meta-Analysis of Postlaryngectomy Pharyngocutaneous Fistula', *Archives of Otolaryngology – Head and Neck Surgery*, 132:1, 67–72.

Peat, B. G., Albery, E. H., Jones, K. and Pigott, R. W. (1994), 'Tailoring Velopharyngeal Surgery: The Influence of Aetiology and Type of Operation', *Plastic and Reconstructive Surgery*, 93:5, 948–53.

Pedersen, P. M., Jorgensen, H. S., Kammersgaard, L. P., Nakayama, H., Raaschou, H. O. and Olsen, T. S. (2001), 'Manual and Oral Apraxia in Acute Stroke, Frequency and Influence on Functional Outcome: The Copenhagen Stroke Study', *American Journal of Physical Medicine and Rehabilitation*, 80:9, 685–92.

Pellowski, M. W. and Conture, E. G. (2002), 'Characteristics of Speech Disfluency and Stuttering Behaviors in 3- and 4-Year-Old Children', *Journal of Speech, Language, and Hearing Research*, 45:1, 20–34.

Pennington, L., Goldbart, J. and Marshall, J. (2004), 'Interaction Training for Conversational Partners of Children with Cerebral Palsy: A Systematic Review', *International Journal of Language and Communication Disorders*, 39:2, 151–70.

Peppard, R. C. (1996), 'Management of Functional Voice Disorders in Adolescents', *Language, Speech, and Hearing Services in Schools*, 27:3, 257–70.

Perez, K. S., Ramig, L. O., Smith, M. E. and Dromey, C. (1996), 'The Parkinson Larynx: Tremor and Videostroboscopic Findings', *Journal of Voice*, 10:4, 354–61.

Perkins, L. (1995), 'Applying Conversation Analysis to Aphasia: Clinical Implications and Analytic Issues', *European Journal of Disorders of Communication*, 30:3, 372–83.

Perkins, L., Whitworth, A. and Lesser, R. (1997), *Conversation Analysis Profile for People with Cognitive Impairment* (CAPPCI), London: Whurr.

Perkins, L., Crisp, J. and Walshaw, D. (1999), 'Exploring Conversation Analysis as an Assessment Tool for Aphasia: The Issue of Reliability', *Aphasiology*, 13:4–5, 259–81.

Perkins, W. H. and Kent, R. D. (1986), *Textbook of Functional Anatomy of Speech, Language and Hearing*, London: Taylor & Francis.

Persson, C., Lohmander, A., Jönsson, R., Óskarsdóttir, S. and Söderpalm, E. (2003), 'A Prospective Cross-Sectional Study of Speech in Patients with the 22q11 Deletion Syndrome', *Journal of Communication Disorders*, 36:1, 13–47.

Peters, C. M., Gartner, C. E., Silburn, P. A. and Mellick, G. D. (2006), 'Prevalence of Parkinson's Disease in Metropolitan and Rural Queensland: A General Practice Survey', *Journal of Clinical Neuroscience*, 13:3, 343–8.

Peterson, P., Carta, J. J. and Greenwood, C. (2005), 'Teaching Enhanced Milieu Language Teaching Skills to Parents in Multiple Risk Families', *Journal of Early Intervention*, 27:2, 94–109.

Petinou, K., Schwartz, R. G., Mody, M. and Gravel, J. S. (1999), 'The Impact of Otitis Media with Effusion on Early Phonetic Inventories: A Longitudinal Prospective Investigation', *Clinical Linguistics and Phonetics*, 13:5, 351–67.

Phelps-Terasaki, D. and Phelps-Gunn, T. (1992), *Test of Pragmatic Language*, San Antonio, TX: Psychological Corporation.

Pignataro, L., Peri, A., Pagani, D., Iudica, F. and Scaramellini, G. (2006), 'Cricoid Chondrosarcoma Coexisting with a Thyroid Mass: Case Report and Review of the Literature', *Tumori*, 92:3, 257–9.

Pilcher, E. S. (1998), 'Dental Care for the Patient with Down Syndrome', *Down Syndrome Research and Practice*, 5:3, 111–16.

Pinder, G. L. and Faherty, A. S. (1999), 'Issues in Pediatric Feeding and Swallowing', in A. Caruso and E. Strand (eds), *Clinical Management of Motor Speech Disorders in Children*, New York: Thieme Medical, pp. 281–318.

Piven, J., Arndt, S., Bailey, J. and Andreasen, N. (1996), 'Regional Brain Enlargement in Autism: A Magnetic Resonance Imaging Study', *Journal of the American Academy of Child and Adolescent Psychiatry*, 35:4, 530–6.

Pohjasvaara, T., Erkinjuntti, T., Vataja, R. and Kaste, M. (1997), 'Dementia Three Months after Stroke', *Stroke*, 28:4, 785–92.

Pollock, K. E. and Hall, P. K. (1991), 'An Analysis of the Vowel Misarticulations of Five Children with Developmental Apraxia of Speech', *Clinical Linguistics and Phonetics*, 5:3, 207–24.

Pothier, D. D., Bredenkamp, C. -L. and Monteiro, P. (2006), 'Is Speech Therapy Really Preventing Recovery in Stutterers?', *International Journal of Language and Communication Disorders*, 41:5, 591–2.

Poulos, M. G. and Webster, W. G. (1991), 'Family History as a Basis for Subgrouping People who Stutter', *Journal of Speech and Hearing Research*, 34:1, 5–10.

Pourmand, R. (1997), 'Myasthenia Gravis', *Disease-a-Month*, 43:2, 70–109.

Powell, G. and Clibbens, J. (1994), 'Actions Speak Louder Than Words: Signing and Speech Intelligibility in Adults with Down's Syndrome', *Down Syndrome Research and Practice*, 2:3, 127–9.

Powell, J. E., Edwards, A., Edwards, M., Pandit, B. S., Sungum-Paliwal, S. R. and Whitehouse, W. (2000), 'Changes in the Incidence of Childhood Autism and Other Autistic Spectrum Disorders in Preschool Children from Two Areas of the West Midlands, UK', *Developmental Medicine and Child Neurology*, 42:9, 624–8.

Powell, T. W., Miccio, A. W., Elbert, M., Brasseur, J. A. and Strike-Roussos, C. (1999), 'Patterns of Sound Change in Children with Phonological Disorders', *Clinical Linguistics and Phonetics*, 13:3, 163–82.

Power, M. L., Fraser, C. H., Hobson, A., Singh, S., Tyrell, P., Nicholson, D. A., Turnbull, I., Thompson, D. G. and Hamdy, S. (2006), 'Evaluating Oral Stimulation as a Treatment for Dysphagia after Stroke', *Dysphagia*, 21:1, 49–55.

Prasher, V. and Smith, B. (2002), *Down Syndrome and Health Care*, Kidderminster: BILD.

Preus, A. (1996), 'Cluttering Upgraded', *Journal of Fluency Disorders*, 21:3–4, 349–57.

Pribuisiene, R., Uloza, V., Kupcinskas, L. and Jonaitis, L. (2006), 'Perceptual and Acoustic Characteristics of Voice Changes in Reflux Laryngitis Patients', *Journal of Voice*, 20:1, 128–36.

Proctor-Williams, K., Fey, M. E. and Loeb, D. F. (2001), 'Parental Recasts and Production of Copulas and Articles by Children with Specific Language Impairment and Typical Language', *American Journal of Speech-Language Pathology*, 10:2, 155–68.

Prosiegel, M., Holing, R., Heintze, M., Wagner-Sonntag, E. and Wiseman, K. (2005), 'Swallowing Therapy – A Prospective Study on Patients with Neurogenic Dysphagia due to Unilateral Paresis of the Vagal Nerve, Avellis' syndrome, Wallenberg's Syndrome, Posterior Fossa Tumours and Cerebellar Hemorrhage', *Acta Neurochirurgica*, Supplement 93, 35–7.

Prutting, C. A. and Kirchner, D. M. (1987), 'A Clinical Appraisal of the Pragmatic Aspects of Language', *Journal of Speech and Hearing Disorders*, 52:2, 105–19.

Pryce, M. (1994), 'The Voice of People with Down's Syndrome: An EMG Biofeedback Study', *Down Syndrome Research and Practice*, 2:3, 106–11.

Rakowicz, W. P. and Hodges, J. R. (1998), 'Dementia and Aphasia in Motor Neuron Disease: An Underrecognised Association?', *Journal of Neurology, Neurosurgery and Psychiatry*, 65:6, 881–9.

Ramig, L. O., Sapir, S., Fox, C. and Countryman, S. (2001), 'Changes in Vocal Loudness Following Intensive Voice Treatment (LSVT®) in Individuals with Parkinson's Disease: A Comparison with Untreated Patients and Normal Age-Matched Controls', *Movement Disorders*, 16:1, 79–83.

Ramritu, P., Finlayson, K., Mitchell, A. and Croft, G. (2000), *Identification and Nursing Management of Dysphagia in Individuals with Neurological Impairment: A Systematic Review, Number 8*, Adelaide: Joanna Briggs Institute for Evidence Based Nursing and Midwifery.

Ramruttun, B. and Jenkins, C. (1998), 'Prelinguistic Communication and Down Syndrome', *Down Syndrome Research and Practice*, 5:2, 53–62.

Ramsden, R. T. and Axon, P. R. (2001), 'Objective Audiometry', in J. Graham and M. Martin (eds), *Ballantyne's Deafness*, London: Whurr, pp. 102–16.

Ramsey, D. J. C., Smithard, D. G. and Kalra, L. (2003), 'Early Assessments of Dysphagia and Aspiration Risk in Acute Stroke Patients', *Stroke*, 34:5, 1252–7.

Ranta, R. (1990), 'Orthodontic Treatment Alternatives for Unilateral Cleft Lip and Palate Patients', in J. Bardach and H. L. Morris (eds), *Multidisciplinary Management of Cleft Lip and Palate*, Philadelphia, PA: W.B. Saunders, pp. 637–41.

Rao, P. R. (1991), 'Neurogenic Stuttering as a Manifestation of Stroke and a Mask of Dysphonia', *Clinics in Communication Disorders*, 1:1, 31–7.

Rapin, I. and Allen, D. A. (1983), 'Developmental Language Disorders: Nosologic Considerations', in U. Kirk (ed.), *Neuropsychology of Language, Reading, and Spelling*, New York: Academic, pp. 155–84.

Rasmussen, P., Borjesson, O., Wentz, E. and Gillberg, C. (2001), 'Autistic Disorders in Down Syndrome: Background Factors and Clinical Correlates', *Developmental Medicine and Child Neurology*, 43:11, 750–4.

Raven, J. C. (1986), *Raven's Progressive Matrices and Vocabulary Scales*, London: Lewis.

Reddy, U. M., Fry, A., Pass, R. and Ghidini, A. (2004), 'Infectious Diseases and Perinatal Outcomes', *Emerging Infectious Diseases* (website: http://www.cdc.gov/ncidod/EID/vol10no11/04-0623_10.htm).

Redmond, S. M. and Rice, M. L. (2001), 'Detection of Irregular Verb Violations by Children with and without SLI', *Journal of Speech, Language, and Hearing Research*, 44:3, 655–69.

Remacle, M. (1996), 'The Contribution of Videostroboscopy in Daily ENT Practice', *Acta Otorhinolaryngologica Belgica*, 50:4, 265–81.

Remington, B. and Clarke, S. (1993a), 'Simultaneous Communication and Speech Comprehension. Part I: Comparison of Two Methods of Teaching Expressive Signing and Speech Comprehension Skills', *Augmentative and Alternative Communication*, 9:1, 36–48.

Remington, B. and Clarke, S. (1993b), 'Simultaneous Communication and Speech Comprehension. Part II: Comparison of Two Methods of Overcoming Selective Attention During Expressive Sign Training', *Augmentative and Alternative Communication*, 9:1, 49–60.

Renfrew, C. (1995), *Word Finding Vocabulary Test*, London: Winslow.

Rescorla, L. and Ratner, N. B. (1996), 'Phonetic Profiles of Toddlers with Specific Expressive Language Impairment (SLI-E)', *Journal of Speech and Hearing Research*, 39:1, 153–65.

Reynell, J. (1985), *Reynell Developmental Language Scales – Revised*, Windsor: NFER-Nelson.

Ribeiro, B. T. (1994), *Coherence in Psychotic Discourse*, New York: Oxford University Press.

Rice, M. L., Cleave, P. L. and Oetting, J. B. (2000), 'The Use of Syntactic Cues in Lexical Acquisition by Children with SLI', *Journal of Speech, Language, and Hearing Research*, 43:3, 582–94.

Rice, M. L., Haney, K. R. and Wexler, K. (1998), 'Family Histories of Children with SLI who Show Extended Optional Infinitives', *Journal of Speech, Language, and Hearing Research*, 41:2, 419–32.

Rice, M. L. and Wexler, K. (1996), 'Toward Tense as a Clinical Marker of Specific Language Impairment in English-Speaking Children', *Journal of Speech and Hearing Research*, 39:6, 1239–57.

Rice, M. L., Wexler, K. and Cleave, P. L. (1995), 'Specific Language Impairment as a Period of Extended Optional Infinitive', *Journal of Speech and Hearing Research*, 38:4, 850–63.

Rice, M. L., Wexler, K. and Hershberger, S. (1998), 'Tense Over Time: The Longitudinal Course of Tense Acquisition in Children with Specific Language Impairment', *Journal of Speech, Language, and Hearing Research*, 41:6, 1412–31.

Rice, M. L., Wexler, K., Marquis, J. and Hershberger, S. (2000), 'Acquisition of Irregular Past Tense by Children with Specific Language Impairment', *Journal of Speech, Language, and Hearing Research*, 43:5, 1126–45.

Richards, R. G., Sampson, F. C., Beard, S. M. and Tappenden, P. (2002), 'A Review of the Natural History and Epidemiology of Multiple Sclerosis: Implications for Resource Allocation and Health Economic Models', *Health Technology Assessment*, 6:10.

Richardson, J. E., Blackmore, C. and Atkin, A. (2007), 'Arguing with Asperger Syndrome' in F. H. van Eemeren, J. A. Blair, C. A. Willard and A. F. Snoeck Henkemans (eds), *Proceedings of the Sixth Conference of the International Society for the Study of Argumentation*, Amsterdam: Sic Sat, pp. 1141–6.

Riches, N. G., Tomasello, M. and Conti-Ramsden, G. (2005), 'Verb Learning in Children with SLI: Frequency and Spacing Effects', *Journal of Speech, Language, and Hearing Research*, 48:6, 1397–411.

Rigueiro-Veloso, M. T., Pego-Reigosa, R., Branas-Fernandez, F., Martinez-Vazquez, F. and Cortes-Laino, J. A. (1997), 'Wallenberg Syndrome: A Review of 25 Cases', *Revista de Neurología*, 25:146, 1561–4.

Riley, G. D. (1972), 'A Stuttering Severity Instrument for Children and Adults', *Journal of Speech and Hearing Disorders*, 37:3, 314–22.

Riley, G. D. (1994), *Stuttering Severity Instrument for Children and Adults*, Austin, TX: Pro-Ed.

Rinehart, N. J., Bradshaw, J. L., Brereton, A. V. and Tonge, B. J. (2001), 'Movement Preparation in High-Functioning Autism and Asperger Disorder: A Serial Choice Reaction Time Task Involving Motor Reprogramming', *Journal of Autism and Developmental Disorders*, 31:1, 79–88.

Ringholz, G. M., Appel, S. H., Bradshaw, M., Cooke, N. A., Mosnik, D. M. and Schulz, P. E. (2005), 'Prevalence and Patterns of Cognitive Impairment in Sporadic ALS', *Neurology*, 65:4, 586–90.

Robbins, J., Gangnon, R. E., Theis, S. M., Kays, S. A., Hewitt, A. L. and Hind, J. A. (2005), 'The Effects of Lingual Exercise on Swallowing in Older Adults', *Journal of the American Geriatrics Society*, 53:9, 1483–9.

Roberts, J., Rescorla, L., Giroux, J. and Stevens, L. (1998), 'Phonological Skills of Children with Specific Expressive Language Impairment (SLI-E): Outcome at Age 3', *Journal of Speech, Language, and Hearing Research*, 41:2, 374–84.

Robertson, A., Singh, R. H., Guerrero, N. V., Hundley, M. and Elsas, L. J. (2000), 'Outcomes Analysis of Verbal Dyspraxia in Classic Galactosemia', *Genetics in Medicine*, 2:2, 142–8.

Robertson, S. J. (1987), *Dysarthria Profile*, Tucson, AZ: Communication Skill Builders.

Robin, D. A. (1992), 'Developmental Apraxia of Speech: Just Another Motor Problem', *American Journal of Speech-Language Pathology*, 1:3, 19–22.

Robinson, P. J., Lodge, S., Jones, B. M., Walker, C. C. and Grant, H. R. (1992), 'The Effect of Palate Repair on Otitis Media with Effusion', *Plastic and Reconstructive Surgery*, 89:4, 640–5.

Robinson, R. J. (1991), 'Causes and Associations of Severe and Persistent Specific Speech and Language Disorders in Children', *Developmental Medicine and Child Neurology*, 33:11, 943–62.

Robinson, R. O., Baird, G., Robinson, G. and Simonoff, E. (2001), 'Landau-Kleffner Syndrome: Course and Correlates with Outcome', *Developmental Medicine and Child Neurology*, 43:4, 243–7.

Robson, J., Marshall, J., Chiat, S. and Pring, T. (2001), 'Enhancing Communication in Jargon Aphasia: A Small Group Study of Writing Therapy', *International Journal of Language and Communication Disorders*, 36:4, 471–88.

Robson, J., Pring, T., Marshall, J. and Chiat, S. (2003), 'Phoneme Frequency Effects in Jargon Aphasia: A Phonological Investigation of Nonword Errors', *Brain and Language*, 85:1, 109–24.

Rodriguez-Ferrera, S., McCarthy, R. A. and McKenna, P. J. (2001), 'Language in Schizophrenia and its Relationship to Formal Thought Disorder', *Psychological Medicine*, 31:2, 197–205.

Roh, J. L., Kim, A. Y. and Cho, M. J. (2005), 'Xerostomia Following Radiotherapy of the Head and Neck Affects Vocal Function', *Journal of Clinical Oncology*, 23:13, 3016–23.

Rondal, J. A. and Comblain, A. (1996), 'Language in Adults with Down Syndrome', *Down Syndrome Research and Practice*, 4:1, 3–14.

Rondal, J. A. and Edwards, S. (1997), *Language in Mental Retardation*, London: Whurr.

Roper, N. (2003), 'Melodic Intonation Therapy with Young Children with Apraxia', *Bridges*, 1:8, 1–7.

Rosamond, W. D., Folsom, A. R., Chambless, L. E., Wang, C. H., McGovern, P. G., Howard, G., Copper, L. S. and Shahar, E. (1999), 'Stroke Incidence and Survival among Middle-Aged Adults: 9-Year Follow-Up of the Atherosclerosis Risk in Communities (ARIC) Cohort', *Stroke*, 30:4, 736–43.

Rosen, K. M., Kent, R. D., Delaney, A. L. and Duffy, J. R. (2006), 'Parametric Quantitative Acoustic Analysis of Conversation Produced by Speakers with Dysarthria and Healthy Speakers', *Journal of Speech, Language and Hearing Research*, 49:2, 395–411.

Rosenbek, J. C., Robbins, J. A., Willford, W. O., Kirk, G., Schiltz, A., Sowell, T. W., Deutsch, S. E., Milanti, F. J., Ashford, J., Gramigna, G. D., Fogarty, A., Dong, K., Rau, M. T., Prescott, T. E., Lloyd, A. M., Sterkel, M. T. and Hansen, J. E. (1998), 'Comparing Treatment Intensities of Tactile-Thermal Application', *Dysphagia*, 13:1, 1–9.

Rosenhall, U., Nordin, V., Sandström, M., Ahlsén, G. and Gillberg, C. (1999), 'Autism and Hearing Loss', *Journal of Autism and Developmental Disorders*, 29:5, 349–57.

Rosenvinge, S. K. and Starke, I. D. (2005), 'Improving Care for Patients with Dysphagia', *Age and Ageing*, 34:6, 587–93.

Rosin, P. and Swift, E. (1999), 'Communication Interventions: Improving the Speech Intelligibility of Children with Down Syndrome', in J. F. Miller, M. Leddy and L. A. Leavitt (eds), *Improving the Communication of People with Down Syndrome*, Baltimore, MD: Paul H. Brookes, pp. 133–54.

Ross, A., Winslow, I., Marchant, P. and Brumfitt, S. (2006), 'Evaluation of Communication, Life Participation and Psychological Well-Being in Chronic Aphasia: The Influence of Group Intervention', *Aphasiology*, 20:5, 427–48.

Rossi, P. G., Parmeggiani, A., Pasar, A., Scaduto, M. C., Chiodo, S. and Vatti, G. (1999), 'Landau–Kleffner Syndrome (LKS): Long-Term Follow-Up and Links with Electrical Status Epilepticus during Sleep (ESES)', *Brain and Development*, 21:2, 90–8.

Rossiter, D. (1998), 'Workforce Planning', *RCSLT Bulletin*, 578, 13–15.

Rossiter, D. (2000), 'Leaving the Profession', *RCSLT Bulletin*, 576, 11–13.

Rossiter, D. (2002), 'Why SLT is a Shortage Profession', *RCSLT Bulletin*, 604, 8–10.

Roy, N., Merrill, R. M., Gray, S. D. and Smith, E. M. (2005), 'Voice Disorders in the General Population: Prevalence, Risk Factors, and Occupational Impact', *Laryngoscope*, 115:11, 1988–95.

Roy, N., Merrill, R. M., Thibeault, S., Parsa, R. A., Gray, S. D. and Smith, E. M. (2004), 'Prevalence of Voice Disorders in Teachers and the General Population', *Journal of Speech, Language, and Hearing Research*, 47:2, 281–93.

Royal College of Speech and Language Therapists (1996), *Communicating Quality 2*, London: RCSLT.

Royal College of Speech and Language Therapists (2005), *Clinical Guidelines*, Oxon: Speechmark.

Rudert, H. (1979), 'First Experiences with Voice-Rehabilitative Laryngectomy, as Described by Staffieri and Amatsu', *Laryngologie, Rhinologie, Otologie*, 58:6, 476–81.

Ruigendijk, E. and Bastiaanse, R. (2002), 'Two Characteristics of Agrammatic Speech: Omission of Verbs and Omission of Determiners, Is There a Relation?', *Aphasiology*, 16:4–6, 383–95.

Russell, V. J. and Harding, A. (2001), 'Speech Development and Early Intervention', in A. C. H. Watson, D. A. Sell and P. Grunwell (eds), *Management of Cleft Lip and Palate*, London: Whurr, pp. 191–209.

Rutter, M., Bailey, A., Bolton, P. and Le Couteur, A. (1994), 'Autism and Known Medical Conditions: Myth and Substance', *Journal of Child Psychology and Psychiatry*, 35:2, 311–22.

Rvachew, S. and Grawburg, M. (2006), 'Correlates of Phonological Awareness in Preschoolers with Speech Sound Disorders', *Journal of Speech, Language, and Hearing Research*, 49:1, 74–87.

Rvachew, S., Nowak, M. and Cloutier, G. (2004), 'Effect of Phonemic Perception Training on the Speech Production and Phonological Awareness Skills of Children with Expressive Phonological Delay', *American Journal of Speech-Language Pathology*, 13:3, 250–63.

Rvachew, S., Ohberg, A., Grawburg, M. and Heyding, J. (2003), 'Phonological Awareness and Phonemic Perception in 4-Year-Old Children with Delayed Expressive Phonology Skills', *American Journal of Speech-Language Pathology*, 12:4, 463–71.

Rvachew, S., Rafaat, S. and Martin, M. (1999), 'Stimulability, Speech Perception Skills, and the Treatment of Phonological Disorders', *American Journal of Speech-Language Pathology*, 8:1, 33–43.

Ryan, B. P. (1992), 'Articulation, Language, Rate, and Fluency Characteristics of Stuttering and Nonstuttering Preschool Children', *Journal of Speech and Hearing Research*, 35:2, 333–42.

Sakai, K., Furui, E., Komai, K., Notoya, M. and Yamada, M. (2002), 'Acquired Stuttering as an Early Symptom in a Patient with Progressive Supranuclear Palsy', *Rinsho Shinkeigaku*, 42:2, 178–80.

Salter, K., Jutai, J., Foley, N., Hellings, C. and Teasell, R. (2006), 'Identification of Aphasia Post Stroke: A Review of Screening Assessment Tools', *Brain Injury*, 20:6, 559–68.

Saltuklaroglu, T. and Kalinowski, J. (2005), 'How Effective Is Therapy for Childhood Stuttering? Dissecting and Reinterpreting the Evidence in Light of Spontaneous Recovery Rates', *International Journal of Language and Communication Disorders*, 40:3, 359–74.

Saltuklaroglu, T. and Kalinowski, J. (2006), 'Is Speech Therapy Really Preventing Recovery in Stutterers? A Reply to Pothier, Monteiro and Bredencamp?', *International Journal of Language and Communication Disorders*, 41:5, 593–5.

Samson-Fang, L., Butler, C. and O'Donnell, M. (2003), 'Effects of Gastrostomy Feeding in Children with Cerebral Palsy: An AACPDM Evidence Report', *Developmental Medicine and Child Neurology*, 45:6, 415–26.

Sandage, M. J. and Zelazny, S. K. (2004), 'Paradoxical Vocal Fold Motion in Children and Adolescents', *Language, Speech, and Hearing Services in Schools*, 35:4, 353–62.

Sandberg, A. D. (1998), 'Reading and Spelling among Nonvocal Children with Cerebral Palsy: Influence of Home and School Literacy Environment', *Reading and Writing*, 10:1, 23–50.

Sandberg, A. D., Ehlers, S., Hagberg, B. and Gillberg, C. (2000), 'The Rett Syndrome Complex: Communicative Functions in Relation to Developmental Level and Autistic Features', *Autism*, 4:3, 249–67.

Sapienza, C. M., Ruddy, B. H. and Baker, S. (2004), 'Laryngeal Structure and Function in the Pediatric Larynx: Clinical Applications', *Language, Speech, and Hearing Services in Schools*, 35:4, 299–307.

Sapir, S., Spielman, J., Ramig, L. O., Hinds, S. L., Countryman, S., Fox, C. and Story, B. (2003), 'Effects of Intensive Voice Treatment (The Lee Silverman Voice Treatment [LSVT]) on Ataxic Dysarthria: A Case Study', *American Journal of Speech–Language Pathology*, 12:4, 387–99.

Sargent, L. A. (1999), *The Craniofacial Surgery Book*, Chattanooga, TN: Williams.

Sarimski, K. (2002), 'Analysis of Intentional Communication in Severely Handicapped Children with Cornelia-de-Lange Syndrome', *Journal of Communication Disorders*, 35:6, 483–500.

Savvopoulos, S., Golaz, J., Bouras, C., Constantinidis, J. and Tissot, R. (1990), 'Huntington Chorea: Anatomoclinical and Genetic Study of 17 Cases', *Encephale*, 16:4, 251–9.

Sawyer, J. and Yairi, E. (2006), 'The Effect of Sample Size on the Assessment of Stuttering Severity', *American Journal of Speech-Language Pathology*, 15:1, 36–44.

Scheffer, I. E., Jones, L., Pozzebon, M., Howell, R. A., Saling, M. M. and Berkovic, S. F. (1995), 'Autosomal Dominant Rolandic Epilepsy and Speech Dyspraxia: A New Syndrome with Anticipation', *Annals of Neurology*, 38:4, 633–42.

Scherer, N. J. and D'Antonio, L. L. (1995), 'Parent Questionnaire for Screening Early Language Development in Children with Cleft Palate', *Cleft Palate-Craniofacial Journal*, 32:1, 7–13.

Schindler, A., Bottero, A., Capaccio, P., Ginocchio, D., Adorni, F. and Ottaviani, F. (2008), 'Vocal Improvement after Voice Therapy in Unilateral Vocal Fold Paralysis', *Journal of Voice*.

Schroer, R. J., Phelan, M. C., Michaelis, R. C., Crawford, E. C., Skinner, S. A., Cuccaro, M., Simensen, R. J., Bishop, J., Skinner, C., Fender, D. and Stevenson, R. E. (1998), 'Autism and Maternally Derived Aberrations of Chromosome 15q', *American Journal of Medical Genetics*, 76:4, 327–36.

Schuele, C. M. and Hadley, P. A. (1999), 'Potential Advantages of Introducing Specific Language Impairment to Families', *American Journal of Speech–Language Pathology*, 8:1, 11–22.

Schuler, A. L. (2003), 'Beyond Echoplaylia: Promoting Language in Children with Autism', *Autism*, 7:4, 455–69.

Schultz, R. T. (2001), 'The Neural Basis of Autism', in N. J. Smelser and P. B. Baltes (eds), *International Encyclopedia of the Social and Behavioral Sciences*, New York: Elsevier Science, pp. 983–7.

Schultz, R. T. (2005), 'Developmental Deficits in Social Perception in Autism: The Role of the Amygdala and Fusiform Face Area', *International Journal of Developmental Neuroscience*, 23:2–3, 125–41.

Schultz, R. T., Gauthier, I., Klin, A., Fulbright, R. K., Anderson, A. W., Volkmar, F., Skudlarski, P., Lacadie, C., Cohen, D. J. and Gore, J. C. (2000), 'Abnormal Ventral Temporal Cortical Activity during Face Discrimination among Individuals with Autism and Asperger Syndrome', *Archives of General Psychiatry*, 57:4, 331–40.

Schultz, R. T., Grelotti, D. J., Klin, A., Kleinman, J., Van der Gaag, C., Marois, R. and Skudlarski, P. (2003), 'The Role of the Fusiform Face Area in Social Cognition: Implications for the Pathobiology of Autism', *Philosophical Transactions of the Royal Society London*, 358:1430, 415–27.

Schultz, R. T., Grelotti, D. J. and Pober, B. (2001), 'Genetics of Childhood Disorders: XXVI. Williams Syndrome and Brain-Behavior Relationships', *Journal of the American Academy of Child and Adolescent Psychiatry*, 40:5, 606–9.

Schultz, R. T., Romanski, L. M. and Tsatsanis, K. (2000), 'Neurofunctional Models of Autistic Disorder and Asperger Syndrome: Clues from Neuroimaging', in A. Klin,

F. R. Volkmar and S. S. Sparrow (eds), *Asperger Syndrome*, New York: Guilford, pp. 172–209.

Schweckendiek, W. (1978), 'Primary Veloplasty: Long-Term Results without Maxillary Deformity. A Twenty-Five Year Report', *Cleft Palate Journal*, 15:3, 268–74.

Schwemmle, C. and Ptok, M. (2007), 'Bamboo Nodes as the Cause of Dysphonias in Autoimmune Diseases', *HNO*, 55:7, 564–8.

Sebastian, C. S. (2002), *Mental Retardation*, USA:eMedicine.com (website: http://www.emedicine.com/med/topic3095.htm).

Seddoh, S. A. K., Robin, D. A., Sim, H. S., Hageman, C. and Moon, J. B. (1996), 'Speech Timing in Apraxia of Speech Versus Conduction Aphasia', *Journal of Speech and Hearing Research*, 39:3, 590–603.

Seifert, E. and Kollbrunner, J. (2006), 'An Update in Thinking about Nonorganic Voice Disorders', *Archives of Otolaryngology – Head and Neck Surgery*, 132:10, 1128–32.

Seinsch, W. (2001), 'Laryngectomy – A Treatment on the Way Out? Voice Restoration, Quo Vadis?', *Laryngo-Rhino-Otologie*, 80:11, 674–6.

Sell, D. A. and Grunwell, P. (2001), 'Speech Assessment and Therapy', in A. C. H. Watson, D. A. Sell and P. Grunwell (eds), *Management of Cleft Lip and Palate*, London: Whurr, pp. 227–57.

Sell, D., Harding, A. and Grunwell, P. (1994), 'GOS.SP.ASS. A Screening Assessment of Cleft Palate Speech', *European Journal of Disorders of Communication*, 29, 1–15.

Sell, D., Harding, A. and Grunwell, P. (1998), *Training Video GOS.SP.ASS (98): Speech Assessment Profile for Children with Cleft Palate and/or Velopharyngeal Dysfunction*, London: Department of Medical Illustration, Great Ormond Street NHS Trust.

Sell, D., Harding, A. and Grunwell, P. (1999), 'Revised GOS.SP.ASS (98): Speech Assessment for Children with Cleft Palate and/or Velopharyngeal Dysfunction', *International Journal of Disorders of Communication*, 34:1, 7–33.

Sellars, C., Hughes, T. and Langhorne, P. (2005), 'Speech and Language Therapy for Dysarthria due to Non-Progressive Brain Damage', *Cochrane Database of Systematic Reviews*, Issue 3, Art. No.: CD002088.DOI: 10.1002/14651858. CD002088. pub 2.

Semb, G. and Schwartz, O. (1997), 'The Impacted Tooth in Patients with Alveolar Clefts', in J. O. Andreasen, J. K. Petersen and D. M. Laskin (eds), *Textbook and Color Atlas of Tooth Impactions: Diagnosis, Treatment, Prevention*, Copenhagen: Munksgaard, pp. 331–48.

Semb, G. and Shaw, W. C. (2001), 'Orthodontics', in A. C. H. Watson, D. A. Sell and P. Grunwell (eds), *Management of Cleft Lip and Palate*, London: Whurr, pp. 299–325.

Semel, E., Wiig, E. H. and Secord, W. (1980), *Clinical Evaluation of Language Fundamentals – Revised (CELF-R)*, San Antonio: Psychological Corporation.

Semel, E., Wiig, E. H. and Secord, W. A. (2003), *Clinical Evaluation of Language Fundamentals-Fourth Edition*, Australia: Psychological Corporation.

Sengupta, D. K., Grevitt, M. P. and Mehdian, S. M. (1999), 'Hypoglossal Nerve Injury as a Complication of Anterior Surgery to the Upper Cervical Spine', *European Spine Journal*, 8:1, 78–80.

Setzen, M., Cohen, M. A., Perlman, P. W., Belafsky, P. C., Guss, J., Mattucci, K. F. and Ditkoff, M. (2003), 'The Association between Laryngopharyngeal Sensory Deficits, Pharyngeal Motor Function, and the Prevalence of Aspiration with Thin Liquids', *Otolaryngology – Head and Neck Surgery*, 128:1, 99–102.

Sewall, G. K., Jiang, J. and Ford, C. N. (2006), 'Clinical Evaluation of Parkinson's-Related Dysphonia', *Laryngoscope*, 116:10, 1740–4.

Sharkawi, A. E., Ramig, L., Logemann, J. A., Pauloski, B. R., Rademaker, A. W., Smith, C. H., Pawlas, A., Baum, S. and Werner, C. (2002), 'Swallowing and Voice Effects of Lee Silverman Voice Treatment (LSVT®): A Pilot Study', *Journal of Neurology, Neurosurgery and Psychiatry*, 72:1, 31–6.

Sharples, P. M., Storey, A., Aynsley-Green, A. and Eyre, J. A. (1990), 'Causes of Fatal Childhood Accidents Involving Head Injury in Northern Region, 1979–86', *British Medical Journal*, 301:6762, 1193–7.

Shaw, D. W., Williams, R. B., Cook, I. J., Wallace, K. L., Weltman, M. D., Collins, P. J., McKay, E., Smart, R. and Simula, M. E. (2004), 'Oropharyngeal Scintigraphy: A Reliable Technique for the Quantitative Evaluation of Oral-Pharyngeal Swallowing', *Dysphagia*, 19:1, 36–42.

Sheinkopf, S. J., Mundy, P., Oller, D. K. and Steffens, M. (2000), 'Vocal Atypicalities of Preverbal Autistic Children', *Journal of Autism and Developmental Disorders*, 30:4, 345–54.

Shewell, C. (1998), 'The Effect of Perceptual Training on Ability to Use the Vocal Profile Analysis Scheme', *International Journal of Language and Communication Disorders*, 33: Supplement, 322–6.

Shields, J., Varley, R., Broks, P. and Simpson, A. (1996), 'Hemispheric Function in Developmental Language Disorders and High-Level Autism', *Developmental Medicine and Child Neurology*, 38:6, 473–86.

Shipster, C., Hearst, D., Dockrell, J. E., Kilby, E. and Hayward, R. (2002), 'Speech and Language Skills and Cognitive Functioning in Children with Apert Syndrome: A Pilot Study', *International Journal of Language and Communication Disorders*, 37:3, 325–43.

Shott, S. R., Myer, C. M., Cotton, R. T. (1989), 'Surgical Management of Sialorrhea', *Otolaryngology – Head and Neck Surgery*, 101:1, 47–50.

Shprintzen, R. J. (2000), *Syndrome Identification for Speech–Language Pathology*, San Diego, CA: Singular.

Shprintzen, R. J., Siegel-Sadewitz, V. L., Amato, J. and Goldberg, R. B. (1985), 'Retrospective Diagnoses of Previously Missed Syndromic Disorders among 1,000 Patients with Cleft Lip, Cleft Palate, or Both', *Birth Defects: Original Article Series*, 21:2, 85–92.

Shriberg, L. D. (1994), 'Developmental Phonological Disorders: Moving Toward the 21st Century – Forwards, Backwards, or Endlessly Sideways?', *American Journal of Speech-Language Pathology*, 3:3, 26–8.

Shriberg, L. D., Aram, D. M. and Kwiatkowski, J. (1997a), 'Developmental Apraxia of Speech: I. Descriptive and Theoretical Perspectives', *Journal of Speech, Language, and Hearing Research*, 40:2, 273–85.

Shriberg, L. D., Aram, D. M. and Kwiatkowski, J. (1997b), 'Developmental Apraxia of Speech: II. Toward a Diagnostic Marker', *Journal of Speech, Language and Hearing Research*, 40:2, 286–312.

Shriberg, L. D., Aram, D. M. and Kwiatkowski, J. (1997c), 'Developmental Apraxia of Speech: III. A Subtype Marked by Inappropriate Stress', *Journal of Speech, Language, and Hearing Research*, 40:2, 313–37.

Shriberg, L. D., Campbell, T. F., Karlsson, H. B., Brown, R. L., McSweeny, J. L. and Nadler, C. J. (2003a), 'A Diagnostic Marker for Childhood Apraxia of Speech: The Lexical Stress Ratio', *Clinical Linguistics and Phonetics*, 17:7, 549–74.

Shriberg, L. D., Flipsen, P., Kwiatkowski, J. and McSweeny, J. L. (2003b), 'A Diagnostic Marker for Speech Delay Associated with Otitis Media with Effusion: The Intelligibility-Speech Gap', *Clinical Linguistics and Phonetics*, 17:7, 507–28.

Shriberg, L. D., Green, J. R., Campbell, T. F., McSweeny, J. L. and Scheer, A. R. (2003c), 'A Diagnostic Marker for Childhood Apraxia of Speech: The Coefficient of Variation Ratio', *Clinical Linguistics and Phonetics*, 17:7, 575–95.

Shriberg, L. D. and Kwiatkowski, J. (1980), *Natural Process Analysis: A Procedure for Phonological Analysis of Continuous Speech Samples*, New York: Macmillan.

Shriberg, L. D., Kwiatkowski, J. and Rasmussen, C. (1990), *The Prosody-Voice Screening Profile*, Tucson, AZ: Communication Skill Builders.

Shriberg, L. D., Lewis, B. A., Tomblin, J. B., McSweeny, J. L., Karlsson, H. B. and Scheer, A. R. (2005), 'Toward Diagnostic and Phenotype Markers for Genetically Transmitted Speech Delay', *Journal of Speech, Language, and Hearing Research*, 48:4, 834–52.

Shriberg, L. D., Paul, R., McSweeny, J. L., Klin, A., Cohen, D. J. and Volkmar, F. R. (2001), 'Speech and Prosody Characteristics of Adolescents and Adults with High-Functioning Autism and Asperger Syndrome', *Journal of Speech, Language, and Hearing Research*, 44:5, 1097–115.

Shriberg, L. D., Tomblin, J. B. and McSweeny, J. L. (1999), 'Prevalence of Speech Delay in 6-Year-Old Children and Comorbidity with Language Impairment', *Journal of Speech, Language, and Hearing Research*, 42:6, 1461–81.

Shuster, L. I. and Wambaugh, J. L. (2000), 'Perceptual and Acoustic Analyses of Speech Sound Errors in Apraxia of Speech Accompanied by Aphasia', *Aphasiology*, 14:5–6, 635–51.

Sigafoos, J., O'Reilly, M. F., Seely-York, S., Weru, J., Son, S. H., Green, V. A. and Lancioni, G. E. (2004), 'Transferring AAC Intervention to the Home', *Disability and Rehabilitation*, 26: 21–2, 1330–4.

Simms, M. D. and Schum, R. L. (2000), 'Preschool Children who Have Atypical Patterns of Development', *Pediatrics in Review*, 21:5, 147–58.

Sinha, G., Corry, P., Subesinghe, D., Wild, J. and Levene, M. I. (1997), 'Prevalence and Type of Cerebral Palsy in a British Ethnic Community: The Role of Consanguinity', *Developmental Medicine and Child Neurology*, 39:4, 259–62.

Sitnikova, T., Salisbury, D. F., Kuperberg, G. and Holcomb, P. J. (2002), 'Electrophysiological Insights into Language Processing in Schizophrenia', *Psychophysiology*, 39:6, 851–60.

Skinder-Meredith, A. E. (2001), 'Differential Diagnosis: Developmental Apraxia of Speech and Phonologic Delay', *Augmentative Communication News*, 14:2&3, 5–8.

Skuse, D. H. (2000), 'Imprinting, the X-Chromosome, and the Male Brain: Explaining Sex Differences in the Liability to Autism', *Pediatric Research*, 47:1, 9–16.

SLI Consortium (2002), 'A Genomewide Scan Identifies Two Novel Loci Involved in Specific Language Impairment', *American Journal of Human Genetics*, 70:2, 384–98.

Sliwinska-Kowalska, M., Niebudek-Bogusz, E., Fiszer, M., Los-Spychalska, T., Kotylo, P., Sznurowska-Przygocka, B. and Modrzewska, M. (2006), 'The Prevalence and Risk Factors for Occupational Voice Disorders in Teachers', *Folia Phoniatrica et Logopaedica*, 58:2, 85–101.

Smith, M. (1991), 'Assessment of Interaction Patterns and AAC Use: A Case Study', *Journal of Clinical Speech and Language Studies*, 1:1, 76–102.

Smith, M. C. and Hoeppner, T. J. (2003), 'Epileptic Encephalopathy of Late Childhood: Landau–Kleffner Syndrome and the Syndrome of Continuous Spikes and Waves During Slow-Wave Sleep', *Journal of Clinical Neurophysiology*, 20:6, 462–72.

Smith, R., Malee, K., Charurat, M., Magder, L., Mellins, C., Macmillan, C., Hittleman, J., Lasky, T., Llorente, A. and Moye, J. (2000), 'Timing of Perinatal Human Immunodeficiency Virus Type 1 Infection and Rate of Neurodevelopment', *Pediatric Infectious Disease Journal*, 19:9, 862–71.

Smith Hammond, C. A. and Goldstein, L. B. (2006), 'Cough and Aspiration of Food and Liquids Due to Oral-Pharyngeal Dysphagia: ACCP Evidence-Based Clinical Practice Guidelines', *Chest*, 129:1, 154S–168S.

Sohner, L. and Mitchell, P. (1991), 'Phonatory and Phonetic Characteristics of Prelinguistic Vocal Development in Cri du Chat Syndrome', *Journal of Communication Disorders*, 24:1, 13–20.

Solot, C. B., Knightly, C., Handler, S. D., Gerdes, M., McDonald-McGinn, D. M., Moss, E., Wang, P., Cohen, M., Randall, P., Larossa, D. and Driscoll, D. A. (2000), 'Communication Disorders in the 22q11.2 Microdeletion Syndrome', *Journal of Communication Disorders*, 33:3, 187–204.

Speyer, R., Speyer, I. and Heijnen, M. A. (2008), 'Prevalence and Relative Risk of Dysphonia in Rheumatoid Arthritis', *Journal of Voice*.

Spiegler, D., Malin, H., Kaelber, C. and Warren, K. (1984), 'Perspectives in Disease Prevention and Health Promotion Fetal Alcohol Syndrome: Public Awareness Week', *Morbidity and Morality Weekly Report*, 33:1, 1–2.

Spinelli, M., Rocha, A. C., Giacheti, C. M. and Richieri-Costa, A. (1995), 'Word-Finding Difficulties, Verbal Paraphasias, and Verbal Dyspraxia in Ten Individuals with Fragile X Syndrome', *American Journal of Medical Genetics*, 60:1, 39–43.

Springer, J. A., Binder, J. R., Hammeke, T. A., Swanson, S. J., Frost, J. A., Bellgowan, P. S. F., Brewer, C. C., Perry, H. M., Morris, G. L. and Mueller, W. M. (1999), 'Language Dominance in Neurologically Normal and Epilepsy Subjects', *Brain*, 122:11, 2033–46.

Square, P. A. (1994), 'Treatment Approaches for Developmental Apraxia of Speech', *Clinics in Communication Disorders*, 4:3, 151–61.

Square, P. A., Goshulak, D., Bose, A. and Hayden, D. (2000), 'The Effects of Articulatory Subsystem Treatment for Developmental Neuromotor Speech Disorders', *Paper presented at the 10th Biennial Conference on Motor Speech Disorders and Speech Motor Control*, San Antonio, TX.

St Louis, K. O. (1996), 'A Tabular Summary of Cluttering Subjects in the Special Edition', *Journal of Fluency Disorders*, 21:3–4, 337–43.

St Louis, K. O. and Hinzman, A. R. (1986), 'Studies of Cluttering: Perceptions of Cluttering by Speech–Language Pathologists and Educators', *Journal of Fluency Disorders*, 11:2, 131–49.

St Louis, K. O. and Myers, F. L. (1995), 'Clinical Management of Cluttering', *Language, Speech, and Hearing Services in Schools*, 26:2, 187–95.

St Louis, K. O., Myers, F. L., Cassidy, L. J., Michael, A. J., Penrod, S. M., Litton, B. A., Coutras, S. W., Olivera, J. L. R. and Brodsky, E. (1996), 'Efficacy of Delayed Auditory Feedback for Treating Cluttering: Two Case Studies', *Journal of Fluency Disorders*, 21:3–4, 305–14.

St Louis, K. O., Myers, F. L., Faragasso, K., Townsend, P. S. and Gallaher, A. J. (2004), 'Perceptual Aspects of Cluttered Speech', *Journal of Fluency Disorders*, 29:3, 213–35.

Stager, S. V., Calis, K., Grothe, D., Bloch, M., Berensen, N. M., Smith, P. J. and Braun, A. (2005), 'Treatment with Medications Affecting Dopaminergic and Serotonergic Mechanisms: Effects on Fluency and Anxiety in Persons Who Stutter', *Journal of Fluency Disorders*, 30:4, 319–35.

Stansfield, J. (1990), 'Prevalence of Stuttering and Cluttering in Adults with Mental Handicaps', *Journal of Mental Deficiency Research*, 34:4, 287–307.

Stengelhofen, J. (1993), 'The Nature and Causes of Communication Problems in Cleft Palate', in J. Stengelhofen (ed.), *Cleft Palate: The Nature and Remediation of Communication Problems*, London: Whurr, pp. 1–30.

Stengelhofen, J. (1999), *Working with Cleft Palate*, Oxon: Winslow.

Stevens, T. and Karmiloff-Smith, A. (1997), 'Word Learning in a Special Population: Do Individuals with Williams Syndrome Obey Lexical Constraints?', *Journal of Child Language*, 24:3, 737–65.

Stewart, T. and Birdsall, M. (2001), 'A Review of the Contribution of Personal Construct Psychology to Stammering Therapy', *Journal of Constructivist Psychology*, 14:3, 215–25.

Stoel-Gammon, C. (2001), 'Down Syndrome Phonology: Developmental Patterns and Intervention Strategies', *Down Syndrome Research and Practice*, 7:3, 93–100.

Stoel-Gammon, C. and Dunn, C. (1985), *Normal and Disordered Phonology in Children*, Baltimore: University Park Press.

Stoel-Gammon, C., Stone-Goldman, J. and Glaspey, A. (2002), 'Pattern-Based Approaches to Phonological Therapy', *Seminars in Speech and Language*, 23:1, 3–13.

Stone, W. L., Ousley, O. Y., Yoder, P. J., Hogan, K. L. and Hepburn, S. L. (1997), 'Nonverbal Communication in Two- and Three-Year-Old Children with Autism', *Journal of Autism and Developmental Disorders*, 27:6, 677–96.

Storkel, H. L. (2004), 'The Emerging Lexicon of Children with Phonological Delays: Phonotactic Constraints and Probability in Acquisition', *Journal of Speech, Language, and Hearing Research*, 47:5, 1194–212.

Strand, E. A. (1995), 'Treatment of Motor Speech Disorders in Children', *Seminars in Speech and Language*, 16:2, 126–39.

Strand, E. A. and McNeil, M. R. (1996), 'Effects of Length and Linguistic Complexity on Temporal Acoustic Measures in Apraxia of Speech', *Journal of Speech and Hearing Research*, 39:5, 1018–33.

Strand, E. A. and Skinder, A. (1999), 'Treatment of Developmental Apraxia of Speech: Integral Stimulation Methods', in A. J. Caruso and E. A. Strand (eds), *Clinical Management of Motor Speech Disorders in Children*, New York: Thieme Medical, pp. 109–48.

Stratton, K., Gable, A., Shetty, P. and McCormick, M. (2001), *Immunization Safety Review: Measles-Mumps-Rubella Vaccine and Autism*, Washington, DC: National Academy Press.

Strauss, M. and Klich, R. J. (2001), 'Word Length Effects on EMG/Vowel Duration Relationships in Apraxic Speakers', *Folia Phoniatrica et Logopaedica*, 53:1, 58–65.

Strong, C. (1998), *The Strong Narrative Assessment Procedure*, Eau Claire, WI: Thinking Publications.

Stroud, A. E., Lawrie, B. W. and Wiles, C. M. (2002), 'Inter- and Intra-Rater Reliability of Cervical Auscultation to Detect Aspiration in Patients with Dysphagia', *Clinical Rehabilitation*, 16:6, 640–5.

Stuart, A., Kalinowski, J., Rastatter, M. P., Saltuklaroglu, T. and Dayalu, V. (2004), 'Investigations of the Impact of Altered Auditory Feedback In-The-Ear Devices on the Speech of People Who Stutter: Initial Fitting and 4-Month Follow-Up', *International Journal of Language and Communication Disorders*, 39:1, 93–113.

Stuart, A., Kalinowski, J., Saltuklaroglu, T. and Guntupalli, V. K. (2006), 'Investigations of the Impact of Altered Auditory Feedback In-The-Ear Devices on the Speech of People Who Stutter: One-Year Follow-Up', *Disability and Rehabilitation*, 28:12, 757–65.

Stuart, J. M. (1996), 'The Meningitis Scare in Perspective', *Practitioner*, 240:1564, 421–3.

Subramaniam, S., Abdullah, A. H. and Hairuzah, I. (2005), 'Histoplasmosis of the Larynx', *Medical Journal of Malaysia*, 60:3, 386–8.

Sugishita, M., Konno, K., Kabe, S., Yunoki, K., Togashi, O. and Kawamura, M. (1987), 'Electropalatographic Analysis of Apraxia of Speech in a Left Hander and in a Right Hander', *Brain*, 110:5, 1393–417.

Sulica, L. (2005), 'Laryngeal Thrush', *Annals of Otology, Rhinology and Laryngology*, 114:5, 369–75.

Sullivan, P. B., Lambert, B., Rose, M., Ford-Adams, M., Johnson, A. and Griffiths, P. (2000), 'Prevalence and Severity of Feeding and Nutritional Problems in Children with Neurological Impairment: Oxford Feeding Study', *Developmental Medicine and Child Neurology*, 42:10, 674–80.

Sumiyoshi, C., Matsui, M., Sumiyoshi, T., Yamashita, I., Sumiyoshi, S. and Kurachi, M. (2001) 'Semantic Structure in Schizophrenia as Assessed by the Category Fluency Test: Effect of Verbal Intelligence and Age of Onset', *Psychiatry Research*, 105:3, 187–99.

Surveillance of Cerebral Palsy in Europe (2002), 'Prevalence and Characteristics of Children with Cerebral Palsy in Europe', *Developmental Medicine and Child Neurology*, 44:9, 633–40.

Susca, M. (2002), 'Diagnosing Stuttering in the School Environment', *Seminars in Speech and Language*, 23:3, 165–72.

Susca, M. (2006), 'Connecting Stuttering Measurement and Management: II. Measures of Cognition and Affect', *International Journal of Language and Communication Disorders*, 41:4, 365–77.

Sweeney, T., Sell, D. and Grunwell, P. (1999a), 'The Relationship between Perceptual Ratings of Nasality, the Nature of the Speech Sample and Nasometry', Paper presented at the European Craniofacial Meeting, Manchester.

Sweeney, T., Sell, D. and Grunwell, P. (1999b), 'The Relationship between Nasal Airflow Errors and Pressure/Flow Measurements', Paper presented at the European Craniofacial Meeting, Manchester.

Swinburn, K., Porter, G. and Howard, D. (2005), *The Comprehensive Aphasia Test*, Hove: Psychology Press.

Swisher, L., Restrepo, M. A., Plante, E. and Lowell, S. (1995), 'Effect of Implicit and Explicit "Rule" Presentation on Bound-Morpheme Generalization in Specific Language Impairment', *Journal of Speech and Hearing Research*, 38:1, 168–73.

Szatmari, P., Jones, M. B., Zwaigenbaum, L. and MacLean, J. E. (1998), 'Genetics of Autism: Overview and New Directions', *Journal of Autism and Developmental Disorders*, 28:5, 351–68.

Takemura, N., Nakahira, A., Ogawa, M., Uesaka, T., Baba, T., Miura, F. and Nishio, S. (2002), 'Frontal Lobe Hematoma Associated with Transcortical Motor Aphasia: Case Report', *No To Shinkei*, 54:9, 823–6.

Takeoka, M., Riviello, J. J., Duffy, F. H., Kim, F., Kennedy, D. N., Makris, N., Caviness, V. S. and Holmes, G. L. (2004), 'Bilateral Volume Reduction of the Superior Temporal Areas in Landau-Kleffner Syndrome', *Neurology*, 63:7, 1152–3.

Tallal, P., Hirsch, L. S., Realpe-Bonilla, T., Miller, S., Brzustowicz, L. M., Bartlett, C. and Flax, J. F. (2001), 'Familial Aggregation in Specific Language Impairment', *Journal of Speech, Language, and Hearing Research*, 44:5, 1172–82.

Tavares, E. L. M. and Martins, R. H. G. (2007), 'Vocal Evaluation in Teachers with or without Symptoms', *Journal of Voice*, 21:4, 407–14.

Taylor, D. L., Edwards, A. D. and Mehmet, H. (1999), 'Oxidative Metabolism, Apoptosis and Perinatal Brain Injury', *Brain Pathology*, 9:1, 93–117.

Tekin, M. and Bodurtha, J. (2002), *Cornelia De Lange Syndrome*, USA: eMedicine.com (website: http://www.emedicine.com/PED/topic482.htm).

Temple, C. (1997), *Developmental Cognitive Neuropsychology*, Hove: Psychology Press.

Tényi, T., Herold, R., Szili, I. M. and Trixler, M. (2002), 'Schizophrenics Show a Failure in the Decoding of Violations of Conversational Implicatures', *Psychopathology*, 35:1, 25–7.

Thacker, R. C. and De Nil, L. F. (1996), 'Neurogenic Cluttering', *Journal of Fluency Disorders*, 21:3–4, 227–38.

Theodoros, D. G., Murdoch, B. E. and Stokes, P. (1995), 'A Physiological Analysis of Articulatory Dysfunction in Dysarthric Speakers Following Severe Closed-Head Injury', *Brain Injury*, 9:3, 237–54.

Theodoros, D. G., Shrapnel, N. and Murdoch, B. E. (1998), 'Motor Speech Impairment Following Traumatic Brain Injury in Childhood: A Physiological and Perceptual Analysis of One Case', *Pediatric Rehabilitation*, 2:3, 107–22.

Thomas, M. and Karmiloff-Smith, A. (2005), 'Can Developmental Disorders Reveal the Component Parts of the Human Language Faculty?', *Language Learning and Development*, 1:1, 65–92.

Thomas, M. S. C., Grant, J., Barham, Z., Gsödl, M., Laing, E., Lakusta, L., Tyler, L. K., Grice, S., Paterson, S. and Karmiloff-Smith, A. (2001), 'Past Tense Formation in Williams Syndrome', *Language and Cognitive Processes*, 16:2, 143–76.

Thomas, P. (1997), 'What Can Linguistics Tell Us About Thought Disorder?', in J. France and N. Muir (eds), *Communication and the Mentally Ill Patient: Developmental and Linguistic Approaches to Schizophrenia*, London: Jessica Kingsley, pp. 30–42.

Thompson, C. K., Lange, K. L., Schneider, S. L. and Shapiro, L. P. (1997), 'Agrammatic and Non-Brain-Damaged Subjects' Verb and Verb Argument Structure Production', *Aphasiology*, 11:4–5, 473–90.

Thompson, C. K., Shapiro, L. P., Ballard, K. J., Jacobs, B. J., Schneider, S. S. and Tait, M. E. (1997), 'Training and Generalized Production of wh- and NP-Movement Structures in Agrammatic Aphasia', *Journal of Speech, Language, and Hearing Research*, 40:2, 228–44.

Thompson, C. K., Shapiro, L. P., Kiran, S. and Sobecks, J. (2003), 'The Role of Syntactic Complexity in Treatment of Sentence Deficits in Agrammatic Aphasia', *Journal of Speech, Language, and Hearing Research*, 46:3, 591–607.

Thoonen, G., Maassen, B., Gabreels, F. and Schreuder, R. (1994), 'Feature Analysis of Singleton Consonant Errors in Developmental Verbal Dyspraxia (DVD)', *Journal of Speech and Hearing Research*, 37:6, 1424–40.

Thoonen, G., Maassen, B., Gabreels, F., Schreuder, R. and de Swart, B. (1997), 'Towards a Standardised Assessment Procedure for Developmental Apraxia of Speech', *European Journal of Disorders of Communication*, 32:1, 37–60.

Tilton, A. H., Miller, M. D. and Khoshoo, V. (1998), 'Nutrition and Swallowing in Pediatric Neuromuscular Patients', *Seminars in Pediatric Neurology*, 5:2, 106–15.

Timmermans, B., De Bodt, M., Wuyts, F. and Van de Heyning, P. (2003), 'Vocal Hygiene in Radio Students and in Radio Professionals', *Logopedics Phoniatrics Vocology*, 28:3, 127–32.

Tjaden, K., Rivera, D., Wilding, G. and Turner, G. S. (2005), 'Characteristics of the Lax Vowel Space in Dysarthria', *Journal of Speech, Language and Hearing Research*, 48:3, 554–66.

Tohara, H., Saitoh, E., Mays, K. A., Kuhlemeier, K. and Palmer, J. B. (2003), 'Three Tests for Predicting Aspiration without Videofluorography', *Dysphagia*, 18:2, 126–34.

Tomblin, J. B., Records, N. L., Buckwalter, P., Zhang, X., Smith, E. and O'Brien, M. (1997), 'Prevalence of Specific Language Impairment in Kindergarten Children', *Journal of Speech, Language, and Hearing Research*, 40:6, 1245–60.

Tomik, B., Krupinski, J., Glodzik-Sobanska, L., Bala-Slodowska, M., Wszolek, W., Kusiak, M. and Lechwacka, A. (1999), 'Acoustic Analysis of Dysarthria Profile in ALS Patients', *Journal of the Neurological Sciences*, 169:1–2, 35–42.

Tomoda, C., Hirokawa, Y., Uruno, T., Takamura, Y., Ito, Y., Miya, A., Kobayashi, K., Matsuzuka, F., Kuma, K. and Miyauchi, A. (2006), 'Sensitivity and Specificity of Intraoperative Recurrent Laryngeal Nerve Stimulation Test for Predicting Vocal Cord Palsy after Thyroid Surgery', *World Journal of Surgery*, 30:7, 1230–3.

Trail, M., Fox, C., Ramig, L. O., Sapir, S., Howard, J. and Lai, E. C. (2005), 'Speech Treatment for Parkinson's Disease', *NeuroRehabilitation*, 20:3, 205–21.

Trier, E. and Thomas, A. G. (1998), 'Feeding the Disabled Child', *Nutrition*, 14:10, 801–5.

Trost-Cardamone, J. E. (1990), 'Speech in the First Year of Life: A Perspective on Early Acquisition', in D. A. Kernahan and S. W. Rosenstein (eds), *Cleft Lip and Palate: A System of Management*, Baltimore, MD: Williams & Wilkins, pp. 204–13.

Tsao, J. W., Shad, J. A. and Faillace, W. J. (2004), 'Tremor, Aphasia, and Stuttering Associated with Helicobacter Pylori Infection', *American Journal of Medicine*, 116:3, 211–12.

Tsunoda, K., Kondou, K., Kaga, K., Niimi, S., Baer, T., Nishiyama, K. and Hirose, H. (2005), 'Autologous Transplantation of Fascia into the Vocal Fold: Long-Term Result of Type-1 Transplantation and the Future', *Laryngoscope*, 115:12, 1–10.

Tuchman, R. F. (1997), 'Acquired Epileptiform Aphasia', *Seminars in Pediatric Neurology*, 4:2, 93–101.

Turkington, C. and Sussman, A. E. (2004), *The Encyclopedia of Deafness and Hearing Disorders*, New York: Facts on File.

Tutuncuoglu, S., Serdaroglu, G. and Kadioglu, B. (2002), 'Landau-Kleffner Syndrome Beginning with Stuttering: Case Report', *Journal of Child Neurology*, 17:10, 785–8.

Tyler, A. A. and Tolbert, L. C. (2002), 'Speech-Language Assessment in the Clinical Setting', *American Journal of Speech-Language Pathology*, 11:3, 215–20.

Tyler, L. K., Karmiloff-Smith, A., Voice, J. K., Stevens, T., Grant, J., Udwin, O., Davies, M. and Howlin, P. (1997), 'Do Individuals with Williams Syndrome Have Bizarre Semantics? Evidence for Lexical Organization Using an On-Line Task', *Cortex*, 33:3, 515–27.

Ulatowska, H. K., Olness, G. S., Wertz, R. T., Samson, A. M., Keebler, M. W. and Goins, K. E. (2003), 'Relationship Between Discourse and Western Aphasia Battery Performance in African Americans with Aphasia', *Aphasiology*, 17:5, 511–21.

United Cerebral Palsy Research and Educational Foundation (2002), *Diagnosis of Cerebral Palsy: A Research Status Report*, Washington, DC: United Cerebral Palsy.

United Cerebral Palsy Research and Educational Foundation (2003), *Treatment of Cerebral Palsy: A Research Status Report*, Washington, DC: United Cerebral Palsy.

Urban, P. P., Rolke, R., Wicht, S., Keilmann, A., Stoeter, P., Hopf, H. C., Dieterich, M. (2006), 'Left-Hemispheric Dominance for Articulation: A Prospective Study on Acute Ischaemic Dysarthria at Different Localizations', *Brain*, 129:3, 767–77.

Uzgiris, I. and Hunt, J. (1975), *Assessment in Infancy: Ordinal Scales of Psychological Development*, Urbana: University of Illinois Press.

Van Borsel, J., De Grande, S., Van Buggenhout, G. and Fryns, J. P. (2004), 'Speech and Language in Wolf-Hirschhorn Syndrome: A Case-Study', *Journal of Communication Disorders*, 37:1, 21–33.

Van Borsel, J., Dhooge, I., Verhoye, K., Derde, K. and Curfs, L. (1999), 'Communication Problems in Turner Syndrome: A Sample Survey', *Journal of Communication Disorders*, 32:6, 435–46.

Van Borsel, J., Geirnaert, E. and Van Coster, R. (2005), 'Another Case of Word-Final Disfluencies', *Folia Phoniatrica et Logopaedica*, 57:3, 148–62.

Van Borsel, J., Moeyaert, J., Mostaert, C., Rosseel, R., Van Loo, E. and Van Renterghem, T. (2006), 'Prevalence of Stuttering in Regular and Special School Populations in Belgium Based on Teacher Perceptions', *Folia Phoniatrica et Logopaedica*, 58:4, 289–302.

Van Borsel, J., van der Made, S. and Santens, P. (2003), 'Thalamic Stuttering: A Distinct Clinical Entity?', *Brain and Language*, 85:2, 185–9.

Van Borsel, J. and Vanryckeghem, M. (2000), 'Dysfluency and Phonic Tics in Tourette Syndrome: A Case Report', *Journal of Communication Disorders*, 33:3, 227–39.

Van Cauwenberge, P. B., De Moor, S. E. G. and Dhooge, I. (1998), 'Acute Suppurative Otitis Media', in H. Ludman and T. Wright (eds), *Diseases of the Ear*, London: Arnold, pp. 353–60.

Van Dam-Baggen, R. and Kraaimaat, F. W. (1999), 'Assessing Social Anxiety: The Inventory of Interpersonal Situations (IIS)', *European Journal of Psychological Assessment*, 15:1, 25–38.

Van De Beek, D., De Gans, J., Spanjaard, L., Weisfelt, M., Reitsma, J. B. and Vermeulen, M. (2004), 'Clinical Features and Prognostic Factors in Adults with Bacterial Meningitis', *New England Journal of Medicine*, 351:18, 1849–59.

Van Demark, D. R. and Hardin, M. A. (1990), 'Speech Therapy for the Child with Cleft Lip and Palate', in J. Bardach and H. L. Morris (eds), *Multi-disciplinary Management of Cleft Lip and Palate*, Philadelphia, PA: W.B. Saunders, pp. 799–806.

Van Gogh, C. D., Verdonck-de Leeuw, I. M., Boon-Kamma, B. A., Langendijk, J. A., Kuik, D. J. and Mahieu, H. F. (2005), 'A Screening Questionnaire for Voice Problems after Treatment of Early Glottic Cancer', *International Journal of Radiation Oncology, Biology, Physics*, 62:3, 700–5.

Van Riper, C. (1973), *The Treatment of Stuttering*, Englewood Cliffs, NJ: Prentice-Hall.

Vandervelden, M. and Siegel, L. (1999), 'Phonological Processing and Literacy in AAC Users and Students with Motor Speech Impairments', *Augmentative and Alternative Communication*, 15:3, 191–211.

Vanryckeghem, M., Brutten, G. J. and Hernandez, L. M. (2005), 'A Comparative Investigation of the Speech-Associated Attitude of Preschool and Kindergarten Children Who Do and Do Not Stutter', *Journal of Fluency Disorders*, 30:4, 307–18.

Vanryckeghem, M., Brutten, G. J., Uddin, N. and Van Borsel, J. (2004), 'A Comparative Investigation of the Speech-Associated Coping Responses Reported by Adults Who Do and Do Not Stutter', *Journal of Fluency Disorders*, 29:3, 237–50.

Vaughn, T. L. and Brown, K. R. (2003), *Drooling*, USA: eMedicine.com (website: http://www.emedicine.com/ent/topic629.htm).

Velleman, S. L. and Strand, K. (1994), 'Developmental Verbal Dyspraxia', in J. E. Bernthal and N. W. Bankson (eds), *Child Phonology: Characteristics, Assessment, and Intervention with Special Populations*, New York: Thieme Medical, pp. 110–39.

Viswanath, N. S., Rosenfield, D. B., Alexander, J. P., Lee, H. S. and Chakraborty, R. (2000), 'Genetic Basis of Developmental Stuttering – Preliminary Observations', in H.-G. Bosshardt, J. S. Yaruss and H. F. M. Peters (eds), *Fluency Disorders: Theory, Research, Treatment and Self-Help. Proceedings of the Third World Congress on Fluency Disorders*, Nijmegen: Nijmegen University Press, pp. 102–8.

Vogindroukas, I., Papageorgiou, V. and Vostanis, P. (2003), 'Pattern of Semantic Errors in Autism: A Brief Research Report', *Autism*, 7:2, 195–203.

Volden, J. (2004), 'Conversational Repair in Speakers with Autism Spectrum Disorder', *International Journal of Language and Communication Disorders*, 39:2, 171–89.

Volkmar, F. R., Klin, A., Siegel, B., Szatmari, P., Lord, C., Campbell, M., Freeman, B. J., Cicchetti, D. V., Rutter, M., Kline, W., Buitelaar, J., Hattab, Y., Fombonne, E., Fuentes, J., Werry, J., Stone, W., Kerbershian, J., Hoshino, Y., Bregman, J.,

Loveland, K., Szymanski, L. and Towbin, K. (1994), 'Field Trial for Autistic Disorder in DSM-IV', *American Journal of Psychiatry*, 151:9, 1361–7.

Volkmar, F. R., Lord, C., Bailey, A., Schultz, R. T. and Klin, A. (2004), 'Autism and Pervasive Developmental Disorders', *Journal of Child Psychology and Psychiatry*, 45:1, 135–70.

Volterra, V., Capirci, O. and Caselli, C. (2001), 'What Atypical Populations Can Reveal about Language Development: The Contrast between Deafness and Williams Syndrome', *Language and Cognitive Processes*, 16:2–3, 219–39.

Volterra, V., Capirci, O., Pezzini, G., Sabbadini, L. and Vicari, S. (1996), 'Linguistic Abilities in Italian Children with Williams Syndrome', *Cortex*, 32:4, 663–77.

von Tetzchner, S. and Martinsen, H. (1996), 'Words and Strategies: Communicating with Young Children who Use Aided Language', in S. von Tetzchner and M. H. Jensen (eds), *Augmentative and Alternative Communication: European Perspectives*, London: Whurr, pp. 65–88.

von Tetzchner, S. and Martinsen, H. (2000), *Introduction to Augmentative and Alternative Communication*, London: Whurr.

Von Tetzchner, S., Øvreeide, K. D., Jørgensen, K. K., Ormhaug, B. M., Oxholm, B. and Warme, R. (2004), 'Acquisition of Graphic Communication by a Young Girl without Comprehension of Spoken Language', *Disability and Rehabilitation*, 26:21–2, 1335–46.

Wacker, A., Holder, M., Will, B. E., Winkler, P. A. and Ilmberger, J. (2002), 'Comparison of the Aachen Aphasia Test, Clinical Study and Aachen Aphasia Bedside Test in Brain Tumor Patients', *Der Nervenarzt*, 73:8, 765–9.

Wada, Y., Yanagihara, C., Nishimura, Y. and Susuki, K. (2006), 'A Case of Acute Oropharyngeal Palsy with Nasal Voice as Main Symptom', *No To Shinkei*, 58:3, 235–8.

Wakefield, A. J., Murch, S. H., Anthony, A., Linell, J., Casson, D. M., Malik, M. et al. (1998), 'Ileal-Lymphoid-Nodular Hyperplasia, Non-Specific Colitis, and Pervasive Developmental Disorder in Children', *Lancet*, 351:9103, 637–41.

Walder, D. J., Seidman, L. J., Cullen, N., Su, J., Tsuang, M. T. and Goldstein, J. M. (2006), 'Sex Differences in Language Dysfunction in Schizophrenia', *American Journal of Psychiatry*, 163:3, 470–7.

Walker, M. (1978), 'The Makaton Vocabulary', in T. Tebbs (ed.), *Ways and Means*, Basingstoke: Globe Education, pp. 172–83.

Waller, A., Dennis, F., Brodie, J. and Cairns, A. Y. (1998), 'Evaluating the Use of TalksBac, A Predictive Communication Device for Nonfluent Adults with Aphasia', *International Journal of Language and Communication Disorders*, 33:1, 45–70.

Wambaugh, J. L. (2002), 'A Summary of Treatments for Apraxia of Speech and Review of Replicated Approaches', *Seminars in Speech and Language*, 23:4, 293–308.

Wambaugh, J. L. and Doyle, P. J. (1994), 'Treatment for Acquired Apraxia of Speech: A Review of Efficacy Reports', *Clinical Aphasiology*, 22, 231–43.

Wambaugh, J. L., Kalinyak-Fliszar, M. M., West, J. E. and Doyle, P. J. (1998), 'Effects of Treatment for Sound Errors in Apraxia of Speech and Aphasia', *Journal of Speech, Language, and Hearing Research*, 41:4, 725–43.

Wambaugh, J. L. and Martinez, A. L. (2000), 'Effects of Rate and Rhythm Control Treatment on Consonant Production Accuracy in Apraxia of Speech', *Aphasiology*, 14:8, 851–71.

Wang, Y. T., Kent, R. D., Duffy, J. R. and Thomas, J. E. (2005), 'Dysarthria Associated with Traumatic Brain Injury: Speaking Rate and Emphatic Stress', *Journal of Communication Disorders*, 38:3, 231–60.

Warburton, P., Baird, G., Chen, W., Morris, K., Jacobs, B. W., Hodgson, S. and Docherty, Z. (2000), 'Support for Linkage of Autism and Specific Language Impairment to 7q3 from Two Chromosome Rearrangements Involving Band 7q31', *American Journal of Medical Genetics*, 96:2, 228–34.

Ward, D. (1992), 'Outlining Semi-Intensive Fluency Therapy', *Journal of Fluency Disorders*, 17:4, 243–55.

Ward, D. (2006), *Stuttering and Cluttering: Frameworks for Understanding and Treatment*, Hove: Psychology Press.

Warrington, E. K. and James, M. (1991), *The Visual Object and Space Perception Battery*, Bury St Edmunds: Thames Valley Test Company.

Watkin, P. (2001), 'The Causes of Childhood Deafness and its Identification and Confirmation', in J. Graham and M. Martin (eds), *Ballantyne's Deafness*, London: Whurr, pp. 181–206.

Watson, A. C. H. (2001), 'Embryology, Aetiology and Incidence', in A. C. H. Watson, D. A. Sell and P. Grunwell (eds), *Management of Cleft Lip and Palate*, London: Whurr, pp. 3–15.

Watson, D. and Friend, R. (1969), 'Measurement of Social–Evaluative Anxiety', *Journal of Consulting and Clinical Psychology*, 33:4, 448–57.

Watts, C. R., Clark, R. and Early, S. (2001), 'Acoustic Measures of Phonatory Improvement Secondary to Treatment by Oral Corticosteroids in a Professional Singer: A Case Report', *Journal of Voice*, 15:1, 115–21.

Wechsler, D. (1991), *Wechsler Intelligence Scale for Children – Third Edition*, San Antonio, TX: Psychological Corporation.

Wechsler, D. (1992), *Wechsler Individual Achievement Test*, San Antonio, TX: Psychological Corporation.

Weiner, F. F. (1979), *Phonological Process Analysis*, Baltimore: University Park Press.

Weismer, S. E., Evans, J. and Hesketh, L. J. (1999), 'An Examination of Verbal Working Memory Capacity in Children with Specific Language Impairment', *Journal of Speech, Language, and Hearing Research*, 42:5, 1249–60.

Weismer, S. E. and Hesketh, L. J. (1996), 'Lexical Learning by Children with Specific Language Impairment: Effects of Linguistic Input Presented at Varying Speaking Rates', *Journal of Speech and Hearing Research*, 39:1, 177–90.

Werner, E. and Dawson, G. (2005), 'Validation of the Phenomenon of Autistic Regression Using Home Videotapes', *Archives of General Psychiatry*, 62:8, 889–95.

Wertz, R. T., LaPointe, L. L. and Rosenbek, J. C. (1984), *Apraxia of Speech in Adults: The Disorder and Its Management*, Orlando, FL: Grune & Stratton.

West, C., Hesketh, A., Vail, A. and Bowen, A. (2005), 'Interventions for Apraxia of Speech Following Stroke', *Cochrane Database of Systematic Reviews*, Issue 4, Art. No.: CD004298. DOI:10.1002/14651858. CD004298.pub2.

Whitehill, T. L., Ma, J. K-Y. and Lee, A. S-Y. (2003), 'Perceptual Characteristics of Cantonese Hypokinetic Dysarthria', *Clinical Linguistics and Phonetics*, 17:4–5, 265–71.

Whitworth, A., Perkins, L. and Lesser, R. (1997), *Conversation Analysis Profile for People with Aphasia* (CAPPA), London: Whurr.

Wichterle, H., Alvarez-Dolado, M., Erskine, L. and Alvarez-Buylla, A. (2003), 'Permissive Corridor and Diffusible Gradients Direct Medial Ganglionic Eminence Cell Migration to the Neocortex', *Proceedings of the National Academy of Sciences of the United States of America*, 100:2, 727–32.

Wiig, E. H., Secord, W. and Semel, E. (1992), *Clinical Evaluation of Language Fundamentals – Preschool*, San Antonio, TX: Psychological Corporation, Harcourt Brace.

Williams, A. L. (2000a), 'Multiple Oppositions: Theoretical Foundations for an Alternative Contrastive Intervention Approach', *American Journal of Speech–Language Pathology*, 9:4, 282–8.

Williams, A. L. (2000b), 'Multiple Oppositions: Case Studies of Variables in Phonological Intervention', *American Journal of Speech–Language Pathology*, 9:4, 289–99.

Williams, D. F. and Dugan, P. M. (2002), 'Administering Stuttering Modification Therapy in School Settings', *Seminars in Speech and Language*, 23:3, 187–94.

Williams, D. F. and Wener, D. L. (1996), 'Cluttering and Stuttering Exhibited in a Young Professional', *Journal of Fluency Disorders*, 21:3–4, 261–9.

Williams, E., Reddy, V. and Costall, A. (2001), 'Taking a Closer Look at Functional Play in Children with Autism', *Journal of Autism and Developmental Disorders*, 31:1, 67–77.

Williams, K., Glasson, E. J., Wray, J., Tuck, M., Helmer, M., Bower, C. I. and Mellis, C. M. (2005), 'Incidence of Autism Spectrum Disorders in Children in Two Australian States', *Medical Journal of Australia*, 182:3, 108–11.

Williams, N. and Carding, P. (2005), *Occupational Voice Loss*, Boca Raton, FL: Taylor & Francis.

Willinger, U., Volkl-Kernstock, S. and Aschauer, H. N. (2005), 'Marked Depression and Anxiety in Patients with Functional Dysphonia', *Psychiatry Research*, 134:1, 85–91.

Wilson, D. K. (1987), *Voice Problems of Children*, Baltimore, MA: Williams & Wilkins.

Wilson, G. N. and Oliver, W. J. (1988), 'Further Delineation of the G Syndrome: A Manageable Genetic Cause of Infantile Dysphagia', *Journal of Medical Genetics*, 25:3, 157–63.

Wing, L. (1981a), 'Sex Ratios in Early Childhood Autism and Related Conditions', *Psychiatry Research*, 5:2, 129.

Wing, L. (1981b), 'Asperger Syndrome: A Clinical Account', *Psychological Medicine*, 11:1, 115–29.

Wing, L. (1991), 'The Relationship between Asperger's Syndrome and Kanner's Autism', in U. Frith (ed.), *Autism and Asperger Syndrome*, Cambridge: Cambridge University Press, pp. 93–121.

Wing, L. and Gould, J. (1979), 'Severe Impairments of Social Interaction and Associated Abnormalities in Children: Epidemiology and Classification', *Journal of Autism and Developmental Disorders*, 9:1, 11–29.

Wingate, M. E. (2002), *Foundations of Stuttering*, San Diego, CA: Academic Press.

Witt, P. D., D'Antonio, L. L., Zimmerman, G. J. and Marsh, J. L. (1994), 'Sphincter Pharyngoplasty: A Preoperative and Postoperative Analysis of Perceptual Speech Characteristics and Endoscopic Studies of Velopharyngeal Function', *Plastic and Reconstructive Surgery*, 93:6, 1154–68.

Wolfe, V., Presley, C. and Mesaris, J. (2003), 'The Importance of Sound Identification Training in Phonological Intervention', *American Journal of Speech–Language Pathology*, 12:3, 282–8.

Wolk, L. and Edwards, M. L. (1993), 'The Emerging Phonological System of an Autistic Child', *Journal of Communication Disorders*, 26:3, 161–77.

Woodcock, R. W. (1987), *Woodcock Reading Mastery Tests – Revised*, Circle Pines, MN: American Guidance Service.

Woodson, G., Hochstetler, H. and Murry, T. (2006), 'Botulinum Toxin Therapy for Abductor Spasmodic Dysphonia', *Journal of Voice*, 20:1, 137–43.

Woolf, G. (1967), 'The Assessment of Stuttering as Struggle, Avoidance, and Expectancy', *British Journal of Disorders of Communication*, 2:2, 158–71.

World Health Organization (1993), *The ICD-10 Classification of Mental and Behavioural Disorders: Diagnostic Criteria for Research*, Geneva: World Health Organization.

Wright, C. D. and Zeitels, S. M. (2006), 'Recurrent Laryngeal Nerve Injuries after Esophagectomy', *Thoracic Surgery Clinics*, 16:1, 23–33.

Wu, E. Q., Shi, L., Birnbaum, H., Hudson, T. and Kessler, R. (2006), 'Annual Prevalence of Diagnosed Schizophrenia in the USA: A Claims Data Analysis Approach', *Psychological Medicine*, 36:11, 1535–40.

Wu, X., Su, Z. Z., Jiang, A. Y., Lin, A. H., Chai, L. P., Wen, W. P. and Lei, W. B. (2005), 'Analysis of Relevant Factors Causing Laryngeal Stenosis after Partial Laryngectomy', *Chinese Journal of Otorhinolaryngology, Head and Neck Surgery*, 40:12, 929–32.

Yamashita, Y., Fujimoto, C., Nakajima, E., Isagai, T. and Matsuishi, T. (2003), 'Possible Association Between Congenital Cytomegalovirus Infection and Autistic Disorder', *Journal of Autism and Developmental Disorders*, 33:4, 455–9.

Yaruss, J. S., Coleman, C. and Hammer, D. (2006), 'Treating Preschool Children who Stutter: Description and Preliminary Evaluation of a Family-Focused Treatment Approach', *Language, Speech, and Hearing Services in Schools*, 37:2, 118–36.

Yaruss, J. S. and Quesal, R. W. (2004), 'Overall Assessment of the Speaker's Experience of Stuttering (OASES)', in A. Packman, A. Meltzer and H. F. M. Peters (eds), *Theory, Research and Therapy in Fluency Disorders. Proceedings of the Fourth World Congress on Fluency Disorders*, Nijmegen: Nijmegen University Press, pp. 237–40.

Yaruss, J. S. and Quesal, R. W. (2006), 'Overall Assessment of the Speaker's Experience of Stuttering (OASES): Documenting Multiple Outcomes in Stuttering Treatment', *Journal of Fluency Disorders*, 31:2, 90–115.

Yavaş, M. (1998), *Phonology Development and Disorders*, San Diego, CA: Singular.

Yavuzer, G., Güzelküçük, S., Küçükdeveci, A., Gök, H. and Ergin, S. (2001), Aphasia Rehabilitation in Patients with Stroke', *International Journal of Rehabilitation Research*, 24:3, 241–4.

Yeoh, H. K., Lind, C. R. and Law, A. J. (2006), 'Acute Transient Cerebellar Dysfunction and Stuttering Following Mild Closed Head Injury', *Child's Nervous System*, 22:3, 310–13.

Yoder, P. J. and Warren, S. F. (1998), 'Maternal Responsivity Predicts the Prelinguistic Communication Intervention that Increases Generalized Intentional Communication', *Journal of Speech, Language, and Hearing Research*, 41:5, 1207–19.

Yoder, P. J. and Warren, S. F. (1999), 'Maternal Responsivity Mediates the Relationship Between Prelinguistic Intentional Communication and Later Language', *Journal of Early Intervention*, 22:2, 126–36.

Yoder, P. J. and Warren, S. F. (2002), 'Effects of Prelinguistic Milieu Teaching and Parent Responsivity Education on Dyads Involving Children with Intellectual Disabilities', *Journal of Speech, Language, and Hearing Research*, 45:6, 1158–74.

Yoon, B. H., Jun, J. K., Romero, R., Park, K. H., Gomez, R., Choi, J. H. and Kim, I. O. (1997), 'Amniotic Fluid Inflammatory Cytokines (Interleukin-6, Interleukin-1β, and Tumor Necrosis Factor-α), Neonatal Brain White Matter Lesions, and Cerebral Palsy', *American Journal of Obstetrics and Gynecology*, 177:1, 19–26.

Yorkston, K. M. and Beukelman, D. R. (1981), *Assessment of Intelligibility of Dysarthric Speech*, Austin, TX: Pro-Ed.

Yorkston, K. M. and Beukelman, D. R. (2000), 'Dysarthria: An Overview of Treatment', in I. Papathanasiou (ed.), *Acquired Neurogenic Communication Disorders: A Clinical Perspective*, London: Whurr, pp. 149–72.

Yorkston, K. M., Beukelman, D. R., Strand, E. A. and Bell, K. R. (1999), *Management of Motor Speech Disorders in Children and Adults*, Austin, TX: Pro-Ed.

Yorkston, K. M., Beukelman, D. R. and Traynor, C. (1984), *Assessment of Intelligibility of Dysarthric Speech*, Tigard, OR: C.C.

Young, E. C., Diehl, J. J., Morris, D., Hyman, S. L. and Bennetto, L. (2005), 'The Use of Two Language Tests to Identify Pragmatic Language Problems in Children with Autism Spectrum Disorders', *Language, Speech and Hearing Services in Schools*, 36:1, 62–72.

Yunusova, Y., Weismer, G., Kent, R. D. and Rusche, N. M. (2005), 'Breath-Group Intelligibility in Dysarthria: Characteristics and Underlying Correlates', *Journal of Speech, Language and Hearing Research*, 48:6, 1294–310.

Zackheim, C. T. and Conture, E. G. (2003), 'Childhood Stuttering and Speech Disfluencies in Relation to Children's Mean Length of Utterance: A Preliminary Study', *Journal of Fluency Disorders*, 28:2, 115–41.

Zebenholzer, K. and Oder, W. (1998), 'Neurological and Psychosocial Sequelae 4 and 8 Years after Severe Craniocerebral Injury: A Catamnestic Study', *Wiener Klinische Wochenschrift*, 110:7, 253–61.

Zebrowski, P. M. (1991), 'Duration of the Speech Disfluencies of Beginning Stutterers', *Journal of Speech and Hearing Research*, 34:3, 483–91.

Zebrowski, P. M. (1994), 'Duration of Sound Prolongation and Sound/Syllable Repetition in Children who Stutter: Preliminary Observations', *Journal of Speech and Hearing Research*, 37:2, 254–63.

Zeitels, S. M., Akst, L. M., Bums, J. A., Hillman, R. E., Broadhurst, M. S. and Anderson, R. R. (2006), 'Pulsed Angiolytic Laser Treatment of Ectasias and Varices in Singers', *Annals of Otology, Rhinology and Laryngology*, 115:8, 571–80.

Zhang, J., Zhou, Y. and Wang, Y. J. (2006a), 'The Clinical Manifestations and Assessment of Post Stroke Dysphagia', *Zhonghua Nei Ke Za Zhi*, 45:5, 379–81.

Zhang, Y., Wang, Y., Wang, C., Zhao, X., Gong, X., Sun, X., Chen, H. and Wang, Y. (2006b), 'Study on the Pathogenic Mechanism of Broca's and Wernicke's Aphasia', *Neurological Research*, 28:1, 59–65.

Ziatas, K., Durkin, K. and Pratt, C. (2003), 'Differences in Assertive Speech Acts Produced by Children with Autism, Asperger Syndrome, Specific Language Impairment, and Normal Development', *Development and Psychopathology*, 15:1, 73–94.

Zielhuis, G. A., Rach, G. H., Van den Bosch, A. and Van den Broek, P. (1990), 'The Prevalence of Otitis Media with Effusion: A Critical Review of the Literature', *Clinical Otolaryngology*, 15:3, 283–8.

Zimmerman, I. L., Steiner, V. G. and Pond, R. E. (1992), *Preschool Language Scale-3*, San Antonio, TX: Psychological Corporation.

Zuniga, J. (1999), 'ASHA and IAPAC Organize Joint Committee to Identify and Address the Needs of HIV-Infected People with Communication Disorders', *Journal of the International Association of Physicians in AIDS Care*, 5:4, 17–23.

Zwinkels, A., Geusgens, C., van de Sande, P. and Van Heugten, C. (2004), 'Assessment of Apraxia: Inter-Rater Reliability of a New Apraxia Test, Association Between Apraxia and Other Cognitive Deficits and Prevalence of Apraxia in a Rehabilitation Setting', *Clinical Rehabilitation*, 18:7, 819–27.

Index

motor (*cont.*)
    dysfunction, 73, 75–6, 78
    execution, 3–4, 6–7, 9
    fibre, 78, 335
    impairment, 89–92, 107, 179, 183, 197
    learning, 101–2, 255, 259–60, 264–5
    programming, 3–4, 6–7, 145, 256–7, 263, 332
    skill, 95–7, 111n, 165, 179, 183–4, 194, 196, 207, 235n, 281
    speech production, 328, 340
    speech (programming) disorder, 194, 245, 310, 328, 331–2, 338, 340; *see also* disorder (speech), impairment (speech)
motor neurone disease (MND), 14, 18, 22, 25n, 310–14, 317–18, 329, 344, 349, 357, 370n; *see also* amyotrophic lateral sclerosis
mucus, 96; *see also* dysphagia, swallowing
multiple sclerosis (MS), 14, 310–13, 317–18, 344, 349, 357–8, 370n, 375n, 408
muscle, 36, 73, 101–3, 150, 303n, 318, 362, 383, 418
    atrophy, 258, 336
    cricopharyngeal, 358
    levator veli palatini, 41, 62, 117n
    palatal, 51
    paralysis, 338
    pterygoid, 79
    tensor veli palatini, 51, 117n
    tone, 72, 120n, 167, 258, 336, 361
    weakness, 235n, 258, 314, 336
muscular dystrophy, 124n, 142
myasthenia gravis, 14, 315–16, 357–8, 408
myelin, 312
myoclonus, 104
myopia, 73
myringotomy, 51, 55; *see also* grommet, ventilating (tube)

nares/nostrils, 43, 46, 361, 371n
narrative, 158–9, 205, 293, 306n, 330, 345–6, 351–2, 399
nasal
    (air) emission/escape, 40, 44–5, 47–8, 50, 62, 84, 262, 371n; *see also* cleft
    ala(e), 33–4, 37
    bridge, 33, 222n
    cavity, 6, 33, 40, 48, 124n, 361
    grimace, 40; *see also* cleft
    pit, 30; *see also* cleft, embryology
    polyp, 6, 405
    process, 29–31, 33; *see also* cleft, embryology
    reflux/regurgitation, 40–1, 44; *see also* cleft
    septum, 33, 35, 37
    tip, 34, 112n, 371n
    turbulence, 50; *see also* cleft
nasalisation, 48, 63, 84
nasality, 47, 84, 313
nasendoscopy, 46–7
nasometry, 47, 325
nasopharynx, 51, 55, 62, 79, 361
nausea, 140–1, 376n
neologism, 345, 365–6, 374n; *see also* aphasia, schizophrenia
neonate, 71–2, 119n, 134–6, 138
nerve, 38, 99, 122n, 312
    acoustic, 53, 88
    auditory, 88, 151
    cranial, 6, 13, 41, 53, 77–8, 80–1, 121n, 122n, 124n, 125n, 141

fibre, 99, 120n
    hypoglossal, 316–17, 322
    optic, 312
    recurrent laryngeal, 316–17, 409, 421n
    superior laryngeal, 377n
nervous system, 13, 70, 72, 119n, 121n, 122n, 137, 221n
    central, 13, 40, 70, 73, 75, 77, 121n, 134, 136, 192, 312, 344
    peripheral, 13, 121n
    tumour, 222n
neurodegenerative disease/disorder, 314–15, 329, 343, 357
neurodevelopment, 13, 15, 70, 75, 119n, 133
neurofibromatosis, 193–4
neurogenic speech disorder, 142; *see also* disorder (speech), impairment (speech)
neurological
    damage, 6, 13, 27, 40, 45, 71, 129
    disease, 14, 283, 315, 317, 331, 357, 401n
    disorder, 14, 124n, 310, 313, 317, 331, 404, 406, 408
    examination, 301, 316
    impairment, 18, 40–1, 77, 100, 126n, 134–5, 139, 141, 265, 281, 327–9
    injury, 89, 310, 331, 357
    status, 321–2
neurology, 12–14, 17, 239n, 350
neuromuscular
    impairment, 245, 338
    junction, 316
    transmission, 315–16, 357–8
noun, 9–10, 290, 353, 366
nucleus, 77, 121n
    brainstem, 122n
    caudate, 246
    cerebellar, 122n
    cochlear, 87, 121n, 122n, 151
    cranial nerve, 122n, 313
    facial nerve, 122n
    motor, 77
    olivary, 122n
    subthalamic, 122n

obstruent, 84, 143; *see also* consonant
obturator, 45, 103; *see also* lift (palatal)
occlusion, 114n, 146, 416; *see also* malocclusion
occupational
    therapist, 16–17, 76, 97, 210, 218–19
    therapy, 86, 218
    voice disorder, 406; *see also* voice disorder
odynophagia, 140; *see also* dysphagia, swallowing
oesophageal
    dysmobility/dysmotility, 139, 222n
    reflux, 405
    speech, 415, 421n; *see also* laryngectomy
    sphincter, 80, 124n, 223n
    voice, 22, 415–16; *see also* laryngectomy
oesophagectomy, 317, 415
oesophagus, 79–80, 223n, 415–16
olfactory pit, 30; *see also* cleft, embryology
olfactory placode, 29–30; *see also* cleft, embryology
oral
    cavity, 6, 13, 33–4, 44, 48, 77–8, 93, 95–8, 102, 123n, 139, 146, 258, 359, 411; *see also* buccal cavity
    examination, 36, 44, 49–50, 272, 359
    hypersensitivity, 45, 94, 102
    intake, 363–4; *see also* dysphagia, swallowing